The term dementia embraces a wide range of diseases leading to progressive cognitive decline, of which Alzheimer's disease is the commonest. Diagnosis in such cases is based on a combination of clinical findings and the appearance of tissue obtained by biopsy during life or post-mortem. Within this volume, Drs Esiri and Morris and their team of international experts provide a uniquely comprehensive account of the neuropathology of diseases causing dementia. Nineteen cross-referenced chapters cover individual or groups of conditions causing dementia and provide detailed advice about not only the steps needed to make a diagnosis but also the important differential diagnoses to consider. In addition to the very practical nature of each chapter, a vast factual resource is provided with concise yet comprehensive accounts of the current clinical understanding of each disease including its aetiology and pathogenesis. The text is yet further enhanced by both careful referencing to original literature and extensive high quality illustration throughout. In addition to the focus on individual conditions, both introductory and appendix chapters cover more general practical issues involved in diagnosis and tissue studies including safety aspects, morphometry and tissue sources.

The neuropathology of dementia

The neuropathology of dementia

Edited by

MARGARET M. ESIRI
and
JAMES H. MORRIS
Department of Neuropathology,
Radcliffe Infirmary, Oxford, UK

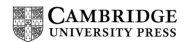

PUBLISHED BY THE PRESS SYNDICATE OF THE UNIVERSITY
OF CAMBRIDGE
The Pitt Building, Trumpington Street, Cambridge CB2 1RP,
United Kingdom

CAMBRIDGE UNIVERSITY PRESS
The Edinburgh Building, Cambridge CB2 2RU, United Kingdom
40 West 20th Street, New York, NY 10011-4211, USA
10 Stamford Road, Oakleigh, Melbourne 3166, Australia

First published 1997

Printed in the United Kingdom at the University Press, Cambridge

Typeset in Times 10/12 pt

A catalogue record for this book is available from the British Library

Library of Congress Cataloguing in Publication data

The neuropathology of dementia / edited by Margaret M. Esiri
   and James H. Morris
      p.   cm.
   Includes bibliographical references and index.
   ISBN 0 521 43311 8 (hardback)
   1. Dementia Pathogenesis.   2. Postmortem changes.   3. Autopsy.
   I. Esiri, Margaret M.   II. Morris, James H.
      [DNLM: 1. Dementia – pathology.   2. Dementia – etiology.
   3. Dementia – complications.   WM 220 N4918 1997]
   RC521.N475   1997
   616.8′3 – dc20
   DNLM/DLC
   for Library of Congress   96-27783 CIP

ISBN 0 521 43311 8 hardback

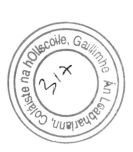

Contents

Contributors   *page* x
Foreword   xi
Preface   xiii

1   **Definition, clinical features and
    neuroanatomical basis of dementia**   1
    T. J. Grabowski and A. R. Damasio
    Introduction   1
    Clinical aspects of dementia   2
    Dementias due to degenerative pathology   2
    The neuroanatomical basis of dementia   4
    Dysfunction in the neural systems marked by
        neurofibrillary lesions may explain the
        neuropsychological manifestations of
        Alzheimer's disease   4
    Pathological hallmarks of Alzheimer's disease   5
    Spatial and temporal distribution of Alzheimer
        changes   7
    Clinical correlates of regional and laminar
        specific pathology   9
    Conclusions   14

2   **Practical approach to the pathological
    diagnosis of dementia: important anatomical
    landmarks in the brain in dementia**   21
    M. M. Esiri and J. H. Morris
    Cerebral cortex   21
    Cerebral white matter   28
    Amygdala   28
    Nucleus basalis of Meynert (basal nucleus)   29
    Basal ganglia   29
    Thalamus and hypothalamus   31
    Brainstem   32
    The cerebellum   33

3   **Practical approach to pathological diagnosis**   36
    M. M. Esiri and J. H. Morris
    The post-mortem examination in cases of
        dementia   36
    Brain biopsies in patients with dementia   59
    Ageing changes in the brain compatible with
        normal mental function   60

4a **Alzheimer's disease**   70
    J. H. Morris
    Historical   70
    Epidemiology   71
    Neuroimaging   75
    Gross findings   76
    Microscopic appearance   80
    Pattern of development of AD changes and their
        relation to the symptoms of dementia   93
    Diagnostic criteria   95
    Staging the severity of AD pathology   97
    Pathogenesis of Alzheimer's disease   101

4b **Neuropathological changes of Alzheimer's
    disease in persons with Down's syndrome**   122
    D. M. A. Mann
    Introduction   122
    Gross changes in the brain in Down's
        syndrome   122
    Neuronal fallout in Down's syndrome   123
    Neurochemical changes in elderly persons with
        Down's syndrome   124
    The prevalence and distribution of senile
        plaques and neurofibrillary tangles in the
        brain in Down's syndrome   124
    The morphological and immunohistochemical
        appearance of SP and NFT in Down's
        syndrome   126
    Conclusion   128
    Chronological studies of the time course of
        pathological events in DS   129

5   **Vascular dementia**   137
    J. H. Morris
    Introduction   137
    How frequent is vascular dementia?   138
    How does cerebrovascular disease produce
        dementia?   144
    Aetiology of vascular dementia   160
    Neuropathological criteria for vascular dementia   166

6 **Parkinson's disease and dementia**   174
   M. M. Esiri and R. H. McShane
   Problems of clinical ascertainment of dementia   174
   Problems of clinical ascertainment of Parkinson's
       disease (PD)   175
   Prevalence and incidence of dementia in clinical
       Parkinson's disease   175
   Clinical correlates of dementia in Parkinson's
       disease   176
   Neuropsychology of Parkinson's disease   177
   Alzheimer's disease and extrapyramidal signs and
       dementia   177
   Pathology of classical Parkinson's disease   178
   Prevalence of Lewy body pathology   180
   Neurochemical findings in Parkinson's disease   181
   Pathological correlates of dementia in
       Parkinson's disease   182
   Cortical Lewy body disease   182
   Towards a clinico-pathological definition of
       cortical Lewy body disease (CLBD)   186
   Aetiological considerations   187
   Pathological differential diagnosis   187

7 **Amyotrophic lateral
   sclerosis/parkinsonism-dementia complex
   of Guam**   194
   D. P. Perl
   Introduction   194
   Neuropathologic features   195
   Aetiology   199
   Summary   201

8 **Pick's disease**   204
   J. H. Morris
   Introduction   204
   Clinical manifestations   204
   Pathological findings   205
   Neurochemistry   210
   Problems in Pick's disease   211
   Related conditions   213

9 **Huntington's disease**   219
   J. P. G. Vonsattel, P. Ge and L. Kelley
   Introduction   219
   Neuropathological history   219
   Epidemiology   220
   Anatomy and nomenclature of the basal ganglia   220
   Physiological considerations   221
   Clinical aspects   221
   Neuropathology   222
   CAG repeats – neuropathology – gene expression   232
   Concomitant neuropathological findings   233
   Clinicopathological discrepancies and differential
       diagnosis   233

10 **Other neurodegenerative diseases causing
   dementia**   241
   M. M. Esiri
   Progressive supranuclear palsy (PSP)   241
   Non-specific frontal lobe dementia   245
   Dementia with motor neuron disease   250
   Thalamic degeneration and dementia   252
   Progressive subcortical gliosis (of Neumann)   253
   Corticobasal degeneration   254
   Dementia with argyrophilic grains   255
   Neurofibrillary tangles with calcification   255
   Dentatorubro pallidoluysian degeneration
       (atrophy)   256
   Multiple system atrophies and dementia   256

11 **Familial cerebral amyloid angiopathies**   260
   G. T. Plant and M. M. Esiri
   Introduction   260
   Historical review   262
   Hereditary cerebral haemorrhage with
       amyloidosis – Icelandic type (HCHWA-I)   262
   Hereditary cerebral haemorrhage with
       amyloidosis – Dutch type (HCHWA-D)   263
   Familial CAA with non-neuritic plaque
       formation   266
   Familial CAA with deafness and ocular
       haemorrhage (Danish type)   270
   Other familial amyloid angiopathies   271
   Hereditary multi-infarct dementia   272
   Differential diagnosis and neuropathological
       recommendations   272

12 **Human prion diseases**   277
   K. Hsiao
   Introduction   277
   Clinical syndromes: infectious, inherited and
       sporadic prion diseases   277
   Diagnosing human prion diseases   283

13 **Alcoholism and dementia**   294
   C. Harper and D. Corbett
   Introduction   294
   Primary alcoholic dementia   294
   The Wernicke–Korsakoff syndrome   296
   Hepatic encephalopathy   301
   Pellagra   303

14 **Dementia due to other metabolic diseases
   and toxins**   307
   M. M. Esiri
   Conditions associated with hypoxia   309
   Haematological conditions   311

Chronic renal failure   311
Hepatic disease   311
Pancreatic disorders   313
Vitamin B$_{12}$ and folate deficiencies   315
Porphyria   315
Alexander's disease   315
Adult polyglucosan body disease (Lafora disease)   316
Kuf's disease (adult onset neuronal ceroid
   lipofuscinosis)   316
Cerebrotendinous xanthomatosis   316
Polycystic lipomembranous osteodysplasia with
   sclerosing leukoencephalopathy   316
Hypocalcaemia with calcification of the basal
   ganglia   316
Neuronal intranuclear inclusion disease   317
Adrenoleukodystrophy   317
GM$_1$ and GM$_2$ gangliosidosis   317
Gaucher's disease, type 1   318
Niemann–Pick disease   318
Mucopolysaccharidosis type IIIB (San-filippo's
   disease)   319
Mitochondrial disorders   319
Leigh's encephalopathy   321
Metachromatic leukodystrophy   322
Fabry's disease   323
Krabbe's disease (globoid cell leukodystrophy)   323
Effects of drugs   324
Effects of environmental toxins   326

15 **Hydrocephalus and dementia**   332
    M. M. Esiri
    Introduction   332
    Cerebrospinal fluid hydrodynamics and normal
       pressure hydrocephalus   332
    Classification, prevalence, natural history and
       clinical features of NPH   334
    Neuropathological findings in NPH   335
    Recommended procedure for diagnosis of NPH   339

16 **Head injury and dementia**   344
    C. J. Bruton
    Dementia pugilistica   344
    Memory loss and dementia: boxing, acute head
       injury and Alzheimer's disease   351

17 **Infectious diseases causing dementia**   357
    F. Scaravilli and M. J. G. Harrison
    Introduction   357
    Herpes simplex encephalitis   357
    Subacute sclerosing panencephalitis (SSPE)   362
    Progressive multifocal leukoencephalopathy
       (PML)   366
    Encephalitis lethargica and post-encephalitic

    parkinsonism   369
    The acquired immune deficiency syndrome (AIDS)   372
    Neurosyphilis   378

18 **Schizophrenia and its dementia**   385
    P. J. Harrison
    Macroscopic brain changes in schizophrenia   385
    Microscopic brain changes in schizophrenia   386
    The nature of the disease process: the
       neurodevelopmental model   390
    The dementia of schizophrenia and its
       neuropathological basis   391
    Suggestions for the neuropathological
       study of schizophrenia   392
    Conclusions   393

19 **Other diseases that cause dementia**   398
    M. M. Esiri
    Space-occupying lesions   398
    Inflammatory conditions   401
    Consequences of cerebral irradiation   405
    Multiple sclerosis   405
    Epilepsy   408
    Superficial haemosiderosis of the central nervous
       system   410
    Whipple's disease   411
    Other obscure conditions   412

    **Appendix 1: Morphometric methods and
    dementia**   415
    J. M. Anderson
    Introduction   415
    Assessment of tissue volumes   415
    Assessment of microscopical changes   420
    Some practical aspects   424

    **Appendix 2: Addresses of dementia brain
    banks**   429
    M. M. Esiri and J. H. Morris

    **Appendix 3: Safety precautions in laboratories
    involved with dementia
    diagnosis and research**   434
    M. M. Esiri and J. H. Morris

    Index   436

Contributors

J. M. Anderson, Department of Histopathology, Ninewells Hospital and University of Dundee, UK

C. J. Bruton, Curator of the Corsellis Collection, Department of Neuropathology, Runwell Hospital, Wickford, Essex, UK

D. Corbett, Royal Prince Alfred Hospital, Camperdown, NSW 2050, Australia

A. R. Damasio, Department of Neurology, Division of Behavioral Neurology and Cognitive Neuroscience, University of Iowa, College of Medicine, Iowa City, IA, USA

M. M. Esiri, Neuropathology Department and University Department of Clinical Neurology, Radcliffe Infirmary, Oxford OX2 6HE, UK

P. Ge, Department of Neuropathology, Warren 3, Massachusetts General Hospital, Fruit St., Boston, Massachusetts, MA 02114, USA

T. J. Grabowski, Department of Neurology, University of Iowa, 200 Hawkins Drive, 2007 RCP, Iowa City, IA 52242, USA

C. Harper, Neuropathology Unit, Department of Pathology, University of Sydney, NSW 2006, Australia *and* Royal Prince Alfred Hospital, Camperdown, NSW 2050, Australia

M. J. G. Harrison, Department of Clinical Neurology, University College London, Medical School, Middlesex Hospital, Mortimer Street, London W1N 8AA, UK

P. J. Harrison, University Department of Psychiatry, Warneford Hospital, Oxford, and University Department of Clinical Neurology (Neuropathology), Radcliffe Infirmary, Oxford, UK

K. Hsiao, Department of Neurology, University of Minnesota, Minneapolis, MN 55455, USA

L. Kelley, Department of Neuropathology, Warren 3, Massachusetts General Hospital, Fruit St, Boston, Massachusetts MA 02114, USA

D. M. A. Mann, Department of Pathological Sciences, Division of Molecular Pathology, University of Manchester, Oxford Road, Manchester M13 9PT, UK

R. H. McShane, Section of Old Age Psychiatry, Warneford Hospital, Oxford OX3 7JX, UK

J. H. Morris, Department of Neuropathology, Radcliffe Infirmary, Oxford OX2 6HE, UK

D. P. Perl, Department of Neuropathology, Mount Sinai School of Medicine, New York, NY 10029, USA

G. T. Plant, Department of Neurology, National Hospital for Nervous Diseases, Queen Square, London WC1N 3BG, UK

F. Scaravilli, Department of Neuropathology, Institute of Neurology, The National Hospital, Queen Square, London WC1N 3BG, UK

J. P. G. Vonsattel, Department of Neuropathology, Warren 3, Massachusetts General Hospital, Fruit Street, Boston, Massachusetts, MA 02114, USA

Foreword

Professor Sir Bernard Tomlinson

For anyone who has to deal frequently with cases of dementia, or has a special interest in the subject, a comprehensive text on the neuropathology has been needed for many years. The last ten years has made that urgent, for the growth of publications and knowledge has made it impossible for any individual to keep track of all the new information, or even where it is to be found. This book, by Margaret Esiri and James Morris, in collaboration with international colleagues, is the most thorough attempt, to my knowledge, to fill the gap; it will have required much effort, skill and determination; in my view, it has largely succeeded.

Margaret Esiri and James Morris have extensive experience of the main causes of dementia and have made many important contributions to research. Alone, together, or with other collaborators, they provide two-thirds of the text. Chapters by other pathologists, neurologists, gerontologists and psychiatrists complete the volume, mostly writing on topics on which they are acknowledged experts.

The book is logically assembled. It starts with an excellent definition of dementia and a summary of its clinical features and neuroanatomical basis. Analyses of the types and distribution of the morphological lesions in Alzheimer's disease are used to advance the view that the disruption of specific neural systems is the best explanation for the cognitive defects which characterize the disorder. This is followed by two chapters on the practical approach to the pathological diagnosis of dementia, and the neuroanatomical structures to which attention must be paid, the latter being clearly diagrammatically illustrated; this is complemented by detailed guidance on the conduct of the post-mortem in cases of dementia, the observations to be made on the unfixed brain, the detailed treatment and histological analysis of the fixed brain, the problems of mixed pathology and the brain changes which may occur in elderly non-demented subjects. These accounts alone will be of immense value to those, particularly pathologists, starting to deal with cases of dementia, and very helpful to many who are already experienced in the pathological diagnosis of dementia or engaged in research.

Major chapters on Alzheimer's disease, and the pathological changes in Down's syndrome, are followed by a profusely illustrated account of vascular dementia in all its forms and a discussion on the difficulties of interpreting the significance of lesions found in some cases in relation to the clinical diagnosis. These, and a chapter on Parkinson's disease and the dementias associated with more widespread Lewy body formation and their relatively frequent association with some of the stigmata of Alzheimer's disease, complete the account of the two (or three) causes of dementia which are responsible for up to 90% of all cases in adults.

The remainder, roughly the second half of the book, is concerned with the very numerous other causes of dementia, many of which are rare. All are important in that their study may advance understanding of the mechanisms which lead to dementia. Some, such as normal pressure hydrocephalus and subdural haematoma are potentially treatable, whilst others, for example, dementia due to excess alcohol, are preventable. A number of primary dementing disorders, the amyotrophic lateral sclerosis/Parkinson's dementia complex of Guam, Pick's disease and Huntington's disease, merit separate chapters, as does human prion disease. Other conditions less constantly associated with dementia are given similar treatment; these are the cerebral amyloid angiopathies, alcoholism, hydrocephalus, head injury and achizophrenia. All are likely to be seen by neuropathologists at some time and may present difficulties in interpreting the lesions found in relation to dementia. The clear, up-to-date account of cognitive decline in schizophrenia makes it apparent that anything beyond an examination for the more common causes of dementia, particularly Alzheimer's disease, should be left to those involved with research in that disorder.

Four chapters each deal with multiple disorders within particular categories. That on infectious diseases covers five viral infections, including AIDS, and briefly neurosyphilis, the latter a reminder that we have not yet seen the last of that former scourge, despite the fact that many pathologists up to middle age may not have encountered a case in the UK. A chapter on 'Other neurodegenerative diseases' describes rare conditions, some of which will have excited considerable neurological interest and will present specific neuropathological features. A chapter on dementia due to metabolic diseases and toxins includes many rare disorders, some of which will nevertheless have a clinical diagnosis attached. The final chapter describes some relatively common disorders such as epilepsy and multiple sclerosis in which varying degrees of dementia may be found, and a small group, including coeliac disease, where dementia may be a rare complication.

Three appendices conclude the text. The first is a highly valuable account of morphometric methods of use in dementia research. The second lists the addresses of dementia brain banks worldwide, and the third the

safety precautions necessary in laboratories dealing with cases of dementia.

The above summary, in my view, amply justifies my earlier statement on the comprehensive nature of the text on the neuropathology of dementia. Perhaps some rare or obscure conditions have escaped notice, but so far I have not identified them. Doubtless, also, some will disagree with the space accorded to different conditions; it could not be otherwise.

Overall, however, the principal authors have, through their own clear accounts, their perceptive insight into pathologists' needs, and their persuasive powers in enlisting authoritative collaborators, produced a book which will be a most welcome addition, and perhaps a treasure, in many laboratories, clinical libraries and personal collections.

I believe it deserves success and I am honoured to be associated with its first edition.

Preface

This book has been written primarily to assist the pathologist faced with the task of determining the cause of dementia in cases requiring post-mortem diagnosis of this all-too-common condition. We have attempted to provide what we hope will prove to be useful guidelines to recognizing and distinguishing between the many different pathological causes of dementia, and to distinguishing these from the normal effects of ageing on the brain. With the help of an international team of authors, we also provide concise but comprehensive accounts of current understanding of the diseases themselves.

Despite considerable recent advances in the clinical investigation of patients with dementia, a well-informed pathologist remains the person best qualified to discover the cause of someone's cognitive decline. However, his or her task is not an easy one. There are practical difficulties: falling autopsy rates in many countries as financial and social conditions increasingly dictate a policy of caring for demented patients in the community; techniques of neuropathological diagnosis that are specialized, time-consuming, labour-intensive and therefore also relatively expensive; and frequent demands for justification of procedures in terms of improved patient care – justification which, in the short term, is hard to provide. Yet, if we take only a slightly longer-term view, the pathological basis of dementia demands most urgent consideration as we near the end of this century with rapidly escalating numbers of afflicted patients and families. For too long, throughout the first half of this century, we lived in ignorance that Alzheimer's disease was the commonest cause of progressive dementia in the elderly, for want of performing large numbers of careful autopsy examinations in such cases. Even now that the need for such autopsies is more widely recognized, not only by clinicians but also by better informed families of those affected, neuropathologists with the appropriate expertise to reach the correct diagnosis remain scarce. All too often, general histopathologists find themselves required to distinguish between one form of dementia and another. This is an undertaking made all the harder when it is realized that there is no absolute dividing line between, for example, the pathological features of Alzheimer's disease or ischaemic dementia and normal ageing or ischaemic changes compatible with normal mental function. Further difficulties have arisen in the last decade as new, unfamiliar diseases such as AIDS and iatrogenically transmitted spongiform encephalopathy have sprung up as causes of dementia in a younger age group.

We believe, therefore, that a book such as this is timely and necessary. We are deeply grateful to the authors who have contributed their time and expertise to assist us. Their prompt writing as well as the publisher's efforts on our behalf, have ensured that the accounts of rapidly advancing research into many of the diseases described here are up-to-date and authoritative. We are also indebted to our clinical colleagues who have done so much to stimulate our own interest in dementia. We hope this volume will ease the pathologists' task and provide enlightenment not only to pathologists but to all those interested in dementia, by enhancing understanding of these fascinating diseases.

Margaret M. Esiri
James H. Morris

CHAPTER ONE

Definition, clinical features and neuroanatomical basis of dementia

T. J. Grabowski and A. R. Damasio

Introduction
Clinical aspects of dementia
Dementias due to degenerative pathology
The neuroanatomical basis of dementia
Dysfunction in the neural systems marked by neurofibrillary lesions may explain the neuropsychological manifestations of Alzheimer's disease
Pathological hallmarks of Alzheimer's disease
Spatial and temporal distribution of Alzheimer changes
Clinical correlates of regional and laminar specific pathology
Conclusions

INTRODUCTION

Decisive contributions to the investigation of Alzheimer's disease have frequently resulted from careful observation of its pathological hallmarks. By painstakingly quantitating the number of senile plaques in the brains of demented and non-demented elderly persons, Blessed and colleagues brought attention to the direct relationship between the specific pathological features of Alzheimer's disease and the accompanying dementia (Blessed et al., 1968). This observation, and that of Corsellis, who recognized the identity of the neuropathology of Alzheimer's presenile dementia and common senile dementia (Corsellis, 1962), led to the realization that half or more cases of dementia are caused by this one disease. The societies of several developed nations, with their expanding elderly populations, placed a high priority on its investigation and, as a consequence, a wealth of evidence has been accumulated regarding the clinical and neurobiological aspects of this disease. One important line of investigation, involving fine-grained neuroanatomical analysis of the distribution of the pathological hallmarks of Alzheimer's disease, has revealed striking regional, cellular and laminar specificities. Meanwhile, investigation of human cognition in focally brain-damaged patients has led to a clearer understanding of the way in which cognitive function maps onto brain structure. These two approaches have matured to a point where it is possible to consider some of the neuropsychological manifestations of the disease in terms of the neural systems which it compromises.

The clearest example of this sort of clinical–pathological correlation is the functional isolation of the hippocampal formation in Alzheimer's disease, to which many investigators attribute the early and prominent amnesia which characterizes the disease. In this chapter, the data supporting this conclusion will be examined in some detail. Since the delineation of this disconnection, there have been numerous contributions in a similar spirit, which will be reviewed next. The few reported exceptions to the usual distribution of Alzheimer's disease pathology assume disproportionate importance because of their predictably altered clinical correlates. Finally, important converging evidence is also now available from the field of functional neuroimaging. Lesion–deficit correlation is a promising approach in the study of other degenerative diseases, such as the lobar atrophies, Lewy body dementia, and Parkinson's disease, although in no other dementing illness is the analysis yet as well developed as in Alzheimer's disease.

CLINICAL ASPECTS OF DEMENTIA

Dementia is an acquired and persistent impairment of intellectual faculties, in an alert individual, affecting several cognitive domains, and of sufficient severity to impair the patient's capacity for personal or social responsibility. This definition is clinical and pragmatic. It says nothing about the pathological correlates of dementia. Indeed, it does not insist on the presence of structural alterations in the brain and thus allows for functional aetiologies of dementia unrelated to recognized structural damage (i.e. depression). Nor does it insist on other attributes that are usually connoted by the term dementia, namely that the process is progressive and that it includes a prominent or disproportionate disorder of memory (e.g. the definition of the DSM-IV). Dementia may be a relatively static condition, as after cumulative large vessel cerebral infarcts, head injury, or herpes simplex encephalitis. In some cases, memory disturbance may not be prominent or may appear later in the course of the illness (for example, in Pick's disease or in certain variants of Alzheimer's disease).

Several aspects of the definition deserve emphasis. First, dementia implies a decline from a previously attained level of intellectual function, therefore excluding developmental encephalopathies. Secondly, dementia implies dysfunction in several aspects of mental function (e.g. memory, language, visuospatial abilities, insight, emotion, reasoning, etc). It excludes cases in which these impairments occur as focal abnormalities (amnesia, aphasia, visual agnosia, etc). Thirdly, the definition excludes the sort of fluctuating encephalopathy which alters the level of consciousness and is known as the 'confusional state' (such fluctuating conditions are usually due to a metabolic disturbance).

The first task of a clinician confronted with a patient with presumed dementia is to establish that the patient's intellectual ability has become diminished relative to its prior level, and that the decline is not 'focal', but rather affects several aspects of cognition. The clinician must also establish that there is no impairment in the patient's level of consciousness.

At this juncture the evaluation of dementia often takes a decidedly prudent turn. The differential diagnosis is potentially vast, but the majority of possible conditions are neither reversible nor treatable, given our current knowledge. Therefore, the clinician often concentrates on potentially treatable causes of dementia rather than adopting the wider point of view necessary to achieve a precise diagnosis. It is important to consider the 'functional' aetiologies of dementia. Some of these are com-

mon and treatable with a high degree of efficacy. These include primary affective disorders, especially major depression ('pseudodementia of depression') and medication encephalopathy. Metabolic disorders (thyroid disease, hypovitaminosis B_{12}, hypercalcaemia, etc), alcoholism, neurosyphilis, and certain structural alterations (chronic subdural haematoma, normal pressure hydrocephalus, brain tumours) are also sought.

It is at this point that the patient may first come to the attention of a neurologist or other specialist. In general, cases of dementia in this referred population are due to progressive structural alterations in the central nervous system. These disorders, and Alzheimer's disease in particular, are the focus of the remainder of this chapter.

It is fundamental to appreciate that, in dementia, neither the pathology nor the cognitive deficits are truly global or diffuse. Every pathological entity causing dementia has a predilection for certain parts of the nervous system, and most dementia syndromes have relative neuropsychological focality, at least in their early stages. Thus, there are two major sources of data that inform the clinical analysis of these cases: the pattern of structural alteration in the brain, which is discerned from the neurological examination and ancillary studies (particularly neuroimaging), and the pattern of neuropsychological impairment, as discerned from the neurological examination and from expert evaluation with standardized neuropsychological instruments (Grant & Adams, in press).

An overview of the degenerative disorders which cause dementia follows. The reader is referred to the appropriate chapters in this volume for a full consideration of these topics.

DEMENTIAS DUE TO DEGENERATIVE PATHOLOGY

Dementia characterized by a prominent anterograde amnesia and the presence of agnosia, aphasia, impaired insight, and other higher-order cognitive impairments, in the *absence* of defects in primary sensory and motor function is usually due to Alzheimer's disease or cortical Lewy body disease. In these cases, cortical atrophy affects all lobes of the cerebral cortex, and especially the mesial temporal lobes.

Alzheimer's disease (AD) (Chapter 4 and below) is the most prevalent disorder of this type. The first recognized case was that of a 55 year-old woman with presenile dementia, described by Alois Alzheimer in 1907. Using the recently developed silver stains to identify the characteristic neurofibrillary tangles and neuritic plaques, Alzheimer established the pathological benchmarks of the disease (Alzheimer, 1907).

The inaugural manifestation of Alzheimer's disease is, almost always, memory impairment, but more precisely an insidious anterograde amnesia for factual material. Some perceptive families also note, in retrospect, that some patients had subtle alterations in personality and affective symptoms. Once manifest, the disease pursues a slowly progressive but relentless course over 8–12 years. There are no remissions. Memory difficulty becomes more pronounced. Visuospatial disorientation, dyscalculia, and impaired lexical access appear within the first 3 years or so. Numerous apraxic, agnosic, and aphasic deficits ensue, combined with a striking lack of insight into them (anosognosia). Severe rigidity and paraplegia in flexion do not appear until the final stage of the disease, when cognitive dysfunction is very severe.

The disease is equally notable for what it spares: patients have no elementary motor or sensory deficits. It is as if all higher-ordered mental functions are singled out. Social graces are usually preserved for quite a while, giving way later to profound alteration in personality and sometimes psychosis, such as that manifested by Alzheimer's original case (Adams & Victor, 1989; Cummings & Benson, 1992).

Although the above description is appropriate for the majority of patients with AD, documentation of variant presentations is accumulating. Some patients, for example, have early and prominent extrapyramidal signs or myoclonus; these patients tend to decline more rapidly (Mayeux, Stern & Spanton, 1985). Some patients have relatively greater language disturbance at the onset (Chui et al., 1985). The pattern of pathology in these patients has yet to be discovered. A very important variant with a distinctive pattern of pathology is that subset of patients presenting with prominent higher order visual impairment. This group will be considered later in this discussion.

Patients with dementia of the Lewy body type (Chapter 6) have a similar pattern of cognitive impairment, but may have prominent and sustained fluctuations in performance, salient hallucinations and/or extra-pyramidal signs. The pathological and clinical overlaps of this disorder with AD have seemed considerable, but nevertheless it is beginning to be clinically distinguished from AD in ante-mortem studies (McKeith et al., 1994).

Another set of conditions produce *lobar* cortical atrophy, that is, atrophy which is disproportionately severe in one or more lobes of the cerebrum. The most important example is Pick's disease (Chapter 8), which is usually marked by temporopolar and/or relatively circumscribed basal frontal and frontopolar atrophy. Again, there is usually a paucity of elementary neurological signs. The neuropsychological profile is often marked by defective executive function and social misconduct which are out of proportion to defects in memory and visuospatial function (Tissot, Constantinidis & Richard, 1985; Knopman et al., 1989), but the clinical distinction from AD can be difficult. Circumscribed frontal atrophy with a similar neuropsychological profile and a rapid course is occasionally associated with motor neuron disease (Neary et al., 1990, Peavy et al., 1992) (Chapter 10). Pronounced left anterior temporal atrophy can occur in association with an isolated progressive disturbance of language dysfunction, usually manifested as dysnomia, dysfluency, and impaired auditory verbal comprehension. These patients sometimes later develop more generalized cognitive defects. These cases are pathologically heterogeneous, but are usually due to Pick's disease or focal spongiform change (Graff-Radford et al., 1990; Snowden et al., 1992). Circumscribed parietal atrophy is a feature of corticobasal degeneration, in which cognitive changes are usually also focal (limited to apraxia and 'cortical' sensory loss). Extrapyramidal signs are usually salient (Gibb, Luthert & Marsden, 1989). We know of no reported cases of focal occipital atrophy.

Several dementing conditions are associated with degeneration in subcortical nuclei, particularly the neostriatum and substantia nigra (Albert, Feldmann & Willis, 1974). These conditions are attended by defects in skeletal and ocular motor control and by gait disorders. The movement disorder may be hyperkinetic or hypokinetic, depending on the pattern of involvement of the basal ganglia and may dominate the clinical picture. These disorders tend to be characterized neuropsychologically by alteration in drive (abulia), personality, emotion (apathy), and by executive dysfunction. Disorders in this category include Huntington's disease (Chapter 9), Parkinson's disease (Chapter 6), progressive supranuclear palsy, and the Shy–Drager syndrome (Chapter 10). Although frontal atrophy may not be disproportionate, functional imaging studies have documented frontal hypometabolism in many of these cases (e.g. Johnson et al., 1992).

The neuropsychological picture of hydrocephalic dementia has much in common with that of the frontal lobar atrophies and with the subcortical dementias, because the ventricular enlargement is most pronounced in the frontal horns of the lateral ventricles, resulting in damage to the deep white matter of the frontal lobe (Chapter 15). The disorder is marked by a prominent gait impairment, urinary incontinence, and dementia (Katzman, 1977), the latter characterized by abulia, apathy and memory disturbance (Cummings and Benson, 1992).

Frontal dysfunction is also inferred in the cases described by Neary *et al.* (1988) and Knopman *et al.* (1990) as 'frontal lobe dementia' and 'dementia lacking distinctive histology', respectively (Chapter 10). The salient clinical features were alteration in personality, mutism, irritability and social misconduct. Prominent dysarthria and dysphagia occurred in many cases. The pattern of brain atrophy was variable; sometimes a frontal predominance was evident, but in most cases, atrophy affected the cortex more generally.

Vascular dementia (Chapter 5) is pathologically heterogeneous. The term embraces dementia due to cumulative large vessel infarcts, cumulative small vessel infarcts (*état lacunaire*), Binswanger encephalopathy (although a vascular aetiology has not been firmly established)(Fisher, 1989), and the sequelae of subarachnoid haemorrhage. The history usually suggests apoplectic events or stepwise decline (Hachinski *et al.*, 1975), and neurological examination and neuroimaging studies usually demonstrate that the process respects vascular territories. The neuropsychological findings are also heterogeneous, but tend to reflect focal deficits and focal sparing that are atypical for the common degenerative conditions.

THE NEUROANATOMICAL BASIS OF DEMENTIA

We have asserted that the degenerative disorders manifesting as dementia are not diffuse processes, either in pathological or neuropsychological terms. The question arises whether the selective distribution of pathological changes can explain the clinical manifestations of dementia. Put another way, the question is: how well does the pattern of neuropsychological deficit correspond to the set of neural systems which are degenerating in the illness in question? Such a correspondence is not obligatory; for example, the pathological hallmarks of a disease could perhaps cause little dysfunction in the tissue; the dysfunction could instead arise from a process that does not alter macroscopic structure (e.g. a neurotransmitter deficiency.)

We were impelled to consider a structural explanation because the manifestations of Alzheimer's disease resemble some of the focal cognitive syndromes that have

been observed in subjects with single stable brain lesions. We have evolved the hypothesis that this principle may have general applicability.

A wealth of information has been obtained concerning the nature of the mapping of cognitive function onto brain structure, principally from the lesion method. (Functional neuroimaging is beginning to make a contribution as well, but as yet has made few fundamental contributions.) Space will not permit a careful treatment of the lesion method and the privileged view of brain function which it has provided, but one of the striking conclusions in this field, that unfolds after the examination of relatively few cases, is that cognitive function is regionalized at systems level (Damasio & Damasio, 1989).

Based on systematic evaluation of the effects of brain lesions, Damasio has proposed a model of neural architecture, known as the convergence zone framework, that is capable of supporting the processes of learning, recall, and recognition. In essence, the model postulates that the mechanism for conscious recall is the reconstruction of the dynamic representation of an entity in topographically mapped early sensorimotor cortices. The components which collectively represent an entity are not spatially but temporally bound, being synchronously activated from convergence zones located in higher-order cortex (or in subcortical nuclei) (Damasio, 1989; Damasio & Damasio, 1994). We have used this framework to explain aspects of amnesia, agnosia, and aphasia. Since some of these syndromes occur in the dementias, it may also prove suitable for the discussion of the neuropsychological phenomena of dementia.

Having explained the rationale for this thesis, we will devote the remainder of the chapter to a consideration of neuropsychological and pathological correlations in AD.

DYSFUNCTION IN THE NEURAL SYSTEMS MARKED BY NEUROFIBRILLARY LESIONS MAY EXPLAIN THE NEUROPSYCHOLOGICAL MANIFESTATIONS OF ALZHEIMER'S DISEASE

The Cholinergic Hypothesis

In the wake of Alzheimer's descriptive paper, two misconceptions became prevalent. First, AD was felt to be relatively uncommon, as only those cases presenting in the presenium were classified as AD. Secondly, the disease was commonly considered to be a 'global' encephalopathy. The idea that the pathology was vascular, or that ageing itself was in some way responsible for the disease, fostered the concept of truly diffuse degenerative pathology.

In the 1960s, the prevalence of AD came to be appreciated (Corsellis, 1962). The second misconception was dispelled by the quantitative work of Blessed and colleagues, who correlated the number of senile plaques (SPs) in elderly subjects with a quantitative index of their degrees of dementia (Blessed, Tomlinson & Roth, 1968), and concluded that the dementia of Alzheimer's type bears a specific relationship to the peculiar pathology of the disease. An appreciation of the significance of the uneven distribution of this pathology was slower in coming, however.

The disproportionate impairment of memory in AD was clearly perceived from the beginning. Although the selective involvement of some neuropsychological functions might have indicated that some cortical neural systems were more vulnerable than others in AD, the focal memory deficit came to be explained by a subcortical abnormality under the 'cholinergic hypothesis' (Bartus et al., 1982). The backdrop that set the stage for the acceptance of this account included the following observations: 1) that there was a cholinergic deficiency in the brain tissue of affected patients (Perry et al., 1977; White et al., 1977, Davies & Maloney 1976); 2) that presynaptic cholinergic markers were severely depleted in the hippocampus and cerebral cortex; 3) that the predominant source of cortical cholinergic afferents, the basal nucleus of Meynert, undergoes marked changes in Alzheimer's disease; and 4) that neuritic plaques are rich in cholinesterase activity, suggesting that the degenerating nerve terminals are the projections of cholinergic neurons (Perry et al., 1981). Because anticholinergic pharmaceuticals, such as scopolamine, cause significant memory impairment, it was reasoned that a deficiency of cholinergic neural transmission in the cortex, resulting from cholinergic deafferentation, might underly the amnesia of AD. The cholinergic hypothesis appealed to the clinical sense of many investigators, who realized that cholinergic drugs were available for the treatment of Alzheimer's disease. There have now been numerous trials of several cholinergic medications in AD, which have, unfortunately, met with very limited success (Growdon, 1992). Although the observations on which the cholinergic hypothesis was founded endure, it has not proved adequate to explain the symptoms of AD or to formulate a successful treatment.

Not until a careful account of the distribution of the pathological hallmarks of Alzheimer's disease was made

did a well-founded alternative to the cholinergic hypothesis become available. This account first focused on mesial temporal limbic structures, as attention had been directed there by a new paradigm for amnesia: the bilateral hippocampal formation lesion.

PATHOLOGICAL HALLMARKS OF ALZHEIMER'S DISEASE

The pathology of Alzheimer's disease is characterized by the accumulation of insoluble fibrous material in intracellular and extracellular locations. The intracellular pathology consists of granulovacuolar change (GVC), Hirano bodies, and neurofibrillary tangles (NFTs). The extracellular (amyloid) deposits are senile plaques (SPs). We will briefly survey these lesions.

Granulovacuolar Change (Fig. 7.4)

Granulovacuolar change was originally described by Simchowicz in 1911 (Simchowicz, 1911). At the light microscopic level, GVC manifests as small inclusions, 3–5 μm in diameter, found primarily in pyramidal neurons of the hippocampal formation and only rarely in other limbic structures. The vacuoles appear clear except for centrally located argyrophilic and basophilic granules (Tomlinson & Kitchener, 1972; Ball & Lo, 1977). Electron microscopy shows these inclusions to be membrane bounded and the core granules to be electron dense. These granules contain epitopes recognized by antibodies to tubulin (Price, Struble & Altschuler, 1985), neurofilaments, tau, and ubiquitin. The pattern of tau immunoreactivity is altered relative to wild-type tau: antibodies to epitopes in the amino terminus, midregion, and carboxy-terminus of tau most often stain only the periphery of the GVC, but antibodies to a phosphorylated exon 2 peptide (E2p) sequence consistently stain the interior. Whether the remainder of tau is masked or has been catabolized is speculative (Dickson et al., 1993). The leading theory of the nature and significance of GVC is that it represents a type of autophagosome (Okamoto et al., 1991). Why the autophagy is evidently limited to the pyramidal cell layer of the hippocampus remains obscure.

Another pathological feature of AD that is limited to the hippocampus is the Hirano body, an eosinophilic, hyaline inclusion body (Fig. 7.3). These have been shown to contain actin and actin-associated proteins (Goldman, 1983). Their pathophysiological role is, however, even less well understood than GVC.

Because of their restricted distribution and because they appear to be playing a secondary pathophysiological role (i.e. the catabolism of the predominant neuropathological elements), GVC and Hirano bodies have not figured prominently in theoretical treatments of AD. We will have little more to say about them here.

Neurofibrillary tangles and neuropil threads (Figs. 3.14b, d, 3.17, 4a.9, 4a.12, 4a.15–20) (see also p. 82)

Neurofibrillary tangles are insoluble intracellular structures composed primarily of accumulations of paired 10 nm helical filaments (PHFs) with a characteristic periodicity, a structure first noted by Kidd (Kidd, 1963). NFTs also contain some straight filaments (structural variants of PHFs) (Goedert, 1993) and amorphous deposits. In molecular terms, NFTs appear to be composed predominantly, if not exclusively, of the microtubule associated protein tau (Goedert, 1993). Tau in its normal state is thought to have the effect of stabilizing microtubule interactions, promoting their assembly. Paired helical filament tau is hyperphosphorylated, proteolysed, ubiquitinated, and cross-linked. The ubiquitination suggests that neurons recognize NFTs as abnormal but fail to catabolize them. Varying degrees of phosphorylation and post assembly processing result in several intermediate manifestations of tau, e.g. 'stage zero tangles' (Bancher et al., 1989), dispersed filaments (Goedert, 1993). Some of these forms of tau present antigenic determinants not found in PHF tau, such as the epitope bound by the monoclonal antibody Alz-50. Alz-50 recognizes a soluble 68 kD form of tau (also known as A68). Originally, Alz-50 was described as co-localizing with NFTs, but recognizing a soluble antigen (Wolozin, Pruchnicki & Dickson, 1986). It failed to co-stain some neurons which lack Nissl substance, and which therefore may lack viable cytoplasm (i.e. 'tombstone neurons') (Hyman, Kromer & Van Hoesen, 1988). It also recognized some tangle-free neurons in regions and laminae that are frequently affected in AD. Accordingly, Alz-50 was felt to recognize a cytoplasmic (possibly cytoskeletal) change that preceded frank tangle formation (Wolozin et al., 1986; Tabaton et al., 1988), although Alz-50 does not bind it in this form. Other investigators have adduced evidence for the accumulation of abnormally phosphorylated tau before the formation of NFTs (Bancher et al., 1989). Alz-50 also recognizes the dystrophic neurites which surround senile plaques and neuropil threads. These neuropil threads are frequently the distal dendrites of tangle-containing neurons (Braak & Braak, 1988). In some cases, the dystrophic neurites are found to localize to the predicted projection zone of tangle-containing neurons (Hyman et

al., 1988). Alz-50 histochemistry can therefore be useful to mark the projections of affected neurons. The neurofibrillary pathology of AD is therefore tripartite: NFTs, neuropil threads, and dystrophic neurites. Despite morphological dissimilarity, these are immunohistochemically similar lesions. Moreover, NFTs and neuropil threads occur in the same pool of neurons. Whether dystrophic neurites colocalize with the other two manifestations of neurofibrillary pathology remains to be seen. There is some preliminary information that dystrophic neurites appear to be more widely distributed than either SPs or NFTs (Kowall & Kosik, 1987).

NFTs are recognized in clinical histologic sections with sensitive silver stains, such as the Bielschowsky stain, or with Thioflavine S. Immunohistochemical techniques have become the mainstay of research studies, however. Antibodies to ubiquitin are also useful in delineating the extent of NFTs in Alzheimer brains.

Neurofibrillary tangles are known to be features of other neurological diseases, for example Pick' disease, progressive supranuclear palsy, dementia pugilistica, Down' syndrome, the Parkinson–dementia complex of Guam, and post-encephalitic parkinsonism. The tau epitope has been detected in Pick's disease, PSP, and Down' syndrome. Some investigators have accordingly proposed that tangle formation is a stereotype cellular reaction that may be initiated by diverse pathophysiological mechanisms (Wisniewski et al., 1979).

Senile plaques (Figs. 3.14b,c, 4a.7–9, 11 and 12) (see also p. 80)

The second major manifestation of AD is the senile or neuritic plaque (SP). Blocq and Marinesco gave the first description of this lesion (Blocq & Marinesco, 1928). Simchowicz coined the term 'senile plaque' and recognized a quantitative relationship between the number of SPs and the severity of the degenerative process (Simchowicz, 1911), a crucial observation that was later rediscovered by Blessed and colleagues (Blessed et al., 1968).

Senile plaques in fully developed form are characterized by a focal spherical deposit of fibrillary amyloid surrounded by dystrophic neurites, reactive astrocytes and some microglia. Plaque cores are composed of the beta amyloid protein, a hydrophobic fragment of a transmembrane glycoprotein known as the beta amyloid precursor protein. Monoclonal antibodies against beta amyloid have been used to demonstrate widely distributed non-neuritic plaques, known as A4- or diffuse plaques. These diffuse plaques are not surrounded by dystrophic neurites. Beta amyloid is also found in leptomeningeal vessels (congophilic amyloid angiopathy, CAA). CAA correlates with numbers of senile plaques containing amyloid cores and is structurally indistinguishable from the amyloid in those structures (Vinters, 1986). Senile plaques are detected clinically with a variety of staining techniques, including with Congo red, Thioflavin S, sensitive silver stains, or antibodies to beta amyloid.

Neuronal loss

In addition to these major pathological features of AD, there is a striking loss of neurons in AD. Gross atrophy and thinning of the cortical ribbon are seen in advanced cases. Terry and colleagues found that the major component of neuronal loss is large neurons, especially those in layer III (Terry, Gonatas & Weiss, 1964). No loss of small neurons could be identified. The neuronal dropout has been correlated with reductions in synaptic immunostaining (DeKosky & Scheff, 1990; Masliah et al., 1991). Neuronal loss appears to occur in the same cell populations that are vulnerable to NFT formation. Hypomyelinization of the periventricular white matter has also been noted by some investigators (Brun & Englund, 1986).

SPATIAL AND TEMPORAL DISTRIBUTION OF ALZHEIMER CHANGES

Despite the amount of descriptive information available regarding the composition of SPs and NFTs, their pathophysiological significance and their relationship to one another have remained controversial. Some insight into this problem is available however from the spatial and temporal distribution of these lesions. They are not distributed uniformly throughout the cerebrum (Mutrux, 1947). Rather, they exhibit characteristic regional, cellular and laminar specificities. Moreover, the distribution of SPs is very different from that of NFTs.

In cases of full-blown Alzheimer's disease, investigators have documented the most severe changes in the hippocampus and in the association cortices, and the least severe changes in primary sensory and motor cortices (Brun & Gustafson, 1976). In their comprehensive survey of the cerebral cortex in AD, Arnold and colleagues found NFTs in greatest numbers in limbic periallocortex (area 28) and allocortex (subiculum, area 51). Corticoid areas (accessory basal nucleus of amygdala, basal nucleus of Meynert) were somewhat less involved. In the neocortex, tangles became progressively

less numerous in the following order: proisocortex (areas 11, 12, 23, 24, 35, 38 and anterior insula), nonprimary association cortex (areas 9, 32, 36, 37, 39, 46, superior temporal sulcus, posterior hippocampus), and primary association cortex (areas 7, 18, 19, posterior 20, posterior 21, posterior 22). Primary motor and sensory cortices were largely spared (Arnold et al., 1991). The only fields with consistently more than 50 NFTs/1.6 mm^2 were the entorhinal cortex and the subiculum/CA1 zone of the hippocampus. In the cerebral cortex, the NFTs predominantly affected layers III and V (Pearson et al., 1985, Lewis et al., 1987; Arnold et al., 1991); in entorhinal cortex, it is layers II and IV that are affected.

Arnold and colleagues have also specifically examined the proisocortical temporal pole in cases of Alzheimer's disease. AD patients showed severe involvement of this region, a multimodal association cortex with widespread connectivity. Neuronal loss was worst in layers II and V and to a lesser degree in layers II and VI. NFTs were very numerous in layers II, III, and V, especially layer V. SPs were more homogeneous in distribution, but tended to be more prominent in layer III (Arnold, Hyman & Van Hoesen, 1994).

Arnold and colleagues' findings are consistent with the findings of several other investigators (Brun & Gustafson, 1976; Pearson et al., 1985; Lewis et al., 1987; Braak & Braak, 1991).

Chu and colleagues have recently extended the study of Arnold to include fine-grained analysis of ventromedial frontal structures (areas 11, 12, 24, 25, 32, posterior orbito-frontal cortex, and anterior insula). These cortices comprise allocortex, agranular and dysgranular paralimbic cortex, and association isocortex. To date, their findings include: 1) NFTs in (periallocortical) area 25 occur mostly in layer V, while layer III is largely spared; 2) In area 11 (isocortex) and the anterior insula (periallocortex), both layers III and V are affected; 3) The highest density of NFTs was observed in a narrow strip of agranular periallocortex along the posteriomedial margin of the orbitofrontal cortex, with only slightly lower counts in the dysgranular (proisocortical) sector anterior to it; 4) The density of NFTs decreased both anteriorly and laterally in the anterolateral granular orbitofrontal (association) cortex (Chu, Van Hoesen & Damasio, 1992; Chu, Flory & Van Hoesen, 1993). These findings indicate that the distribution of NFTs in frontal cortices conforms to the same hierarchical pattern seen in medial temporal and posterior sensory association cortices.

NPs are found in a much different distribution. They are relatively uncommon in limbic periallocortex and allocortex. They tend to be distributed more evenly throughout the cerebral cortex than NFTs. Although NPs are found infrequently in primary sensory cortex, diffuse, or primitive, plaques are found commonly there, as well as in other areas, such as the striatum (Braak & Braak, 1990*a*) and the cerebellum (Joachim, Mori & Selkoe, 1989) where both NPs and NFTs are not found. Most investigators have reported that NPs have less specific regional and laminar distribution patterns than NFTs, though they tend to be more numerous in cortical layers III and IV (Duyckaerts *et al.*, 1986; Arnold *et al.*, 1991; Braak & Braak, 1991; Hof *et al.*, 1992).

A consideration of the temporal distribution of Alzheimer pathology begins with the observation that all the lesions reported in AD have been observed (in much lower numbers) in the brains of nondemented elderly individuals (Blessed *et al.*, 1968; Dayan, 1970; Tomlinson, Blessed & Roth, 1970; Miller *et al.*, 1984; Ulrich, 1985; Crystal *et al.*, 1988; Bouras *et al.*, 1994). The pathological distinction of AD from ageing is based on quantitative criteria (Khachaturian, 1985; Mirra *et al.*, 1991). The presence of Alzheimer pathology in nondemented elderly subjects has been studied carefully by Arriagada and colleagues, who found that, in this population, NFTs occur most frequently in the perirhinal cortex, entorhinal cortex, and CA1/subiculum. A few tangles may also be found in neocortical areas. The rank order of involvement was highly consistent across individuals: entorhinal cortex > perirhinal cortex > CA1 > amygdala > nucleus basalis of Meynert > area 20 > parasubiculum > 21 > CA3/4, dentate gyrus, presubiculum, area 21 and area 41. The entorhinal cortex was involved in 24 of 25 cases, with laminae II and IV predominantly affected. In perirhinal cortex, lamina III was the affected layer. In hippocampus, CA1/subiculum was the only significantly affected area. The number of NFTs, but not SPs, correlated with increasing patient age. SPs that are Alz-50 immunoreactive were found only in those areas which are also invested with NFTs or Alz-50 immunoreactive neurons. SPs that were beta amyloid immunoreactive were found more extensively in the neocortex, and much less frequently in those limbic cortices where NFTs were found (Arriagada *et al.*, 1992*b*). This spatial pattern of Alzheimer pathology in elderly persons is strikingly similar to the reported distribution of the lesion burden in AD (Pearson *et al.*, 1985; Hyman, Van Hoesen & Damasio, 1990; Arnold *et al.*, 1991; Braak & Braak, 1991; Arriagada *et al.*, 1992*a,b*). Arriagada and colleagues concluded that elderly nondemented individuals and Alzheimer patients display

the same hierarchical pattern of selective vulnerability, differences between these populations being quantitative rather than qualitative.

Braak and Braak have devised a staging system for Alzheimer-related pathology (Braak & Braak, 1991). They found the pattern of development of NFTs to be much more consistent and useful for staging than the distribution of SPs. In their hands, there is a stage of transentorhinal (perirhinal) involvement that precedes involvement of the entorhinal cortex proper. They distinguish two transentorhinal stages, followed by two 'limbic' stages, and finally two stages with progressively severe isocortical involvement. Their study did not involve correlation of pathological stage with clinical assessment of dementia. Which pathological stage might correspond to the earliest manifestation of dementia therefore is unclear. At an earlier date, Braak and Braak reported six cases of demented individuals with neurofibrillary pathology limited to layer II of the entorhinal cortex and the pre-alpha layer of the transentorhinal lesion. The patients also had widespread nonneuritic senile plaques. The authors discussed the possibility that this pattern may represent an initial stage of clinical AD (Braak & Braak, 1990*b*).

Hof and colleagues reported pathological findings in an 82 year-old subject who was felt to have had incipient dementia at the time of death. No neuropsychological data had been obtained, but unusually reliable collateral historical data was available (Hof *et al.*, 1992). In this patient, NFT counts similar to those of AD patients were found only in the perirhinal cortex, layers II and IV of the entorhinal cortex, and subiculum. NFTs were found in lesser numbers in hippocampal sectors and in the layers V and VI of the inferior temporal cortex. The nucleus basalis of Meynert had low NFT density but higher SP density. SPs were found throughout the neocortex.

Hyman and colleagues have reported another patient whose neuropsychological examination disclosed evidence of Alzheimer's disease. Autopsy 7 weeks after the examination showed NFTs in the entorhinal cortex, hippocampus, amygdala, dorsal raphe, and inferior temporal gyrus. Alz-50 positive SPs were limited to limbic areas; beta-amyloid immunoreactive SPs were widespread in the association cortex and amygdala (Hyman *et al.*, 1991*a,b*). Taken together, these cases suggest that the minimal lesion which can cause dementia in AD encompasses area 28, CA1, and probably the neocortex of the inferior temporal gyrus. At this stage, neuritic plaques may be limited to limbic structures.

Bouras and colleagues have recently buttressed this hypothesis with data from a large number of unselected autopsies performed at a geriatric hospital (Bouras *et al.*, 1994). Their cases, for which premorbid MMSE and clinical data were available, suggested that 'mild cognitive impairment and disorientation' was the maximal deficit seen in patients in whom NFTS did not yet invest the inferior temporal cortex.

CLINICAL CORRELATES OF REGIONAL AND LAMINAR SPECIFIC PATHOLOGY

We will consider the specificity of Alzheimer pathology in regard to three brain regions: 1) temporal lobe limbic structures; 2) association cortex in general; 3) ventromedial frontal lobe.

The medial temporal lobe and anterograde memory

The association of bilateral mesial temporal lesions with amnesia was first reported by Glees and Griffith (1952). In 1953, patient H.M. underwent bilateral mesial temporal lobe resection for the treatment of intractable epilepsy and developed a profound and irrevocable anterograde amnesic syndrome (Corkin, 1984). The case of H.M. became the paradigm of the amnesic syndrome. Numerous subsequent lesion studies have confirmed the inevitable correlation of bilateral hippocampal formation lesions with anterograde amnesia. The most focal and perhaps the most instructive case is that of Zola-Morgan and Squire's patient, R.B., who became amnesic as a result of an hypoxic-ischaemic intra-operative event. When he died 5 years later, an autopsy disclosed that the loss of neurons was limited to field CA1 of the hippocampus (Zola-Morgan, Squire & Amaral, 1986). Though the nature of the operations it accomplishes is debated, the hippocampal formation is established solidly as an essential neural substrate for the acquisition of new factual memory. The predilection in AD for early NFT formation in structures related to the hippocampus offers an alternative explanation to the cholinergic hypothesis for the early amnesia of Alzheimer's disease.

Fine-grained neuroanatomical analysis of the distribution of lesions in AD makes it clear that the hippocampus must be functionally disconnected from the cerebral cortex and amygdala in AD. We will now consider this evidence in some detail.

Anatomy of medial temporal limbic structures

The entorhinal cortex (EC, Brodmann's area 28) is a relatively large field of periallocortex that occupies the anterior part of the parahippocampal gyrus. It is composed of six layers, but it is atypical in several ways. Layer II contains large stellate neurons which are assembled in a complex mosaic that is interspersed with a fibre plexus. These clusters of neurons appear as intracortical cellular islands in cortical cross-sections. Layer III has pyramidal neurons that resemble those in isocortex. However, its deeper portion is acellular and packed densely with cell processes (the lamina dessicans). Layer IV is formed by a population of large multipolar neurons. Layers V and VI are not well defined and are composed of many different cell types. The transition from entorhinal cortex to temporal isocortex occurs as interdigitations of allo- and isocortical laminae rather than as a smooth transition (Braak & Braak, 1985). At the entorhinal border of this perirhinal or 'transentorhinal' cortex (Brodmann's area 35), the cellular islands of layer II amalgamate (Braak's pre-alpha layer). The pre-alpha layer gradually moves obliquely through the outer cellular layers to lie in a deeper position at the isocortical border of this zone. The connectivity of the neurons of the pre-alpha layer is not known.

The entorhinal cortex sits at the apex of an orderly system of feedforward and feedback connections from the occipital, parietal, temporal, and limbic lobes (Van Hoesen *et al.*, 1986; Jones & Powell, 1970; Seltzer & Pandya, 1978; Pandya & Yeterian, 1985). Primary sensory cortices project (primarily via pyramids in layer III) to the surrounding early association cortices. These connections are reciprocated, primarily by pyramids in layer V (Rockland & Pandya, 1979; Barbas, 1986). Early association cortices (e.g. Brodmann areas 18, 19) project to higher order cortices; these connections are also reciprocated. Eventually the polymodal sensory association cortices converge on the entorhinal cortex (Kosel, Van Hoesen & Rosene, 1982; Van Hoesen, 1982). There are also afferents to the EC from limbic (cingulate gyrus) and unimodal sensory association cortices. The EC is essentially the only cortical portal into the hippocampus. The main cortical afferent tract to the hippocampus, the perforant pathway, has its cell bodies in layer II and the superficial portion of layer III of the entorhinal cortex. The perforant pathway 'perforates' the subiculum and crosses the hippocampal fissure to terminate in the outer two-thirds of the molecular layer of the dentate gyrus, synapsing there with the outer dendritic branches of the dentate granule cells.

The hippocampus proper is the rolled up edge of the medial temporal lobe. It is an allocortical structure with distinct subfields. Area CA4 (CA = cornu ammonis,

Ammon's horn) is found within the hilus of the dentate gyrus. Proceeding around Ammon's horn to the subiculum, one sequentially encounters the fields CA3, CA2, and then CA1. The subiculum itself has recognized subdivisions which are interposed between the hippocampus and the entorhinal cortex: presubiculum, prosubiculum, parasubiculum.

Although the hippocampus projects to several structures, including the amygdala and the hypothalamus, it has essentially only one cortical projection: via the subiculum, to layer IV of the entorhinal cortex. Thus, anatomical evidence strongly suggests that the entorhinal cortex is in a strategic location with respect to hippocampal–cortical interactions, as all direct communication between these structures bottlenecks there. Moreover, the close proximity of the neurons of the afferent and efferent arms of this reciprocal projection affords an opportunity for the hippocampal formation to modulate its own activity.

The amygdala is a conspicuous subcortical limbic structure which lies immediately anterior to the hippocampus. It has connections with several structures related to memory: entorhinal cortex, hippocampus, basal nucleus of Meynert, dorsomedial nucleus of the thalamus. Like the entorhinal cortex, it is also an area of convergence of multimodal information from all sensory modalities. There are major connections from the amygdala to the hypothalamus and to the autonomic centres of the brainstem. Although the role of the amygdala in memory is not fully understood, it is fair to say this structure is indispensable in the processing of stimuli with affective significance.

Early pathological changes in AD isolate the hippocampus

The earliest Alzheimer changes may occur in the pre-alpha layer of area 35. Although it is noteworthy that lesions of the perirhinal and entorhinal cortex in animals lead to amnesia (Zola-Morgan et al., 1989), it is difficult to predict the consequences of the selective loss of the transentorhinal pre-alpha neurons, given their unknown connectivity. Another reason to be circumspect about correlating perirhinal pathology with memory impairment is that patients presenting the earliest signs of AD have pathology that has moved beyond the transentorhinal stage to also involve the entorhinal cortex, CA1, and the inferior temporal isocortex.

Layers II and IV of the entorhinal cortex are some of the very earliest affected structures in AD. Layer II contains most of the cells of origin of the strategic

perforant pathway, and layer IV receives the subicular afferents that constitute the only cortical projection of the hippocampus. Hyman and colleagues have convincingly demonstrated the invariable involvement of the perforant pathway's cells of origin (Hyman, Van Hoesen & Damasio, 1986) and projections (Hyman et al., 1988a,b) in AD. In the hippocampus proper, the CA1/subicular zone and especially the prosubiculum is invariably heavily involved with SPs and NFTs in AD. It is this hippocampal zone that sends the projection to the entorhinal cortex. By precluding hippocampal–cortical interaction, these early changes of AD are likely to contribute to the early and prominent amnesia so characteristic of AD. The hippocampus is functionally isolated from the cerebral cortex.

Changes in amygdala

Although the structural-functional correlation is seen with greatest clarity in the hippocampal–entorhinal relationship, AD affects numerous other temporal and neocortical structures that make a contribution to memory function. It is likely that many of these lesions take their toll.

In a study in which they examined the temporal lobes of 20 persons with AD, Kromer Vogt, Hyman and others found that in all cases there were NFTs and senile plaques in the amygdala (Kromer-Vogt et al., 1990). Certain nuclei of this complex structure are severely and consistently affected. The most severely affected nuclei, in terms of numbers of NFTs, are the accessory basal and cortical nuclei. The mediobasal nucleus is moderately affected and the medial, lateral, laterobasal and central nuclei are relatively spared. SPs are found in a somewhat different distribution: Accessory basal and medial basal > cortical, lateral, latero-basal, and medial nuclei (Hyman et al., 1990). Of the nuclei which project heavily to the hippocampus, accessory basal, and lateral, the accessory basal is severely affected with NFTs. The accessory basal nucleus is also one of the major sources of afferents to the entorhinal cortex, which terminate in layer III. βA4 amyloid protein deposition in this layer has been demonstrated. Hippocampal and entorhinal projections to the amygdala arise from EC layer IV and from the CA1/subiculum zone, both of which are severely affected by AD and contain numerous NFTs. Olfactory connections to the amygdala are affected inconsistently. Connections with the basal nucleus of Meynert (via laterobasal nucleus) are relatively spared (Kromer-Vogt et al., 1990).

In summary, the cells of origin of most of the interconnecting projections of the EC, the hippocampal formation, and the amygdala are vulnerable to NFT formation. Specifically, disruption of the perforant pathway, the projection from EC layer IV to amygdala, and the projections of the prosubiculum to the entorhinal cortex and amygdala are all affected.

Pathological changes in isocortex

The general pattern of cognitive impairment of moderately advanced Alzheimer's disease (e.g. Braaks' first isocortical stage) might also have been predicted from the hierarchical vulnerability of the neocortical association cortices. The pattern of impairment of factual knowledge in AD can be understood in terms of the convergence zone framework, which has been developed to account for the pattern of deficits observed in human subjects with acquired focal brain lesions (Damasio & Damasio 1994; Damasio, 1989). Some important aspects of this framework are: 1) damage to early association cortices compromises the retrieval of entity features (e.g. colour); 2) damage to intermediately placed cortices leaves the retrieval of features intact, but compromises the retrieval of knowledge for non-unique entities, sometimes in a category-specific manner; 3) damage to the anteriormost cortices compromises retrieval of unique entities and events. For example, patients with lesions in the left temporal pole can have defective retrieval of the word forms for proper nouns but not common nouns (Graff-Radford et al., 1990). Patients with bilateral lesions of both inferotemporal cortices cannot access the unique knowledge pertinent to a visual entity, such as a face (Damasio et al., 1990).

The neuropsychological profile of the patient known as Boswell is instructive. This patient suffered selective, bilateral destruction of the following brain structures due to herpes simplex encephalitis: entorhinal cortex, hippocampus, amygdala, temporal pole (BA 38), anterolateral and anteroinferior temporal cortices (BA 20, 21, anterior 22, portions of 37), the entire basal forebrain (septum, nucleus basalis of Meynert, nucleus accumbens) and the posterior orbitofrontal cortex. The pattern of involvement in Boswell is therefore strikingly analogous to the regional pattern of involvement in Alzheimer's disease, in which the mesial temporal structures and temporal pole are severely affected, the area known as IT (areas 20, 21, and 37) and the posterior orbitofrontal cortex are also affected, though less severely, and the early sensory and motor cortices are relatively spared. Boswell's cognitive impairments include: complete anterograde amnesia for factual knowledge,

retrograde amnesia for all unique entities and events, and a deficit of knowledge for certain categories of non-unique factual knowledge. Boswell's ability to learn motor skills, his basic perceptual and motor abilities, his ability to sustain attention, and categorical knowledge are unimpaired.

There is a striking overall correspondence between Boswell's deficits and those of Alzheimer patients. AD patients are, as a rule, free of elementary motor and sensory impairments, as might be expected from the virtual sparing of primary sensory and motor cortices. Like Boswell, these patients have a relatively intact capacity for the acquisition of perceptuomotor skills whose retrieval does not require the generation of a conscious internal representation (i.e. procedural or motor learning). Finally, AD patients display defective knowledge of unique objects and events, while manifesting relative sparing of categorical knowledge. They fail to recognize faces of family members and forget their names, but have no difficulty recognizing the gender of faces, for example. AD patients manifest higher order sensory and motor impairments (agnosia and apraxia), consistent with the involvement of the highest order association cortices. Indeed, Alzheimer's disease appears to affect selectively the very neurons upon which large-scale cortico-cortical interconnectivity depends. NFTs are found primarily in the large pyramids of layer III, which feed forward to higher order association cortices, and in the large pyramids of layer V, which feed back to earlier association cortices (Rockland & Pandya, 1979).

Data supporting the presence of a vulnerable subpopulation of neurons that respects the hierarchical arrangement of corticocortical connectivity has also been recently marshalled by De Lacoste and White (1993; see also the commentary which follows).

Ventromedial frontal cortex

Chu and colleagues have related the laminar pattern of NFT formation in ventromedial frontal cortices to abnormalities of autonomic function in Alzheimer patients. For example, area 25, the posterior orbito-frontal cortices, and the anterior insula are important in central autonomic regulation, via afferents from layer V. These connections are disrupted by the neurofibrillary pathology in layer V (Chu et al., 1992). Chu has found that AD patients fail to develop sympathetic skin conduction responses to emotionally charged visual stimuli, as do patients with focal lesions in these same cortices (Chu, 1994). These same patients exhibit defective personal and social decision-making as their prominent behavioural abnormality. This is in keeping with the somatic marker hypothesis advanced by Damasio and colleagues, which postulates the reactivation of visceral and musculoskeletal states as a component in the process of normal personal and social decision-making (Damasio, Tranel & Damasio, 1991).

Are plaques or tangles better correlated with clinical symptoms of Alzheimer's disease?

Which manifestation of AD, NFTs or SPs, is more directly related to AD's clinical symptoms? If the amnesia of AD is any indication, it appears that the distribution of the neurofibrillary changes provides a good correlate to the neuropsychological impairments of AD patients, at least in the early stages of AD. The following facts also support this conclusion: 1) There are well-documented cases of non-demented elderly individuals with extensive SPs in neocortex. 2) The distribution of NFTs in AD is highly stereotyped and hierarchical, making staging of the disease possible, whereas SPs are distributed less specifically and less consistently. 3) A recent quantitative study failed to establish a significant correlation between SP burden and severity of dementia, whereas the correlation between NFT burden and severity of dementia was highly significant (Arriagada *et al.*, 1992*a*). Wilcock and Esiri (1982) and Bouras *et al.*, (1994) have reported similar findings. This last finding is discrepant in relation to the seminal work of Tomlinson, Blessed, and colleagues, the first to show a relationship between SPs and dementia by regression analysis. One explanation for this discrepancy might be the inclusion of non-demented individuals in the sample in Blessed's series. When only affected individuals are considered, a trend is present but correlation does not reach statistical significance (Terry *et al.*, 1991; Arriagada *et al.*, 1992*b*). Moreover, these investigators did not attempt to correlate tangles with dementia. Some investigators have called attention to a poorer correlation between plaques and tangles and cognitive impairment in the later stages of AD (Terry *et al.*, 1991). These investigations demonstrated that neuronal and synaptic loss made a better correlate (Neary 1986) of global neuropsychological indices in these cases. This possibly reflects the failure of NFTs and plaques to accumulate with time in association cortex (Mann *et al.*, 1988); whereas in medial temporal structures, degenerated neurons are marked with tombstone tangles, in the isocortex tombstone neurons are rare. Another possibility is that not all neurons destined to degenerate develop NFTs. Never-

theless, it appears to be the population of cells which is marked by NFT formation which drops out.

But these facts, intriguing as they are, do not fully answer the question of which lesion type is most closely related to the *aetiology* of AD. While one may reason that the initial pathological manifestations of a disease most likely reflect the primary insult, it is possible that NFT formation is a sort of stereotyped cellular reaction to the disease which is maladaptive and leads to the cognitive dysfunction as a secondary phenomenon. It is possible that only a certain class of neurons, large cortico-cortical projecting pyramidal cells, react in this characteristic way. The state of understanding of the aetiology and pathogenesis of AD has recently become, if anything, less clear by virtue of the recent development of several vigorous and as yet unharmonized lines of investigation (Yankner *et al.*, 1990; Selkoe, 1991; Nitsch *et al.*, 1992; Strittmatter, Saunders & Schmechel, 1993; Schmechel & Milner, 1957). Although tangle formation is only one aspect of a complex pathophysiological process, the correlations we and others have enumerated make it plausible that therapy aimed at interrupting the process leading to NFT formation in this vulnerable neuronal subpopulation could ameliorate the clinical course of Alzheimer's disease.

Additional evidence to support this interpretation of the literature relating Alzheimer pathology to clinical deficits comes from atypical presentations of AD, to which we now turn.

Variant cases of Alzheimer's disease: pathological correlations

A small number of pathologically verified cases of Alzheimer's disease present with visual disturbances, rather than with amnesia (Cogan, 1985; Hof *et al.*, 1989, 1990*a*; Levine, Lee & Fisher, 1993). The even smaller number of such cases in which systematic neuropathological observations have been made contribute substantially to the confidence with which neuropsychological deficits can be correlated with regional Alzheimer lesion burden.

Levine and colleagues (Levine *et al.*, 1993) reported the case of a 59 year-old executive whose first difficulty was reading. At the time of his first neurological examination, two years later, problems in locating and identifying objects by sight dominated the neuropsychological profile. Although the history indicated subtle memory difficulty, no objective memory impairment was detected by the examiners. His illness pursued a 12-year, relentlessly progressive course which was remarkable for progressive visual dysfunction and the relatively late development of marked amnesia and aphasia. Careful neuropsychological and psychophysical observations were made during his illness. At autopsy, striking occipitoparietal atrophy was found. NFTs were abundant in the primary (area 17) and association (areas 18 and 20) visual cortices, the posterior cingulate gyrus, hippocampus, amygdala, and temporal isocortex. There were far fewer tangles in the frontal lobes than in the parietal and occipital lobes, which is the reverse of the usual pattern. Beta-amyloid immunoreactive plaques were most numerous in visual association cortex and frontal cortex, but neuritic plaques made up high percentages of the plaques in primary visual cortex and visual association cortex. The unusual occurrence of large numbers of NFTs and NPs in the primary visual cortex, and the disproportionate numbers of NFTs and NPs in the visual association cortices in this case correlate extraordinarily well with the patient's well-documented clinical course.

Hof and colleagues reported eight cases pathologically similar to the case of Levine et al. (1993). Although far less clinical information was available for these cases, they were all said to have Balint's syndrome. The pathological findings were homogeneous (Hof, Cox & Morrison, 1990b): 1) Brodmann's areas 17, 18, 19 had much higher numbers of NFTs and NP than did typical AD control cases. In the deep layers of area 17, the number of NFTs was 63-fold higher than AD controls. Moreover, there was a striking dropout of Meynert cells in layers V and VI of the primary visual cortex, cells which are normally not affected in AD. 2) There were greatly increased numbers of NFTs in the superior colliculus, relative to AD controls. 3) There were significantly fewer NFTs in prefrontal cortices (areas 9, 45, 46) relative to AD controls. 4) Parietal area 7b and the posterior cingulate (area 23) had higher incidences of NPs than AD controls. The hippocampus was severely affected in all subjects. This group had previously shown that the affected pyramidal cells in the occipital cortex in AD are those giving rise to long corticocortical connections (Hof & Morrison, 1990).

Hof and Bouras (1991) have also reported a case of an 89 year-old Alzheimer patient who was found to have a prominent defect in visual object recognition at the time of diagnosis, in the context of 'slight memory disturbances and disorientation'. Tactile agnosia and prosopagnosia occurred later in the course. At autopsy, disproportionate occipito-temporal atrophy was found. The distribution of NFTs was similar to Hof's cases of AD-Balints, with the following exceptions. In the middle temporal gyrus (BA 21), this case had more NFTs than AD controls and in the posterior parietal cortex (BA 7b), strikingly fewer NFTs than controls (Hof & Bouras, 1991). The authors interpret their findings to represent relative interruption of the ventral visual stream in the case of AD-visual agnosia, and relative interruption of the dorsal stream in AD-Balints. Although cases with careful ante-mortem neuropsychological testing will be required to put this interpretation on solid footing, their cases do help to establish the visual variant of Alzheimer disease.

Yet another unusual Alzheimer variant was reported by Jagust and colleagues (Jagust et al., 1990). This patient manifested a clinical course that was generally typical for Alzheimer's disease, but was exceptional because of a progressive left hemiparesis associated with signs of corticospinal tract dysfunction. At autopsy, in addition to advanced and classically distributed AD pathology, there was focally severe atrophy of the right post-central gyrus (BAs 3,1,2). This area was invested with numerous NFTs. As with the visual variant cases, the exception proves the rule: atypical clinical findings were explained by an atypical distribution of pathology.

Crystal and colleagues reported a case of a woman presenting with left-sided astereognosis and pseudo-athetosis and preserved memory, in whom a right frontal biopsy revealed Alzheimer's disease. A CT scan showed cortical atrophy which was worse on the right side. Further pathological data was not obtained (Crystal et al., 1982).

The well-documented cases of variant Alzheimer presentations are significant mainly for reinforcing the idea that the cognitive impairments in AD can be related directly to the distribution of cortical pathology. Although cases such as these are rare (Hof culled the eight cases of AD-Balints from 2500 autopsies), minor differences in cognitive profiles between AD patients are common, and potentially amenable to clinico-pathologic correlation using quantitative approaches. For example, early onset AD may feature disproportionate language disturbance (Sevush, Leve & Brickman, 1993). Functional imaging, which can identify metabolic asymmetries in these subjects, can provide converging evidence in this sort of endeavour. Several investigators have reported that in some cases of AD, parietal hypometabolism is asymmetric and that this correlates with neuropsychological findings (Foster et al., 1983). For example, Haxby and colleagues reported a longitudinal study of 11 demented subjects. Right–left asymmetries of parietal glucose metabolism, identified with positron emission tomography, correlated significantly with neuropsychological discrepancies between visuospatial and language abilities in these patients. The detected asymmetries were stable over time, indeed tending to become more pronounced (Haxby *et al.*, 1990).

CONCLUSIONS

Since Alzheimer's disease respects regional and laminar structure in the brain and because of the relatively stereotyped evolution of the burden of lesions, it is possible to attempt deficit–lesion correlation. The indispensable role of the hippocampal formation in anterograde memory, the anatomy of the entorhinal–hippocampal connections, and the characteristically limited extent of the lesion burden in incipient Alzheimer's disease, when amnesia in the overriding deficit, made it possible to establish the first clinical–pathological correlation in AD. Careful inventory of the brain regions affected by NFTs and, to a lesser extent, SPs, also explains the characteristic sparing of elementary motor and sensory function in AD. Other efforts have followed in a similar spirit, including important observations in the brains of patients with the visual variant of Alzheimer's disease.

The realization that the distribution of pathology in AD harmonizes and converges with evidence from the lesion literature constitutes a significant departure from previous attempts to account for the neuropsychological deficits found in patients with AD, which have largely been attributed to a neurochemical deficiency resulting from the degeneration of subcortical nuclei. We believe that the cognitive deficits which characterize this disease can best be explained in terms of selective disruption of certain neural systems.

ACKNOWLEDGEMENTS

Supported by a grant from Kiwanis International (Illinois-Eastern Iowa District) and Spastic Paralysis Research Foundation and from the Iowa Scottish Rite Charitable and Educational Foundation.

REFERENCES

Adams RD, Victor M (1989) *Principles of Neurology* 4th edn., McGraw-Hill, New York.

Albert ML, Feldman RG, Willis AL (1974) The 'subcortical dementia' of progressive supranuclear palsy. *J Neurol, Neurosurg, Psychiat* 37: 121–30.

Alzheimer A (1907) On a peculiar disease of the cerebral cortex. *Allg Zeit Psychiat Psych-gericht Med* 64: 146.

American Psychiatric Association Task Force on Nomenclature and Statistics. (1994). *Diagnostic and Statistical Manual of Mental Disorders*, 4th edn, revised.

Armstrong RA (1993) Is the clustering of neurofibrillary tangles in Alzheimer's patients related to the cells of origin of specific cortico-cortical projections? *Neurosci Lett* 160: 57–60.

Arnold SE, Hyman BT, Flory J, Damasio AR, Van Hoesen GW (1991) The topographical and neuroanatomical distribution of neurofibrillary tangles and neuritic plaques in the cerebral cortex of patients with Alzheimer's disease. *Cerebral Cortex* 1: 103–16.

Arnold SE, Hyman BT, Van Hoesen GW (1994) Neuropathologic changes of the temporal pole in Alzheimer's disease and Pick's disease. *Neurol* 51: 145–50.

Arriagada PV, Growdon JH, Hedley-Whyte ET, Hyman BT (1992a). Neurofibrillary tangles but not senile plaques parallel duration and severity of Alzheimer's disease. *Neurology* 42: 631–9.

Arriagada PV, Hyman BT (1990) Predominance of A-4 over Alz-50 positive plaques in demented elderly (abstract). *Neurobiol Aging*, 11.

Arriagada PV, Marzloff K, Hyman BT (1992b) Distribution of Alzheimer-type pathologic changes in nondemented elderly individuals matches the pattern in Alzheimer's disease. *Neurology* 42: 1681–8.

Ball MJ (1978) Topographic distribution of neurofibrillary tangles and granulovacuolar degeneration in hippocampal cortex of aging and demented patients. *Acta Neuropath* 42: 73–80.

Ball MJ, Lo P (1977) Granulovacuolar degeneration in aging brain and in dementia. *J Neuropath Exp Neurol* 36: 474–87.

Ball MJ, Fisman M, Hachinski V, Blume W, Fox A, Kral VA, Kirshen AJ, Fox H (1985) A new definition of Alzheimer's disease: a hippocampal dementia. *Lancet* i: 14–16.

Ball MJ, Vis CL (1978) Relationship of granulovacuolar degeneration in hippocampal neurones to aging and to dementia in normal-pressure hydrocephalus. *J Gerontol* 33: 815–24.

Bancher C, Brunner C, Lassmann H, Budka H, Jellinger K, Wiche G, Seitelberger F, Grundke-Iqbal I, Iqbal K, Wisniewski HM (1989) Accumulation of abnormally phosphorylated tau precedes the formation of neurofibrillary tangles in Alzheimer's disease. *Brain Res* 477: 90–9.

Barbas H (1986) Pattern in the laminar origin of corticocortical connections. *J Comp Neurol* 252: 415–22.

Barcikowska M, Wisniewski HM, Bancher C, Grundke-Iqbal I (1989) About the presence of paired helical filaments in dystrophic neurites participating in the plaque formation. *Acta Neuropath* 78: 225–31.

Bartus RT, Dean RL III, Beer B, Lippa AS (1982) The cholinergic hypothesis of geriatric memory dysfunction. *Science* 217: 408–14.

Bell MA & Ball MJ (1990) Neuritic plaques and vessels of the visual cortex in aging and Alzheimer's dementia. *Neurobiol Aging* 11: 359–70.

Benson DF, Davis RJ, Snyder BD (1988) Posterior cortical atrophy. *Arch Neurol* 45: 789–93.

Benton JS, Bowen DM, Allen SJ, Haan EA, Davison AN, Neary D, Murphy RP, Snowden JS (1982) Alzheimer's disease as a disorder of the isodendritic core. *Lancet* i, 456.

Blessed G, Tomlinson BE, Roth M (1968) The association between quantitative measures of dementia and of senile change in the cerebral grey matter of elderly subjects. *Br J Psychiat* 114: 797–811.

Blocq P, Marinesco G (1928) Sur les lésions et le pathogénie de l'epilepsie dite essentielle. *Sem Med (Paris)* 12: 445–6.

Bouras C, Hof PR, Giannakopoulos P, Michel J-P, Morrison JH (1994) Regional distribution of neurofibrillary tangles and senile plaques in the cerebral cortex of elderly patients: a quantitative evaluation of a one-year autopsy population from a geriatric hospital. *Cerebral Cortex* 4: 138–50.

Braak H, Braak E (1985) On areas of transition between entorhinal allocortex and temporal isocortex in the human brain. Normal morphology and lamina-specific pathology in Alzheimer's disease. *Acta Neuropath* 68: 325–32.

Braak H, Braak E (1988) Neuropil threads occur in dendrites of tangle-bearing nerve cells. *Neuropath Appl Neurobiol* 14: 39–44.

Braak H, Braak E (1990a) Alzheimer's disease: striatal amyloid deposits and neurofibrillary changes. *J Neuropath Exp Neurol* 49: 215–24.

Braak H, Braak E (1990b) Neurofibrillary changes confined to the entorhinal region and an abundance of cortical amyloid in cases of senile and presenile dementia. *Acta Neuropath* 80: 479–86.

Braak H, Braak E (1991) Neuropathological staging of Alzheimer-related changes. *Acta Neuropath* 82: 239–59.

Braak H, Braak E, Grundke-Iqbal I, Iqbal K (1986) Occurrence of neuropil threads in the senile human brain and in Alzheimer's disease: a third location of paired helical filaments outside of neurofibrillary tangles and neuritic plaques. *Neurosci Lett* 65: 351–5.

Brayne C, Calloway P (1988) Dogma disputed. *Lancet* 337: 1265–7.

Brun A, Englund E (1986) A white matter disorder in dementia of the Alzheimer type: a pathoanatomical study. *Ann Neurol* 19: 253–62.

Brun A, Gustafson L (1976) Distribution of cerebral degeneration in Alzheimer's disease. *Acta Psychiat Nervenkr* 223: 15–33.

Cabalka LM, Hyman BT, Goodlett CR, Ritchie TC, Van Hoesen GW (1992) Alteration in the pattern of nerve terminal protein immunoreactivity in the perforant pathway in Alzheimer's disease and in rats after entorhinal lesions. *Neurobiol Aging* 13: 283–91.

Chu C-C (1994) Pathology in the autonomic-related limbic cortices in Alzheimer's disease and its possible behavioral roles. (Dissertation, University of Iowa).

Chu C-C, Flory J, Van Hoesen GW (1993) Orbitofrontal pathology in Alzheimer's disease. *Soc Neurosci Abst* 19: 190.

Chu C-C, Tranel D, Damasio AR (1994) Impaired autonomic responses to emotionally significant stimuli in Alzheimer's disease. *Soc Neurosci Abst*, 20.

Chu C-C, Van Hoesen GW, Damasio AR (1992) Cellular specific pathology alters probable cortico-autonomic afferents in Alzheimer's disease. *Soc Neurosci Abst* 18: 735.

Chui HC, Teng EL, Henderson VW, Moy AC (1985) Clinical subtypes of dementia of the Alzheimer type. *Neurology* 35: 1544–50.

Cogan DG (1985) Visual disturbances with focal progressive dementing disease. *Am J Ophthalmol* 100: 68–72.

Corkin S (1984) Lasting consequences of bilateral medial temporal lobectomy: Clinical course and experimental findings in HM. *Semin Neurol* 4: 249–59.

Corsellis JAN (1962) *Mental Illness and the Aging Brain: the Distribution of Pathological Change in a Mental Hospital Population.* Oxford University Press, London.

Crystal H, Dickson D, Fuld P, Masur D, Scott R, Mehler M, Masdeu J, Kawas C, Aronson M, Wolfson L (1988) Clinicopathologic studies in dementia: nondemented subjects with pathologically confirmed Alzheimer's disease. *Neurology* 38: 1682–7.

Crystal HA, Horoupian DS, Katzman R, Jotkowicz S (1982) Biopsy-proved Alzheimer disease presenting as a right parietal syndrome. *Ann Neurol* 12: 186–8.

Cummings JL, Benson DF (1992) *Dementia: A Clinical Approach.* Butterworth-Heinemann, Boston.

Damasio AR (1989) The brain binds entities and events by multiregional activation from convergence zones. *Neur Comput* 1: 123–32.

Damasio AR, Damasio H (1994) Cortical systems for retrieval of concrete knowledge: the convergence zone framework. In Koch C (ed) *Large-Scale Neuronal Theories of the Brain*, MIT Press, Cambridge.

Damasio AR, Damasio H, Tranel D, Brandt JP (1990) Neural regionalization of knowledge access: preliminary evidence. In *Quantitative Biology*. Cold Spring Harbor, New York.

Damasio AR, Tranel D (1991) Disorders of higher brain function. In Rosenberg RN (ed) *Comprehensive Neurology*, New York: Raven Press, New York, pp. 639–57.

Damasio AR, Tranel D, Damasio H (1990) Face agnosia and the neural substrates of memory. *Ann Rev Neurosci* 13: 89–109.

Damasio AR, Tranel D, Damasio H (1991) Somatic markers and the guidance of behavior: theory and preliminary testing. In Levin HS, Eisenberg HM, Benton AL (eds) *Frontal Lobe Function and Dysfunction*, Oxford University Press, New York, pp 217–99.

Damasio AR, Van Hoesen GW, Hyman BT (1990) Reflections on the selectivity of neuropathological changes in Alzheimer's disease. In Schwartz MF (ed) *Modular Deficits in Alzheimer-Type Dementia*, MIT Press, Cambridge, MA, pp 83–99.

Damasio H, Damasio AR (1989) *Lesion Analysis in Neuropsychology*. Oxford University Press, New York.

Davies L, Wolska B, Hilbich C, Multhaup G, Martins R, Simms G, Beyreuther K, Masters CL (1988) A4 amyloid protein deposition and the diagnosis of Alzheimer's disease. *Neurology* 38: 1688–93.

Davies P, Maloney AJF (1976) Selective loss of central cholinergic neurons in Alzheimer's disease. *Lancet* ii: 1403.

Davis PC, Gray L, Albert M, Wilkinson W, Hughes J, Heyman A, Gado M, Kumar AJ, Destian S, Lee C, Duvall E, Kido D, Nelson MJ, Bello J, Weathers S, Jolesz F, Kikinis R, Brooks M (1992) The consortium to establish a registry for Alzheimer's disease (CERAD). Part III. Reliability of a standardized MRI evaluation of Alzheimer's disease. *Neurology* 42: 1676–80.

Dayan AD (1970) Quantitative histological studies on the aged human brain. *Acta Neuropath* 16: 95–102.

De Lacoste M-C, White CL (1993) The role of cortical connectivity in Alzheimer's disease pathogenesis: a review and model system. *Neurobiol of Aging* 14: 1–16.

De Renzi E (1986) Slowly progressive visual agnosia or apraxia without dementia. *Cortex* 22: 171–80.

DeKosky ST, Scheff SW (1990) Synapse loss in frontal cortex biopsies in Alzheimer disease: correlation with cognitive security. *Ann Neurol* 27: 457–64.

Delacourte A, Flament S, Dibe EM, Hublau P, Sablonniere B, Hemon B, Sherrer V, Defossez A (1990) Pathological proteins Tau 64 and 69 are specifically expressed in the somatodendritic domain of the degenerating cortical neurons during Alzheimer's disease. *Acta Neuropath* 80: 111–17.

Delaere P, Duyckaerts C, Brion JP, Poulain V, Hauw JJ (1989) Tau, paired helical filaments and amyloid in the neocortex: a morphometric study of 15 cases with graded intellectual status in aging and senile dementia of Alzheimer type. *Acta Neuropath* : 645–53.

Di Patre PL (1991) Cytoskeletal alterations might account for the phylogenetic vulnerability of the human brain to Alzheimer's disease. *Med Hypotheses* 34: 165–70.

Dickson DW, Liu WK, Kress Y, Ku J, DeJesus O, Yen SHC (1993) Phosphorylated tau immunoreactivity of granulovacuolar bodies (GVB) of Alzheimer's disease: localization of two amino terminal tau epitopes in GVB. *Acta Neuropath* 85: 463–70.

Duyckaerts C, Hauw JJ, Bastenaire F, Piette F, Poulain C, Rainsard V, Javoy-Agid Berthaux P (1986) Laminar distribution of neocortical senile plaques in senile dementia of the Alzheimer type. *Acta Neuropath* 70: 249–56.

Emson PC, Lindvall O (1986) Neuroanatomical aspects of neurotransmitters affected in Alzheimer's disease. *Br Med Bull* 42: 57–62.

Esiri MM, Pearson RCA, Steele JE, Bowen DM, Powell TPS (1990) A quantitative study of the neurofibrillary tangles and the choline acetyltransferase activity in the cerebral cortex and the amygdala in Alzheimer's disease. *J Neurol, Neurosurg Psychiat* 53: 161–5.

Fisher CM (1989) Binswanger's encephalopathy: a review. *J Neurol* 236: 65–79.

Foster NL, Chase TN, Fedio P, Patronas NJ, Brooks RA, Di Chiro G (1983) Alzheimer's disease: focal cortical changes shown by positron emission tomography. *Neurology* 33: 961–5.

Foster NL, Chase TN, Mansi L, Brooks R, Fedio P, Patronas NJ, Di Chiro G (1984) Cortical abnormalities in Alzheimer's disease. *Ann Neurol* 16: 649–54.

Freedman L, Selchen DH, Black SE, Kaplan R, Garnett ES, Nahmias C (1991). Posterior cortical dementia with alexia: neurobehavioural, MRI, and PET finding. *J Neurol, Neurosurg, Psychiat* 54: 443–8.

Gibb, WRG, Luthert PJ, Marsden CD (1989) Corticobasal degeneration. *Brain* 112: 1171–92.

Glees P, Griffith HB (1952) Bilateral destruction of the hippocampus (cornu ammonis) in a case of dementia. *Monatssch Psychiat Neurol* 123: 193–204.

Goedert M (1993) Tau protein and the neurofibrillary pathology of Alzheimer's disease. *Trends Neurosci* 16: 460–5.

Goldman JE (1983) The association of actin with Hirano bodies. *J Neuropath Exp Neurol* 42: 146–52.

Graff-Radford NR, Damasio AR, Hyman BT, Hart MN, Tranel D, Damasio H, Van Hoesen GW, Rezai K (1990) Progressive aphasia in a patient with Pick's disease: a neuropsychological, radiologic, and anatomic study. *Neurology* 40: 620–6.

Grant I, Adams KM (1994) *Neuropsychological Assessment of Neuropsychiatric Disorders*. Oxford University Press, New York (in press).

Growdon JH (1992) Treatment for Alzheimer's disease. *New Eng J Med* 327: 1306–8.

Hachinski VC, Iliff LD, Zilhka E, Du Boulay GH, McAllister VL, Marshall J, Russell RWR, Symon L (1975) Cerebral blood flow in dementia. *Arch Neurol* 32: 632–7.

Hansen LA, Masliah E, Quijada-Fawcett S, Rexin D (1991) Entorhinal neurofibrillary tangles in Alzheimer disease with Lewy bodies. *Neurosci Lett* 129: 268–72.

Haxby JV, Grady CL, Koss E, Horwitz B, Heston L, Schapiro M, Friedland RP, Rapoport SI (1990) Longitudinal study of cerebral metabolic asymmetries and associated neuropsychological patterns in early dementia of the Alzheimer type. *Arch Neurol* 47: 753–60.

Hof PR, Bierer LM, Perl DP, Delacourte ABL, Bouras C, Morrison JH (1992) Evidence for early vulnerability of the medial and inferior aspects of the temporal lobe in an 82 year old patient with preclinical signs of dementia. *Arch Neurol* 49: 946–53.

Hof PR, Bouras C (1991) Object recognition deficit in Alzheimer's disease: possible disconnection of the occipito-temporal component of the visual system. *Neurosci Lett* 122: 53–6.

Hof PR, Bouras C, Constantinidis J, Morrison JH (1989) Balint's syndrome in Alzheimer's disease: specific disruption of the occipito-parietal visual pathway. *Brain Res* 493: 368–75.

Hof PR, Bouras C, Constantinidis J, Morrison JH (1990*a*) Selective disconnection of specific visual association pathways in cases of Alzheimer's disease presenting with Balint's syndrome. *J Neuropath Exp Neurol* 49: 168–84.

Hof, PR, Cox K, Morrison JH (1990*b*) Quantitative analysis of a vulnerable subset of pyramidal neurons in Alzheimer's disease: I. Superior frontal and inferior temporal cortex. *J Comp Neurol* 301: 44–54.

Hof PR, Morrison JH (1990) Quantitative analysis of a vulnerable subset of pyramidal neurons in Alzheimer's disease: II. Primary and secondary visual cortex. *J Comp Neurol* 301: 55–64.

Hubbard BM, Fenton GW, Anderson JM (1990) A quantitative histological study of early clinical and preclinical Alzheimer's disease. *Neuropath Appl Neurobiol* 16: 111–21.

Hyman BT (1992) Down syndrome and Alzheimer disease. *Prog Clin Biol Res* 379: 123–42.

Hyman BT, Arriagada PV, McKee AC, Ghika J, Corkin S, Growdon JH (1991*a*) The earliest symptoms of Alzheimer disease: anatomic correlates. *Soc Neurosci Abst*, 352.

Hyman BT, Damasio AR, Van Hoesen GW, Barnes CL (1984) Alzheimer's disease: cell specific pathology isolates the hippocampal formation. *Science* 225: 1168–70.

Hyman BT, Flory JE, Arnold SE, Van Hoesen GW, Schelper RL, Ghanbari H, Haigler H (1991*b*) Quantitative assessment of ALZ-50 immunoreactivity in Alzheimer's disease. *J Geriat Psychiat Neurol* 4: 231–5.

Hyman BT, Kromer LJ, Van Hoesen GW (1988*a*) A direct demonstration of the performant pathway terminal zone in Alzheimer's disease using the monoclonal antibody Alz-50. *Brain Res* 450: 392–7.

Hyman BT, Marzloff K, Wenniger JJ, Dawson TM, Bredt DS, Snyder SH (1992*a*) Relative sparing of nitric oxide synthase-containing neurons in the hippocampal formation in Alzheimer's disease. *Ann Neurol* 32: 818–20.

Hyman BT, Tanzi RE (1992) Amyloid, dementia and Alzheimer's disease. *Curr Opin Neurol Neurosurg* 5: 88–93.

Hyman BT, Tanzi RE, Marzloff K, Barbour R, Schenk D (1992*b*) Kunitz protease inhibitor-containing amyloid beta protein precursor immunoreactivity in Alzheimer's disease. *J Neuropath Exp Neurol* 51, 76–83.

Hyman BT, Van Hoesen GW, Damasio AR (1986) Glutamate depletion of the perforant pathway terminal zone in Alzheimer's disease. *Soc Neurosci Abstr* 11: 458.

Hyman BT, Van Hoesen GW, Damasio AR (1990) Memory-related neural systems in Alzheimer's disease: an anatomic study. *Neurology* 40: 171–30.

Hyman BT, Van Hoesen GW, Kromer LJ, Damasio AR (1986) Perforant pathway changes and the memory impairment of Alzheimer's disease. *Ann Neurol* 20: 472–81.

Hyman BT, Van Hoesen GW, Masters CL, Beyreuther K (1989) A4 amyloid protein immunoreactivity in neurofibrillary tangles and terminal zones of the hippocampal formation in Alzheimer's disease. *Soc Neurosci Abstr* 15: 1378.

Hyman BT, Van Hoesen GW, Wolozin BL, Davies P, Kromer LJ, Damasio AR (1988*b*) Alz-50 antibody recognizes Alzheimer-related neuronal changes. *Ann Neurol* 23: 371–9.

Hyman BT, Wenniger JJ, Tanzi RE (1993) Nonisotopic *in situ* hybridization of amyloid beta protein precursor in Alzheimer's disease: expression in neurofibrillary tangle bearing neurons and in the microenvironment surrounding senile plaques. *Brain Res Mol Brain Res* 18: 253–8.

Jagust WJ, Davies P, Tiller-Borcich JK, Reed BR (1990) Focal Alzheimer's disease. *Neurology* 40: 14–19.

Joachim CL, Mori H, Selkoe DJ (1988) Amyloid B-protein deposition in tissues other than brain in Alzheimer disease. *Nature* 341: 226–30.

Joachim CL, Morris JH, Selkoe DJ (1989) Diffuse senile plaques occur commonly in the cerebellum in Alzheimer's disease. *Am J Path* 135: 309–19.

Johnson KA, Sperling RA, Holman BL, Nagel JS, Growdon JH (1992) Cerebral perfusion in progressive supranuclear palsy. *J Nucl Med* 33: 707–9.

Jones EG, Powell TPS (1970) An anatomical study of converging sensory pathways within the cerebral cortex of the monkey. *Brain* 93: 793–820.

Jorm AF (1985) Subtypes of Alzheimer's dementia: a conceptual analysis and critical review. *Psychiat Med* 15: 543–53.

Katzman R (1977) Normal pressure hydrocephalus. In Wells CE (ed) *Dementia*, 2nd edn., FA Davis, Philadelphia, pp 69–92.

Katzman R, Terry RD (1983) *The Neurology of Aging. American Academy of Neurology*, Washington DC.

Katzman R, Terry R, DeTeresa R, Brown T, Davies P, Fuld P, Renbing X, Peck A (1988) Clinical, pathological, and neurochemical changes in dementia: a subgroup with preserved mental status and numerous neocortical plaques. *Ann Neurol* 23: 138–44.

Khachaturian ZS (1985) Diagnosis of Alzheimer's disease. *Arch Neurol* 42: 1097–105.

Kidd M (1963) Paired helical filaments in electron microscopy of Alzheimer's disease. *Nature* 197: 192–3.

Knopman DS, Christensen KJ, Schut LJ, Harbaugh RE, Reeder T, Ngo T, Frey W (1989) The spectrum of imaging and neuropsychological findings in Pick's disease. *Neurology* 39: 362–8.

Knopman DS, Mastri AR, Frey WH, Sung JH, Rustann T (1990) Dementia lacking distinctive histologic features: a common non-Alzheimer degenerative dementia. *Neurology* 40: 251–6.

Kosel KC, Van Hoesen GW, Rosene DL (1982) Nonhippocampal cortical projections from the entorhinal cortex in the rat and rhesus monkey. *Brain Res* 244: 202–14.

Kowall NW, Kosik KS (1987) Axonal disruption and aberrant localization of Tau protein characterize the neuropil pathology of Alzheimer's disease. *Ann Neurol* 22: 639–43.

Kromer-Vogt LJ, Hyman BT, Van Hoesen GW, Damasio AR (1990) Pathological alterations in the amygdala in Alzheimer's disease. *Neuroscience* 37: 377–85.

Kuljis RO (1994) Lesions in the pulvinar in patients with Alzheimer's disease. *J Neuropath Exp Neurol* 53: 202–11.

Lee VM-Y, Balin BJ, Otvos L, Trojanowski JQ (1991) A68: A major subunit of paired helical filaments and derivatized forms of normal tau. *Science* 251: 675–8.

Levine DN, Lee JM, Fisher CM (1993) The visual variant of Alzheimer's disease: A clinicopathologic case study. *Neurology* 43: 305–13.

Lewis DA, Campbell MJ, Terry RD, Morrison JH (1987) Laminar and regional distributions of neurofibrillary tangles and neuritic plaques in Alzheimer's disease: a quantitative study of visual and auditory cortices. *J Neurosci* 7 1799–08.

Lippa CF, Smith TW, Swearer JM (1994) Alzheimer's disease and Lewy body disease: a comparative clinicopathological study. *Ann Neuro* 35: 81–8.

Lowe J, Mayer RJ (1990) Ubiquitin, cell stress and diseases of the nervous system. *Neuropath Appl Neurobiol* 16 281–91.

Mann DMA, Brown AMT, Prinja D, Jones D, Davies CA (1990) A morphological analysis of senile plaques in the brains of nondemented persons of different ages using silver, immunocytochemical and lectin histochemical staining techniques. *Neuropath Appl Neurobiol* 16: 17–25.

Mann DMA, Esiri MM (1988) The site of the earliest lesions of Alzheimer's disease. *N Engl J Med* 318: 78–90.

Mann DMA, Marcyniuk B, Yates PO, Neary D, Snowden JS (1988) The progression of the pathological changes of Alzheimer's disease in frontal and temporal neocortex examined both at biopsy and at autopsy. *Neuropath Appl Neurobiol* 14: 177–95.

Marsden CD (1978) The diagnosis of dementia. In Isaacs AD, Post F (eds) *Studies of Geriatric Psychiatry*, John Wiley, Chichester, pp. 95–118.

Marsden CD (1985) Assessment of dementia. In Frederiks JAM (ed.) *Handbook of Clinical Neurology*, Elsevier, Amsterdam, pp. 221–32.

Masliah E, Terry RD, Alford M, DeTeresa R, Hansen LA (1991) Cortical and subcortical patterns of synaptophysin-like immunoreactivity in Alzheimer's disease. *Am J Path* 138: 235–46.

Mayeux R, Stern Y, Spanton S (1985) Heterogeneity in dementia of the Alzheimer type: evidence of subgroups. *Neurology* 35: 453–61.

McKee AC, Kosik KS, Kowall NW (1991) Neuritic pathology and dementia in Alzheimer's disease. *Ann Neurol* 30: 156–65.

McKeith IG, Fairbairn AF, Bothwell RA, Moore PB, Ferrier IN, Thompson P, Perry RH (1994) An evaluation of the predictive validity and inter-rater reliability of clinical diagnostic criteria for senile dementia of Lewy body type. *Neurology* 44: 872–7.

McKhann G, Drachmann D, Folstein M, Katzman R, Price D, Stadlan EM (1984) Clinical diagnosis of Alzheimer's disease: Report of the NINCDS-ARRDA Work Group under the auspices of Dept. of Health & Human Services Task Force on Alzheimer's Disease. *Neurology* 34: 940.

Merske H, Ball MJ, Blume WT, Fox AJ, Fox H, Hersch EL, Kral VA, Palmer RB (1980) Relationships between psychological measurements and cerebral organic changes in Alzheimer's disease. *Can J Neurol Sci* 7: 45–9.

Miller FD, Hicks SP, D'Amato CJ, Landis JR (1984) A descriptive study of neuritic plaques and neurofibrillary tangles in an autopsy population. *Am J Epidemiol* 120: 331–41.

Mirra SS, Heyman A, McKeel D, Sumi SM, Crain, BJ, Brownlee LM, Vogel FS, Hughes JP, van Belle G, Berg L (1991) The consortium to establish a registry for Alzheimer's disease (CERAD). Part II. Standardization of the neuropathologic assessment of Alzheimer's disease. *Neurology* 41: 479–86.

Moossy J, Zubenko GS, Martinez J, Rao GR (1988) Bilateral symmetry of morphologic lesion in Alzheimer's disease. *Arch Neurol* 45: 251–4.

Morris JC, Edland S, Clark C, Galasko D, Koss E, Mohs R, van Belle G. Fillenbaum G, Heyman A (1993) The consortium to establish a registry for Alzheimer's disease (CERAD). Part IV. Rates of cognitive change in the longitudinal assessment of probable Alzheimer's disease. *Neurology* 43: 2457–65.

Morris JC, Heyman A, Mohs RC, Hughes JP, van Belle G, Fillenbaum G, Mellits ED, Clark C (1989) The consortium to establish a registry for Alzheimer's disease (CERAD). Part I. Clinical and neuropsychological assessment of Alzheimer's disease. *Neurology* 39: 1159–65.

Morris JC, McKeel DW, Storandt M, Rubin EH, Price JL, Grant EA, Ball MJ, Berg L (1991) Very mild Alzheimer's disease: informant-based clinical, psychometric, and pathologic distinction from normal aging. *Neurology* 41: 469–78.

Mutrux S (1947) Diagnostic différentiel histologique de la maladie d'Alzheimer et de la démence Sénile. *Monatssch Psychiat Neurol* 113: 114–17.

Neary D, Snowden JS, Mann DMA, Bowen DM, Sims NR, Northen B, Yates PO, Davison AN (1986) Alzheimer's disease: a correlative study. *J Neurol, Neurosurg, Psychiat* 49: 229–37.

Neary D, Snowden JS, Mann DMA, Northen B, Goulding PJ, Macdermott N (1990) Frontal lobe dementia and motor neuron disease. *J Neurol, Neurosurg, Psychiat* 53: 23–32.

Neary D, Snowden JS, Northen B, Goulding P (1988) Dementia of frontal lobe type. *J Neurol, Neurosurg, Psychiat* 51: 353–61.

Nitsch, RM, Blusztajn JK, Pittas AG, Slack BE, Growdon JH, Wurtman RJ (1992) Evidence for a membrane defect in Alzheimer disease brain. *Proc Sci, USA* 89: 1671–5.

Okamoto K, Hirai S, Iizuka T, Yanigisawa T, Watanabe M (1991) Reexamination of granulovacuolar degeneration. *Acta Neuropath* 82: 340–5.

Pandya DN, Yeterian EH (1985) Architecture and connections of cortical association areas. In Peters A, Jones EG (eds) *Cerebral Cortex*, vol. 4, Plenum Press, New York.

Pearson RCA, Esiri MM, Hiorns RW, Wilcock GK, Powell TPS (1985) Anatomical correlates of the distribution of the pathological changes in the neocortex in Alzheimer disease. *Proc Nat Acad Sci* 82: 4531–4.

Peavy GM, Herzog AG, Rubin NP, Mesulam M-M (1992) Neuropsychological aspects of dementia of motor neuron disease: a report of two cases. *Neurology*, 1004–8.

Perry EK (1986) The cholinergic hypothesis – ten years on. *Br Med Bull* 42: 63–9.

Perry EK, Perry RH, Blessed G, Tomlinson BE (1977) Necropsy evidence of central cholinergic deficits in senile dementia. *Lancet* i: 189.

Perry EK, Tomlinson BE, Blessed G, Bergmann K, Gibson PH, Perry RH (1978) Correlation of cholinergic abnormalities with senile plaques and mental test scores in senile dementia. *Br Med J* 2: 1457–9.

Perry RH, Blessed G, Perry EK, Tomlinson BE (1981) Histochemical observations on cholinesterase activities in the brains of elderly normal and demented (Alzheimer type) patients. *J Neurol Sci* 51: 279–87.

Price DL, Struble RG, Altschuler RJ (1985) Aggregation of tubulin in neurons in Alzheimer's disease. *Am Ass Neuropath*, 178.

Price JL, Davis PB, Morris JC, While DL (1991). The distribution of tangles, plaques and related immunohistochemical markers in healthy aging and Alzheimer's disease. *Neurobiol Aging* 12: 295–312.

Rebeck GW, Hyman BT (1993) Neuroanatomical connections and specific regional vulnerability in Alzheimer's disease. *Neurobiol Aging*, 14: 45–7, discussion 55–6.

Rebeck GW, Marzloff K, Hyman BT (1993) The pattern of NADPH-dipahorase staining, a marker of nitric oxide synthase activity, is altered in the perforant pathway terminal zone in Alzheimer's disease. *Neurosci Lett* 152: 165–8.

Rockland KS, Pandya DN (1979) Laminar origins and terminations of cortical connections of the occipital lobe in the rhesus monkey. *Brain Res* 179: 3–20.

Rogers J, Morrison JH (1985) Quantitative morphology and regional and laminar distributions of senile plaques in Alzheimer's disease. *J Neurosci* 5: 2801–8.

Rosenberg RN (1993) A causal role for amyloid in Alzheimer's disease: the end of the beginning. *Neurology* 43: 851–6.

Roth M, Tomlinson BE, Blessed G (1966) Correlations between scores for dementia and counts of 'senile plaques' in cerebral grey matter of elderly subjects. *Nature* 209: 109–10.

Scheff SW, Sparks DL, Price DA (1993) Quantitative assessment of synaptic density in the entorhinal cortex in Alzheimer's disease. *Ann Neurol* 34: 356–61.

Schmechel WB, Milner B (1957) Loss of recent memory after bilateral hippocampal lesions. *J Neurol, Neurosurg Psychiat* 20: 11.

Selkoe DJ (1991) The molecular pathology of Alzheimer's disease. *Neuron* 6: 487–98.

Selkoe DJ (1993) Physiological production of the β-amyloid protein and the mechanism of Alzheimer's disease. *Trends Neurosci* 16: 403–9.

Selkoe DJ, Pdolisny MB, Joachim CL, Vickers EA, Lee G, Fritz LC, Oltersdorf T (1988) β-Amyloid precursor protein of Alzheimer's disease occurs as 110- to 135-kilodalton membrane-associated proteins in neural and nonneural tissues. *Proc Nat Acad Sci USA* 85: 7341–5.

Seltzer B, Pandya DN (1978) Some cortical projections to the parahippocampal area in the rhesus monkey. *Exp Neuro* 50: 146–60.

Sevush S, Leve N, Brickman A (1993) Age at disease onset and pattern of cognitive impairment in probable Alzheimer's disease. *J Neuropsychiat* 5: 66–72.

Simchowicz T (1911) Hitologiesche studien uber die senile demenz. *Hitog Histopath Arbeit Grobhirn* 4 267–444.

Snowden JS, Neary D, Mann DMA, Goulding PJ, Testa HJ (1992) Progressive language disorder due to lobar atrophy. *Ann Neurol* 31: 174–83.

Strittmatter WJ, Saunders AM, Schmechel DE (1993) Apolipoprotein E: high avidity binding to β-amyloid and increased frequency of type 4 allele in late-onset familial Alzheimer disease. *Proc Nat Acad Sci USA* 90: 1977–81.

Tabaton M, Whitehouse PJ, Perry G, Davies P, Autilio-Gambetti L, Gambetti P (1988) Alz-50 recognizes abnormal filaments in Alzheimer's disease and progressive supranuclear palsy. *Ann Neurol* 24: 407–13.

Tanzi RE, Hyman BT (1991) Studies of amyloid beta-protein precursor expression in Alzheimer's disease. *Ann N Y Acad Sci* 640: 149–54.

Tanzi RE, Vaula G, Romano DM, Mortilla M, Huang TL, Yupler RG, Wasco W, Hyman BT, Haines JL, Jenkins BJ *et al* (1992) Assessment of amyloid beta-protein precursor gene mutations in a large set of familial and sporadic Alzheimer disease cases. *Am J Hum Genet* 51: 273–82.

Tanzi RE, Wenniger JJ, Hyman BT (1993) Cellular specificity and regional distribution of amyloid beta protein precursor alternative transcripts are unaltered in Alzheimer hippocampal formation. *Brain Res Mol Res* 18: 246–52.

Terry R, Masliah E, Salman D, Butters N, DeTeresa R, Hansen L, Katzman R (1990) Structure–function correlations in Alzheimer disease (abstract). *J Neuropath Exp Neuerol* 49: 318.

Terry RD, Gonatas NK, Weiss M (1964) Ultrastructural studies in Alzheimer's presenile dementia. *Am J Path* 44: 269–97.

Terry RD, Hansen LA, DeTeresa R, Davies P, Tobias H, Katzman R (1987) Senile dementia of the Alzheimer type without neocortical neurofibrillary tangles. *J Neuropath Exp Neurol* 46: 262–8.

Terry RD, Katzman R (1983) Senile dementia of the Alzheimer type. *Ann Neurol* 14: 497–506.

Terry RD, Masliah E, Salmon DP, Butters N, DeTeresa R, Hill R, Hansen LA, Katzman R (1991) Physical basis of cognitive alterations in Alzheimer's disease: synapse loss is the major correlate of cognitive impairment. *Ann Neurol* 80.

Terry RD, Peck A, DeTeresa R, Schechter R, Horoupian DS (1981) Some morphometric aspects of the brain in senile dementia of the Alzheimer type. *Ann Neurol* 10: 194–92.

Tissot R, Constantinidis J, Richard J (1985) Pick's disease. In *Handbook of Clin Neurology*, vol. 2, Fredericks JAM (ed), Elsevier Science Publishers, Amsterdam, pp 46.

Tomlinson BE, Blessed G, Roth M (1970) Observations on the brains of demented old people. *J Neurol Sci* 11: 205–42.

Tomlinson BE, Kitchener D (1972) Granulovacuolar degeneration of hippocampal pyramidal cells. *J Pathol* 106: 165–85.

Tourtellotte WW, Van Hoesen GW, Hyman BT, Tikoo RK, Damasio AR (1990) Alz-50 immunoreactivity in the thalamic reticular nucleus in Alzheimer's disease. *Brain Res* 515: 227–34.

Ulrich J (1985) Alzheimer changes in nondemented patients younger than sixty five: a possible early stage of Alzheimer's disease and senile dementia of Alzheimer's type. *Ann Neurol* 17: 273–7.

Van Essen DC (1985) Functional organization of primate visual cortex. In *Cerebral Cortex*, Peters A, Jones EG, Plenum Press, New York, pp 259–330.

Van Hoesen GW (1982) The primate parahippocampal gyrus: New insights regarding its cortical connections. *Trends Neurosci*, 5: 345–50.

Van Hoesen GW, Damasio AR (1987) Neural correlates of cognitive impairment in Alzheimer's disease. In Mountcastle VB (ed) *Handbook of Physiology*, American Psychological Society, Bethesda.

Van Hoesen GW, Hyman BT (1990) Hippocampal formation: anatomy and the patterns of pathology in Alzheimer's disease. *Prog Brain Res*, 83: 445–57.

Van Hoesen GW, Hyman BT, Damasio AR (1986) Cell-specific pathology in neural systems of the temporal lobe in Alzheimer's disease. In *Progress in Brain Research*, Swaab DF, Fliers M, Mirmiran WA, Van Gool WA, Van Haaren F, Elsevier, Amsterdam.

Van Hoesen GW, Hyman BT, Damasio AR (1991) Entorhinal cortex pathology in Alzheimer's disease. *Hippocampus* 1: 1–8.

Vinters HV (1986) Cerebral amyloid angiopathy, a critical review. *Stroke* 18: 311–24.

Vinters HV, Miller BL, Pardridge WM (1988) Brain amyloid and Alzheimer disease. *Ann Int Med* 109: 41–54.

Welsh K, Butters N, Hughes J, Mohs R, Heyman A (1991) Detection of abnormal memory decline in mild cases of Alzheimer's disease using CERAD neuropsychological measures. *Arch Neurol* 48: 278–81.

Welsh KA, Butters N, Hughes JP, Mohs RC, Heyman A (1992) Detection and staging of dementia in Alzheimer's disease: use of the neuropsychological measures developed for the consortium to establish a registry for Alzheimer's disease. *Arch Neurol* 49: 448–52.

White P, Hilley CR, Goodhardt MJ, Carrasco LH, Keet JP, Williams IEI, Bowen DM (1977) Neocortical cholinergic neurons in elderly people. *Lancet* i: 668–70.

Whitehouse PJ, Price DL, Struble RG, Clark AW, Coyle JT, DeLong MR (1982) Alzheimer's disease and senile dementia: loss of neurons in the basal forebrain. *Science* 215: 1237–9.

Wilcock GK, Esiri MM (1982) Plaques, tangles and dementia. A quantitative study. *J Neurol Sci* 56: 343–56.

Wisniewski K, Jervis GA, Moretz RC, Wisniewski HM (1979) Alzheimer neurofibrillary tangles in diseases other than senile and presenile dementia. *Ann Neurol* 5: 288–94.

Wolozin BL, Pruchnicki A, Dickson DW (1986) A neuronal antigen in the brains of Alzheimer patients. *Science* 232: 648–50.

Wright C, Geula C, Mesulam M-M (1993) Neuroglial cholinesterases in the normal brain and in Alzheimer's disease: relationship to plaques, tangles, and patterns of selective vulnerability. *Ann Neurol* 34: 373–84.

Yamaguchi H, Hirai S, Morimatsu M, Shoji M, Harigaya Y (1988) Diffuse type of senile plaques in the brains of Alzheimer-type dementia. *Acta Neuropath* 77: 113–19.

Yankner BA, Duffy LK, Kirschner DA (1990) Neurotrophic and neurotoxic effects of amyloid B protein: reversal by tachykinin neuropeptides. *Science* 250: 279–82.

Yoshimura N (1989) Topography of Pick body distribution in Pick's disease: a contribution to understanding the relationship between Pick's and Alzheimer's disease. *Clin Neuropath* 8: 1–6.

Zola-Morgan A, Squire LR, Amaral D (1986) Human amnesia and the medial temporal region: enduring memory impairment following a bilateral lesion limited to the CAI field of the hippocampus. *J Neurosci* 6: 2950–67.

Zola-Morgan S, Squire LR, Amaral DG, Suzuki WA (1989) Lesions of perirhinal and parahippocampal cortex that spare the amygdala and hippocampal formation produce severe memory impairment. *J Neurosci* 9: 4355–70.

CHAPTER TWO

Practical approach to the pathological diagnosis of dementia: important anatomical landmarks in the brain in dementia

M. M. Esiri and J. H. Morris

Cerebral cortex
Cerebral white matter
Amygdala
Nucleus basalis of Meynert (basal nucleus)
Basal ganglia
Thalamus and hypothalamus
Brainstem
The cerebellum

In this chapter we summarize the more important structures in the brain with which it is essential to be familiar when studying the pathological basis of dementia. As described in Chapter 3, many dementing conditions are impossible to distinguish on naked eye examination of the brain since they do not display gross regional pathology. In order to reach the correct diagnosis, it is necessary to select the appropriate areas for more detailed examination. To do that requires knowledge of the parts of the brain that are significant in the particular context of dementia. For more detailed information textbooks of neuroanatomy such as Paxinos (1990), Carpenter and Sutin (1983), Nieuwenhuys Voogd & van Huijzen (1988) or Heimer (1995) should be consulted.

CEREBRAL CORTEX

Chapter 1 has already emphasized the crucial importance of the cerebral cortex for the cognitive functions which deteriorate in dementia. The cerebral cortex can be divided anatomically into a phylogenetically older and simpler *allocortex* consisting of the *hippocampus* and closely related *entorhinal cortex*, *subiculum* and olfactory regions, and the remaining, much more voluminous and phylogenetically more recent, *neocortex*.

Hippocampus, subiculum and entorhinal cortex (archicortex, allocortex)

These structures have already been mentioned in Chapter 1 but, because of their importance, it is worth providing a brief supplementary account here. Excellent recent reviews of the structure of the human hippocampus and related cortex can be found in Amaral and Insausti (1990) and Duvernoy (1988).

The entorhinal cortex lies in the uncus and anterior para-hippocampal gyrus and forms an intermediate type of cortex between the complex six-layered neocortex of the temporal lobe and the simpler, basically three-layered, cortex of the hippocampus. Entorhinal cortex, parasubiculum, presubiculum and subiculum lie in continuity with each other in the medial temporal lobe ribbon of cortex seen in coronal slices of the brain, curving dorsally and then laterally to join the curled-up structure of the hippocampus in the floor of the inferior horn of the lateral ventricle (Fig. 2.1). The hippocampus has a head, a body and a tail and extends 4–4.5 centimetres in an antero-posterior direction from just behind the amygdala to the splenium of the corpus callosum. Anteriorly, the hippocampus is relatively expanded (the head) (Fig. 2.2), whereas more posteriorly it is compact, as seen at the level of the lateral geniculate body (the body) (Fig. 2.3).

The hippocampus contains two interlocked, cortical ribbons. One, the *cornu ammonis*, which is a continuation from the subiculum, is enclosed at its termination in a second, the *dentate fascia* (Fig. 2.1). The hippocampus contains pyramidal and non-pyramidal cells like the neocortex, but here they form one main layer sandwiched between two cell-sparse layers. In the cornu ammonis the three layers are made up of a deep *molecular layer*, largely devoid of cell bodies, but containing dendrites and axons, in which three strata can be distinguished – the *strata radiatum, lacunosum and moleculare*. Adjacent to this is the *stratum pyramidale* layer of large pyramidal neurons. The pyramidal cells show regional variations in the arrangement which provides the main basis for dividing the cornu ammonis (CA) into four subdivisions – CA1-4 (Lorente de No 1934) (Figs. 2.4 and 2.6). CA1 is the largest zone, extending from the subiculum as a broad band of triangular-shaped, well-spaced neurons to the point where the band of cells narrows abruptly and the cell bodies become more oval in shape in CA2. CA3 neurons are slightly more widely dispersed than those of CA2 and they curve in a band to

enter the region bounded by the dentate fascia. CA4 refers to the area containing widely scattered, large neurons enclosed by the dentate fascia granule cells. This region is sometimes also referred to as the *end folium*. (Alternative terminologies have been put forward by Rose (1927) and Vogt and Vogt (1937), their H1 zone being equivalent to CA1, H2 to CA2 and CA3 and H3 to CA4). The third, outer, layer of the cornu ammonis, called the *stratum oriens* contains a few scattered interneurons, but consists mainly of the basal dendrites and axons of the pyramidal cells. The axons collect up into a fibre tract called the *alveus* (Fig. 2.4). This is the chief efferent outflow tract from the hippocampus and it sweeps over its ventricular surface to form a delicate, compact tract, the *fimbria*. The fimbria arches from the posterior hippocampus superiorly and medially to form the *fornix*, which lies beneath the corpus callosum, directed rostrally. At the genu of the corpus callosum it bends downwards and back as the column of the fornix (Fig. 2.5). The efferent hippocampal fibres in the fornix, derived principally from the large hippocampal and subicular pyramidal cells, are distributed to the lateral septal region in the basal forebrain, mamillary bodies of the hypothalamus and anterior nucleus of the thalamus.

The *dentate fascia* (Fig. 2.4) also contains three main layers, one richly and two sparsely populated with neurons: the innermost *polymorphic layer* containing mainly the axons of the granule cells, next to this the *granule cell layer* containing tightly packed small neurons and the outermost *molecular layer* containing axons and dendrites.

Connections of the hippocampus (Fig. 2.6)

One source of afferent fibres to the hippocampus is the medial septal nucleus via the fimbria to the pyramidal cells of the cornu ammonis and the granule cells of the dentate fascia. This is a cholinergic supply. There are also a few commissural fibres derived from the contralateral hippocampus also via the fornix and fimbria. However, the chief afferent connections of the hippocampus are derived from the nearby entorhinal area via the *perforant path* which crosses the subiculum and ends chiefly on the dendrites of the granule cells in the molecular layer of the dentate fascia. There is a lesser perforant path projection from entorhinal cortex to subiculum and the strata moleculare and lacunosum of CA1 and CA3 regions of the hippocampus. This is a glutamatergic projection. Connections then run via the axons of the granule cells of the dentate fascia, which traverse the polymorphic layer to end on dendrites of

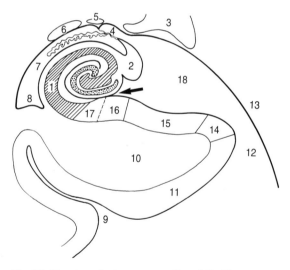

Fig. 2.1. Drawing of a transverse section of the hippocampus and adjacent cortex. (Modified from Duvernoy, 1988.) Arrow indicates the hippocampal sulcus. 1: hippocampus, 2: fimbria, 3: lateral geniculate body, 4: choroid fissure and tela choroidea, 5: stria terminalis, 6: tail of caudate nucleus, 7: temporal horn and choroid, plexus, 8: collateral eminence, 9: collateral sulcus, 10: parahippocampal gyrus, 11: entorhinal area, 12: ambient cistern, 13: mesencephalon, 14: parasubiculum, 15: presubiculum, 16: subiculum proper, 17: prosubiculum, 18: transverse fissure.

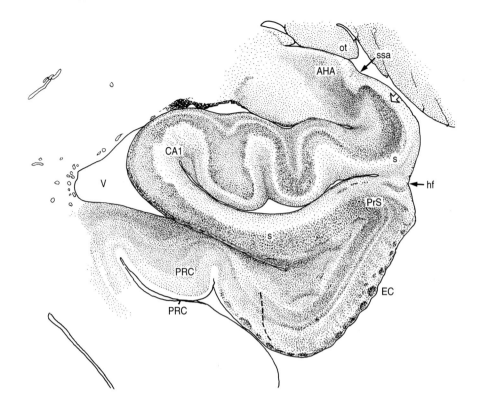

Fig. 2.2. Drawing of a transverse section of the head of the hippocampus. AHA: amygdala hippocampal area, CA1: CA1 field of hippocampus, EC: entorhinal cortex, hf: hippocampal fissure, ot: optic tract, PRC: perirhinal cortex, PrS: presubiculum, s: subiculum, ssa: sulcus semiannularis, V: inferior horn of ventricle.

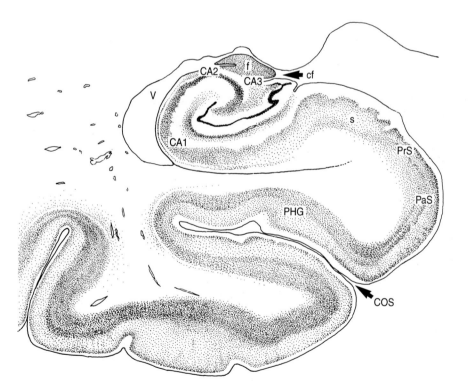

Fig. 2.3. Drawing of a transverse section of the body of the hippocampus. CA1: CA1 field of hippocampus, CA2: CA2 field of hippocampus, CA3: CA3 field of hippocampus, cf: choroidal fissure, COS: collateral sulcus, f: fimbria, PaS: parasubiculum, PrS: presubiculum, PHG: parahippocampal gyrus, V: inferior horn of ventricle.

pyramidal cells in the molecular layer of CA3 and CA4 (Fig. 2.7). The granule cell axons, known as *mossy fibres*, are also glutamatergic and have an exceptionally high level of zinc in their endings. Axons of CA3/4 neurons enter the alveus, but before doing so give off prominent collateral branches known as *Schaffer collaterals*, which run in the strata radiatum and lacunosum of the cornu ammonis and synapse there with CA1 pyramidal cell apical dendrites. Axons of CA1 neurons enter the alveus from whence they are distributed via collaterals to the subiculum as well as via the fimbria to its terminations in the lateral septal region, mamillary bodies and thalamus.

The large pyramidal cells, particularly those of CA1, of the hippocampus are highly susceptible to neurofibrillary tangle formation, granulovacuolar degeneration and Hirano body formation in normal aging (see Chapter 3) and even more in Alzheimer's disease (Chapter 4). The small pyramidal cells of the dentate fascia granule cell layer as well as the large pyramidal cells, are susceptible to Pick body formation in Pick's disease (Chapter 8). The whole hippocampus and adjacent temporal lobe, amygdala and interconnected cingulate gyrus are liable to be destroyed in herpes simplex encephalitis (Chapter 17).

Neocortex

The neocortex is built on a common structural plan, being composed of about 3–500 μm diameter columns of neurons of many different types (Fig. 2.8). Each column lies perpendicular to the surface and functions as a unit, but has intimate connections with many other units (Fig. 2.8b). Allocortex shows more variable arrangements of neurons. Between allo- and neo-cortex there are transitional zones.

At current levels of understanding of dementing processes it is helpful to distinguish between two main categories of cortical neurons: *pyramidal* and *non-pyramidal* (Jones, 1986). Many of the cellular pathological changes characteristic of degenerative disease are found in pyramidal cells. *Pyramidal cells* have a triangular-shaped cell body, a long axon arising from the base of the pyramid, and a long apical dendrite extending towards the pial surface of the cortex. They outnumber non-pyramidal cells but the proportions are not constant

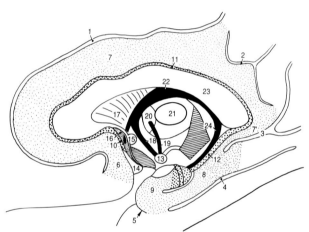

Fig. 2.5. Diagram to show the connections of the hippocampus with the limbic system with the fornix and mamillothalamic tract shown in black. (Redrawn from Duvernoy, 1988.) The limbic sulcus is divided into: 1: cingulate sulcus. 2: subparietal sulcus, 3: anterior calcarine sulcus, 4: collateral sulcus, 5: rhinal sulcus. The limbic gyrus (fine dots) is divided into: 6: subcallosal gyrus, 7: cingulate gyrus, 7′: isthmus, 8: parahippocampal gyrus, 9: anterior segment of the uncus. The intralimbic gyrus (with large dots) is divided into: 10: prehippocampal rudiment (precommissural hippocampus), 11: indusium griseum (supracommissural hippocampus), 12: hippocampus (retrocommissural hippocampus), 13: mamillary body, 14: anterior perforated substance, 15: anterior commissure, 16: septal nuclei covered by the paraterminal gyrus, 17: precommissural fornix, 18: postcommissural fornix (anterior column), 19: mamillothalamic tract, 20: anterior thalamic nucleus, 21: medial thalamic nucleus, 22: body of fornix, 23: corpus callosum, 24: crus of fornix.

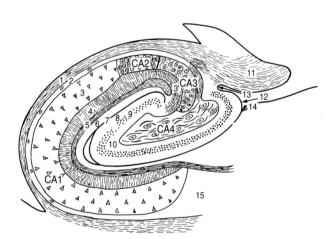

Fig. 2.4. Close-up drawing of a transverse section of the body of the hippocampus. (Redrawn from Duvernoy, 1988.)
CA1–CA4: fields of the hippocampus (cornu ammonis), 1: alveus, 2: stratum oriens, 3: stratum pyramidale, 4: stratum radiatum, 5: stratum lacunosum, 6: stratum moleculare, 7: hippocampal sulcus, 8: stratum moleculare of dentate gyrus, 9: stratum granulosum of dentate gyrus, 10: polymorphic layer of dentate gyrus, 11: fimbria, 12: margo denticulatus, 13: fimbriodentate sulcus, 14: hippocampal sulcus, 15: subiculum.

either regionally or throughout the depth of the six-layered columns. Pyramidal cells are particularly prominent in motor cortex, where the largest of them form the Betz cells. In all regions pyramidal cells are concentrated in cortical layers 2, 3, 5 and 6. Most vary in approximate diameter from 10–50 μm, but the Betz cells measure up to 120 μm.

The efferent and afferent connections of the cortex have been deduced principally in laboratory animals including primates, but the essential features are probably applicable to man. These studies have shown that pyramidal cells are the main, though not the only, source of efferent axons from the neocortex. Depending on their origin, the efferent axons are directed towards one or more of four target tissues: 1) other areas of cortex via ipsilateral and contralateral (callosal) connections; 2) the amygdala and basal ganglia (chiefly claustrum, caudate nucleus and putamen); 3) the specific and non-specific nuclei of the thalamus and 4) the brainstem and spinal cord. Pyramidal cells release excitatory neurotransmitters at their terminals, particularly glutamate and aspartate. In addition to having a wide influence on other regions of the brain, pyramidal cells are also subject to a wide variety of inputs from their rich afferent supply. The afferents are derived from: 1) other distant and more local cortical pyramidal cells; 2) local non-pyramidal cells and 3) subcortical neurons. The latter include cholinergic afferents from the nucleus basalis of Meynert (excitatory), noradrenergic afferents from the locus ceruleus (excitatory) and serotonergic afferents from the raphe nuclei (excitatory) (see below). Given the key role of these cells in linking parts of the cortex together, it is not difficult to understand that their degeneration results in dementia.

Non-pyramidal cells are distributed in all layers of the cortex, but are particularly numerous in layer 4. They take a variety of forms but they are generally of small size, 5–15 μm. Most of them are interneurons with

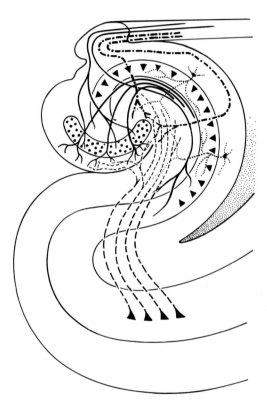

Fig. 2.6. Diagram of the main connections of the hippocampus. Pyramidal neurons of the cornu ammonis send efferent fibres into the alveus (top, dash-dot lines). Afferent fibres arriving via the alveus from septal nuclei and contralateral hippocampus are indicated by solid lines. Afferent fibres from entorhinal cortex are indicated by dashed lines. Connections of basket interneurons are indicated by fine dotted lines. Processes of the dentate fascia neurons forming mossy fibres are indicated by solid lines. (Redrawn and modified from Williams & Warwick, 1980.)

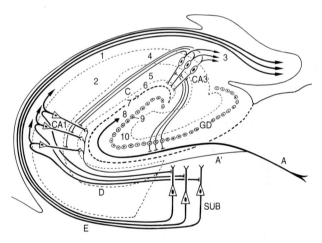

Fig. 2.7. Diagram of the internal connections of the subiculum and hippocampus. (Redrawn from Duvernoy, 1988.) ABCDE are parts of the sequential chains forming the principal pathways. A': these perforant fibres join the apical dendrites of the pyramidal neurons directly. Cornu ammonis: 1: alveus, 2: stratum pyramidale, 3: axon of pyramidal neurons, 4: Schaffer collateral, 5: stratum radiatum and lacunosum, 6: stratum moleculare, 7: hippocampal sulcus. 8: stratum moleculare, 9: stratum granulosum, 10: polymorphic layer, GD: gyrus dentatus, CA3, CA1: fields of the cornu ammonis, SUB: subiculum.

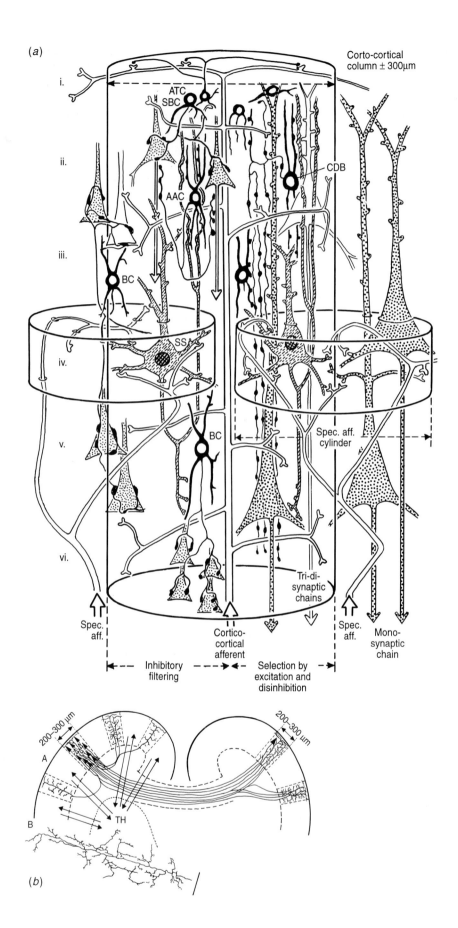

(a)

Corto-cortical
column ± 300μm

i.

ATC
SBC

ii.

CDB

AAC

iii.

BC

iv.

SS

Spec. aff.
cylinder

v.

BC

vi.

Tri-di-
synaptic
chains

Spec.
aff.

Cortico-
cortical
afferent

Selection by
excitation and
disinhibition

Spec.
aff.

Mono-
synaptic
chain

Inhibitory
filtering

(b)

200–300 μm

A

200–300 μm

B

TH

Fig. 2.8. Drawings to illustrate the principles of cortical neuronal connectivity. (a) The internal connectivity in a cortical column outlined by the cylinder. The discs in layer IV (SPEC. AFF CYLINDER) indicate the sites of arborization of specific afferents which this column of neurons shares with adjacent columns. Corticocortical afferents (arrow bottom, centre) terminate at all levels of the column and, in layer I, beyond it. Pyramidal neurons (punctate shading) provide the efferent outflow from the column and are illustrated on the right. Interneurons of excitatory type (spiny stellate = SS, dashed shading) and inhibitory type (basket cells = BC in lower laminae, small basket cells = SBC in lamina II, axonal tuft cells = ATC and axoaxonic cells = AAC) are illustrated on the left side. CDB (= cellule à double bouquet) cells, inhibitory interneurons that act specifically on inhibitory interneurons and therefore have a disinhibitory effect, are shown on the right-hand side.

(b) 'A' shows the manner in which cortical columns such as that shown in (a) interact with other columns. Ipsilateral connections are derived mainly from pyramidal neurons in lamina III (shown left in outline) and contralateral connections from pyramidal neurons in layers II–VI (shown left in black) TH = thalamus. 'B' illustrates a single, Golgi-stained corticocortical afferent orientated as in the left-hand column of 'A', but at higher magnification to show the profuse branching in all laminae. ((a) and (b) modified and redrawn from Szentágothai, 1978, 1979 and Eccles, 1984.)

connections chiefly confined to their near vicinity particularly, though not exclusively, within their own column of neurons and the columns immediately adjacent. They employ a variety of neurotransmitters including acetylcholine (ACh), γ-amino butyric acid (GABA) and the neuropeptides somatostatin, substance P, enkephalins, calcitonin gene-related peptide, corticotrophin releasing factor, VIP, bombasin and neurotensin and their influence is thought to be predominantly inhibitory. Most studies of dementing diseases have so far found less pathology in these neuronal populations than in pyramidal cells, though loss of non-pyramidal cells occurs even in normal ageing and can be severe (Braak & Braak 1986). An important exception is the large stellate cells found in clusters in layer 2 of the entorhinal cortex (see below). These are highly susceptible to neurofibrillary tangle formation in normal ageing as well as in Alzheimer's disease.

Regional sub-division of the cerebral cortex
Brodmann in 1909 described regional sub-divisions of the cerebral cortex which remain widely used and are based on slight differences in the laminar architecture (Figs 2.9 and 2.10). Although other maps were subsequently produced and some controversies persist, subsequent anatomical and physiological studies have generally underlined the functional significance and anatomical value of these Brodmann maps of the cortex. In sampling the cerebral cortex for the purpose of identifying microscopical changes characteristic of different

dementing conditions, some Brodmann areas are much more useful than others. The aim is to sample regions with high selectivity and sensitivity for the pathological changes under consideration. In Alzheimer's disease, neurofibrillary tangles are readily found in the temporal lobe neocortex of Brodmann areas 22 and 38, areas that do not normally contain tangles in normal ageing. These are therefore suitable areas to sample when considering a diagnosis of Alzheimer's disease. In contrast, frontal (e.g. areas 9 and 46), parietal (e.g. area 7) and occipital (e.g. areas 18 and 19) association cortex, though regularly affected by tangle formation in younger cases of Alzheimer's disease, may have few or no tangles in the very elderly cases and so are less sensitive areas to sample than the temporal lobe areas. On the other hand, some areas of the temporal lobe, such as periamygdaloid cortex of the uncus (area 34) and parahippocampal gyrus (area 28), may contain at least a *few* tangles even in normal undemented elderly people, so these areas lack selectivity for Alzheimer's disease. Some areas (e.g. primary motor-cortex (area 4), primary somatosensory (area 1–3), primary visual (area 17) and primary auditory (area 41) cortices lack tangles even in severe, young cases of the disease and are therefore unsuitable for sampling (Pearson *et al.*, 1985; Esiri *et al.*, 1990). To take other examples: Pick's disease most commonly affects frontal and temporal poles (areas 8–12 and 38) and diffuse Lewy body disease affects the anterior cingulate cortex (area 24), insula (area 16) and parahippocampal gyrus (area 28), so these are good areas to sample to confirm the presence of these respective diseases.

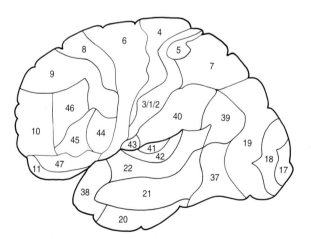

Fig. 2.9. Brodmann (1909) map of the medial surface of the human cerebral hemisphere. Numbering indicates Brodmann's subdivisions.

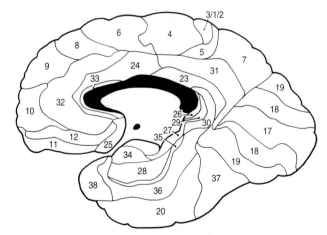

Fig. 2.10. Brodmann (1909) map of the lateral surface of the human cerebral hemisphere. Numbering indicates Brodmann's subdivisions.

Glial cells and vascular supply of cortex

Scattered in the neocortex and archicortex are many astrocytes, satellite oligodendroglial and microglial cells, the latter being members of the macrophage lineage of cells. The vascular supply of the neocortex comes from inwardly directed arterioles given off from leptomeningeal branches of the three main cerebral arteries – anterior, middle and posterior. The hippocampus derives its blood supply chiefly from the anterior and posterior choroidal arteries.

Venous drainage from the neocortex is chiefly via superficial veins to the nearby venous sinuses. From the hippocampus small veins enter the vein of Galen and straight sinus via the basilar vein.

CEREBRAL WHITE MATTER

The main cerebral white matter occupies much of each cerebral hemisphere. It contains myelinated fibres passing to the cerebral cortex from other parts of the cortex, thalamus and brainstem, and reciprocal fibres passing in the reverse direction. Some of these fibres are collected into more or less compact tracts such as the pyramidal tract and the corpus callosum. Others run more diffusely, criss-crossing each other in the centrum semiovale (Fig 2.11). Cortico-cortical fibres that are distributed locally run in immediately sub-cortical fibre bundles. Scattered between the myelinated fibres are glial cells of all three main types – astrocytes, oligodendrocytes and microglia, with oligodendrocytes predominating. Much

of the blood supply to the white matter is carried in long arterioles which course, unbranching, through the cortex before breaking up in the sub-cortical and deep white matter to supply a coarser network of capillaries than is found in the cortex. The venous drainage of the white matter is chiefly towards the ventricles where there are subependymal tributaries of the deep cerebral veins, which join the vein of Galen and drain into the straight sinus.

The cerebral white matter is affected in a variety of different dementing diseases most notably some forms of ischaemic dementia (Chapter 5), AIDS (Chapter 17) and progressive multifocal leukoencephalopathy (Chapter 17). If the main cerebral white matter is extensively demyelinated in other white matter diseases such as multiple sclerosis or leukodystrophy dementia also results. Cerebral white matter is also much reduced in volume in many degenerative conditions including Pick's disease, Alzheimer's disease, Huntington's disease, in alcoholic brain damage or after severe head injury. This loss of white matter in neurodegenerative diseases probably mainly reflects Wallerian degeneration due to loss of neurons. Periventricular white matter is at risk of damage in normal pressure hydrocephalus.

AMYGDALA

This subcortical collection of grey matter lies just in front of the hippocampus and the inferior horn of the lateral ventricle, in the dorsomedial portion of the deep temporal lobe (Figs 2.12 and 2.13). It has a number of constituent nuclei which can be considered here to form two main groups: the basolateral and cortico-medial nuclei. Seen in cross-section in a coronal slice through the mamillary bodies, the amygdala appears as an almond-shaped structure separated on its medial and inferior aspect by a thin layer of white matter from the neighbouring peri-amygdaloid cortex of the uncus. The *cortico-medial nuclei* have close afferent connections with the olfactory system via the lateral olfactory stria, and with the hypothalamus, brainstem, nucleus of the horizontal limb of the diagonal band and bed nucleus of the stria terminalis. Their neurons project to other nuclei in the amygdala, medial frontal cortex, dorsomedial thalamus and hypothalamus.

The basolateral nuclei receive fibres from the substantia innominata, the thalamus, hypothalamus, brainstem and cerebral cortex, including allocortex. They project back to many of these regions and to the bed nucleus of the stria terminalis and striatum. There are large, me-

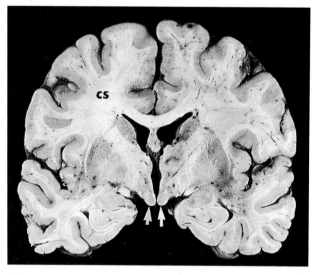

Fig. 2.11. Coronal slice across the cerebral hemispheres at the level of the mamillary bodies (arrows). CS = centrum semiovale.

dium and small-sized neurons in the amygdala, some of them pyramidal-like. The latter, particularly in the cortico-medial nuclei, are susceptible to neurofibrillary tangle formation in Alzheimer's disease (Chapter 4) and to Lewy body formation in diffuse Lewy body disease (Chapter 6).

NUCLEUS BASALIS OF MEYNERT (BASAL NUCLEUS)

A great deal has been written in the last 12 years or so about the basal nucleus of Meynert (see review by Saper 1990). The reason for this recent interest is that animal studies in the 1970s established it as the source of most of the acetylcholine in the cerebral cortex (the remainder coming from local interneurons) (Mesulam & van Hoesen 1976), a transmitter that was found at about the same time to be selectively depleted in the cortex in Alzheimer's disease (Bowen et al., 1977; Davies, 1979). The basal nucleus forms a collection of large multipolar neurons in the substantia innominata strung out from the level of the optic chiasm rostrally to the mamillary bodies caudally. The cell group merges anteriorly with similar cholinergic cells in the nuclei of the vertical and horizontal limbs of the diagonal band. Its anterior part lies ventral to the anterior commissure, a discrete band of transversely running myelinated fibres, while its posterior part lies ventral to the globus pallidus (Figs 2.13 and 3.10). Its cells are predominantly cholinergic

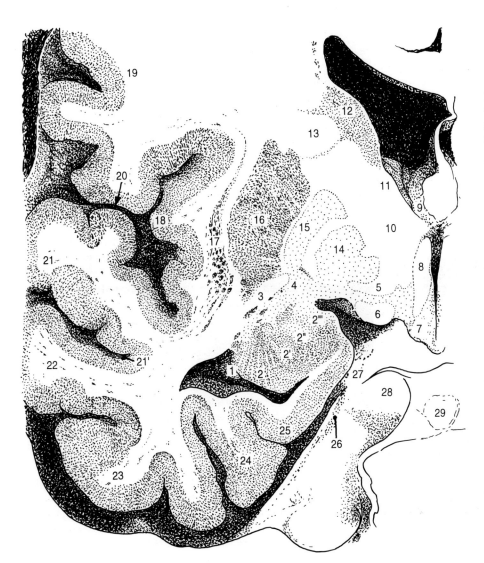

Fig. 2.12. Drawing of a coronal slice through the anterior temporal lobe, amygdala and basal ganglia. (Redrawn from Duvernoy, 1988.) 1: hippocampal head (digitationes hippocampi), 2: lateral nucleus of the amygdala, 2': basal nucleus of the amygdala, 2": accessory basal nucleus of the amygdala, 2''' cortical nuclei of the amygdala, 3: anterior commissure, 4: anterior perforated substance, 5: ansa lenticularis, 6: optic tract, 7: hypothalamus, 8: anterior column of fornix, 9: interventricular foramen, 10: ventral anterior thalamic nucleus, 11: anterior thalamic nucleus, 12: caudate nucleus, 13: genu of internal capsule, 14: globus pallidus, pars medialis, 15: globus pallidus, pars lateralis, 16: putamen, 17: Claustrum, 18: insula, 19: precentral gyrus, 20: lateral sulcus, 21: superior temporal gyrus, 21': superior temporal sulcus, 22: middle temporal gyrus, 23: inferior temporal gyrus, 24: gyrus fusiformis, 25: parahippocampal gyrus, 26: tentorium cerebelli, 27: posterior cerebral artery, 28: internal carotid artery within the cavernous sinus, 29: hypophysis (posterior lobe).

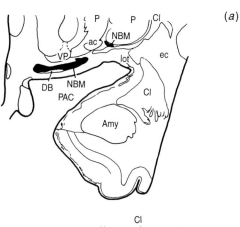

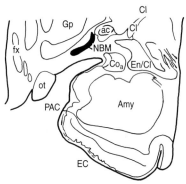

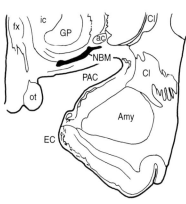

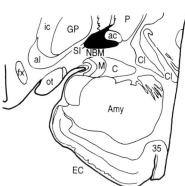

(b)

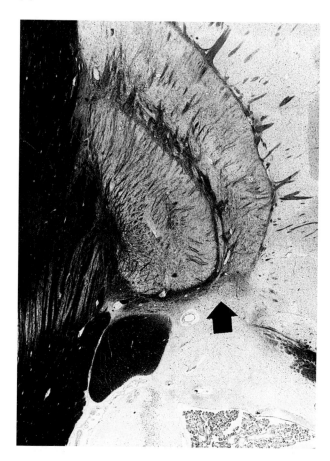

Fig. 2.13. Nucleus basalis of Meynert. (a) Diagrams showing the position of the nucleus (in black) at different antero-posterior levels of the human ventral forebrain. (b) Photograph of a luxol fast-blue/cresyl violet stained section of the basal ganglia. An arrow points to the nucleus basalis.
(c) Photomicrograph of a Nissl-stained section of the basal nucleus to show the large, multipolar neurons that characterize it. ac: anterior commissure, al: ansa lenticularis, Amy: amygdala, C: central nucleus of the amygdala, Cl: claustrum, Co_a anterior cortical nucleus of the amygdala, DB: diagonal band, EC: entorhinal cortex, ec: external capsule, fx: fornix, GP: globus pallidus, ic: internal capsule, lot: lateral olfactory tract, NBM: nucleus basalis of Meynert, ot: optic tract, P: putamen, PAC: periamygdaloid cortex, Sl: substantia innominata, 35: Cortical area 35 of Brodmann.

and project widely to all parts of the hemisphere. The nucleus basalis is involved in the pathology of both Alzheimer's disease (Chapter 4) and Parkinson's disease (Chapter 6).

BASAL GANGLIA

The number of different nuclei that are included among the basal ganglia is somewhat variable, but here we shall consider the following: caudate nucleus, putamen, globus pallidus and sub-thalamic nucleus (Figs 2.12, 3.11 and 10.2). These heterogeneous masses of grey matter contain nerve cells of varying size, shape and connectivity, together with glial cells, bundles of interspersed myelinated fibres and blood vessels. The caudate nucleus and putamen, referred to collectively as the striatum, are functionally and structurally similar and perform important tasks related to the control of movement. They receive a massive afferent input from the cerebral cortex (glutamatergic) and additional afferents from the intra laminar thalamic nuclei, the substantia nigra (dopaminergic) and brain stem raphe nuclei (serotonergic). Their afferent connections are with the globus pallidus and substantia nigra and, via connections of these structures with the thalamus and motor parts of the cerebral cortex.

The most abundant cell type, accounting for more than 90% of cells in the caudate and putamen, is a small neuron with spiny dendrites that contains the neurotransmitter gamma amino butyric acid (GABA). There are additional separate populations of large (cholinergic) interneurons and somatostatin-immunoreactive neurons.

The globus pallidus consists of two parts, the external and internal segments, both of which receive their main afferents from the striatum. Most efferents from the internal segment project to the ventral thalamus and (c) corticomedian nucleus of the thalamus, while those from the external segment are directed towards the sub-thalamic nucleus, where connections are made with the substantia nigra and back to the globus pallidus.

THALAMUS AND HYPOTHALAMUS

The thalamus and hypothalamus are further heterogeneous collections of subcortical grey matter nuclei that need to be considered in a few dementing diseases. They form the walls of the third ventricle, the hypothalamus lying ventral to the thalamus which forms a very large mass of grey matter medial to the internal capsule and ventral and partly posterior to the basal ganglia. The major groups of thalamic nuclei can be recognized, separated from each other by narrow bands of white matter – the internal medullary lamina – the median, lateral and anterior groups. The nuclei within the thalamus that are of particular interest in dementia are the dorsomedial nucleus, the anterior nucleus and some of the intralaminar nuclei (Fig. 2.14). The dorsomedial nucleus forms part of a circuit involving the pre-frontal cortex (to which it projects) and the amygdala (which

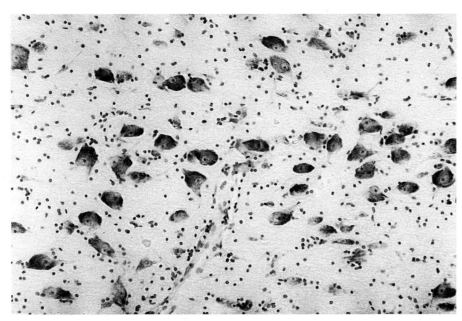

Fig. 2.13 (c)

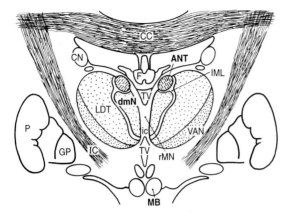

Fig. 2.14. Drawing of a transverse section through the thalamus at the level of the mamillary bodies (MB). ANT: anterior nucleus of thalamus, cc: corpus callosum, CN: caudate nucleus, dmN: dorso-medial nucleus of thalamus, F: fornix, GP: globus pallidus, IC: internal capsule, ic: interthalamic connection, IML: intra-medullary lamina and nuclei of thalamus, LDT: lateral dorsal nucleus of thalamus, P: putamen, rMN: midline nuclei of thalamus, TV: third ventricle, VAN: ventral anterior nucleus of thalamus.

projects to it). The anterior nuclear complex, like the dorsomedial nucleus, forms part of the limbic system, and projects to cingulate cortex, entorhinal cortex and subiculum as well as to non-limbic cortex, receiving reciprocal connections from most of these areas and from the mamillary bodies. The intralaminar nuclei divide the medial nuclei from the lateral and ventral nuclei and include rostral and caudal groups. The dorsomedial and anterior nuclei are closely involved in memory function and in the pathology of Alzheimer's disease. The dorsomedial nucleus is also often affected in Wernicke's encephalopathy (Chapter 13) and in dementia associated with thalamic degeneration (Chapter 10).

The hypothalamus contains many nuclei that exert central control over the autonomic nervous system. However, some of its nuclei are prominently involved in dementing processes – the mamillary bodies (Figs 2.11 and 2.14), lateral hypothalamic area (Fig. 2.15) and the less readily identified suprachiasmatic nucleus, for example (Braak & Braak 1987).

BRAINSTEM

Structures that are of chief interest in the *mid-brain* are the substantia nigra, the raphe nuclei, the superior corpora quadrigemina, the red nuclei and the periaquaductal grey matter (Fig. 2.16). The darkly pigmented dopaminergic

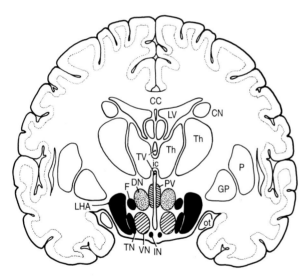

Fig. 2.15. Drawing of a transverse section of the cerebral hemispheres showing the position of some hypothalamic nuclei. (Redrawn and modified from Snell, 1992.) CC: corpus callosum, LV: lateral ventricle, CN: caudate nucleus, Th: thalamus, ic: interthalamic connection, P: putamen, GP: globus pallidus, ot: optic tract, IN: infundibular nucleus, TN: tuberomammillary nuclei, VN: ventromedial nucleus, LHA: lateral hypothalamic, F: fornix, DN: dorsomedial nucleus, PV: paraventricular nucleus, TV: third ventricle.

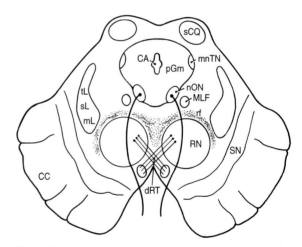

Fig. 2.16. Drawing of a transverse section of the upper midbrain. (Redrawn and modified from Snell, 1992.) sCQ: superior corpora quadrigemina, CA: cerebral aqueduct, pGm: periaqueductal grey matter, mnTN: mesencephalic nucleus of trigeminal nerve, nON: nucleus of oculomotor nerve, MLF: medial longitudinal fasciculus, rf: reticular formation, RN: red nucleus, SN: substantia nigra, dRT: decussation of rubrospinal tracts, CC: crus cerebri, mL: medial lemniscus, sL: spinal lemniscus, tL: trigeminal lemniscus.

neurons of the *substantia nigra* are readily seen in a transverse cut across the mid-brain at the level of the corpora quadrigemina, lying ventral and lateral to the red nuclei and dorsal to the cerebral peduncles (Fig. 2.16). There are two parts to the substantia nigra which lie side-by-side: the ventrolateral pars reticularis and the dorsomedial pars compacta. The cells of the pars compacta are selectively damaged in Parkinson's disease, and form one of the sites of pathology in progressive supranuclear palsy and some forms of multiple system atrophy. The large serotonergic cells of the *dorsal and median raphe* form two large midline nuclei lying one above the other in the mid-brain and pons (Fig. 2.17). They are involved in the pathology of Alzheimer's disease, Parkinson's disease and progressive supranuclear palsy. The *superior corpora quadrigemina*, the more rostral pair of dome-like protuberances on the dorsal surface of the mid-brain (Fig. 2.16), are damaged in progressive supranuclear palsy. The *periaqueductal* grey matter (Fig. 2.16) is at risk of damage in Wernicke's encephalopathy and progressive supranuclear palsy. The *superior cerebellar peduncles* (Fig. 2.17) lying to either side of the upper end of the fourth ventricle in the lower mid-brain, are often atrophied in progressive supranuclear palsy.

In the *pons* the noradrenergic pigmented nucleus, the *locus ceruleus*, lying just ventral to the lateral angle of the floor of the lower aqueduct and rostral part of the fourth ventricle, is at risk in Alzheimer's disease and Parkinson's disease, while the tegmental nuclei and medial longitudinal fasciculus (Figs. 2.16–18) are damaged in progressive supranuclear palsy. The pontine nuclei are damaged in the pontocerebellar variety of multiple system atrophy (Fig. 2.17) (Chapter 10), and the median raphe in Parkinson's disease (Chapter 6).

The *medulla* (Fig. 2.18) is less obviously affected than the more rostral parts of the brainstem, the pons and mid-brain, in dementing diseases. However, it is worth noting here the positions of the pigmented dorsal vagal nuclei, damaged in Parkinson's disease, the inferior olives which suffer secondary retrograde degeneration if the Purkinje cells of the cerebellum are destroyed by disease, and the hypoglossal nucleus and medullary pyramids which degenerate in some cases of motor neuron disease with dementia (Chapter 10).

THE CEREBELLUM (Fig. 2.19)

The division of the cerebellum into midline vermis and lateral hemispheres is worth noting. Certain diseases,

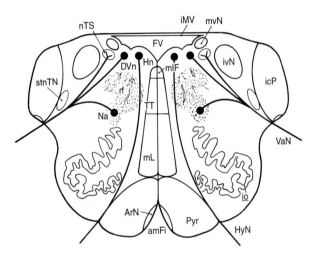

Fig. 2.18. Drawing of a transverse section of the medulla (Redrawn and modified from Snell, 1992). iMV: inferior medullary vellum, FV: cavity of fourth ventricle, mvN: medial vestibular nucleus, ivN: interior vestibular nucleus, icP: inferior cerebellar peduncle, VaN: vagus nerve, io: inferior olive, HyN: hypoglossal nerve, Pyr: pyramid, ArN: arcuate nuclei, amFi: anterior median fissure, mL: medial lemniscus (see Figure 2.15 also), TT: tectospinal tract, Na: nucleus ambiguus, StnTN: spinal tract and nucleus of trigeminal nerve, rf: reticular formation, nTs: nucleus of tractus solitarius, DVn: dorsal vagal nucleus, Hn: hypoglossal nucleus, mlF: medial longitudinal fasciculus.

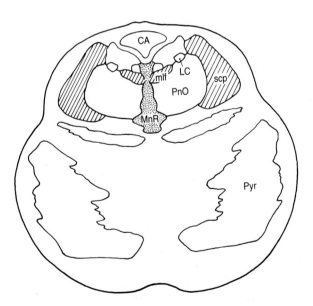

Fig. 2.17. Drawing of the upper pons to show the position of the median raphe (MnR) superior cerebellar peduncles (SCP) and locus ceruleus (LC). PnO: pontine reticular nucleus, Pyr: pyramidal tract, mlf: median longitudinal fasciculus, CA: cerebral aqueduct. The pontine nuclei lie between the pyramidal tract fibre bundles.

particularly alcoholic cerebellar degeneration, affect the vermis more than the hemispheres. Widespread cerebellar cortical damage occurs in Creutzfeldt–Jakob disease, Gerstmann Sträussler syndrome (Chapter 12), ponto-cerebellar atrophy and paraneoplastic disease (Chapter 19). The deep cerebellar white matter may share in the pathology of white matter diseases such as progressive multi-focal leukoencephalopathy and AIDS. The dentate nucleus of the cerebellum, forming a wavy band of large, deeply situated neurons above the roof of the fourth ventricle, is selectively damaged in progressive supranuclear palsy. If cells from the dentate nuclei are lost, their outflow tracts in the superior cerebellar peduncles, whose position has already been noted lateral to the fourth ventricle, in the upper pons and mid-brain, become atrophic.

REFERENCES

Amaral DC, Insausti R (1990) Hippocampal formation. In Paxinos G (ed) *The Human Nervous System*. Academic Press, New York, pp 711–56.

Bowen DM, Smith CB, White P, Flack RHA, Carrasco LH, Gedge JL, Davison AN (1977) Chemical pathology of the organic dementia. II Quantitative estimation of cellular changes in post mortem brains. *Brain* 100: 427–53.

Braak H, Braak E (1986) Ratio of pyramidal cells versus non-pyramidal cells in the human frontal isocortex and changes in ratio with ageing and Alzheimer's disease. *Progr. Brain Res* 70: 185–212.

Braak H, Braak E (1987) The hypothalamus of the human adult: chiasmatic region. *Anat Embryol* 176: 315–30.

Brodmann K (1909) *Vergleichende Lokalisation lehre der Gross Hirnrinde in ihren Prinzipiem dargestellt auf Gruand des Zellenbaues*. J A Barth, Leipzig.

Carpenter MB, Sutin J (1983) *Human Neuroanatomy*. Williams and Wilkins 3rd edn.

Davies P (1979) Neurotransmitter-related enzymes in senile dementia of the Alzheimer type. *Brain Res* 171: 319–27.

Duvernoy HM (1988) *The Human Hippocampus*. Bergmann Verlag, Munich.

Eccles JC (1984) The cerebral cortex: a theory of its operation. In Jones EG, Peters A (eds) *Cerebral Cortex Vol 2 Functional Properties of Cortical Cells*. Plenum Press, Mass. pp 1–36.

Esiri MM, Pearson RCA, Steele JE, Bowen DM, Powell TPS (1990) A quantitative study of the neurofibrillary tangles and the choline acetyltransferase activity in the cerebral cortex and the amygdala in Alzheimer's disease. *J Neurol Neurosurg Psychiat* 53: 161–5.

Heimer L (1995) The human brain and spinal cord. *Functional Neuroanatomy and Dissection Guide*. 2nd edn. Springer, Berlin.

Jones EG (1986) Neurotransmitters in the cerebral cortex. *J Neurosurg* 65: 135–53.

Lorente de No (1934) Studies on the structure of the cerebral cortex II. Continuation of the study of the Ammonic system. *J Psychol Neurol* 46: 113–77.

Mesulam M-M, van Hoesen GW (1976) Acetylcholinesterase-rich projections from basal forebrain of the rhesus monkey to neocortex. *Brain Res* 109: 152–7.

Nieuwenhuys R, Voogd J, van Huijzen C (1988) *The Human Central Nervous System. A Synopsis and Atlas*. 2nd edn. Springer, Berlin.

Paxinos G (ed) (1990) *The Human Nervous System*. Academic Press, New York.

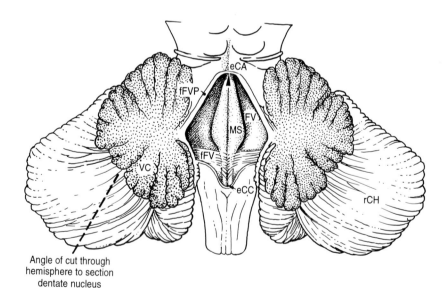

Fig. 2.19. Drawing of the cerebellum from above, with the vermis bisected and the hemispheres displaced laterally. (Redrawn and modified from Snell, 1992.) eCA: entrance into cerebral aqueduct, FV: cavity of the fourth ventricle, MS: median sulcus, rCH: right cerebellar hemisphere, eCC: entrance into central canal, fFV: floor of fourth ventricle formed by medulla oblongata, VC: vermis of cerebellum, fFVP: floor of fourth ventricle formed by pons.

Pearson RCA, Esiri MM, Hiorns RW, Wilcock GK, Powell TPS (1985) Anatomical correlates of the distribution of the pathological changes in the neocortex in Alzheimer's disease. *Proc Natl Acad Sci (USA)* 82: 4531–4.

Rose M (1927) Allocortex bei Tier und Mensch die sogennante Richrinde beim Menschem und beim Affen. *J Psychol Neurol* 34: 261–401.

Saper CB (1990) Cholinergic system. In Paxinos G (ed) *The Human Nervous System*. Academic Press, New York, pp. 1095–1114.

Snell RS (1992) *Clinical Neuroanatomy for Medical Students*. 3rd edn. Little, Brown and Co.

Szentágothai J (1979) Local neuron circuits of the neocortex. In Schmitt FO, Worden FG (eds) The Neuroscience fourth study program. MIT Press, Cambridge, Mass. pp. 399–415.

Szentágothai J (1978) The neuron network of the cerebral cortex: a functional interpretation. *Proc. Roy Soc Lond Ser B*. 201: 219–48.

Vogt C, Vogt O (1937) *Sitz und Wesen der Krankheiten in Lichte der topistischen Hirnforschung und des Variereus der Tiere, erster Teil*. Barth, Leipzig, p. 457.

Williams PL, Warwick R (1980) *Gray's Anatomy*. 36th Edn. Churchill Livingston, London.

CHAPTER THREE

Practical approach to pathological diagnosis

M. M. Esiri and J. H. Morris

The post-mortem examination in cases of dementia
Brain biopsies in patients with dementia
Ageing changes in the brain compatible with normal mental function

THE POST-MORTEM EXAMINATION IN CASES OF DEMENTIA

It has been said, with a good deal of truth, that the answer to every question in medicine is in three parts: first, take a history, secondly, make a physical examination, and thirdly, perform the relevant special tests and investigations. For the pathologist, the first two parts of this rubric are fulfilled by reading the patient's chart. The third is the performance of what, in at least one sense, is the ultimate diagnostic test, the post-mortem examination.

History and examination

The clinical information available to the pathologist called upon to perform an autopsy examination on a case of dementia is extraordinarily variable. At one extreme is the patient who has been studied over an extended period where the quality and exent of cognitive failure has been documented and, often, a presumptive pathological diagnosis is made. This type of history is often supplemented by more or less objective tests of intellectual function and the results of numerous investigations. Patients submitted to this degree of investigative rigour are often seen in centres that have a particular interest or active research programme into dementia. In these circumstances it can (we hope) be assumed that there is good liaison between the clinical service and the pathology department and the cases will be dealt with according to protocol.

The opposite end of this particular spectrum is the patient coming to autopsy examination who is reported to have an unspecified degree of cognitive decline, variously described in imprecise terms. In such cases recourse to considerable ingenuity is required to form an idea of the nature and severity of the decline. Clues can sometimes be gleaned from the nursing notes or even the patient's address. Residents of nursing homes are often more disabled than those living in the community, and the nursing home itself offers a source of an experienced assessment of the ability to perform the activities of daily living in a community.

Whatever information is available, it should be carefully studied before the autopsy is commenced. It may well contain useful pointers to the type of disease present and indicate aspects of the general autopsy that require particular attention. It is unwise to place too great a reliance on the diagnosis made during life since clinical accuracy in the diagnosis of the cause of dementia is not always very high (Gilleard *et al.*, 1992) (Table 3.1). However, the pathologist has at his disposal the additional important fact that the patient has died. The length of the history may have significant safety implications for the performance of the post mortem, most particularly in relation to the diagnosis of Creutzfeldt–Jakob disease and other prion diseases.

Prion diseases

The possible presence of a prion disease (Chapter 12) in cases of dementia should be a sufficient stimulus to ensure careful scrutiny of the patient's notes before performing an autopsy on a patient with dementia. Special safety requirements need to be fulfilled before performing an autopsy on a case of suspected Creutzfeldt–Jakob disease, Gerstmann-Sträussler syndrome, fatal familial insomnia (Medori *et al.*, 1992) or any other suspected prion disease (HMSO, 1992, ANA, 1986; Bell & Ironside, 1993, Budka *et al.*, 1995). (Methods for handling this material are discussed in Appendix 3.)

Table 3.1. *Accuracy of clinical diagnosis of Alzheimer's disease*

Study	Type	Criteria	n	AD (%)	AD only (%)
Non-systematic diagnosis					
Todorov & Go (1975)	R	Less established	273	220(81)	149(56)
Sulkava et al. (1983)	P	Less established	27	22(81)	22(81)
Perl, Pendlebury & Bird (1984)	R	Limited information	26	21(81)	9(35)
Mölsä et al. (1985)	P	Less established	28	23(82)	20(71)
Neary et al. (1986)	P	Less established	24	18(75)	—
Kokmen, Offord & Okazaki (1987)	R	Less established	32	23(72)	20(63)
Wade et al. (1987)	R	Less established	39	35(90)	28(72)
Homer et al. (1988)	P	Consensus	13	6(46)	6(46)
Joachim, Morris & Selkoe (1988)	R	Limited information	150	127(90)	105(74)
Ettlin et al. (1989)	P	Less established	13	12(92)	7(54)
Mendez et al. (1992)	R	Variable	650	505(78)	390(60)
			1275	1012(79)	726(60)
Systematic diagnosis					
Müller & Schwartz (1978)	R	ICDA-8	41	37(90)	—
Alafuzoff et al. (1987)	R	DSM III	32	26(81)	17(53)
Martin et al. (1987)	P	NINCDS–ADRDA	11	11(100)	—
Morris et al. (1988)	P	NINCDS–ADRDA	26	26(100)	16(62)
Crystal et al. (1988)	P	NINCDS and DSM III	13	11(85)	—
Tierney et al. (1988)	P	NINCDS–ADRDA	22	18(82)	17(77)
Boller, Lopez & Moossy (1989)	R	NINCDS–ADRDA	44	35(80)	—
Jellinger et al. (1990)	R	NINCDS, DSMIII, ICD9	273	246(90)	236(86)
Risse et al. (1990)	P	NINCDS and DSM III	25	17(68)	16(64)
Burns et al. (1990)	P	NINCDS and ADRDA	50	42(84)	34(68)
			537	469(87)	336(78)

R (retrospective), P (prospective).
Adapted from Mendez et al., 1992.

The most likely prion disease to be encountered is Creutzfeldt–Jakob disease (CJD), and the notes should be looked through to see if this diagnosis has been considered. It should be specifically considered in cases with a rapidly progressive course and death from natural causes within a year or less of onset of dementia. It is our practice to regard anyone who becomes severely demented and dies in a year or less to have CJD unless there is good reason to think otherwise. In this context it is worth remembering that 50% of cases of pathologically confirmed CJD die within 4 months and 90% within a year of onset. Two years after onset, 95% of all cases of CJD will have died (Brown et al., 1986, Brown, 1988a). By contrast, less than 10% patients with Alzheimer's disease have died within a year of presentation to a psychiatrist or geriatrician, and approximately 40% are still alive 5 years later. The insidiousness of the onset of symptoms in Alzheimer's disease, in fact, means that survival from the time of onset of symptoms is considerably longer than these figures suggest, with an estimated 50% survival of 8.1 years (Barclay et al., 1985).

Although the '1 year rule' will certainly catch most cases of Creutzfeldt–Jakob disease, it is not foolproof, as approximately 5% of patients survive for more than 2 years following diagnosis (Brown et al., 1984, 1986, 1987) and there is one report of survival for as long as 16 years (Cutler et al., 1984). As a group, these long survivors tend to have a higher frequency of familial incidence, younger age at onset and a lower frequency of accompanying myoclonus (see below). The longer survival cases may have a clinical course not dissimilar from Alzheimer's disease from which they cannot be reliably distinguished on clinical grounds. It is not necessarily a great comfort to know that these cases are usually very easy to recognize on microscopic examination as they have prominent spongiform change.

As well as rate of progression, another pointer in the history to the possible presence of prion disease is the occurrence of adventitious movements. In Creutzfeldt–Jakob disease there is typically a marked startle myoclonus, that comes on during the course of the disease. Even if the diagnosis of CJD has not apparently been considered by the patient's medical advisors, the prudent pathologist should consider it in cases of a progressive dementia with abnormal movements. However, 'en medecin, comme l'amour, pas de jamais, pas de toujour', for myoclonus is a rather common occurence and occurs in a large number of neurological conditions, including, as might be surmised, some cases of Alzheimer's disease (Haltia et al., 1994).

Parenthetically, although usually thought of as a dementing disease, CJD has other guises. It has been our experience that 'pareneoplastic syndrome' is one of the most frequent suggested clinical diagnoses in atypical cases that prove to have CJD on pathological examination. Like CJD, paraneoplastic disease is subacutely progressive and may affect grey matter in both the cerebellum and cerebral hemispheres. It is particularly likely to cause confusion with those cases of CJD where the cerebrellar symptoms predominate in the early clinical stages. Prion disease, in addition to causing difficulty by masquerading as other neurological conditions in its clinical expression, may also be cryptic in its pathological expression. As the report by Collinge and colleagues (Collinge et al., 1990) demonstrates, prion disease is not always, or necessarily, accompanied by spongiform change when the brain is examined microscopically.

Currently therefore, we are in the unfortunate situation of not knowing the full range of either the clinical or the pathological expression of the prion diseases. The council of perfection in this circumstance would be to perform all autopsies as if they were possible cases of prion disease but this is hardly a practicable course of action. In our view, while it is very necessary to take appropriate precautions, it is also important not to overreact to the possible risks of exposure to prions. The infectivity of prions, although demonstrable, is not high, and the only established cases of nosocomial transmission to humans have been from corneal transplants (Duffy et al., 1974), contaminated stereotactic electrodes, cadaver-derived dural implants (Center for Disease Control, 1987), and cadaver-derived human growth and gonadotropin hormone administration (Brown et al., 1988b, Centers for Disease Control, 1985). In this context it is appropriate to remember that numerous autopsies were performed on patients with prion diseases before the 'infective' nature of prions was demonstrated. Given the comparatively cavalier way in which these autopsies were conducted and the brain tissue handled, mortuary technicians and neuropathologists should have been at a substantial risk of contracting prion disease if performance of an autopsy was a significant exposure. The risk, if there is one, is probably in handling the tissue in the histology laboratory where at least one histology technician who was known to have handled cases of CJD has died of CJD, although there is no evidence that demonstrated that the disease was contracted by exposure to the tissue (Miller, 1988). This potential risk can, however, be removed by treatment of tissue to be processed by formic acid (Brown, Wolff & Gajdusek, 1990) which effectively eliminates infectivity from tissue specimens (see Appendix 3).

Returning to the history, in patients who have not been well investigated and who have uncharacterized cognitive decline, perhaps the first question to be asked is whether the patient has a true dementia or a confusional state brought about by metabolic derangments. Pointers to a confusional state are a marked variability in the degree of impairment, and usually, relatively short duration.

It is always helpful to establish if possible the length of time for which the patient has been cognitively impaired. A sense of the rate and character of the progression of the decline is also very informative. For example, a patient with a cognitive decline that does not seem to have undergone significant progression for several years is not, in general, likely to be suffering from a neurodegenerative disease since, once symptomatic, these tend to be progressive.

The manner of the presentation can also be relevant. It is commonplace that the symptoms that first bring a patient to medical attention markedly influence the manner of the patient's progression through the medical establishment, and also the way in which they are investigated. Patients with Alzheimer's disease who present with alteration in mood or affect are much more likely to find their way to a psychiatrist, while those with, for example, language disorders, are usually referred to a neurologist. It is revealing of the state of medical practice that the outcome, in terms of history taken, character of the physical examination and investigations performed, is often very different in these two groups of patients.

A formal neurological examination is always useful, as it will almost always include some assessment of the mental state. Within the neurological examination, it is worthwhile looking for any evidence of focal neurological signs and symptoms, and their temporal relationship, if any, to the onset and/or progression of the decline in cognitive function. Myoclonus and cerebellar symptoms have already been mentioned in relation to prion diseases, but parkinsonian symptoms, choreiform movements, and signs of upper and lower motor neurone loss are all encountered in different forms of dementia. Stroke syndromes are also important, whether they be fixed impairments or transient ischaemic attacks. Bilaterally upgoing plantar responses as an isolated neurological sign are, in general, not a useful observation, as they have no localizing value and do not differentiate between structural and metabolic disease.

Another aspect of the history which is worth specific attention is the family history. There are a number of dementing diseases that are familial, Huntington's disease, for example, and many of the degenerative and other forms of dementia have a familial component. Both Alzheimer's and Pick's disease have a familial representation, as does Creutzfeldt-Jakob disease. However, it has to be admitted that this is usually one of the least well-documented aspects of a patient's history.

Investigations
NEUROIMAGING
Of all the investigations, neuroradiological imaging studies probably have the most immediate and direct value and should be looked for specifically. The quality of neuroimaging now available makes it perfectly feasible to make a reasonable assessment of the degree and distribution of, for example, brain atrophy, in life. Indeed, it is probably quite reasonable to suppose that neuroimaging, particularly MRI, is able to provide at least as good an estimate of the degree of atrophy as neuropathological examination. The potential of MRI for functional studies of the nervous system is only just beginning to be exploited, and it is likely that more advanced forms of electronic manipulation of MRI-derived information will be a fruitful field of investigation of many forms of neurological disease in the relatively near future. Our personal experience of correlations of hippocampal size between CT and pathology in Alzheimer's disease (Jobst et al., 1992, 1994) and MRI and pathology in temporal lobe epilepsy indicates that imaging and pathology findings give very good correlation in both ventricular size and severity of pathology.

Correlation between imaging and pathology, is not, however, always this good or this simple. The situation in vascular disease for example is very different. Neuro-radiological phenomena such as the so-called 'unidentified bright objects' (UBOs) and leukoaraiosis, have a less consistent association with either pathology or clinical phenomenology, so that neuroimaging findings should not be accepted uncritically.

In some circumstances more arcane forms of neuroimaging may also be available. The most notable are single photon emission computed tomography (SPECT) which gives an indication of the distribution of blood flow in the brain, and positron emission tomography (PET) which gives information about the patterns of metabolic activity. Although these imaging methods are not commonly available (particularly the very expensive PET scanning), patterns of activity in different diseases are beginning to be recognized which are suggestive of specific pathological diagnoses.

The post-mortem examination
EXAMINING THE EXTRA-CRANIAL ORGANS
Pathological processes that cause dementia are rarely the direct cause of death. Most patients with progressive dementia die as a result of complications of their inactive, often terminally mute, and unresponsive state with bronchopneumonia, pulmonary embolism, urinary tract infections or terminal septicaemia. A few die as a result of the direct systemic effects of the primary disease, such as pneumocystis pneumonia in AIDS or complications of liver cirrhosis in alcoholics or subjects with Wilson's disease. Cardiac deaths are also common in demented subjects, particularly in those with ischaemic dementia.

In addition to providing a cause of death, the systemic autopsy examination may also show other findings significantly related to the dementing process. Where particular types of pathological process are suspected, the following aspects of the general autopsy examination require particular attention.

Vascular dementia: state of the heart (particularly valves, sources of emboli in left atrium and ventricle, patency of foramen ovale) and great vessels (particularly the aorta, internal carotid arteries in the neck and the vertebral arteries); sources of fat emboli; sources of emboli from leg veins if foramen ovale patent; evidence of infarction in other organs, especially the kidneys and spleen; evidence of widespread vasculitis and/or renal lesions of systemic lupus erythematosus; evidence of neoplasia (carcinoma, lymphoma); evidence of sickle cell anaemia.

Infective causes: fungal or tuberculous infections in lungs/paranasal sinuses; Whipple's disease; syphilis; systemic features of AIDS or another cause of immunosuppression such as sarcoidosis or lymphoma; parasitic infestations such as toxoplasmosis or cysticercosis.

Intracerebral tumour or hydrocephalus: extra-cerebral neoplasia; Paget's disease.

Alcoholic intoxication: evidence of repeated trauma, liver cirrhosis, peripheral neuropathy.

Dialysis dementia: renal disease and aluminium deposits in bones.

Other metabolic disease: liver disease (hepatic encephalopathy, Wilson's disease); pancreatic or extra pancreatic insulinomia (hypoglycaema); adrenal atrophy (adrenoleukodystrophy); mitochondrial myopathy, cardiomyopathy (mitochondrial cytopathies); peripheral neuropathy (vitamin deficiencies, some storage disorders, porphyria).

Paraneoplastic disease: small cell lung carcinoma, ovarian carcinoma in women, lymphoma.

The spinal cord should be removed for later examination if the following are suspected: Gerstmann–Sträussler syndrome, familial amyloid angiopathy, motor neuron disease with dementia, metabolic storage disorders, adrenoleukodystrophy, multiple system atrophy, Hallervorden–Spatz disease, infective conditions, multiple sclerosis, vitamin deficiencies, cases with clinical evidence of peripheral neuropathy, paraneoplastic syndrome. In the latter two conditions samples of sensory and autonomic ganglia should also be removed for microscopic examination. Samples of peripheral nerves and muscles should also be removed from cases of suspected motor neuron disease, metabolic storage diseases, adrenoleukodystrophy, vitamin deficiency, peripheral neuropathy and paraneoplastic syndrome.

Examination of fresh brain

For the pathologist with little experience in examining demented brains, a systematic approach to the examination of the brain is the most effective way of building the familiarity that will permit reliable differentiation between the, in some cases very wide, range of normal appearances and genuine pathology. If a number of cases are to be examined and compared, it is almost essential that they be handled in a similar and systematic fashion. Where rare conditions are to be studied, it is usually necessary to collect material from a number of different sources and this sort of study is made either difficult or impossible if the brain has been handled in very different ways. As will be seen in relation to a number of causes of dementia, the lack of systematic examination and recording is a considerable handicap to progress in understanding.

The foregoing can be read as a plea for neuropathologists to abandon subsidiarity and relinquish a little of their sovereignty to adopt a common minimum standard or protocol for the examination of the brain in cases of dementia. It is our opinion that, for the examination of cases of dementia, there is a very good product already available. Under the leadership and guidance of Drs Al Heyman and Sue Mirra, the consortium to establish a registry for Alzheimer's disease (CERAD) has performed the invaluable service of producing a neuropathology assessment instrument (Mirra *et al.*, 1991) that, although concentrating on Alzheimer's disease, is specifically applicable to all causes of dementia and which is subject to continual review and periodic updating. The CERAD protocol is essentially a research tool and, properly applied, is too detailed for what might be called routine diagnostic use, but its outline and principles are entirely applicable to a standard diagnostic approach. On pages 52–3 we reproduce a scaled-down version of CERAD that we recommend to readers for this purpose.

After opening the skull, the following features should be sought before removing the brain

Chronic or acute subdural haematomas (small subdural haematomas are not uncommon as a consequence of brain atrophy or in the presence of an intra-ventricular shunt; occasionally large subdural haematomas are a cause of dementia).

Meningeal thickening (though in chronic meningitis this may be more evidenced at the base of the brain than over the vertex).

Cerebrospinal fluid: This may be readily removed if required from the pre-pontine cisterns during removal of the brain from the cranial cavity.

The brain should then be removed carefully and attention paid particularly to avoiding tears of the mid-brain after the cerebral hemispheres have been freed but the contents of the posterior fossa are still anchored.

After removal, the brain should be weighed and placed in a bowl to allow its natural shape to be retained. The main cerebral vessels at the base should be carefully examined and the extent of atheroma and any sites of arterial stenosis or occlusion noted. Aneurysms should be sought at branch points on the circle of Willis and middle cerebral arteries and any fresh subarachnoid haemorrhage or rusty discolouration of leptomeninges, either generalized or localized, suggestive of old subarachnoid haemorrhage, described. A search should also be made for old contusions suggestive of head injury, particularly on the inferior surfaces of the frontal and inferolateral surfaces of the temporal lobes. Any surface softenings or tumours should be delineated and described. Frequently the cerebral gyri appear atrophied and the extent of such atrophy and its distribution should be documented. Atrophy may be more readily appreciated if the leptomeninges are stripped from the surface. The cerebellar folia and brainstem should also be examined for evidence of atrophy.

At this stage a strong lead as to the cause of the patient's dementia may have been obtained. For example, Creutzfeldt–Jakob disease is very likely if the history of dementia was very short, perhaps two to three months, from normal mental state to mute and unresponsive, no abnormalities were found in the general autopsy examination other than a cause of death such as bronchopneumonia or pulmonary embolism, and the brain appears normal or shows only slight generalized cerebral atrophy. With the same post-mortem findings but a long history, measured in years, Alzheimer's or Parkinson's disease is possible; if there was a small cell lung carcinoma and a normal appearing brain, paraneoplastic syndrome is very likely; if the lymph nodes appeared lymphomatous and the brain unremarkable, progressive multifocal leukoencephalopathy is possible. If there is gross atrophy, particularly confined to temporal and frontal poles, the diagnosis is almost certainly Pick's disease. However, it is equally possible that no clear lead may emerge at this stage or indeed until the microscopy is available.

RETENTION OF FRESH FROZEN BRAIN SAMPLES

It may frequently be advisable to retain fresh samples of brain or cerebrospinal fluid for microbiological, molecular biological, biochemical or frozen section analysis before proceeding to fix the brain. Many centres undertaking research on dementia have defined requirements

for fresh frozen tissue. The addresses of brain banks receiving fresh tissue in the UK and elsewhere are listed in Appendix 2. In some centres, one-half of the brain or one cerebral hemisphere may be removed and frozen intact, or after slicing to allow gross pathology to be identified first. In most degenerative diseases the pathological changes are more or less symmetrically distributed and it is a likely safe assumption, at least to a first approximation, that the frozen tissue contains the same pathology as the equivalent area of the fixed hemisphere. However, if a precise match of pathology and frozen tissue analysis is essential, it is necessary to take immediately adjacent small samples for this purpose. Some pathological processes are not symmetrical and freezing half a brain or hemisphere in such cases is more problematic. This is particularly true of ischaemic dementia, some infective causes of dementia and neoplasias. Since these causes may be impossible to exclude at this stage there is a case for limiting removal of fresh samples to small blocks (1 to 5 grams) of cerebral cortex from most cases since this will suffice for many research requirements.

When any necessary fresh samples have been removed from the brain and any external features of interest noted and photographed, the remainder should be fixed by suspension from the basilar artery in a large closed container of fixative (commonly neutral 10% formalin). After three to four weeks the fixed brain will be ready for slicing.

Examination of fixed brain

Before slicing the brain, the formalin should be poured out of its container and replaced with water for one to two days to avoid excessive exposure to formalin vapour.

WEIGHT AND VOLUME CHANGES IN NORMAL AND DEMENTED BRAINS

There is a concept that might be called 'spurious precision' where a parameter is measured with great precision but can be interpreted only very approximately (the measurement of lactic dehydrogenase (LDH) springs to mind as a good example). So it is with brain weight; although easily measured to the nearest tenth of a gram, the range of normal values is so wide that it is impossible to interpret with equivalent precision. Any value between 1000 and 1500 g could be within the normal range or indicate a significant degree of atrophy. The very great variation in brain size that this difference in weights implies is illustrated in Fig. 3.1.

Several autopsy studies indicate that there are modest reductions in brain weight and volume, particularly in the cerebrum, in old age. Computerized tomography scan on healthy old people confirm these changes. They start about the age of 50 years and amount to a loss of weight and volume of the cerebral hemispheres of about 2–3% per decade (Davis & Wright 1977; Miller, Alston & Corsellis, 1980). Compared to the brain of a young person, the brain from an elderly person thus shows some slight narrowing of the cortical gyri and widening of the sulci (Fig. 3.2), and there is also slight collagenous thickening of the leptomeninges. Brain weights in those 70–80 years average 1344 g for men and 1213 g for women (Dekaban & Sadowsky, 1978). Comparable average brain weights in young adults are 1450 g for men and 1290 g for women (Dekaban & Sadowsky, 1978) (Fig. 3.16). Loss of volume of brain substance in old age is generally greater for white matter (11% loss between 70 and 85 years) than grey matter (2–3% loss between 70 and 85 years), but the greatest loss in one study was in the subiculum of the hippocampus (28% between 70 and 85 years) (Anderson *et al.*, 1983).

OTHER EXTERNAL FEATURES
The external configuration of the brain can reveal generalized or focal atrophy or focal lesions. The assessment of the degree of atrophy cannot be complete before the brain is sliced, but some brains show clear evidence of widening of the sulci (Figs. 3.3 and 3.4) that is usually easiest to see in the frontal and temporal lobes. If it is important to define or document the distribution and degree of sulcal widening, it is often helpful to strip off the leptomeninges (Fig. 3.5). Although this has the advantage of revealing the configuration of the gyri more clearly, it also removes most of the arterial supply to the cortex and it may be appropriate to strip the meninges from one hemisphere only. The absence of significant atrophy can also be important information. In a rapidly progressive dementia such as CJD, the external appearance of the brain is usually normal. External inspection of the fixed brain will also confirm the features identified when it was fresh. Sometimes areas of softening that were overlooked at an earlier stage become evident since fixation accentuates the difference in consistency between normal and softened brain. The vascular anatomy should also be noted and any softening should be related to the arterial territories of supply. Occasionally softening may be due to necrotizing encephalitis, for example, due to toxoplasmosis or herpes simplex encephalitis. In these cases the softened areas will not conform to arterial territories or boundary zones. Failure to conform to arterial boundaries is also found in diffuse ischaemia where the parasagittal and lateral occipital arterial boundary zones are the most vulnerable to grossly visible damage.

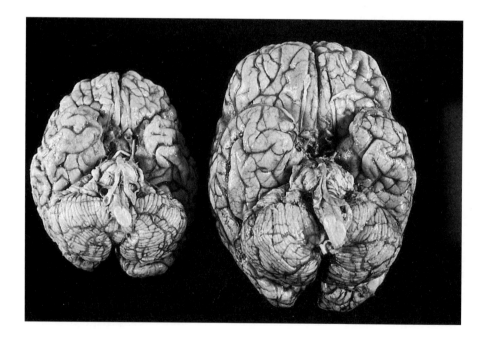

Fig. 3.1. Variation in size of non-atrophic brains. Both these patients were considered in life to be neurologically normal. The brain on the left weighed 860 g, and that on the right 1760 g.

EXAMINATION OF BRAIN SLICES

This is best done systematically, and as an aid to this there is considerable merit in laying the slices out on a tray which enables an overall impression to be gained and encourages the sequential examination of the slices.

At this stage the hind brain can be separated from the cerebrum by slicing through the mid-brain. The conventional manner of slicing the fixed cerebrum from cases of dementia is at 1 cm intervals in the coronal plane. Unless there is a need to compare horizontal slices with CT scan

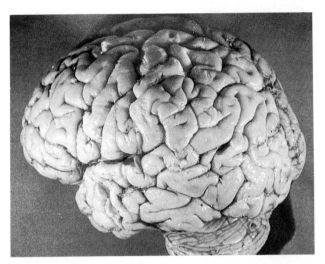

(a)

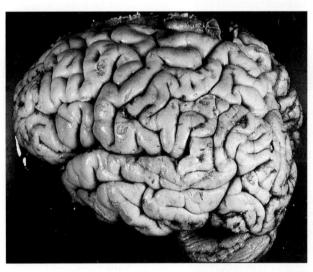

(b)

Fig. 3.2. Comparison of a young (a) and an aged normal (b) brain. There is slight widening of the sulci in the aged normal, but the changes are quite inconspicuous.

appearances, coronal slices are recommended because the hippocampal formation is better seen in this plane. The first slice is taken through the mamillary bodies which are readily identified at the base of the brain. When the hemispheres have been sliced in this manner the deep aspects – cerebral white matter and deep grey matter as well as the hippocampus, insula and ventricles – can be examined for the first time. Assessment of ventricular size provides useful diagnostic information, focal areas of deep softening or focal atrophy can be identified, and the features of interest photographed and reported. The hind brain is similarly examined in slices transverse to the brainstem with the cerebellum attached. Alternatively, the cerebellum can be removed by slicing through the cerebellar peduncles which affords an opportunity for making a midline cut through the vermis of the cerebellum and an oblique lateral cut through the hemispheres and dentate nuclei,

Cerebral atrophy

VENTRICULAR SYSTEM

Assessment of ventricular size and configuration is an important part of the estimation of the degree of atrophy (Fig. 3.6). The range of normal variation in the size of the lateral ventricles within the older population is considerable, and only major degrees of ventricular enlargement can be unequivocally interpreted. The conventional places to examine are the angle and curvature between the head of the caudate and the internal capsule of the frontal poles, and, in particular, the volume of the temporal horn. The normal variation in the width of the third ventricle is less than that seen in the lateral ventricles, and a significantly barrel shaped third ventricle is almost always an indication of atrophy. Ventricular dilatation can also be seen in brains sectioned in the CT plane (Fig. 3.7), but it is difficult to compare the degree of ventricular dilatation in brains sectioned in a CT plane with that seen in brains sectioned in the coronal plane. One caveat in the examination of ventricular size and configuration is that the brain should have been properly suspended during fixation. All too often, asymmetric flattening of the gyri over the convexities indicates not a focal mass lesion but the distortion that comes from sitting on the bottom of a bucket. When this has occurred, there will usually be considerable distortion of the ventricular configuration.

One aspect of atrophy as manifested by ventricular dilatation that can be assessed on gross examination of brain slices is its distribution. Atrophy is rarely entirely uniform, and differences in the relative dilatation of the frontal, temporal and occipital poles of the lateral ventricles is sometimes conspicuous. Pick's disease is a good example, there being cases where the frontal and temporal lobes can be affected to quite different degrees, producing quite different degrees of dilatation of the frontal and temporal horns. Asymmetric atrophy, and indeed asymmetry in general, should also be looked for.

The fourth ventricle is not often significantly enlarged in dementia, except in those diseases that affect the cerebellum and where there is usually a significant history of ataxia. One condition where gross examination of the fourth ventricle can be very helpful is in progressive supranuclear palsy, a condition that can be mistaken for Parkinson's disease. In both conditions there is degeneration and depigmentation of the sub-

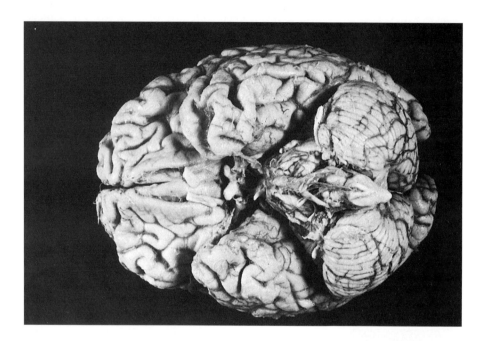

Fig. 3.3. Ventral view of a moderately atrophic brain. The conspicuous feature is the widening of the sulci towards the temporal poles. There is also some expansion of the sulci at the frontal poles.

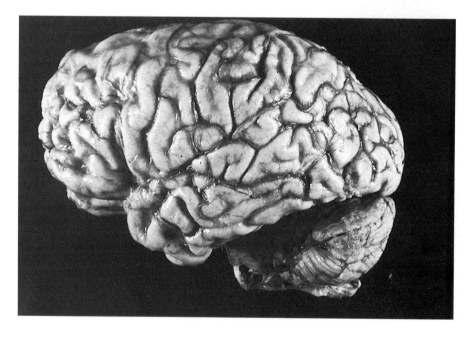

Fig. 3.4. A lateral view of the same brain as Fig. 3.3. Widening of the sulci is apparent in both the frontal and temporal lobes.

stantia nigra, but in PSP, there is also degeneration of the deep grey nuclei of the cerebellum which results in degeneration of the superior cerebellar peduncle. This results in a marked relative expansion of the superior end of the fourth ventricle where it merges with the aqueduct of Sylvius that can be seen on gross inspection of brain slices (Fig. 10.1a).

EXAMINATION OF THE BRAIN PARENCHYMA

Within each slice we have found it helpful to examine the cortical ribbon, white matter and deep grey nuclei separately. It has to be admitted that, with most cases of degenerative dementia, the gross examination of brain slices is seldom decisive. In cerebrovascular disease by contrast, the gross examination can be very important and in this circumstance it can be very helpful to have some sort of proforma of brain slices on which to record the observations (see Chapter 5).

Cerebral cortex: Many, if not most, of the causes of dementia affect the cerebral cortex and its assessment is therefore a very important part of the examination of the brain in cases of dementia.

Cortical atrophy

In most cases of dementia secondary to degenerative disease the cortical ribbon is not visibly attenuated or narrowed and the cortical degeneration is reflected only in the widening of the cortical sulci and expansion of the ventricles. However, when there is severe atrophy, the cortical ribbon can be seen to be reduced in thickness and altered in character even when examined by the naked eye. Grossly visible cortical atrophy is particularly easy to see in Pick's disease because of the focal nature of the atrophy and is particularly noticeable in the contrast between the preservation of the cortex of the posterior superior temporal gyrus and the atrophic cortex of the adjacent middle temporal gyrus and insula.

Other cortical changes

Those that can be assessed are predominantly vascular. Focal infarcts can, of course, generally be seen, and their pattern is sometimes very informative (and occasionally misleading). One pattern that can stand out is that associated with the so-called 'watershed' or 'boundary-zone' lesions that are prominent parasagittally and tend to expand over the lateral occipital gyri. This pattern is usually quite recognizable and is associated with generalized reductions in cerebral perfusion and, in long-term survivors, widespread cortical damage and cognitive impairment.

However, too much reliance should not be put on apparent distribution, we have had the experience of diagnosing probable boundary zone infarction by gross inspection only to discover on microscopic examination that the appearance was a result of myriad micro-atheroemboli, which, because of their very small size had

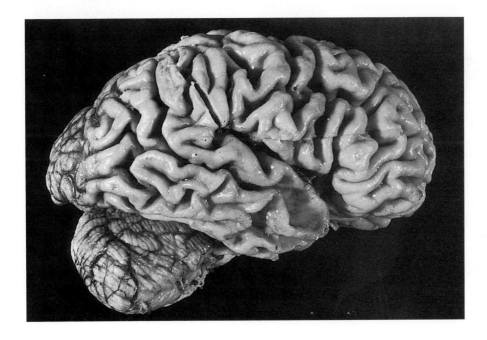

Fig. 3.5 Removal of the meninges permits a more accurate estimation of the degree of cortical atrophy. In this case, where the atrophy is more severe than in Fig. 3.4, there is marked widening of the sulci in the frontal, temporal and parietal lobes. In this case, in which a diagnosis of Alzheimer's disease was made on microscopic examination, there is no obvious sparing of the primary cortex bordering the Rolandic sulcus.

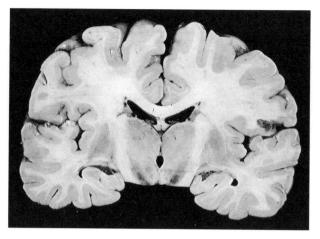

(a)

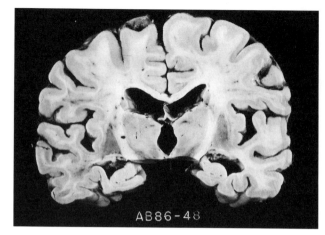

(d)

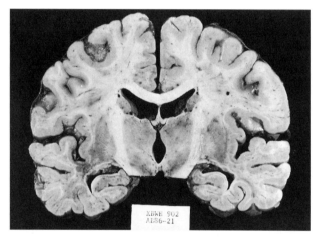

(b)

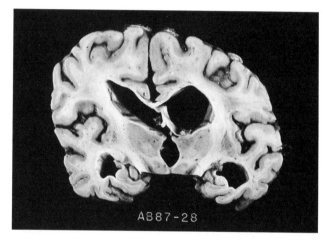

(e)

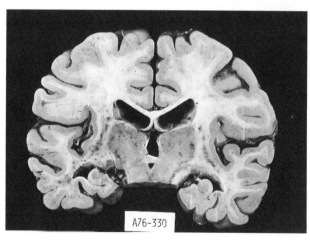

(c)

Fig. 3.6. Variations in ventricular size (a)–(e). Progressive expansion of the cerebral ventricles. (a) Normal brain. (b) Mild expansion of the third ventricle and the Sylvian fissure. (b) Widening of the angle of the lateral ventricles and the beginnings of expansion of the temporal horns of the lateral ventricles. (c) Further widening of the angles of the lateral ventricles with more pronounced barrel shaped expansion of the third ventricle and significant expansion of the temporal horns of the lateral ventricles. (d), (e) Marked expansion of the temporal horns of the lateral ventricles with obvious atrophy of the hippocampi. There is also gross expansion of the remainder of the lateral ventricles.

impacted in the most distal arterial branches. In another case, the distribution of the cortical and white matter damage superficially appeared to be consistent with boundary zone ischaemia, but microscopy showed the presence of chronic progressive multifocal leukoencephalopathy (PML).

Hippocampus and amygdala: The hippocampus should always be examined specifically. In Alzheimer's disease, for example, both hippocampi are often atrophic (Fig. 3.8). However, asymmetries are always worth looking for, and, if visible on macroscopic examination, are very likely to be pathologically significant. Imaging and tissue studies have shown that there is very little differ-

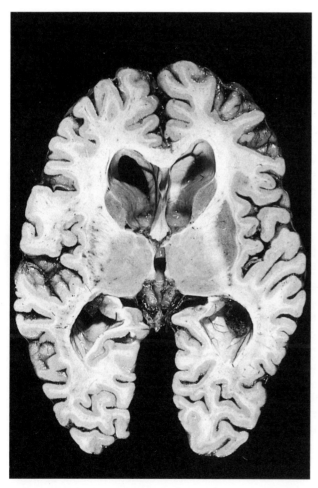

Fig. 3.7. Ventricular enlargement is also apparent in a CT plane brain slice. In this example, the expansion of the temporal horns of the lateral ventricles is particularly conspicuous.

ence in size between the left and right hippocampi in normals. Where there is a detectable difference in size, microscopic examination of both hippocampi is recommended.

Although strictly a subcortical grey nucleus, it is convenient to examine the amygdala at the same time as the hippocampus since the anterior hippocampus is coextensive with the amygdala which, at least grossly, merges with the entorhinal cortex of the uncus of the temporal horn. Atrophy of the amygdala is most easily detected by the expansion of the anterior extent of the temporal horn of the lateral ventricle that is its result (Fig. 3.8). In the cortical dementias the degree of amygdala atrophy is variable, but is usually very noticeable in Pick's disease when the temporal lobe is affected and it is also often affected in Alzheimer's disease.

White matter: Specific features of the white matter that are relevant in the examination of the brain from a patient with dementia are: (1) volume, (2) appearance, and (3) texture.

Volume: The white matter volume is really an aspect of atrophy and is most easily assessed as an inverse reflection of ventricular size. In patients with severe cortical disease there is almost always a correspondingly severe loss of white matter most marked in the affected lobes. As with cortical atrophy this is most easily seen in one of the focal atrophies, Pick's disease again being the most dramatic. However, there are a few situations, such as for example Binswanger's subcortical leukoencephalopathy, where the white matter may be disproportionately reduced in volume and the grey matter relatively preserved. This usually produces a picture of atrophy where the ventricular enlargement is out of proportion to the sulcal widening. In this circumstance making an assessment of the thickness of the anterior corpus callosum is sometimes helpful. In patients with not much apparent cortical atrophy, significant attenuation of the anterior corpus callosum may be a good indicator of severe white matter damage,

Appearance: Linear streaks of tissue infarction along the course of a long penetrating artery, the presence of lacunar infarction and a peppering with tiny holes (cribriform state) may all be indicators of the presence of diffuse vascular disease in the white matter. Other white matter lesions are the characteristic sharp-edged irregular, grey, translucent plaques of multiple sclerosis or the tiny punctate lesions coalescing almost imperceptibly into larger translucent areas of demyelination of PML (a rare cause of cognitive impairment). Occasionally, much more dramatic findings crop up; we have seen subacute cognitive decline as a result of bihemispheric radiation/chemotherapy leukoencephalopathy, and almost total hemispheric demyelination in a patient carrying a clinical diagnosis of schizophrenia with a 'degenerative neurological disease' which proved to be adreno-leukodystrophy. The vital clue here was the observation in the general autopsy of very small adrenal glands!

Texture: Normal white matter of the fixed brain is firm but not rubbery. Focal necrotizing lesions produce marked local softening that is easily detected by running

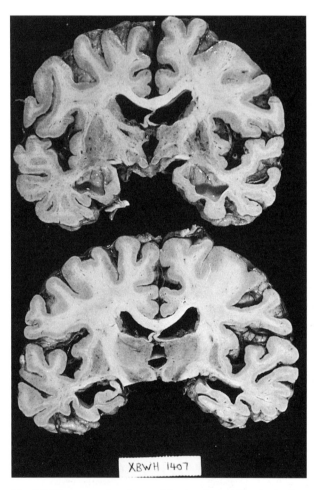

Fig. 3.8. Hippocampal and amygdala atrophy in AD: a brain slice at the level of the posterior thalamus showing marked hippocampal atrophy and accompanying expansion of the temporal horns of the lateral ventricles. In the more anterior slice, above, there is marked expansion of the temporal horn of the lateral ventricle anterior to the hippocampus in the normal location of the amygdala.

a gloved finger lightly over the cut surface of the brain. Sometimes the edge of these lesions is particularly easy to detect. With diffuse white matter loss, such as that seen in subcortical leukoencephalopathy (Binswanger's disease) the white matter has a much more rubbery texture, a finding that is usually accompanied by the 'pockmarked' appearance of the cribriform state.

Basal ganglia: The basal ganglia consist chiefly of the caudate, putamen and globus pallidus. Gross examination will reveal atrophy, and, often some indication of any degree of vascular disease. Atrophy of the caudate/putamen is most conspicuous in conditions such as Huntington's disease and other diseases principally affecting the extrapyramidal motor system. However, it is important to remember that it can also occur in Alzheimer's and, particularly, Pick's disease, in which latter association it can be as dramatic as Huntington's disease. In Pick's disease, the presence of the associated lobar atrophy serves to distinguish it from Huntington's disease. In hypertensive vascular disease, the expansion of the Virchow-Robin spaces around the lenticulo-striate arteries that supply the caudate/putamen can sometimes be very conspicuous (and may be misidentified as lacunes by inexperienced pathologists and by neuroradiologists interpreting scans) (Fig. 3.9). Small vessel vascular disease in the basal ganglia often produces a slightly pockmarked appearance of these nuclei (and also of the thalamus as all the deep grey nuclei tend to be affected by vascular disease to a similar extent (something that is not true of degenerative disease where the atrophy tends to be focal and affect specific nuclei leaving others relatively intact).

The basal nucleus of Meynert cannot be evaluated effectively by gross examination, and it must therefore be sampled microscopically. The easiest way to locate it is to find the anterior commissure and sample the rectangular block of tissue that extends underneath the putamen/globus pallidus (lentiform nucleus) immediately inferior and posterior to the commissure (Fig. 3.10).

Thalamus, hypothalamus and subthalamus: One of the rarer associations of dementia is with damage to or degeneration of the thalamus and this may be reflected in bilateral thalamic changes. The syndrome of thalamic dementia has been described in association with a number of different causes of bilateral thalamic damage including prion disease, ischaemia and infarction secondary to occlusion to thalamic perforating arteries, tumour infiltration, trauma, and necrotizing infection.

These processes may all have manifestations elsewhere in the brain, but from the perspective of the dementia, the thalamic damage may be the most significant and therefore the thalamus merits a specific evaluation on gross examination of the brain.

Within the hypothalamus, one of the most readily evaluable structures relevant to patients with dementia are the mamillary bodies. These may be atrophic and discoloured in the amnestic dementia (Korsakoff's psychosis) most especially associated with alcoholism. The dorsomedial thalamus also usually shows marked neuronal loss and consecutive gliosis, but this cannot be appreciated on gross examination of the brain.

In the subthalamus, the subthalamic nucleus (body of

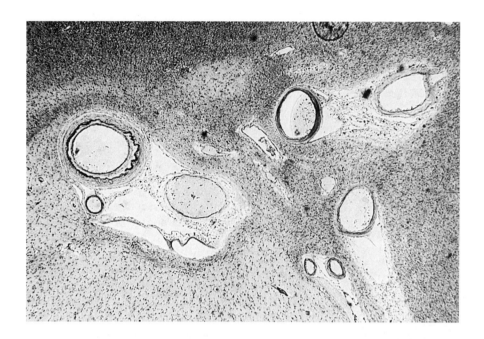

Fig. 3.9. Dilatation of the perivascular Virchow–Robin spaces in the basal ganglia. This appearance can sometimes be misinterpreted as lacunar disease on imaging studies, but the presence of an artery within each 'lacune' demonstrates their true nature.

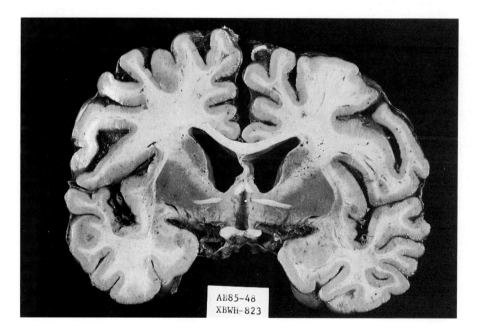

AB85-48
XBWH-823

Fig. 3.10. A section of brain showing the location of the nucleus basalis of Meynert inferior to the anterior commissure. This photograph is almost at its anterior margin and the preferred block would be from the block face posterior to this cut.

Luys) can be seen as a lozenge shaped region just medial to the upper extremity of the substantia nigra (see Fig. 5.11). It is not clearly visible in all sections that include the substantia nigra and a little experience is required to decide whether the nucleus is truly atrophic or the section does not contain a good section of the nucleus. The most important condition in which it is clearly atrophic is progressive supranuclear palsy (PSP) (Fig. 3.11). Atrophy of this region can produce a characteristic pattern of expansion of the third ventricle where the expansion is of the inferior portion of the ventricle (cf. Fig. 3.11 with Fig. 5.11).

Brainstem–Mesencephalon, pons and medulla: The most readily evaluable regions on naked eye examination of the brainstem are the pigmented nuclei, the substantia nigra and the locus ceruleus. Loss of pigmentation in these nuclei occurs in a quite large number of different conditions.

Substantia nigra: The substantia nigra is a major component of the extrapyramidal motor system and the principal source of dopaminergic input to the caudate/putamen. Many of the extrapyramidal syndromes, notably idiopathic Parkinson's disease, multiple system atrophy and progressive supranuclear palsy (Fig. 3.12), with and without dementia exhibit depigmentation of the substantia nigra. However, Alzheimer's disease and Pick's disease, the quintessential cortical dementias, as

well as frontal lobe dementia, have a significant incidence of associated degeneration of the substantia nigra. To reinforce the importance of examining the substantia nigra in cases of dementia, some examples of what appear to be clinically typical cases of Alzheimer's disease, prove on neuropathological examination to have only the changes of idiopathic Parkinson's disease with cortical Lewy bodies (the clue here is often a normal weight brain in a patient with a long history of progressive dementia). Hence, the substantia nigra should always be specifically examined in cases of dementia.

Locus ceruleus: Depigmentation of the locus ceruleus can be seen grossly and is most obvious in cases of idiopathic Parkinson's disease, progressive supranuclear palsy and Alzheimer's disease. Indeed, none of these diseases is likely to be present in a brain with a normally pigmented locus ceruleus.

Cerebellum: Cerebellar changes in patients with decline in cognitive function are seen most often in the amnestic dementia of alcoholism (Korsakoff's syndrome), multiple system atrophy, and progressive supranuclear palsy. Significant folial atrophy is reflected both in the external appearance of the cerebellar hemispheres and by expansion of the fourth ventricle (Fig. 3.13).

In alcoholic cerebellar disease, the ataxia is truncal and the atrophy occurs in the superior vermis. To obtain an adequate section through the tissue, the cerebellum

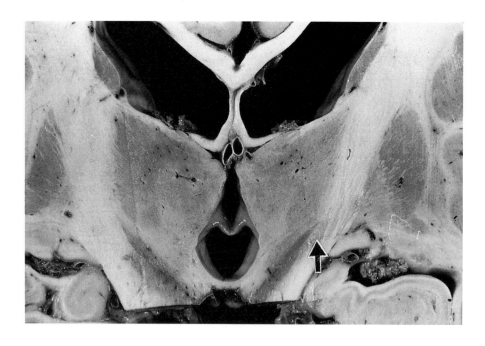

Fig. 3.11. A photograph of the thalamus in a case of progressive supranuclear palsy (PSP). The location of the atrophic subthalamic nucleus is indicated by the arrow. The loss of tissue from the subthalamic region has resulted in dilatation of the inferior part of the third ventricle, while its superior portion is undilated. Comparison with Fig. 3.6(*d*) shows the more conventional 'barrel'-shaped atrophy of the third ventricle with the less selective tissue loss that is seen in Alzheimer's disease.

should be detached from the brain stem and sectioned sagittally, just to one side of the midline. It should be noted that, to the inexperienced eye, the folia of the superior vermis almost always seem to be a little atrophic.

Selection of tissue blocks

In some cases a strong suspicion of the pathological diagnosis will have been formed by the time the fixed brain has been examined with the naked eye. The evidence obtained from the brain slices may have yielded further diagnostic clues, although it is commonly still difficult at this stage to positively identify some diseases, including Alzheimer's disease.

Brain blocks for histological examination should be selected at this stage and should be chosen to display as readily as possible the pathological features of the disease process suspected. Most laboratories now use paraffin embedding exclusively or occasionally supplement this with resin embedding. Because it is essential to be certain that a required structure will be included in the sections taken, it is advisable to mark the block in such a way that the technician knows which surface to cut. In many cases it is necessary, in addition to taking blocks to confirm a suspected non-Alzheimer's disease, to take blocks to see if Alzheimer's disease is also present. This is because Alzheimer's disease is very common, cannot be excluded without histological examination and not infrequently occurs together with other

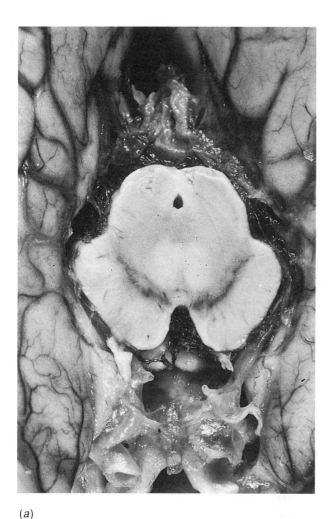

(a)

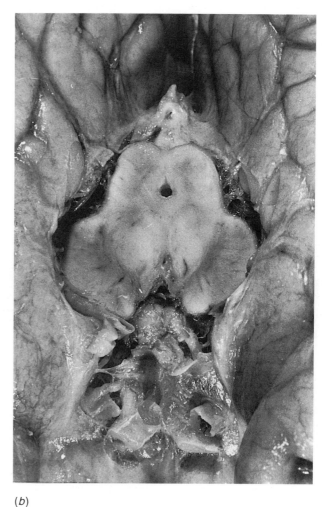

(b)

Fig. 3.12. (a) The pale substantia nigra in a case of idiopathic Parkinson's disease. (b) Normally pigmented mesencephalon.

pathology such as ischaemic dementia or Parkinson's disease.

For the pathologist who is not used to examining the brain, the complexity of the organ seems to produce almost insurmountable problems of obtaining an adequate sample. Compounding this difficulty is the additional problem that, in the neuropathological examination of dementia, there are often no very obvious focal lesions to be seen on macroscopic examination. Fortunately, there are ways in which this problem can be both

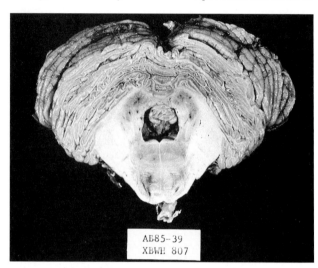

(a)

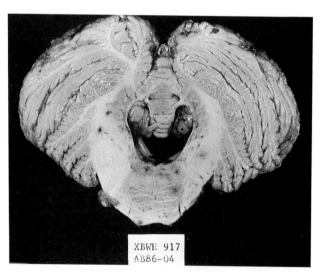

(b)

Fig. 3.13. (a) Normal fourth ventricle. (b) A case of PSP where the fourth ventricle is dilated as a consequence of degeneration and neuronal loss in the deep cerebellar nuclei and atrophy of the outflow fibres in the cerebellar white matter.

simplified and systematized. At the risk of uttering a truism, it is perhaps worthwhile to state that the general principle to follow is to sample the areas that provide diagnostic information. It might also usefully be said that the giant sections so beloved of neuro-pathologists, although pleasing to the eye, and very helpful in the assessment of diffuse white matter loss, are not essential for adequate sampling of the brain in dementia.

SCHEMA OF SELECTION

In this situation, adherence to a protocol, such as that produced by CERAD, for the examination of brains with dementia is very useful because it provides a scheme of tissue block selection.

The sections listed below are based on those recommended by CERAD, augmented to permit the diagnosis of dementing diseases other than Alzheimer's disease. In selecting areas to sample where there are no focal lesions that need to be separately sampled, the brain has been divided into: 1. Cortex and White matter; 2. Deep grey nuclei; 3. Brainstem; and 4. Cerebellum. We have found the following brain samples useful in the diagnosis of dementia:

Cortex and white matter:
1. Middle frontal gyrus.
2. Hippocampus and parahippocampal gyrus: many people sample the posterior hippocampus at the level of the lateral geniculate body.
3. Superior and middle temporal gyri.
4. *Anterior cingulate cortex: a good section to examine for cortical Lewy bodies.
5. *Amygdala and entorhinal cortex: sensitive to early plaque formation.
6. Inferior parietal lobule: the white matter in this plane is particularly sensitive to Binswanger changes.
7. *Occipital cortex including primary optic (striate) cortex.

Deep grey nuclei:
8. Caudate/putamen: just posterior to the anterior commissure. When sampled at this level, a good general impression of the basal nucleus of Meynert can be obtained.
9. Thalamus/subthalamus: at the level of the subthalamic nucleus. Also permits an additional examination of the substantia nigra and the red nucleus, if the latter is not present in the section of mesencephalon.

Brainstem:
10. Mesencephalon: Substantia nigra, periaqueductal grey, raphe nuclei.
11. Pons: Locus ceruleus, raphe nuclei, basis pontis.
12. Medulla: olive, dorsal motor nucleus of vagus.

Cerebellum:
13. Cerebellar hemisphere: a section that includes dentate nucleus.
*Optional

These 13 sections will, in our experience, permit a diagnosis to be made in most cases of dementia. They have the additional merit that if, after looking at them, the diagnosis is still not evident they can be referred to other, and perhaps more experienced, authorities without serious embarrassment as to the adequacy of the sample.

They do not, however, quite cover all possible eventualities and the following additions would be recommended in specific situations.

1. If subcortical leukoencephalopathy is suspected: Deep white matter in the centrum semiovale, parietal lobe and occipital lobe.
2. In amnestic dementia when Korsakoff's psychosis is suspected: hypothalamus through the mamillary bodies.
3. Cerebellar vermis: as above.
4. If there is a suspicion of motor neurone loss the XII nerve nucleus needs to be examined.

Choice of stains: Stains to be used on sections from the blocks selected are, to some extent, the subject of personal preference. Most diagnoses can be made using haematoxylin and eosin alone but the abnormalities can be much more readily discerned in many instances if additional stains are also used. Silver stains are particularly valuable for the argyrophilic plaques and neurofibrillary tangles of Alzheimer's disease, Pick bodies in Pick's disease and axonal pathology.

The selection of a silver stain is markedly influenced by individual laboratory skills and preferences but there are very significant differences in what is revealed by different silver stains (Fig. 3.14). There is, however, wide acceptance of the value of the modified Bielschowsky stain for the demonstration of plaques and tangles that occur in Alzheimer's disease. One feature of silver stains that needs to be recognized (and is well known to all who use them regularly) is the considerable variability in

sensitivity of the different stains, and the influence of variations in staining technique when the same stain is used in different laboratories (and in the same laboratory at different times and by different personnel). This has been demonstrated on a number of occasions (Duyckaerts *et al.*, 1990) and most recently by Dr Mirra and her collaborators in CERAD who submitted sections from eight cases of Alzheimer's disease of varying severity together with two controls to 18 different laboratories in the USA and Canada (Mirra *et al.*, 1994). The different laboratories (and pathologists) were asked to produce quantitative and semi-quantitative measures to assess the cases. The results showed that, while there was good agreement among the centres where semiquantitative measures were used, quantitative measures produced significant differences among the raters that reflected major differences in stain sensitivity and staining technique. These findings must engender a certain caution towards the current tendency to the adoption of purely numerical criteria in the diagnosis of, particularly, Alzheimer's disease.

Myelin stains are very helpful in delineating white matter pathology, Nissl stain for neuron cell bodies, congo red for vascular amyloid deposits, periodic acid Schiff (PAS) in lysosomal storage disorders, a reticulin stain in lesions of Wernicke's encephalopathy and phosphotungstic acid haematoxylin, Holzer or Cajal's gold chloride method for displaying gliosis.

Almost all laboratories supplement these basic tinctures with an increasing variety and range of immunocytochemical stains of significant epitopes in the wide variety of different diseases encountered in patients with dementia. Immunocytochemistry has a very useful place in showing βA4 peptide in congophilic angiopathy (Fig. 3.15) and argyrophilic plaques: prion protein in the non-neuritic plaques of Gerstmann–Sträussler syndrome: the hyperphosphorylated form of the microtubule-associated tau protein to assess neurofibrillary tangles and the neuritic components in Alzheimer's disease plaques: ubiquitin to show cortical Lewy bodies: glial fibrillary acidic protein (GFAP) to show gliosis: and Ricin communis agglutinin–lectin or certain macrophage antibodies such as HAM 56 to show macrophages and microglial cell reactions. Many of the required antibodies are available commercially.

Immunocytochemistry or *in situ* hybridization are also useful for confirming the presence of viral or parasitic organisms such as measles in subacute sclerosing panencephalitis (SSPE), JC virus in progressive multifocal leukoencephalopathy (PML), cytomegalovirus (CMV) in glial nodule encephalitis, human immunodeficiency virus (HIV) in AIDS encephalopathy and toxoplasma in toxoplasmosis.

MICROSCOPIC EXAMINATION

One of the major benefits of using a protocol such as that produced by CERAD for microscopic examination is that it engenders a systematic approach to histological evaluation. Users quite rapidly develop a familiarity with the range of microscopic appearances that are encountered in the different regions of the brain when they are systematically and repeatedly sampled and examined in a standard way. This familiarity noticeably sharpens the ability to detect more subtle microscopic differences which can be of great value in difficult cases. The use of protocols is also very useful in training and helps to inculcate the habit of systematic examination.

The microscopic features characteristic of the individual dementing diseases are described in the chapters to follow. We believe, however, that it may be worth making a few general points about the microscopic examination of the brain in cases of dementia.

First, it is important to know which types of cell and

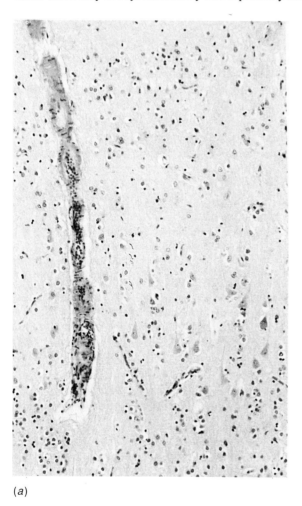

(a)

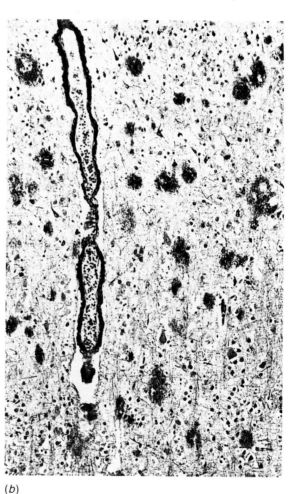

(b)

Fig. 3.14. A comparison of some different staining methods in a case of Alzheimer's disease. (a) A haematoxylin and eosin stained section of cerebral cortex showing prominent pyramidal neurons and a cortical blood vessel that contains amyloid in the wall. × 50 (b) Bielschowsky silver stained adjacent section: in the parenchyma both neuritic plaques and neurofibrillary tangles are stained and the amyloid in the blood vessel shows conspicuous silver staining. × 50 (c) A methenamine silver (MS) stain shows at least as many senile plaques, but does not show clearly the neuritic component of the plaques or the neurofibrillary tangles. × 50 (d) A Cross stain by comparison shows only the neuritic elements of the plaques, the neuropil threads and the neurofibrillary tangles × 50.

their locations are susceptible to developing inclusions characteristic of particular diseases. By searching in the wrong type of neuron, or in the wrong layer of cortex, the relevant findings may be missed. Two examples will suffice. Pick bodies may be difficult to find in the neocortex in some cases of Pick's disease, but are more readily found in the cells of the dentate fascia of the hippocampus; and typical oligodendroglial inclusions of PML are more readily found at, or just beyond, the margins of the demyelinated foci rather than in their centres.

Secondly, it is necessary to be aware of a common tendency to underestimate nerve cell loss in a nucleus in which there is selective loss of only some of the cells; the atrophy that the nucleus may have undergone causes the remaining cells to be more closely crowded together and the overall neuron density may be little altered. This can occur in Huntington's disease in which only small neurons of the caudate nucleus are lost and the large ones are crowded together because of the global atrophy of the whole nucleus. Sometimes the degree of cell loss is better evaluated by examining the size, axonal density or depth of myelin staining in the outflow tract of the relevant nucleus, for example, the superior cerebellar peduncles in the case of the cerebellar dentate nuclei, or the myelinated fibre bundles in the caudate-putamen. Either way, when examining grey matter nuclei or outflow tracts, it is essential to have available for comparison normal brain sections of comparable areas using the same stains. Mild or even moderate nerve cell loss is notoriously difficult to evaluate by simple inspection and resort to morphometric methods may be required (Appendix 1). Useful information may be gleaned from the glial stains which are likely to show definite gliosis in the presence of significant neuron loss (note that the converse is not true: gliosis need not imply local neuron loss since the degeneration of the afferent input to a nucleus may also result in

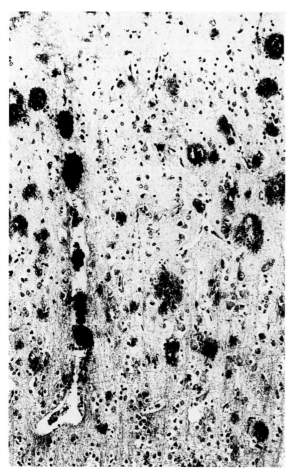

(a)

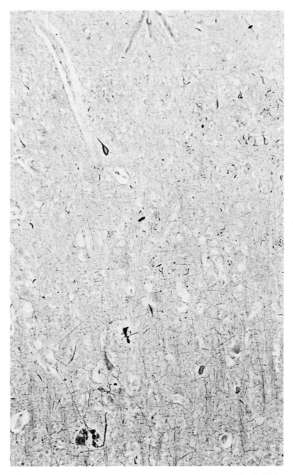

(b)　　　　　　　　　　　　　　　Fig. 3.14 (cont.)

gliosis without the neuron cell bodies themselves being affected).

Thirdly, some of the abnormal cytopathology, particularly that of Alzheimer's disease, commonly needs to be at least crudely quantified, and in some contexts the counting of neurofibrillary tangles or argyrophilic plaques may be necessary. In other contexts, picture matching is a relatively objective method of assessing the number of discrete structures in a microscopic field and one to which the human eye is well attuned.

ARRIVING AT A FINAL PATHOLOGICAL DIAGNOSIS

Some cases of dementia present no problems of pathological diagnosis: such is the case, for example, if there are severe changes of Alzheimer's disease with no other pathology and the clinical history is consonant with this diagnosis; or if there is a strong family history of dementia and the pathology conforms to one of the inherited diseases such as Huntington's disease or Pick's disease; or a small cell lung carcinoma is discovered along with features of paraneoplastic encephalitis, despite this condition not having been clinically considered.

However, in a significant minority of cases there is difficulty at arriving at a final pathological diagnosis. Three dilemmas account for most of such cases: first, there is mixed pathology present and it is uncertain how much weight should be given to each; secondly, there are mild pathological changes but perhaps they are within

normal limits for the age of the patient; or thirdly, there are no pathological features of any dementing disease, yet the patient was clearly clinically demented. A fourth related problem is whether to make a final pathological diagnosis of a dementing disease in the absence of a history of dementia. These situations are briefly discussed in turn below.

THE PROBLEM OF MIXED PATHOLOGY

The most common forms of mixed pathology are the co-existence of Alzheimer's disease with cerebrovascular disease and of Alzheimer's disease with Parkinson's disease. These are discussed below. Alzheimer's disease occurring with Down's Syndrome is a special case and is considered in Chapter 4b. Other combinations occur occasionally: Alzheimer's disease with a cerebral glioma or meningioma; Pick's disease and Alzheimer's disease; multiple sclerosis and Alzheimer's disease; Alzheimer's disease and Creutzfeldt–Jacob disease and cerebrovascular disease with Parkinson's disease. These have all occurred together in our personally studied cases or have been reported together in cases in the literature. Most combined pathology occurs in the elderly, and the commonest diseases are those found together most frequently. This raises the suspicion that their coexistence is often a matter of chance but it may also represent increased susceptibility to one disease in the face of the other. In reporting such cases, it is necessary to try to determine the relative contributions of the two diseases

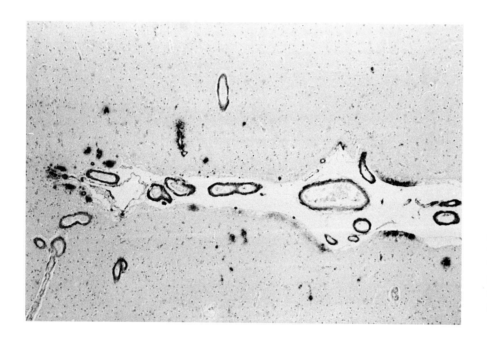

Fig. 3.15. Immunocytochemistry of congophilic angiopathy using a polyclonal antibody raised against vascular amyloid. Many vessels and some plaque cores are conspicuously stained. There is also some subpial amyloid deposition. × 50.

specifically to the clinical dementia, as distinct from other clinical neurological features that may also have been present.

CEREBROVASCULAR DISEASE AND ALZHEIMER'S DISEASE

There are sound reasons for believing that Alzheimer's disease and some forms of cerebrovascular disease are pathogenetically related. Alzheimer's disease is associated with variable amounts of β/A4-amyloid peptide deposited in leptomeningeal and cortical arterioles. When these deposits are extensive they may be associated with diffuse ischaemic changes, falling short of frank infarction, in the white matter. These are attributable to reduction in blood supply in narrowed arterioles that first traverse the cortex before supplying blood to the white matter (Gray, Dubas & Escourolle, 1984, Gray et al., 1985). This form of ischaemic white matter pathology closely resembles that found in other small vessel amyloid angiopathies (Plant et al., 1990) (Chapter 11). Further studies are needed to establish its frequency. The vascular amyloid deposits in Alzheimer's disease are also not infrequently the cause of lobar intracerebral haemorrhages, some of them fatal, as well as of more trivial subarachnoid haemorrhages (Vinters & Gilbert, 1983; Vinters, 1987). The association of Alzheimer's disease with the apolipoprotein Ee4 allele is a further association between the two conditions, since this particular apolipoprotein allele is also associated with an increased risk of cardiovascular disease, and therefore, to some degree, cerebrovascular disease.

Other forms of cerebrovascular disease which are often associated with atheroma of intra- and extra-cranial vessels and arteriolo-sclerosis with hypertension – infarcts, white matter lacunes and état criblé – are not at present clearly linked pathogenetically to Alzheimer's disease, but may nevertheless contribute to dementia, particularly if they are multiple, bilateral and involve parts of the brain which, from animal studies, might be expected to play an important part in cognitive function or interrupt white matter connections between them. Such areas include the hippocampus and frontal, temporal and occipital association cortex, and deep cerebral white matter. It is noteworthy that the hippocampus and substantial parts of the occipital and parietal association cortex and subcortical white matter all fall within the territory of supply of the posterior cerebral arteries which derive most of their blood supply from the vertebrobasilar circulation, whence emboli can be distributed both to right and left cerebral hemispheres. Atheromatous or embolic disease of the vertebrobasilar system would therefore appear well placed to provide a substrate for significant ischaemic dementia (see Chapter 5). Only future carefully performed, community-based, prospective clinico-pathological studies are likely to be able to establish the frequency with which such cerebrovascular disease and Alzheimer's disease coexist and whether such coexistence is a chance association.

In any individual case of Alzheimer's disease the pathologist should try to assess the extent to which β/A4-amyloid angiopathy may have contributed to dementia by producing diffuse white matter ischaemia and, based on their distribution and number, the extent to which any other vascular lesions might have been expected to have contributed to dementia. It is reasonable to expect that, in the presence of both vascular disease and Alzheimer's disease, clinical dementia may supervene at a level of pathology of each disease that is less severe than when dementia is produced by one of the diseases on its own, i.e. the disease processes may summate. The clinico pathological study of del Ser et al. (1990) in which pathological features in demented and undemented subjects with cerebrovascular disease were compared supports this view. This study found a greater frequency of plaques in the demented group even though the number fell short of that generally required to make a diagnosis of Alzheimer's disease.

ALZHEIMER'S DISEASE AND PARKINSON'S DISEASE

Alzheimer's disease and Parkinson's disease are both common neurodegenerative diseases affecting the cytoskeleton of neurons in overlapping parts of the brain: nucleus basalis, locus ceruleus, hypothalamus, raphe nuclei and, if diffuse Lewy body disease is included as part of the spectrum of Parkinson's disease, the cerebral cortex. In patients who present with Parkinsonism, approximately one-third go on to become frankly demented and most of these will be found to have Alzheimer's changes on neuropathological examination. As noted by Katzman (1933a), it is lucky that Martin et al., (1973) reviewed this topic before the advent of L-dopa treatment of Parkinson's disease and found a similar fraction becoming demented so that the dementia cannot be attributed to treatment with L-dopa. Conversely, about 15% of patients with Alzheimer's disease are found to have Parkinsonian changes at post-mortem (Ditter & Mirra, 1987; Gearing et al., 1995) although the extrapyramidal motor symptoms in these patients are often not typical of Parkinson's disease. The prevalence of Lewy bodies in normal-aged patients is not easy to establish with certainty and estimates have ranged between 4.5% and 10.5%. However, Perry and colleagues (1990), in a study that was careful to exclude patients with neuropsychiatric disease concluded that in patients without neuropsychiatric disease the prevalence was only 2.3% (3/131). Despite suggestions that the association is a statistical artefact of chance coexistence of two common diseases (Quinn, Rossor & Marsden, 1986), it seems possible that their coexistence is more than a matter of chance. It has been suggested by Hansen *et al.* (1990) that the combination of Alzheimer's disease and frequent cortical Lewy bodies constitutes a separate clinically and pathologically recognizable entity that they have called the Lewy body variant of Alzheimer's disease. Although the cellular mechanisms for this association are completely unknown, similar pathogenic mechanisms may operate in the two diseases.

At a practical level, pathological changes of the two diseases coexist sufficiently frequently that, when features of one disease are found, features of the other should be looked for. As with Alzheimer's disease and cerebrovascular disease, it is reasonable to expect that, in the presence of both diseases, symptoms of dementia may supervene at a lesser degree of severity of pathology than if each disease was present on its own.

THE PROBLEM OF MILD PATHOLOGICAL CHANGES, PERHAPS WITHIN NORMAL LIMITS FOR AGE

There are no widely accepted criteria for distinguishing categorically between cellular changes of the type found in Alzheimer's disease in normal ageing and Alzheimer's disease itself. Attempts to produce such criteria have been made (Khatchachurian, 1985) but have not been universally accepted. Improved criteria are in the process of being refined (Tierney *et al.*, 1988; Mirra *et al.*, 1991). The present situation is galling enough for neuropathologists who regularly examine brains from patients with dementia, but it is perhaps even more confusing for general pathologists who see far fewer cases. We believe that the most reliable pathological feature of Alzheimer's *disease*, at present, is the presence of neurofibrillary tangles in neocortical association cortex, particularly in the temporal lobe. There is little or no overlap here between ageing and Alzheimer's disease. Picture matching of argyrophilic plaque densities is also considered helpful in distinguishing between normal ageing changes and Alzheimer's disease, but in our

experience the range of plaque densities found in elderly subjects with no prospectively detected dementia can be remarkably wide and substantially overlaps the range seen in Alzheimer's disease. This may reflect variable thresholds before clinical dementia supervenes, these thresholds perhaps being related to previous intellectual performance or cognitive 'reserve' function, although this has not been systematically studied. There is also much variation of the literature in the thoroughness with which intellectual deterioration has been looked for and this will clearly influence the frequency with which such deterioration is found.

As discussed above, the normal thresholds that may be considered to divide Alzheimer change in normal ageing from Alzheimer's *disease* almost certainly need modifying downwards in the face of additional pathology, most commonly cerebrovascular disease or Parkinson's disease. Whether, after applying such modified criteria, one is justified in making a final pathological diagnosis of Alzheimer's disease is, however, open to question.

The two other diagnostic problems that regularly present themselves, are a history without a diagnosis, and its converse, a diagnosis without a history!

THE PROBLEM OF NO PATHOLOGICAL FEATURES TO ACCOUNT FOR CLINCAL DEMENTIA

There can be few, if any, pathologists who claim always to be able to produce a diagnosis in cases of clinical dementia. Almost all the large clinicopathological series of cases of dementia contain a small residuum of cases that have defied the best efforts of the pathologist. In recent series some of which were highly selected, the percentage is very low, varying from 0 to 3.0% (Gearing *et al.*, 1995), but in unselected cases the percentages are almost certainly higher. To account for these undiagnosed cases, it is tempting to envisage a whole world of novel pathological mechanisms of which we are currently entirely ignorant. There may indeed be some such examples within the cases that currently defy diagnosis but there are a number of rather more prosaic explanations.

First, although it is impossible to be certain, it seems likely that the most frequent explanation for the inability to find morphological changes in the brain in a patient with what is clinically described as dementia, is that the patient was suffering not from dementia but from depression. It has been well demonstrated that there are a few cases of clinical dementia which are virtually indistinguishable from depression. In one clinical series the proportion of such cases was put at 8% (Marsden & Harrison, 1972), and the percentage is likely to vary depending on the energy and expertise with which the clinical diagnosis is pursued. Although not currently feasible routinely, it is likely that advances in neurochemical knowledge will allow us to identify this group in the future.

Secondly, it is well recognized that some chronic drug intoxications without described neuropathology can induce a clinical state indistinguishable from organic dementia (Oxbury, 1991). These drugs include tranquillizers, barbiturates, L-dopa, isoniazid, and lithium.

Thirdly, other primarily psychiatric pseudodementias are also rarely encountered.

Fourthly, there are a few families with inherited spongiform encephalopathy in which some demented members have shown no pathological abnormalities despite the presence of clearcut pathology in others (Medori et al., 1992). It may turn out to be the case that further investigation of such cases by screening for a prion disease mutation is worthwhile.

Fifthly, the patient may have been suffering from a rare or undescribed dementing disease that is missed by the pathologist.

Finally, just as the thresholds at which Alzheimer-type changes are considered to be Alzheimer's *disease* are applicable to an *average* population, and a higher burden of such change can probably be carried out by someone of *above* average intellect and education without developing dementia (Katzman, 1993b), so it may be speculated that someone of *below* average intellect or functional reserve may develop dementia while his or her burden of Alzheimer-type change is still within the range of normal.

THE PROBLEM OF WHETHER TO MAKE A FINAL PATHOLOGICAL DIAGNOSIS OF A DEMENTING DISEASE IN THE ABSENCE OF A HISTORY OF DEMENTIA

The converse of the patient with a history but no diagnosis is that of morphological changes of a specific diagnosis in the absence of any history of disease. This situation is probably most frequently encountered in brains containing numerous plaques and tangles that would, with the appropriate history, be confidently diagnosed as Alzheimer's disease.

This problem really occurs in two forms. The more common is that of the patient who has no history because he has not been medically examined, so that the problem is really that of an unknown rather than a definitively negative history. There is no 'right' way to classify such cases, but CERAD adopts the position that all such cases should be classified as possible Alzheimer's disease, no matter how severe the morphological changes.

The other, less common form of this problem is that of the patient with significant morphological findings who has been medically examined and found to be within the normal range of mental function. There are two general reasons that might explain this type of finding. First, there is almost always a time lag between the last mental state examination and the death of the patient, during which significant deterioration in mental function might have taken place. The second possible explanation is that the criteria used for the diagnosis are themselves faulty in that they are not closely related to mental function. This is particularly the case in Alzheimer's disease where total plaque count and amyloid burden, are not closely related to cognitive scores. Hence, making the diagnosis of AD on the basis of plaque counts alone (particularly if 'diffuse' plaques are included) may lead to an inappropriate diagnosis of AD.

The pathologist must be a faithful chronicler of what she or he finds. If well-marked pathological changes are present that warrant the name of a pathological dementing condition, then that name should be applied, albeit with the qualification that it was an incidental finding. We do not favour the application of altered pathological criteria for Alzheimer's disease based on the clinical presence or absence of dementia (Khachaturian, 1985). We are too well aware of how easily dementia can be clinically overlooked or dismissed in elderly subjects for this to be advocated.

BRAIN BIOPSIES IN PATIENTS WITH DEMENTIA

Brain biopsy is rarely resorted to for the diagnosis of the cause of dementia in the very elderly, but is employed to a varying extent in different centres in younger subjects and in patients with rapidly progressive undiagnosed disease. There are several reasons for the sparing use of brain biopsy for the diagnosis of dementia. First, most cases are likely to be due to Alzheimer's disease, a disease for which there is so far no well-founded treatment and most clinicians consider it unethical to undertake an invasive procedure such as brain biopsy, to diagnose a disease for which there is no treatment. Secondly, there are non-invasive diagnostic methods such as single-

Table 3.2. *Dementing conditions diagnosable on brain biopsy*

Condition	Major pathological finding
Alzheimer's disease	Plaques and tangles
Pick's disease	Pick bodies/cells
Creutzfeldt–Jacob disease	Spongiform change
Gerstmann–Sträussler syndrome	Prion amyloid plaques
Cerebral arteritis	Vascular changes
Familial amyloid angiopathies	Specific vascular amyloid
Progressive multifocal leukoencephalopathy	Viral inclusion bodies
Herpes simplex encephalitis	Viral inclusion bodies
Subacute sclerosing panencephalitis	Viral inclusion bodies
Leukodystrophy	White matter changes
Whipple's disease	PAS positive macrophages
Syphilis – general paresis	Inflammation/organisms
Intravascular lymphoma	Perivascular/parenchymal tumour
Diffuse glioma/multiple metastases	Tumour
HIV encephalitis	Multinucleated macrophages and HIV-specific antigens

photon emission tomography (SPET), positron emission tomography (PET), magnetic resonance imaging (MRI) and computerized axial tomography (CT) scanning which have helped to push recent diagnostic accuracy in cases of progressive dementia to 80–90%, at least in Alzheimer's disease (Tierney *et al.*, 1988; Joachim *et al.*, 1988). However, with all the sophistication of modern imaging and investigative techniques, it is important not to forget old fashioned diseases and older simpler methods of diagnosis. One of us has had the experience of diagnosing neurosyphilis on a brain biopsy. The diagnosis had not been considered prior to biopsy, and the serological tests not performed. It is also necessary to be aware that brain biopsy itself may not yield a diagnosis because the small sample of cortex and white matter that is removed may lack specific diagnostic features. Finally, there is a remote but real risk of transmitting Creutzfeldt–Jakob disease by contamination of neurosurgical equipment as a result of performing biopsy, if this is the disease responsible (see Chapter 12). The range of possible pathology to be found in a brain biopsy from a case of progressive dementia is very wide (Table 3.2). Details can be found in appropriate chapters of this book.

If a decision to perform a brain biopsy is made, the biopsy is usually taken from the frontal or temporal lobe cortex of the non-dominant hemisphere. It should include subcortical white matter so that there is an opportunity to diagnose white matter diseases such as

progressive multifocal leukoencephalopathy, multiple sclerosis, a leukodystrophy or HIV encephalopathy as well as predominantly cortical diseases such as Alzheimer's disease, Pick's disease or Creutzfeldt–Jakob disease. The sample should be divided, with a small portion being taken for resin embedding and electron microscopy, another small sample snap frozen for cryostat sectioning and the remainder fixed in neutral, buffered formalin and then embedded in paraffin wax. It is wise to treat the specimens as potentially infective as occasional cases may be due to human immunodeficiency virus infection, progressive multifocal leukoencephalopathy or Creutzfeldt–Jakob disease. Paraffin sections should be stained with haemotoxylin and eosin, a myelin stain, a stain for reactive astrocytes, an axonal stain and methods for showing neurofibrillary tangles, argyrophilic plaques and vascular amyloid deposits. Electron microscopy may be helpful if a viral infection or leukodystrophy is suspected. Cryostat sections are useful for some histochemical, immunocytochemical or nucleic acid hybridization procedures.

AGEING CHANGES IN THE BRAIN COMPATIBLE WITH NORMAL MENTAL FUNCTION

It is important to be aware when examining brains from possible cases of dementia, of common, perhaps universal involutionary changes that take place in most, if not all, brains even those of people whose mental function remains unimpaired on formal intellectual tasks. Some of these changes are directly related to those found in dementing conditions such as Alzheimer's disease, Parkinson's disease and ischaemic dementia. The pathologist needs to be aware of these changes so that features that are found in cases of dementia can be set against those that would be expected in an undemented person of the same age.

Loss of brain weight and volume

Changes in brain weight in normal males and females is illustrated in Fig. 3.16. As is shown there is a slow decline with advancing age, starting at approximately age 40, which produces an approximately 10% loss of brain weight over the succeeding 50 years. As can be seen from the Figure, there is no evidence for an increase in the rate of decline in brain weight in the later decades, and no significant difference between changes in brain weight in males and females.

Loss of nerve cells

Recent attempts to estimate nerve cell numbers with ageing using automatic image analytical techniques have led to some conflicting findings, but there is general agreement that modest nerve cell loss and rather more shrinkage of nerve cells occurs in some, though not all, parts of the brain in old age. The neocortex and

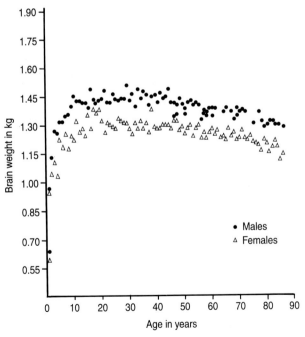

Fig. 3.16. Changes in brain weight with age.

hippocampus participate in these changes as do the substantia nigra, locus ceruleus and raphe nuclei of the brainstem (for review see Tomlinson, 1979; Esiri (1994) (Table 3.3). Some of the apparent loss of large nerve cells is accounted for by shrinkage; for example, Terry, de Teresa & Hansen (1987) found a 'loss' of large cortical neurons in old age that was largely offset by an increase in small neurons. Cell shrinkage is more common after 85 years of age (Meier-Ruge, 1988). Some nuclei, including the nucleus basalis of Meynert, the inferior olives and the raphe nuclei do not show neuron loss with age (Table 3.4).

Intraneuronal alterations

There is *accumulation of lipofuscin* in neurons with age (Mann, Yates & Stamp, 1978; Brizzee & Ordy, 1981), but this is not clearly deleterious as nerve cell populations showing such accumulation: which include the inferior olives and lateral geniculate bodies, do not show obvious loss of neurons with age. There is also a *reduction in nucleolar volume* in some nerve cells with age, a change that is thought to reflect reduced protein synthetic capability (Mann & Sinclair, 1978)). Golgi studies of cortical pyramidal neurons have shown reductions in the length and number of dendrites and a loss of dendritic spines in old age (Scheibel et al., 1975; Nakamura et al., 1985). However, other studies indicate that there are extensions in some parts of the dendritic trees, possibly reflecting an attempt at compensatory regeneration (Buell & Coleman, 1981; Coleman & Flood, 1986).

Neurofibrillary tangles (see Chapters 1 and 4)

These commonly develop in certain neurons in normal old age, most notably in the large stellate cells of the entorhinal cortex and in a few hippocampal pyramidal cells (Fig. 3.17). However, to find neurofibrillary tangles outside these restricted allocortical areas and in any more than modest numbers in prospectively assessed undemented subjects is extremely unusual.

Argyrophilic plaques (see Chapters 1 and 4)

These are extracellular structures that are found with increasing prevalence after the fifth decade in neocortex and hippocampus (Fig. 3.18). There is some overlap in plaque densities between mentally well-preserved subjects and those with Alzheimer's disease – more so than for neurofibrillary tangles.

Hirano bodies (Fig. 7.3), and granulovacuolar degeneration (Fig. 7.4)

These are pathological features that are commonly found in the hippocampus in Alzheimer's disease. Like

Table 3.3. *Sites with significant depletion of nerve cells in normal ageing*

Sites with significant reductions in nerve cells		Reference
Superior frontal gyrus	8% annual loss of neurons over age range studied (41–87 yrs)	Brody, 1970
Pre- and post-central gyrus, superior and inferior temporal gyrus and striate cortex	Approx 50% of neurons in superior temporal gyrus and slightly fewer in other areas lost by age 90 yrs	Brody, 1955
Striate cortex	At least 50% loss of neurons by age 80 yrs	Devaney & Johnson, 1980
Pre- and post-central gyrus, superior and inferior temporal gyri, gyrus rectus	Approx 35% loss of small neurons and 50% loss of large neurons between 20 and 90 yrs	Henderson, Tomlinson & Gibson, 1980
Cortex (areas 11, 22, 24) and subiculum	Approx 15% loss of neurons between 70 and 85 yrs, lost at rate of 1% pa	Anderson *et al.*, 1983
Cortex (areas 8, 9, 20–22, 24, 7, 17)	Trivial differences between those aged less than 80 yrs and more than 80 yrs except in inferior temporal and parietal cortex where cell counts in columns of those over 80 yrs were reduced by 19% and 15%, respectively	Mountjoy *et al.*, 1983
Temporal cortex (area 22)	7.5% reduction in pyramidal neurons in each decade between 50 and 90 yrs	Mann, Yates & Marcyniuk, 1985
Frontal cortex (area 11)	'Fairly constant' number of pyramidal neurons but 47% loss of non-pyramidal neurons between 28 and 96 yrs	Braak & Braak, 1986
Cortex (areas 9, 10, 46, 38, 39, 40)	10–15% loss of neurons between 24 and 100 yrs	Terry *et al.*, 1987
Cortex (areas 9, 10, 46, 38, 39, 40)	Large neurons reduced by 23–39% in those aged 80–100 compared with those aged 50–65 yrs. Larger reductions in superior temporal and inferior parietal than in middle frontal cortex	Hansen *et al.*, 1988
Hippocampus	Approx 27% loss of pyramidal neurons between ages 45 and 95 yrs	Ball, 1977
Hippocampus	20% reduction of neurons after age 68 yrs	Mourizen Dam, 1979
Hippocampus	Loss of pyramidal neurons of 3.6% per decade between 15 and 96 yrs	Miller *et al.*, 1984
Hippocampus	6.2% reduction in pyramidal cells per decade between 50 and 90 yrs	Mann *et al.*, 1985
Cerebellar Purkinje cells	Mean reduction of 2.5% per decade between 0 and 100 yrs	Hall, Miller & Corsellis, 1975
Locus ceruleus	40% reduction in neurons after age 63 yrs	Vijayashankar & Brody, 1977
Locus ceruleus	60–70% reduction in neurons by 8th and 9th decades	Tomlinson, Irving & Blessed, 1981
Locus ceruleus	35–40% reduction in neurons between 11 and 97 yrs	Mann, Yates and Marcyniuk, 1984
Locus ceruleus	27–37% reduction in neurons in old age (8th and 9th decades)	Chan-Palay & Asan, 1989
Dorsal motor nucleus of vagus	35–40% reduction in neurons between 11 and 97 yrs	Mann *et al.*, 1984
Supra chiasmatic nucleus of hypothalamus	54% reduction in neurons in those over 80 yrs compared with those aged 61–80 yrs	Swaab, Fliers & Partiman, 1985
Substantia nigra	35% loss of neurons between 11 and 91 yrs	Mann *et al.*, 1984

Table 3.4. *Sites with no significant reduction of nerve cells in normal ageing*

Site	Reference
Nucleus basalis	Whitehouse *et al.*, 1983; Chiu *et al.*, 1984
Supra optic nucleus of hypothalamus	Fliers *et al.*, 1985
Paraventricular nucleus of hypothalamus	Fliers *et al.*, 1985
Dorsal tegmental nucleus	Mann *et al.*, 1984
Cortex (areas 6, 11, 17, 20)	Haug, 1985
Ventral cochlear nucleus	Konigsmark & Murphy, 1970
Seventh nerve nucleus	van Buskirk, 1945
Deep cerebellar nuclei	Heidary & Tomasch, 1969
Inferior olive	Monagle & Brody, 1974; Moatamed, 1966

argyrophilic plaques and neurofibrillary tangles, they can also be found in small numbers in the hippocampus in normal ageing (Woodward, 1962*b*; Tomlinson & Kitchener, 1972; Ball & Lo, 1977; Gibson & Tomlinson, 1977).

Fig. 3.19 shows the progressive rise in the frequency of neurofibrillary tangles, senile plaques and granulovacuolar degeneration that occurs with advancing age in the hippocampus and neocortex. It emphasizes the very high frequency of neurofibrillary tangles in the hippocampus and senile plaques in the neocortex in patients in their eighth, ninth and tenth decades. Although the series from which these data are derived is unselected, most of the patients in these decades would not have been demented.

Vascular deposits of amyloid

These are composed of β/A4 protein (see chapter 4) and occur in slightly over 30% of brains from elderly undemented subjects (Morimatsu *et al.*, 1975; Esiri & Wilcock, 1986). These deposits are found in the walls of small lepto-meningeal arteries or cortical arterioles. Affected vessels may occasionally leak, giving rise to slight or more extensive subarachnoid or intracerebral haemorrhage. According to Vinters and Gilbert (1983) the prevalence of vascular amyloid deposition rises with age after the sixth decade.

Lewy bodies

These are found in small numbers in pigmented neurons associated with no more than slight loss of such neurons in the substantia nigra in 5–18% of elderly, apparently normal, subjects (Woodard, 1962*a*; Forno, 1969; Gibb & Lees, 1988) though a lower figure of 2.2% was obtained in a recent study in which care was taken to exclude cases of possible Lewy-body related disease (Smith, Irving &

Perry, 1991). Pigmented neurons of the locus ceruleus are similarly affected.

Neuronal spheroids

These consist of focal swellings in axons and occur as the result of many different insults to the nervous system. They are also found in normal old age, particularly in the posterior column nuclei, pars reticularis of the substantia nigra, globus pallidus and spinal anterior horns (Tomlinson, 1979). Neuroaxonal spheroids appear as round, pale hyaline or slightly granular, argyrophilic structures 15–20μm across.

Corpora amylacea

These occur in human brains of all ages but they become more numerous with advancing age. They consist of well-circumscribed round, sometimes laminated, bodies 5–20 μm across, deeply stained purple by haematoxylin and eosin and magenta by periodic-acid Schiff. They are particularly numerous in subependymal and subpial locations and prominent collections may be found around blood vessels. Ultrastructurally they have been localized to astrocytic processes.

Small cerebral infarcts (lacunes) and widened perivascular spaces (*état criblé*)

Foci of old softening suggestive of small infarcts are common in the brains of elderly subjects with no history of strokes. They are particularly liable to occur in the basal ganglia and thalamus (Fig. 5.11). They are commoner in those who have been hypertensive. A similar association with hypertension and hyalinization of small arterioles is found with the occurrence of état criblé (cribriform state) (Fig. 3.20) – a condition in which the perivascular spaces in deep grey and white matter are widened and adjacent neuropil loosened and gliotic.

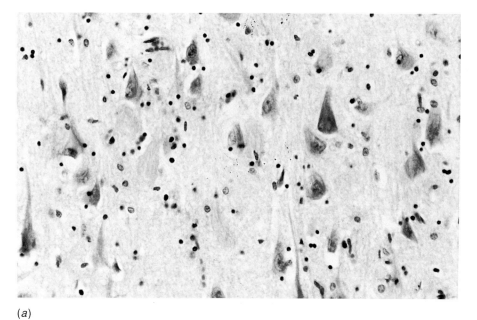

(a)

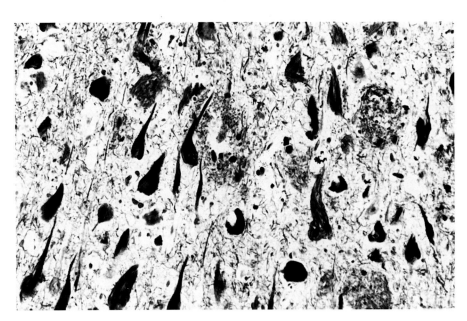

(b)

Fig. 3.17. (a) A Bielschowsky silver stain of an adjacent section of the same hippocampus. The intracellular tangles are densely stained while the 'ghost' tangles are less densely stained and more obviously fibrillar. The silver stain also reveals the presence of neuritic plaques and the numerous neuropil threads scattered throughout the parenchyma between the neurons. × 125 (b) An haematoxylin and eosin stained section of part of the pyramidal cell layer of the hippocampus with numerous intra- and extracellular (ghost or tombstone) neurofibrillary tangles. × 125

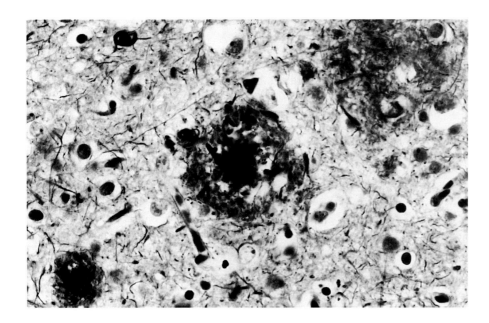

Fig. 3.18. Bielschowsky stain of a classical neuritic plaque with a prominent amyloid core surrounded by as neuritic reaction. This Figure also illustrates the neuropil threads referred to in Fig. 3.17(a) × 250

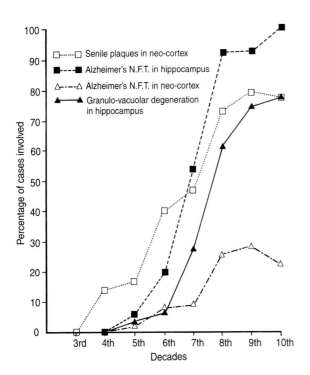

Fig. 3.19. Increasing frequency of plaques, tangles and granulovacuolar degeneration with age. (Redrawn from Tomlinson 1979.)

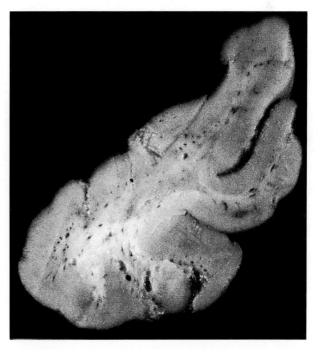

Fig. 3.20. Etat criblé: Anterior temporal lobe showing very marked expansion of the Virchow–Robin spaces that produces the appearance of état criblé.

This is thought to result from chronic damage due to pressure from the expansion of hyalinized vessel walls under increased arterial pressure. The widened perivascular spaces are liable to contain a few hemosiderin-containing macrophages.

REFERENCES

Alafuzoff I, Iqbal K, Frieden H, Adolfson R, Winblad B (1987) Histopathological criteria for progressive dementia disorder. Clinico-pathological correlation and classification by multivariate data analysis. *Acta Neuropathol (Berl)* 74: 209–23.

Anderson JM, Hubbard BM, Coghill GR, Slidders W (1983) The effect of advanced old age on the neurone content of the cerebral cortex. *J Neurol Sci* 58: 233–44.

Ball M (1977) Neuronal loss, neurofibrillary tangles and granulovacuolar degeneration in the hippocampus with ageing and dementia: a quantitative study. *Acta Neuropathol* 37: 111–18.

Ball MJ, Lo P (1977) Granulovacuolar degeneration in the ageing brain and in dementia. *J Neuropathol Exp Neurol* 36: 474–87.

Barclay LL, Zemcov A, Blass JP, Sansone J (1985) Survival in Alzheimer's disease and vascular dementias. *Neurology* 35: 834–40.

Bell JE, Ironside JW (1993) How to tackle a possible Creutzfeldt–Jakob disease necropsy *J Clin Path* 46: 193–7.

Bernoulli C, Seigfried J, Baumgartner G *et al.* (1977) Danger of accidental person-to-person transmission of Creutzfeldt–Jakob disease by surgery. *Lancet* i: 478–9.

Boller F, Lopez OL, Moossy J (1989) Diagnosis of dementia: clinico-pathologic correlations. *Neurology* 39: 76–9.

Braak H, Braak E Ratio of pyramidal cells versus non-pyramidal cells in the human frontal isocortex and changes in ratio with ageing and Alzheimer's disease. *Progr Brain Res.* 1986 70: 185–212.

Brizzee KR, Ordy JM (1981) Age pigments, cell loss and functional implications in the brain. In Sohal (ed) *Age pigments.* Elsevier, Amsterdam pp. 317–34.

Brody H (1955) Organisation of the cerebral cortex III. A study of ageing in the human cerebral cortex. *J Comp Neurol.* 102: 511–56.

Brody H (1970) Structural changes in the aging nervous system. *Interdiscipl Topics Gerontol* 7: 9–21.

Brown P (1988a) The clinical neurology and epidemiology of Creutzfeldt–Jakob disease, with special reference to iatrogenic cases. In Bock G, Marsh J (eds) *Novel Infectious Agents and the Central Nervous System.* Ciba Foundation Symposium 135, John Wiley & Sons, Chichester,

Brown P (1988b) Human growth hormone therapy and Creutzfeldt–Jakob disease: a drama in three acts. *Pediatrics* 81: 85–92.

Brown P, Rodgers-Johnson P, Cathala F, Gibbs CJ, Gajdusek DC (1984) Creutzfeldt–Jakob disease of long duration: clinicopathological characteristics, transmissibility, and differential diagnosis. *Ann Neurol* 16: 295–304.

Brown P, Cathala F, Castaigne P, Gajdusek DC (1986) Creutzfeldt–Jakob Disease: Clinical analysis of a consecutive series of 230 neuropathologically verified cases. *Ann Neurol* 20: 597–602.

Brown P, Cathala F, Raubertas RF, Gajdusek DC, Castaigne, P (1987) The epidemiology of Creutzfeldt–Jakob disease: conclusion of a 15 year investigation in France and review of the world literature. *Neurology* 37: 895–904.

Brown P, Wolff A, Gajdusek DC (1990) A simple and effective method for inactivating virus infectivity in formalin-fixed tissue samples from patients with Creutzfeldt–Jakob disease. *Neurology* 40: 887–90.

Budka H, Aguzzi A, Brown P *et al.* (1995) Tissue handling in suspected Creutzfeldt–Jakob disease and other human spongiform encephalopathies. *Brain Path* 5: 319–22.

Buell SJ, Coleman PD (1981) Quantitative evidence for selective dendritic growth in normal ageing but not in senile dementia. *Brain Res* 214: 23–41.

Burns A, Luthert P, Levy R *et al.* (1990) Accuracy of clinical diagnosis of Alzheimer's disease. *Br Med J* 301: 48.

Carpenter MB, Sutin J (1983) *Human Neuroanatomy.* Williams and Wilkins 3rd edn.

Center for Disease Control (1987) Rapidly progressive dementia in a patient who received a cadaveric dura mater graft. *MMWR* 36: 49–50, 55.

Center for Disease Control (1985) Fatal degenerative neurologic disease in patients who received pituitary-derived human growth hormone. *MMWR* 34: 359–60, 365–6.

Chan-Palay V, Asan E (1989) Quantitation of catecholamine neurons in the locus ceruleus in human brains of normal young and older adults and in depression. *J Comp Neurol* 287: 357–72.

Chiu HC, Bondareff W, Zarrow C, Slager U (1984) Stability of neuronal number in human nucleus basalis of Meynert with age. *Neurobiol Aging* 5: 83–8.

Coleman PD, Flood DG (1986) Denditric proliferation in the ageing brain as a compensatory repair mechanism. *Progr Brain Res* 70: 227–37.

Collinge J, Owen F, Poulter M *et al.* (1990) Prion dementia without characteristic pathology. *Lancet* 336: 7–9.

Committee on Health Care Issues, American Neurological Association (1986) Precautions in handling tissues, fluids and other contaminated mateials from patients with documented or suspected Creutzfeldt-Jakob disease. *Ann Neurol* 19: 75–7.

Crystal H, Dickson D, Fuld P *et al.* (1988) Clinico-pathologic studies in dementia: non-demented subjects with pathologically confirmed Alzheimer's disease. *Neurology* 38: 1682–7.

Cutler NR, Brown PB, Narayan T, Parisi JE, Janota F, Baron H (1984) Creutzfeldt–Jakob Disease: A case of 16 years duration. *Ann Neurol* 15: 107–10.

Davis PJM, Wright EA (1977) A new method for measuring cranial cavity volume and its application to the assessment of cerebral atrophy at autopsy. *Neuropathol Appl Neurobiol* 3: 341–58.

Dekaban AS, Sadowsky D (1978) Changes in brain weights during the span of human life: relation of brain weights to body heights and body weights. *Ann Neurol* 4: 345–56.

del Ser T, Bermejo F, Portera A, Arredondo JM, Bouras C, Constantinidis J (1990) Vascular dementia. A clinico-pathological study. *J Neurol Sci* 96: 1–17.

Devaney KO, Johnson HA (1980) Neuron loss in the ageing visual cortex of man. *J Geront* 35: 836–41.

Ditter SM, Mirra SS (1987) Neuropathologic and clinical features of Parkinson's Disease in Alzheimer disease patients. *Neurology* 37: 754–60.

Duffy PC, Wolf J, Collins G, DeVoe AG, Streeten B, Cowan D (1974) Possible person-to-person transmission of Creutzfeldt–Jakob disease. *N Engl J Med* 290: 692–3.

Duyckaerts C, Delaere P, Hauw JJ *et al.* (1990) Rating of the lesions in senile dementia of the Alzheimer type: concordance between laboratories. A European multi-centre study under the auspices of EURAGE. *J Neurol Sci* 97: 295–326.

Esiri MM (1994) Dementia and normal aging: neuropathology. In Huppert FA, Brayne C, O'Connor DW (eds) *Dementia and Normal Aging* CUP, Cambridge pp. 385–436.

Esiri MM, Wilcock GK (1986) Cerebral amyloid angiopathy in dementia and old age. *J Neurol Neurosurg Psychiat* 49: 1221–6.

Ettlin TM, Staehelin HB, Kischka U *et al.* (1989) Computed tomography, electroencephalography, and clinical features in the differential diagnosis of senile dementia. A prospective clinico-pathologic study. *Arch Neurol* 46: 1217–20.

Fliers E, Swaab DF, Pool CW, Verwer RWH (1985) The vasopressin and oxytocin neurons in the human supra optic and para ventricular nucleus; changes with ageing and in senile dementia. *Brain Res* 342: 45–53.

Forno LS (1969) Concentric hyaline intraneuronal inclusions of Lewy type in the brains of elderly persons (50 accident cases): relationship to Parkinsonism. *J Am Geriat Soc* 17: 557–75.

Gearing M, Mirra SS, Hedreen JC, Sumi SM, Hansen LA, Heyman A (1995) The consortium to establish a registry for Alzheimer's disease (CERAD). Part X. Neuropathology confirmation of the clinical diagnosis of Alzheimer's disease. *Neurology* 45: 461–6.

Gibb WRG, Lees AJ (1988) The relevance of the Lewy body to the pathogenesis of idiopathic Parkinson's disease. *J Neurol Neurosurg Psychiat* 51: 745–52.

Gibson P, Tomlinson BE (1977) The numbers of Hirano bodies in the hippocampus of normal and demented subjects with Alzheimer's disease. *J Neurol Sci.*

Gilleard CJ, Kellett JM, Coles JA *et al.* (1992) The St George's dementia bed investigation study: a comparison of clinical and pathological diagnosis. *Acta Psychiatr Scand* 85: 264–9.

Gray F, Dubas F, Escourolle R (1984) Cerebral amyloid angiopathy and leukoencephalopathy. *J Neuropathol Exp Neurol* 43: 316 (Abstract).

Gray F, Dubas F, Roullet E, Escourolle R (1985) Leukoencephalopathy in diffuse haemorrhagic cerebral amyloid angiopathy. *Ann Neurol* 18: 54–9.

Hall TC, Miller AKH, Corsellis JAN (1975) Variations in the human Purkinje cell population according to age and sex. *Neuropathol Appl Neurobiol* 1: 267–92.

Haltia M, Viitanen M, Sulkava R *et al.* (1994) Chromosome 14-encoded Alzheimer's disease: Genetic and clinico-pathological description. *Ann Neurol* 36: 362–7.

Hansen LA, De Teresa R, Davies P, Terry RD (1988) Neocortical morphometry, lesion counts and choline acetyltransferase levels in the age spectrum of Alzheimer's disease. *Neurology* 38: 48–54.

Hansen L, Salmon D, Galasko D *et al.* (1990) The Lewy body variant of Alzheimer's disease: a clinical and pathological entity. *Neurology* 40: 1–8.

Haug H (1985) Are neurons of the human cerebral cortex really lost during ageing? A morphometric examination. In Traber J, Gispen WH (eds) *Senile Dementia of the Alzheimer Type.* Springer, Berlin, pp. 150–63.

Heidary H, Tomasch J (1969) Neuron numbers and perikaryon areas in the human cerebellar nuclei. *Acta Anat (Basel)*, 74: 290–6.

Henderson G, Tomlinson BE, Gibson PH (1980) Counts in human cerebral cortex in normal adults throughout life using an image analysing computer. *J Neurol Sci* 46: 113–36.

HMSO (1994). *Advisory Committee on Dangerous Pathogens: Precautions for work with human and animal transmissible spongiform encephalopathies.* 1st edn., London.

Homer A, Honavar M, Lantos P, Hastie I, Kellet J, Millard P (1988) Diagnosing dementia: do we get it right? *Br Med J* 297: 894–6.

Jellinger K, Danielczyk W, Fischer P, Gabriel E (1990) Clinicopathological analysis of dementia disorders in the elderly. *J Neurol Sci* 95: 239–58.

Joachim CL, Morris JH, Selkoe DJ (1988) Clinically diagnosed Alzheimer's disease: autopsy results in 150 cases. *Ann Neurol* 24: 50–6.

Jobst KA, Smith AD, Szatmari M *et al.* (1992) Detection in life of confirmed Alzheimer's disease using a simple measurement of medial temporal lobe atrophy by computed tomography. *Lancet* 340: 1179–83.

Jobst KA, Smith AD, Szatmari M *et al.* (1994) Rapidly progressing atrophy of medial temporal lobe in Alzheimer's disease. *Lancet* 343: 829–31.

Katzman R (1993a) Clinical and epidemiological aspects of Alzheimer's disease. *Clin Neurosci* 1: 165–70.

Katzman R (1993b) Education and the prevalence of dementia and Alzheimer's disease. *Neurology* 43: 13–20.

Khatchaturian, ZS (1985) Diagnosis of Alzheimer's disease. *Arch Neurol* 42: 1097–105.

Kokmen E, Offord KP, Okazaki H (1987) A clinical and autopsy study of dementia in Olmsted county, Minnesota, 1980–1981. *Neurology* 37: 426–30.

Konigsmark BW, Murphy EA (1970) Neuronal populations in the human brain. *Nature (Lond)* 228: 1335–6.

Mann, DMA, Sinclair KGA (1978) The quantitative assessment of lipofuscin pigment, cytoplasmic RNA and nucleolar volume in senile dementia. *Neuropathol Appl Neurobiol* 4: 129–35.

Mann DMA, Yates PO, Stamp JE (1978a) The relationship between lipofuscin pigment and ageing in the human nervous system. *J Neurol Sci* 37: 83–93.

Mann DMA, Yates PO, Marcyniuk B (1984) Monoaminergic neurotransmitter systems in presenile Alzheimer's disease and in senile dementia of Alzheimer's type. *Clin Neuropathol* 3: 199–205.

Mann DMA, Yates PO, Marcyniuk B (1985) Some morphometric observations on the cerebral cortex and in hippocampus in Alzheimer's presenile dementia, senile dementia of Alzheimer type and Down's Syndrome in middle age. *J Neurol Sci.* 69, 139–59.

Marsden CD, Harrison MFG (1972) Outcome of investigations of patients with presenile dementia. *Br Med J* 2: 249–52.

Martin WE, Loewenson RB, Resch JA, Baker AB (1973) Parkinson's disease. Clinical analysis of 100 patients. *Neurology* 23: 783–90.

Martin EM, Wilson RS, Penn RD et al. (1987) Cortical biopsy results in Alzheimer's disease: correlation with cortical deficits. *Neurology* 37: 1201–4.

Medori R, Tritschler H-J, LeBlanc A et al. (1992) Fatal familial insomnia, a prion disease with a mutation at codon 178 of the prion protein gene. *N Engl J Med* 326: 444–9.

Meier-Ruge W (1988) Morphometric methods and their potential value for gerontological research. In Ulrich J (ed) *Histology and Histopathology of the Ageing Brain. Interdiscipl Top in Gerontol.* 25. Karger, Basel pp. 90–100.

Mendez MF, Mastri AR, Sung JH, Frey WH (1992) Clinically diagnosed Alzheimer's disease: neuropathologic findings in 650 cases. *Alzheimer Dis Assoc Disord* 6: 35–43.

Miller AKH, Alston RL, Corsellis JAN (1980) Variation with age in the volumes of grey and white matter in the cerebral hemispheres of man. Measurements with an image analyser. *Neuropathol Appl Neurobiol* 6: 119–32.

Miller AK, Alston RL, Mountjoy CQ, Corsellis JA (1984) Automated differential cell counting in a sector of the normal human hippocampus: the influence of age. *Neuropathol Appl Neurobiol* 10: 123–41.

Miller, DC (1988) Creutzfeldt–Jakob disease in histopathology technicians. *N Engl J Med* 318: 853–4.

Mirra SS, Heyman A, McKeel D, Sumi SM et al. (1991) The Consortium to Establish a Registry for Alzheimer's Disease (CERAD). II Standardization of the neuropathologic assessment of Alzheimer's disease. *Neurology* 41: 479–86.

Mirra SS, Gearing M, McKeel DW, Crain BJ, Hughes JP, van Belle G, Heyman A (1994) Interlaboratory comparison of neuropathology assessments in Alzheimer's disease: a study of the Consortium to Establish a Registry of Alzheimer's Disease (CERAD) *J Neuropath Exp Neurol* 53: 303–15.

Moatamed F (1966) Cell frequencies in the human olivary complex. *J Comp Neurol.* 128: 109–16.

Mölsä PK, Paljävi L, Rinne UK, Säkö E (1985) Validity of clinical diagnosis in dementia: a prospective clincopathological study. *J Neurol Neurosurg Psychiat* 48: 1085–90.

Monagle RD, Brody H (1974) The effects of age on the main nucleus of the inferior olive in the human. *J Comp Neurol.* 155: 61–6.

Morimatsu M, Hirai S, Muramatsu A, Yoshikawa M (1975) Senile degenerative brain lesions and dementia. *J Am Geriat Soc* 23: 390–406.

Morris JC, McKeel DW, Fulling K, Torak RM, Berg L (1988) Validation of clinical diagnostic criteria for Alzheimer's disease. *Ann Neurol* 24: 17–22.

Morris JC (1994) Differential diagnosis of Alzheimer's disease. Clin Geriat med 10: 257–76.

Mountjoy CP, Roth M, Evans NJR, Evans H (1983) Cortical neuronal counts in normal elderly controls and demented patients. *Neurobiol Ageing* 4: 1–11.

Mourizen Dam A (1979) The density of neurons in the human hippocampus. *Neuropathol Appl Neurobiol* 5: 249–64.

Müller HF, Schwartz (1978) Electroencephalograms and autopsy findings in geropsychiatry. *J Gerontol* 4: 504–13.

Nakamura S, Akiguclin J, Kameyama M, Mizuno N (1985) Age-related changes of pyramidal changes of pyramidal cell basal dendrites in layers III and V of human motor cortex. A quantitative Golgi study. *Acta Neuropathol* 65: 281–4.

Neary D, Snowden JS, Bowen DM et al (1986) Neuropsychological syndromes in dementia due to cerebral atrophy. *J Neurol Neurosurg Psychiat* 49: 163–74.

Oxbury JM (1991) Dementia In Swash M, Oxbury JM (eds) *Clinical Neurology* Churchill Livingstone, Edinburgh pp 112–19.

Perl DP, Pendlebury WW, Bird ED (1984) Detailed neuropathologic evaluation of banked brain submitted with clinical diagnosis of Alzheimer's disease. In Wurtman R, Corkin S, Growden UJ (eds) *Alzheimer's disease: advances in Basic Research and Therapies.* CBSM, Cambridge, MA, p. 463.

Perry RH, Irving D, Tomlinson BE (1990) Lewy body prevalence in the aging brain: relationship to neuropsychiatric disorders, Alzheimer type pathology and catecholaminergic nuclei. *J Neurol Sci* 100: 223–33.

Plant GT, Révéz T, Barnard RO, Harding AE, Gautier-Smith PC (1990) Familial cerebral amyloid angiopathy with non-neuritic amyloid plaque formation. *Brain* 113: 721–47.

Quinn NP, Rossor MN, Marsden CD (1986) Dementia and Parkinson's disease – pathological and neurochemical considerations. *Br Med Bull* 42: 86–90.

Risse SC, Raskind MA, Nochlin D *et al* (1990) Neuropathological findings in patients with clinical diagnoses of probable Alzheimer's disease. *Am J Psychiat* 147: 168–72.

Scheibel ME, Lindsay RD, Tomiyasu U, Scheibel AB (1975) Progressive dendritic changes in ageing human cortex. *Exp Neurol.* 47: 392–403.

Smith PEM, Irving D, Perry RH (1991) Density, distribution and prevalence of Lewy bodies in the elderly. *Neurosci Res Commun.* 8: 127–35.

Sulkava R, Haltia M, Paetau A *et al* (1983) Accuracy of clinical diagnosis in primary degenerative dementia: correlation with neuropathological findings. *J Neurol Neurosurg Psychiat* 46: 9–13.

Swaab DF, Fliers E, Partiman TS (1985) The suprachiasmatic nucleus of the human brain in relation to sex, age and senile dementia. *Brain Res* 342: 37–44.

Terry RD, de Teresa R, Hansen LA Neocortical cell counts in normal human adult aging. *Ann Neurol* 1987: 21: 530–39.

Tierney MC, Fisher RH, Lewis AJ *et al* (1988) The NINCDS-ADRDA work group criteria for the clinical diagnosis of probable Alzheimer's disease: a clinicopathologic study of 57 cases. *Neurology* 38: 359–64.

Todorov AB, Go RCP, Constantinidis J, Elston RC (1975) Specificity of the clinical diagnosis of dementia. *J Neurol Sci* 26: 81–98.

Tomlinson BE (1979) The ageing brain. In Smith WT, Cavanagh JB (eds) *Rec Advs Neuropathol Vol 1.* Churchill Livingstone, Edinburgh: pp 129–59.

Tomlinson BE, Kitchener D (1972) Granulovacuolar degeneration of hippocampal pyramidal cells. *J Pathol* 106: 165–85.

Tomlinson BE, Irving D, Blessed G (1981) Cell loss in the locus ceruleus in senile dementia of Alzheimer type. *J Neurol Sci* 49: 419–28.

van Buskirk C (1945) The seventh nerve complex. *J Comp Neurol* 82: 303–34.

Vijayashankar N, Brody H (1977) A quantitative study of the pigmented neurons in the nuclei locus ceruleus and subceruleus in man as related to aging. *J Neuropath Exp Neurol* 38: 490–7.

Vinters HV, Gilbert JJ (1983) Cerebral amyloid angiopathy: incidence and complications in the ageing brain. II The distribution of amyloid vascular changes. *Stroke.* 14: 924–8.

Vinters HV (1987) Cerebral amyloid angiopathy: a critical review. *Stroke* 18: 311–24.

Wade JPH, Mirsen TR, Hachinski VC *et al* (1987) The clinical diagnosis of Alzheimer's disease. *Arch Neurol* 44: 24–9.

Whitehouse PJ, Parhad IM, Hedreen JC *et al* (1983) Integrity of the nucleus basalis of Meynert in normal aging. *Neurol Suppl* 2: 33, 159.

Woodward SJ (1962*a*) Concentric hyaline inclusion body formation in mental disease. Analysis of 27 cases. *J Neuropathol Exp Neurol* 21: 442–9.

Woodward SJ (1992*b*) Clinico-pathological significance of granulovacuolar degeneration in Alzheimer's disease. *J Neurol Exp Neurol* 21: 85–91.

Alzheimer's disease

J. H. Morris

Historical
Epidemiology
Neuroimaging
Gross findings
Microscopic appearance
Pattern of development of AD changes and their relation to the symptoms of dementia
Diagnostic criteria
Staging the severity of AD pathology
Pathogenesis of Alzheimer's disease

HISTORICAL

Alzheimer's disease (AD) is the sole cause of about half of the cases of dementia in later life and a significant contributor to cognitive decline in a further quarter (Tomlinson, 1992). It is therefore overwhelmingly the most important factor in what has been called the silent epidemic of dementia that is occurring in societies with ageing populations. Since this includes virtually all of the currently developed world, and because the incidence of AD can be confidently expected to rise in all societies where economic progress leads to increased life expectancy, AD ranks with tuberculosis and malaria in economic and social importance. In part for this reason, an enormous amount of research work has been performed in the last two decades, and significant progress has been made in our understanding of the pathophysiology of Alzheimer's disease. It is true that no cure is yet in sight, but progress has been substantial and there are several avenues of research that might generate significant therapeutic advances within the next few years.

No account of the disease would be complete without some mention of the man himself. Amaducci, Rocca & Schoenberg (1986) in an interesting article have described some aspects of the early history of the definition of the disease. Alois Alzheimer in 1907, when he was working in the Laboratory of Anatomy at the Psychiatric and Neurologic Clinic in Munich, described the clinical and pathologic features of the disease which came to be named for him in a demented patient who had become symptomatic in her early 50s. It was Alzheimer (1907), along with his coworkers, Bonfiglio and Perusini, who first described neurofibrillary tangles.

Senile plaques had been identified much earlier by Blocq and Marinesco (1892). In the same year that Alzheimer described his case, Fischer (1907), who was working with Pick in Prague, reported the presence of senile plaques, then called miliary necrosis or miliary foci, in 12 of 16 cases of what was called senile dementia. Amaducci et al. (1986) suggest that it is 'inexplicable' that the natural connection between the plaques in Fischer's cases and those in Alzheimer's case was not made, but allow that it is just possible that professional and institutional rivalry may have played a role! Whatever the original reason, from this point on until relatively recently a distinction was made between pre-senile 'Alzheimer's disease' occurring in patients under the age of 65, and brains of those of greater age with similar pathological findings that were at first called 'senile dementia'. This distinction resulted, over the succeeding decades, in the publication of a considerable body of work directed at demonstrating similarities or differences between 'Alzheimer's disease' and 'senile dementia'. With the progressive recognition of the impossibility of separating them pathologically, 'senile dementia' metamorphosed first into the rather cumbersome, 'senile dementia of the Alzheimer type' (SDAT) and finally was incorporated into AD proper. This is one of the (few) circumstances when the current vogue for 'political correctness' would be entirely justified in condemning the arbitrary distinction between pre-senile and senile dementia as 'ageist'!! Ironically, this abolition of an essentially arbitrary distinction based entirely on age, has coincided with the recognition of a genuine genetic aetiological heterogeneity in AD that may ultimately be manifested in some real pathological differences among the different genetic types.

Although in the decades following the initial descriptions, there was a considerable body of work published on both AD and senile dementia, for most people of this generation the modern history of AD begins with the series of papers published by Tomlinson and his colleagues starting in 1966 (Roth *et al.*, 1966, Tomlinson, Blessed & Roth, 1968, 1970, Blessed, Tomlinson & Roth, 1968). Part of the impetus behind these studies was the continuing reverberations resulting from the separation of AD from senile dementia that was made on such 'inexplicable' grounds in 1907. In the intervening decades there had been an ongoing debate on the validity of the distinction between the two, the later stages of which are reflected in summaries of work to date in the first two editions of *Greenfield's Neuropathology* (McMenemy, 1958, 1963). This debate effectively received its quietus in the third edition (Corsellis 1976) in part as a result of the expansion of work on AD that occurred in the late 1960s and early 1970s following Tomlinson's publications. However, in the early 1960s there was still a widely held, though by no means universal (Corsellis 1962), belief that there was a poor correlation between the presence of dementia in older people and the concomitant presence of Alzheimer changes. In an interesting pre-echo of the recently kindled debate on the importance of the degree of education in the development of dementia, some of the reported lack of correlation was attributed to factors in the individual's response and the implicit concept of 'reserve capacity' expressed in the thought that a degree of cerebral degeneration that produced dementia in one person might be tolerated in another.

The studies of Tomlinson and his co-workers were centred around the comparison of the neuropathological findings in 50 brains from demented elderly (Tomlinson *et al.*, 1970) to those of 28 undemented controls (Tomlinson *et al.*, 1968). In the paper where they recorded the findings in the brains of 50 demented old people, they made the diagnosis of what was then called senile dementia in 25 of the 50 brains and concluded that the same process played a significant role in approximately a further quarter of the cases. In the 28 control brains, they found markedly lower frequency and den-

sity of Alzheimer changes and concluded that there was in fact a very significant correlation between the presence of Alzheimer changes and the occurrence of dementia in older patients (Roth, Tomlinson & Blessed, 1966; Blessed *et al.*, 1968). The nature and results of their studies effectively set the agenda for much of the work on AD in succeeding decades. Their prescience in identifying so many of the significant problems of dementia in general, and AD in particular, can be illustrated most effectively by listing some of the major findings and discussion points of these seminal papers.

- The essentially quantitative nature of the differences between the degree of Alzheimer change in the demented and non-demented aged;
- The relative significance of plaques and tangles in the causation of the dementia;
- The confusion generated by the use of the term senile dementia in a pathologically imprecise way and the validity or not of its distinction from pre-senile AD;
- The problems of getting a genuinely representative sample of the aged population to estimate the frequency of disease in the community;
- The possibility that Alzheimer change is more frequent in women;
- The difficulty of adequate demonstration that controls have normal mental function;
- The degree and significance of cerebrovascular disease and infarction in the aetiology of dementia;
- Their suggestion that the diagnosis of arteriosclerotic dementia is made more frequently on clinical grounds than can be confirmed pathologically.

As will be seen in subsequent discussion, many of these problems, in some cases hardly changed, are still with us.

EPIDEMIOLOGY

Clinical studies
As will be seen again in relation to dementia in association with cerebrovascular disease, disarmingly simple appearing questions such as 'how common is a disease?' are difficult to answer precisely. AD is no exception to this rule, although it needs to be acknowledged that the purely epidemiological difficulties in establishing the incidence and prevalence of a genetically heterogeneous

disease with a large sporadic component that is predominantly a condition of later life are very considerable (Brayne, 1993). Another of the major reasons for the difficulty in establishing the frequency of AD is that, in most cases, the diagnosis of AD cannot be made unequivocally by clinical means alone and hence a clinical diagnosis of AD has to be confirmed by (usually) post-mortem neuropathological examination (Lopez et al., 1990; Kukull et al., 1990; Galasko et al., 1994). Clinical methods are particularly unreliable in elderly patients with mixed dementias where there is a combination of Alzheimer change with a significant burden of cerebrovascular disease or Parkinsonism (Gilleard et al., 1992). In terms of the incidence and prevalence of AD in the community there is currently no large-scale community study of cognitive decline where the clinical estimates of the frequency of AD are substantiated by subsequent neuropathological examination of the brain in the study patients who die.

In the absence of a pathologically confirmed study of the frequency of AD in an unselected community population, some information can certainly be gathered from the various general surveys of patients with cognitive decline or dementia. There is a considerable body of literature relating to clinical estimates of the incidence and prevalance of cognitive decline and dementia within community populations including populations in France (Dartigues et al., 1991), China (Zhang et al., 1990), Italy (Rocca et al., 1990) and the central (Kokmen et al., 1989) and north-east United States (Framingham) (Bachman, Wolf & Linn, 1992). Although there is some variation in individual percentages, meta-analyses (Jorm, Korten & Henderson, 1987; Hofman et al., 1991) of these and other surveys are united in their agreement that the prevalence and age-specific incidence rates of cognitive decline in the general population approximately doubles with each decade over the age of 60 and reaches a maximum of around 25–35% of the population in those over 85 years of age (Skoog et al., 1993).

One study that produces somewhat different results is the East Boston study (Evans et al., 1989) where more than 3600 people were surveyed (just over 80% of all the age eligible persons in the community population). When fractionated into age cohorts, of those 65–74 years old 3.0% (95% CL 0.8–5.2%) had probable AD, while in the 75–84 year cohort the figures were 18.7% (95% CL 13.2–24.2%) and in the 85–94 year-old group a staggering 47.2% (95% confidence limits 37.0–63.2%) were considered to have probable AD. Katzman (1993a) discussed the possible reasons for the significantly larger

fraction of demented patients in this study, which probably relate, at least in part, to the lack of functional assessment in the estimation of dementia. Although the estimate of an approximately 50% rate for dementia in the over 85s can perhaps be discounted, a rate of 25–35% is still, even given current longevity, a very formidable amount of disease.

There is still controversy over whether the increasing incidence continues into the tenth decade but some studies suggest that above the age of 95 years the rate of dementia stabilizes at about 45% (Wernicke & Reischies, 1994). The difficulty in arriving at a definite conclusion is at least partly a result of the small numbers of nonagenarians and centenarians in most surveys of cognitive decline and partly because of differences in diagnostic criteria adopted, particularly in the way in which mildly affected persons are classified.

Although quite a wide range of ethnic diversity is included in these studies, they seem in general to suggest that different ethnic groups tend to have a generally similar pattern of increase in age-related cognitive decline and the incidence of Alzheimer's disease. An exception to this rule may be African populations. In examining aged populations from Africa, there are considerable methodological difficulties in establishing chronological age, particularly in very old people, although historical event recording and the use of birth records have been used with claimed success. Studies seem to indicate a low incidence of clinically estimated AD in elderly Nigerians (Ogunniyi et al., 1992) and this has been supported by findings of small numbers of neurofibrillary tangles and plaques (Osuntokun, Ogunniyi & Ledwauwa, 1992) and amounts of $\beta A4$ deposition (Osuntokun et al., 1994) in non-demented individuals that are proportionately markedly lower than found in equivalent-aged Australian populations (Davies et al., 1988). Interestingly, this reported low incidence in Africans living in Africa is not replicated in those of African descent living in America (Schoenberg, Anderson & Haerer, 1985; Heyman et al., 1991; Gorelick et al., 1994).

Clinico-patholigical studies

Given these estimates of the clinical prevalence of cognitive decline or clinically diagnosed AD, the question is whether, and to what extent, these clinical rates translate simply into pathological AD. As reported by Mendez et al. (1992) clinico-pathological studies have produced a rather wide range of diagnostic accuracy, that is not greatly improved by the use of more systematic diagnostic criteria (Table 3.1). A significant consideration is at what point in the disease process the clinical diagnosis is made. In patients with late stage advanced dementia that has been progressing for some time, it might be reasonable to expect a considerably greater degree of accuracy in clinical diagnosis than early in the course of the disease, but diagnosis at this time in the disease is significantly less useful to the patient and his family. In studies of small groups of carefully selected patients with clinically typical AD, the accuracy of the clinical diagnosis of AD is usually between 80 and 90% (Sulkava *et al.*, 1983; Wade *et al.*, 1987), and can reach 100% (Martin *et al.*, 1987). However, with less well characterized patients and earlier dementia diagnostic accuracy can fall as low as 50% (Homer 1988).

A useful, though not precisely formulated, type of study is that of Joachim and colleagues (1988), who looked at 150 consecutive brains referred to a major centre for AD research. The brains came from a wide variety of community and hospital sources in New England, but all had a clinical diagnosis of AD. Although not precisely specified, the sample represented the whole spectrum of investigation from tertiary hospital to community nursing home, but probably excluded most patients with severe cerebrovascular disease. As such, it probably represents a broad spectrum of what might be called 'uncharacterized degenerative dementia'. Their findings were that almost 90% of patients with the clinical diagnosis of AD at the time of death met what were then the accepted neuropathological criteria (Khatchaturian, 1985) for the diagnosis.

Two more recent large scale studies are those of Jellinger *et al.* (1990), Mendez *et al.* (1992) (for review see Morris (1994)) which suggest that, in studies of generalized dementia and clinically diagnosed AD, approximately 60% of patient population will have pure AD with a further 15% a combination of AD with either Parkinson's disease or cerebrovascular disease. A few other rarer combinations with AD were also seen. Of the remaining 25%, a significant fraction can be expected to have either Parkinson's disease alone or cerebrovascular disease alone (16% in Jellinger's study of dementia, and 8% in Mendez' study of clinically diagnosed AD), and the remainder a fairly long list of rare causes of dementia, including, of course some cases of Creutzfeldt–Jakob disease. Interestingly, in these large studies, only between 1 and 2% had no reported pathology that could account for the dementia. The most recently published study at the time of writing is that of the consortium to establish a registry for Alzheimer's disease (CERAD)

(Gearing *et al.*, 1995) who, in a survey of 106 patients, attained a diagnostic accuracy of 87%. These patients were assessed by standardized clinical neuro-psychological and imaging tools (Morris *et al.*, 1989; Davis *et al.*, 1992) and were therefore a rather thoroughly investigated group of patients. In this study, those found not to have AD were very heterogeneous in terms of their pathology, which tends to suggest that the clinical diagnostic batteries used for these research studies are becoming quite refined.

To what extent do pathologic studies of this type provide information about the incidence and prevalence of AD in the population at large? As has been described by Brayne (1993) in her review of clinico-pathological studies of the dementias, the interpretation of these studies is complicated by issues relating to the criteria used for the pathological diagnosis of Alzheimer's disease and the clinical diagnosis of AD (Burns *et al.*, 1990; Kellett *et al.*, 1991; Lindley & Dennis, 1991; Manning, 1991, Byrne, 1991; Tozer, 1991; Burns, Levy & Jacoby, 1991). Further, as Brayne notes, almost all of the studies where neuropathologic verification is included also have some degree of institutional bias (for example: Roth *et al.*, 1966; Blessed *et al.*, 1968 – psychiatric/psychogeriatric patients: Wilcock and Esiri, 1982 – hospital inpatients; nursing homes – Katzman *et al.*, 1988) built into them, which makes them unable definitively to answer the simple question we started with.

With all these reservations, it is safe to conclude that, in the dementia of older age, when easily diagnosable cerebrovascular disease has been excluded as the cause of the dementia, the large majority of the remaining cases will be examples of AD. However, in a specific patient there is at present, in most cases, no substitute for pathological examination to establish a diagnosis of AD. This is particularly so if the task is to differentiate AD from other degenerative causes of dementia such as diffuse Lewy body disease and mixed dementia. This is not to say that pathological examination is problem free; the controversies in diagnostic criteria for AD are considered in a later section.

Risk factors

In classical epidemiological terms there are a number of risk factors that are associated with the development of AD and these have been examined in a number of studies (Heyman, Wilkinson & Stafford, 1984; Rocca, Amaducci & Schoenberg, 1986; Prince, Cullen & Mann, 1994) and recently reviewed by Katzman (1993*a*, *b*). One of the

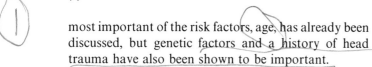

most important of the risk factors, age, has already been discussed, but genetic factors and a history of head trauma have also been shown to be important.

The specific genetic factors that operate in the pathogenesis of AD will be discussed in more detail later but in general terms it has been calculated that genetic factors could play a significant part in at least a quarter of cases (van Duijn *et al.*, 1991), and probably more. It is likely that this is an underestimate of the total genetic influence given that, in families with onset of AD after the age of 65 years, family history will often be negative for parents who have died before they were old enough to have developed the disease.

In practical terms, there is a, relatively small, group of patients with early onset familial AD where a specific gene defect predisposing to the development of AD can be identified by molecular genetic techniques. It is likely that the size of this group will increase as more molecular genetic information becomes available, although the utility of molecular genetics as a diagnostic tool in specific individual cases is likely to be most conspicuous in early onset cases. In the, numerically much larger, group of late onset cases of AD, the poly- genetic nature of the genetic component of most cases suggests that it is unlikely that molecular biological techniques will be the path to routine clinical diagnosis. Thus, for the present, neuropathological examination of the brain, either by biopsy (which is not usually justified), or post-mortem examination is required to confirm a clinical diagnosis in the overwhelming majority of cases. In the consideration of genetic influences, it must be remembered that, as revealed by identical twin studies that are discordant for AD (Jarvik, Ruth & Matsuyama, 1980; Cook, Schenk & Clark, 1981; Kumar *et al.*, 1991; Rapoport, Pettigrew & Schapiro, 1991) there are certainly a large number of genuinely sporadic cases of AD.

Another recognized risk factor for the development of AD is head trauma. An episode of head trauma which causes loss of consciousness or results in admission to hospital is reported to increase the chance of subsequently developing AD by a factor of two (Mortimer *et al.*, 1991; Gentleman & Roberts, 1991). Head injury has been shown to be associated with the acute deposition of β-amyloid protein (β/A4) in the cortical ribbon and increased expression of the β amyloid precursor protein (βAPP) in adjacent cortical neurons (Roberts *et al.*, 1994). It has also been demonstrated convincingly that the repeated head trauma associated with a career in boxing leads to a well-characterized progressive dementing syndrome and the formation of diffuse plaques

and tangles within the brain (Corsellis, Bruton & Freeman-Browne, 1973; Roberts, Allsop & Bruton, 1990; Dale *et al.*, 1991). Roberts *et al.* (1994) also report anecdotally that head trauma can seemingly advance the development of dementia in patients with a βAPP gene mutation that predisposes to dementia. However, although there are tantalizing and very suggestive links between acute head injury, increased β/A4 expression in cells and acute deposition of βA4 in the cortex, it is not at all clear how this could predispose to the development of AD years, or decades, later. One suggestion is that the release of acute-phase reactant proteins in trauma could facilitate the conversion of non-fibrillar β/A4-amyloid peptide to a more stable form and hasten the formation of the compact amyloid that is more likely to stimulate a neuritic reaction (Katzman, 1993*a*). If such a mechanism was operative, it could be argued that the deposition of microscopic quantities of persisting fibrillar amyloid following trauma could act as an inciting nidus to further amyloid deposition many years later. This might effectively advance a process that would otherwise have occurred at a considerably later time.

As eloquently expressed by Katzman (1993*b*), AD has been considered to be a democratic process and no respector of rank or position, affecting university presidents and physicians, mathematicians and musicians as well as those without memorial. However, there are recent studies that seem to indicate that the Alzheimer process is not quite the populist democrat it has been portrayed to be, and that degree of education has a significant influence in the development of symptomatic dementia in AD. Studies from geographical and cultural locations as disparate as Western Europe (Dartigues *et al.*, 1991; Bonaiuto *et al.*, 1990; Frataglioni *et al.*,1991; Sulkava *et al.*, 1985), Israel (Korczyn, Kahana & Galper, 1991) and Shanghai (Zhang *et al.*, 1990; Hill *et al.*, 1993) indicate that there is a protective effect of education, although it should be noted that no such protective effect was observed in Rochester, Minnesota (Beard *et al.*, 1992) or Cambridge, England (O'Connor, Pollit & Treasure, 1991). An idea of the possible extent of this effect is given in the studies of elderly Catholic nuns where those with a bachelor's degree were more than twice as likely to be functionally independent as those without a college education (Snowden, Ostwald & Kane, 1989). Katzman (1993*b*) and Friedland (1993), in their reviews, discuss a number of possible explanations for this effect. In the past few years it has been demonstrated that synaptic density declines in association neocortex in AD (Masliah *et al.*, 1989) and it has recently

Control

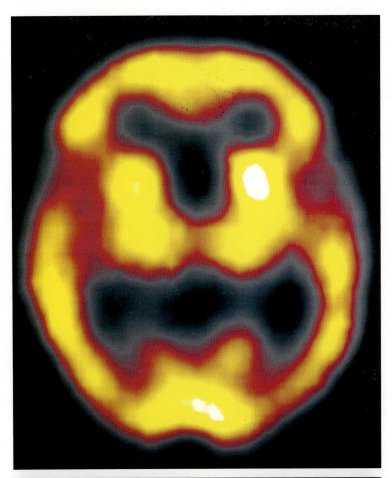

Patient

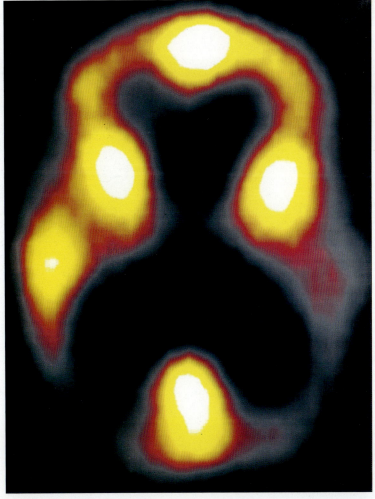

Fig. 4.2(*a*). Single photon emission computerized tomography (SPECT) in AD: SPECT scans of the same control and patient as in Fig. 4.1. The patient with AD shows the bilateral parietal perfusion defects typically seen in AD.

been shown that there is a good correlation between the density of synaptic terminals and MMSE scores (De Kosky & Scheff, 1990; Terry *et al.*, 1991). Katzman advances the possibility that, in those with higher education, there is a greater synaptic density that would provide a reserve synaptic capacity. He considers that this effect might be sufficient to delay the onset of symptoms by up to 5 years and thereby reduce the prevalence of dementia at a given age by up to 50%.

The effects of education described in the previous paragraph fuel the suspicion that, far from being demo-cratic, the Alzheimer process is actually rather élitist, and its democratic credentials are further undermined by indications that it might be sexist as well. In a number of the epidemiological studies of cognitive decline and clinically diagnosed Alzheimer's disease, there is a con-siderably higher age specific prevalence in women (Kok-men *et al.*, 1989; Bachman *et al.*, 1992; Mölsä *et al.*, 1982; Sulkava *et al.*, 1983; Schoenberg, 1987; Zhang *et al.*, 1990), although other studies do not find a significant difference in prevalence (Frataglioni *et al.*, 1991; Hofman *et al.*, 1991; Hachinski *et al.*, 1975; Wernicke & Reischies, 1994). There is rather more uncertainty as to whether there is a gender difference in age specific incidence rates (Katzman *et al.*, 1989; Hagnell, Öjesö & Rorsman, 1992; Prince *et al.*, 1994).

As discussed by Henderson and Buckwalter (1994), the interpretation of such differences is complicated by the fact that there are at least some differences in ways in which men and women perform in cognitive tasks in AD and the possibility that the observed gender differences in prevalence might also reflect some subtle ascertain-ment biases that favour men. A systematic difference in prevalence could be explained by differences in rate of progression or mortality, although there is no evidence to suggest that this is the case. A confounding factor here may also be the apparent importance of duration of education in the development of dementia. It has been suggested that many of the studies showing an excess of women contain large numbers of elderly women with little formal education, and that this might be sufficient to account for the greater prevalence of dementia in women in some studies.

However, the possibility that there may be a real gender difference in susceptibility to the Alzheimer process has been given some indirect support from studies that report improved cognitive performance in women with a clinical diagnosis of AD taking hormone replacement therapy (Henderson *et al.*, 1994). At a pathological level, there has been a report that, in

Down's syndrome, the severity of Alzheimer pathologi-cal change is greater in women than in men (Raghaven *et al.*, 1994). These reports, and the presence of oestrogen receptors on cholinergic neurons of the basal forebrain (Toran-Allerand *et al.*, 1992) have spawned a tentative hypothesis that links lack of oestrogen to reduced cholinergic activity and the possibility of impaired post-menopausal cognitive function (Fillit *et al.*, 1986; Honjo *et al.*, 1989).

Age, genetic factors and head trauma are probably the best recognized risk factors for the development of AD but there are a number of other candidates that have been advanced. These include myocardial infarction (Aronson *et al.*, 1990) and coronary artery disease (Sparks *et al.*, 1990), and it has been suggested that cerebrovascular disease may also be a factor (Jellinger, 1976). Maternal age and hypothyroidism (van Duijn *et al.*, 1991) have also been canvassed as risk factors, but there is no convincing evidence to support them as having a significant role. The role of aluminium is a subject of continuing controversy and another chapter (Chapter 14).

Given the depressing number of adverse factors for the development of AD, it may come as some relief that there is a factor that appears to decrease the risk of developing AD. However, any relief is immediately tempered by the revelation that the factor in question is cigarette smoking (Brenner *et al.*, 1993), since any protective effect of cigarette smoking is bought at a very high price in lung cancer, heart disease (which may increase the risk again!), stroke, and all the other ills rightly condemned by James I. The protective effect against AD is, however, not negligible with unmatched odds ratios of between 0.47 and 0.8. A pooled re-analysis has generated a statistically significant negative associ-ation with an odds ratio of 0.78 (CL: 0.62–0.98) (Graves *et al.*, 1991). To date, no recognized medical authority has had the temerity to suggest that taking up cigarette smoking is a desirable preventive strategy against the development of AD!

NEUROIMAGING

Outside the standard clinical methods of history and examination, the other important clinical tools in at-tempting to make the diagnosis of AD in life are neuroimaging and there have been CT studies that have indicated significant medial temporal lobe atrophy in dementia (De Leon *et al.*, 1989; Kido *et al.*, 1989) (Fig.4a.1). A recent clinico-pathologic study has suggest-ed a high correlation between early medial temporal lobe atrophy as demonstrated by temporal lobe-orientated CT scanning with a subsequent pathologic diagnosis of AD (Jobst *et al.*, 1992, 1994*a* (Fig. 4a.1), and there has been some subsequent confirmation (Pasquier *et al.*, 1994). Similar findings have also been reported using MRI scanning (Erkinjuntti *et al.*, 1993). On serial scans, patients with a subsequent post-mortem diagnosis of AD can be seen to undergo a rapidly progressive atrophy of the medial temporal lobe structures, and detectable atrophy is present quite early in the progression of cognitive decline. This being so, medial temporal atrophy is an early phenomenon as it offers a potentially useful diagnostic examination in patients with cognitive decline. However, although helpful in defining the location of disease, techniques of imaging the temporal lobe are not likely always to be able to distinguish AD from some other possible causes of medial temporal lobe atrophy such as Pick's disease or frontal lobe degeneration.

The other imaging modality that might have a role to play in the pre-mortem diagnosis of AD is single-photon emission computed tomography (SPECT) which measures regional blood flow within the brain. There have been a number of studies of dementia and AD using this scanning modality (for review see Claus *et al.*, 1994), and it is reported that AD often gives a rather characteristic temporo-parietal deficit (Fig. 4a.2; see colour plate). As with many modalities, its sensitivity significantly improved with increasing severity of cognitive decline. In their recent study (Claus *et al.*, 1994), with specificity set at 90%, sensitivity rose from 42% in mild clinically diagnosed AD to 79% in severe cases. One attractive possibility that might enable AD to be distinguished from other causes of temporal lobe atrophy might be to combine the use of temporal lobe-orientated CT/MRI scanning to define focal atrophy with SPECT to see the changes in blood flow (Jobst *et al.*, 1991, 1994*b*). Preliminary results on the OPTIMA study group of patients suggest that this combination offers a significantly higher degree of sensitivity and specificity than either modality used alone.

GROSS FINDINGS

Brain weight
As with other diseases, gross brain weight is not, in individual cases, a very helpful quantity except at the extremes of the weight curve. It is the general experience

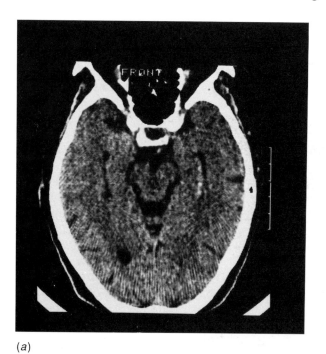
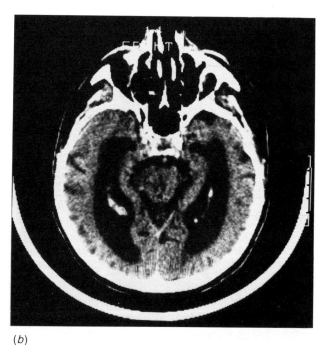

(a)   (b)

Fig. 4a.1. Temporal lobe orientated computerized tomography (CT) in AD: CT scans of a normal control and a patient with AD with the patient positioned in the scanner to obtain a view of the medial temporal lobe. In the patient with AD, the brain is generally atrophic, but the atrophy is particularly marked in the medial temporal lobes.

that, in younger patients with AD, there is likely to be considerably greater atrophy and loss of brain weight than in older patients where both atrophy and brain weight often fall well within accepted norms in the presence of AD. Most brains that are less than 950 grammes in weight will prove, on neuropathological examination, to have some pathological process, but on its own the brain weight is of very little value in identifying the nature of the process.

External appearance

The external appearance of the brain in AD, although sometimes characteristic, is not diagnostic. Particularly in younger patients, there may be obvious atrophy affecting the frontal, temporal and parietal lobes (Fig. 4a.3). In some cases, the degree of atrophy can be sufficiently focal and severe to resemble that seen in Pick's disease (Joachim, Morris & Schoene, 1986). However, many cases that, on microscopic examination prove to have AD, have a most undistinguished external appearance with either mild generalized fronto-temporal atrophy not greater than that seen in a number of aged brains to no detectable atrophy at all. This impression has received numerical support from the study of Hubbard and Anderson (1981a) who showed that, in patients with AD above the age of 80 years, cerebral volume and atrophy were often within the normal range. One of the reasons for younger patients to show more marked atrophy is probably that they tend to have a longer survival and hence a greater chance for atrophy to develop. Although a fronto-temporal bias in the atrophy is very much the usual finding, there are rare but well-described cases of AD where the principal burden of disease falls on the occipital regions and this is reflected in a predominantly parieto-occipital pattern of atrophy (Brun & Englund, 1981; Berthier *et al.*, 1991; Levine, Lee & Fisher, 1993; see also Chapter 1). However, as is the case with the primary progressive aphasias (Chapter 8), this localization of disease, while it has many common features to the associated clinical phenomenology, is pathologically heterogeneous. Victoroff *et al.* (1994) report three cases of what has come to be called posterior cortical atrophy with diagnoses of Alzheimer's disease, Creutzfeldt–Jakob disease and subcortical gliosis.

Brain slices

As with the gross appearance, there are no pathognomonic changes on brain slices. There may be some degree of macroscopically apparent atrophy with widening of the cortical sulci. The cortical ribbon is rarely visibly attenuated, although there may be some narrowing in the most severely affected cases, particularly in the temporal lobe (Hubbard & Anderson 1981b). Conversely, the hippocampal formation is very often visibly atrophic, a feature that is reflected in the frequent expansion of the temporal horns of the lateral ventricle (Fig. 4a.4). It is this frequent grossly apparent atrophy of the hippocampus that is presumably the anatomic basis for the radiological finding of medial temporal lobe atrophy in AD (Fig. 4a.1). The appearance of the

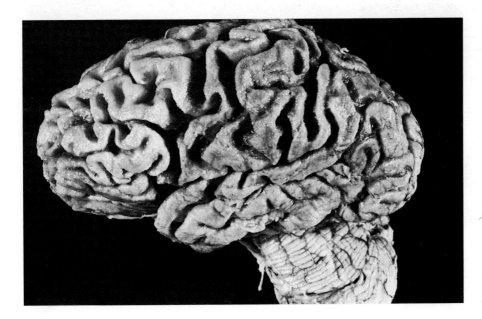

Fig. 4a.3. The most advanced degree of cerebral atrophy, rarely seen in Alzheimer's disease, shows very marked gyral atrophy involving the frontal, temporal and parietal lobes. With this degree of atrophy, even the primary cortex around the Rolandic sulcus shows marked atrophy.

amygdala is very variable. Sometimes it appears to have an almost normal volume while, on other occasions, it is severely atrophic to naked eye inspection. Given its location at the anterior end of the temporal horns of the lateral ventricles, gross atrophy of the amygdala is usually found in those cases with very marked dilatation of the temporal horns of the lateral ventricles (Fig. 3.8). As with the external appearance, very occasionally the cortical changes are sufficiently fronto-temporally local-ized as to resemble the changes in Pick's disease even to the extent of some visible cortical attenuation in the most affected cortical areas (Fig. 4a.5).

Dilatation of the frontal and occipital poles of the lateral ventricles is usually apparent, but, again particularly in older persons, is not invariably obvious and, in some cases, the size can be within the normal limits for age (Tomlinson *et al.*, 1970; Hubbard & Anderson 1981a; Berg *et al.*, 1993). Not infrequently there may be a

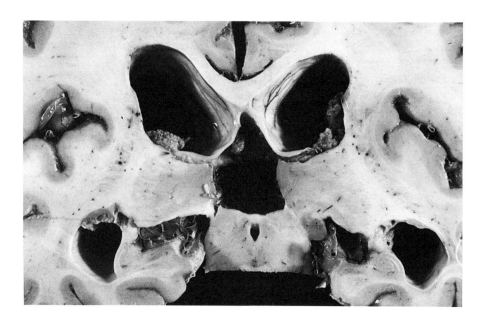

Fig. 4a.4. Part of a brain slice from a case of Alzheimer's disease showing marked hippocampal atrophy with accompanying dilatation of the temporal horns of the lateral ventricles. The parietal lateral ventricles are also considerably dilated, although the dilatation is often most conspicuous in the occipital poles.

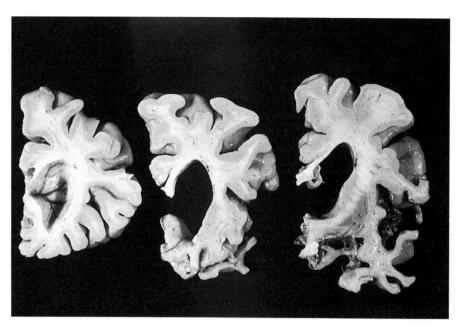

Fig. 4a.5. In some cases of Alzheimer's disease there is very marked atrophy of the temporal lobe as severe as that seen in Pick's disease. In this example, there is no sparing of the superior temporal gyrus that is typically seen in Pick's disease.

discrepancy between apparent cortical atrophy and the degree of ventricular dilatation. In some cases, the ventricles may be quite dilated where the cortical sulci are not strikingly widened. When there is significant atrophy and ventricular dilatation, there is almost always notable expansion of the occipital poles of the lateral ventricles (Fig. 4a.6). Some expansion of the third ventricle is usually evident, and in severe cases it becomes barrel shaped. In contrast, the aqueduct and fourth ventricle are normal sized. Except in those cases with concomitant cerebrovascular disease or severe amyloid angiopathy, the white matter is not usually visibly abnormal in character. As evidenced by the dilatation of the cerebral ventricles that usually accompanies widening of the cortical sulci, there is invariably some reduction in overall volume of white matter which has been reported to vary between 3% and 19% in a quantitative study (de la Monte, 1989).

In the deep grey nuclei of the cerebral hemispheres, atrophy, when it is detectable, is restricted to the caudate and putamen. On CT scans, atrophy of the caudate with proportional expansion of the frontal poles of the lateral ventricles can occasionally be sufficiently marked to be confusable with the appearance of Huntington's disease, although the clinical history will usually be sufficient to give the lie to this. On brain slices, although there may be considerable reduction in the bulk of the caudate (less conspicuous in the putamen), some degree of convex curvature in relation to the lateral ventricle is almost

always retained to distinguish the appearance from that of severe Huntington's disease. The degree of atrophy is almost always symmetrical, and gross asymmetry of cortical atrophy or ventricular dilatation should suggest a search for an alternative diagnosis.

No changes are apparent in the macroscopic appearance of the globus pallidus and thalamus or in the substantia innominata (location of the nucleus basalis of Meynert), even though it is markedly affected in AD. Elsewhere in the brain, the only other consistent macroscopic finding in Alzheimer's disease is loss of pigmentation in the locus ceruleus. The three major causes of macroscopically visible loss of pigmentation in the locus ceruleus are idiopathic Parkinson's disease (Chapter 7), progressive Supranuclear Palsy (PSP) (Chapter 10) and AD. In idiopathic Parkinson's disease the depigmentation of the locus ceruleus is accompanied by depigmentation of the substantia nigra. In PSP there is depigmentation of the substantia nigra and also usually a detectable dilatation of the fourth ventricle that is particularly noticeable superiorly where it merges with the aqueduct. This pattern of dilatation is a result of the degeneration of the dentate nucleus of the cerebellum and atrophy of the superior cerebellar peduncle. Both of the other major causes of depigmentation of the locus ceruleus are accompanied by pallor of the substantia nigra. Consequently, the finding of pallor of the locus caeruleus without depigmentation of the substantia nigra in a patient with dementia is one of the most

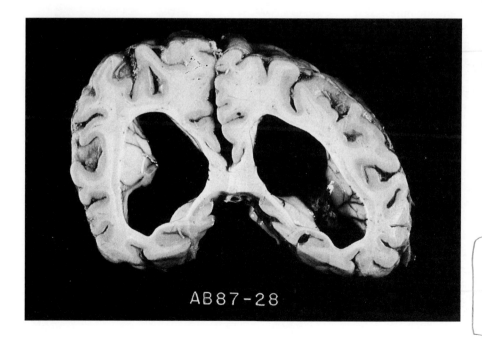

AB87-28

Fig. 4a.6. Dilation of the occipital poles of the lateral ventricles. In some cases of Alzheimer's disease this is the location of the most conspicuous ventricular dilatation.

suggestive gross findings that support a diagnosis of AD.

However, the converse, i.e. depigmentation of both the substantia nigra and the locus ceruleus does not exclude the diagnosis of AD since the combination of AD and idiopathic Parkinson's disease in the same patient is not at all uncommon. There has been quite a wide variation in estimates of the frequency of this combination, but in the series of 150 consecutive cases published by Joachim *et al.* (1988*a*) this combination was present in 11% of cases of AD.

MICROSCOPIC APPEARANCE

The major microscopic findings in AD are well known and have been described frequently and reviewed recently (Tomlinson, 1992). The major pathological features are senile plaques and the various manifestations of neuritic pathology, principally neurofibrillary tangles but also neuropil threads and neuritic plaques. There are also other microscopic features, notably Hirano bodies and granulovacuolar degeneration that have been described in Chapter 1.

Senile plaques

Senile plaques are best visualized by silver stains and/or immunocytochemistry for amyloid protein. However they are visualized, they have a wide range of morphological appearances and with the application of different antibodies and computerized reconstructions the descriptions have become increasingly sophisticated. However, for most practical and diagnostic purposes it is still probably most useful to divide them into the so-called 'diffuse' or 'pre-amyloid' plaques and the 'classical' or 'neuritic' plaques (Figs. 4a.7, 4a.8 and 4a.9).

Diffuse plaques, although they stain with Bielschowsky and MS silver stains and are immunochemically reactive for the amyloid β/A4 protein, have an amorphous irregular configuration and do not stain with Congo red. This pattern of staining implies that, in diffuse plaques, the β/A4 is not in the β-pleated sheet conformation that is characteristic of amyloids of all compositions. Immunochemically, there is also little or no evidence of reactive astrocytic or microglial changes and no neuronal damage. When examined with the electron microscope, the neuropil has a normal appearance, and there are few, if any of the characteristic amyloid filaments.

Morphologically, the neuritic plaque is composed of a central amyloid core surrounded by a halo of distorted neurites that contain the characteristic paired helical filaments found in neurofibrillary tangles and that stain for the tau protein. The amyloid in the core of these plaques is composed of the β/A4 protein that is characteristic of AD, and is similar to the amyloid found in the blood vessels in congophilic angiopathy of AD. Ultrastructurally, the plaque cores show a characteristic appearance with fingers of fibrillar amyloid extending into the surrounding neuropil (Fig. 4a.10).

The feature common to these two types of plaque is the amyloid β/A4 protein (which is a 39 to 43 amino acid protein) derived from a much larger β amyloid precursor protein (βAPP) which occurs in various lengths between 695 to 770 amino acids. The βAPP is a transmembrane protein of currently unknown function and the β/A4 portion is part of the transmembrane region of this protein. The relationship between these two types of

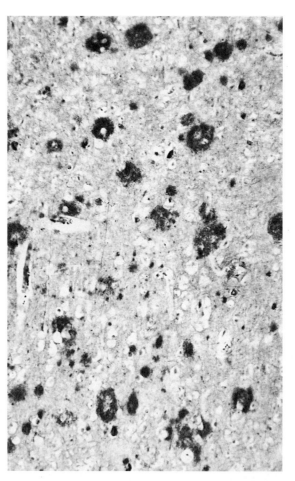

Fig. 4a.7. A low power illustration of cortex containing numerous diffuse plaques showing their characteristic irregular outline. (Bielschowsky × 50)

plaque is not entirely clear. The simple view would be that the diffuse plaque is an antecedent of the neuritic plaque, but it is clearly not that straightforward. Studies of patients with Down's syndrome have shown that the earliest changes in the development of Alzheimer changes are the development of diffuse plaques in the entorhinal regions and that the formation of neuritic plaques is a later event, but there is no convincing evidence that individual diffuse plaques actually evolve into the neuritic variety. One major difference between the two types of plaque is the nature of the amyloid β/A4 protein that is present. Recent studies using end-specific monoclonal antibodies to β/A4 in AD have shown diffuse plaques in cortex and basal ganglia and cerebellum are β/A4–42 (43) positive but β/A41–40 negative, and that the appearance of plaques positive for both β/A41–42 (43) and β/A41–40 was strongly correlated with the presence of mature neuritic plaques (Iwatsubo et al., 1994; Murphy et al., 1994). In patients with Down's syndrome it has been shown that the deposition of

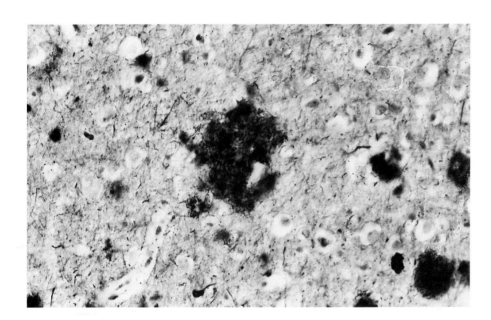

Fig. 4a.8. Typical diffuse plaque with irregular outline and no discernible neuritic reaction. (Bielschowsky × 250)

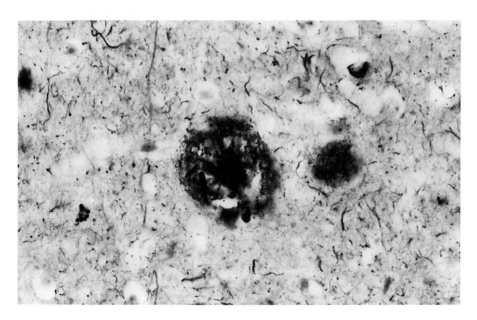

Fig. 4a.9. Mature plaque showing the characteristic central core of amyloid surrounded by a neuritic reaction. Neuropil threads are seen in the surrounding neuropil. (Bielschowsky × 250)

β/A41–42 (43) precedes that of β/A41–40 by about a decade (Iwatsubo *et al.*, 1995). It is not known what factors influence this change of whether it represents *in situ* processing of β/A41–42 (43) into the shorter β/A41–40 or an aggregation of β/A41–40 on to existing deposits of β/A41–42 (43).

It also seems very likely that tissue factors have a considerable influence on the conformation of plaques since there are a number of regions in the brain where diffuse plaques are commonly found but neuritic plaques are invariably absent. The best examples of this are in the caudate/putamen and the cerebellum (Joachim, Morris & Selkoe, 1989) (Fig. 4a.11). In both of these structures, diffuse plaques are common in Alzheimer's disease, but even when there are abundant neuritic plaques in the neocortex, they are not found in these structures. Whatever is spurring the neuritic reaction in the cortex is not present in the caudate/putamen or cerebellum.

Senile plaques may be found in the hippocampal formation and throughout the cortex. In the neocortex they are most frequent in the association areas and there is marked relative sparing of the primary cortical areas (Esiri, Pearson & Powell, 1986). This is most easy to see in the primary optic cortex, probably because it is very easy to identify primary cortex in this situation. In almost all cases of AD, there is a mixture of diffuse and neuritic plaques, and in severe cases very large numbers of plaques are present.

Neurofibrillary changes

As described in Chapter 1 the three expressions of neurofibrillary pathology are neurofibrillary tangles, the dystrophic neurites of neuritic plaques and the so-called neuropil threads which are found scattered in the neuropil (Fig. 4a.12). All represent intracellular accumulations of paired helical filaments (PHF) the basic component of which is hyperphosphorylated tau protein.

In AD, neurofibrillary tangle formation is particularly conspicuous in Sommer's sector of the hippocampus, entorhinal cortex and in the amygdala. However, it has long been recognized that tangles are present in these regions in many older people who are not known to be demented. Ball (1977) has shown that, although neurofibrillary tangles are present in the hippocampus of intellectually intact older people, they are at a lower density than in patients with AD. This observation is also implicit in the staging system of Braak and Braak (1991) (see below) where tangles may be present in hippocampus and entorhinal cortex in 'presymptomatic' disease. For this reason, it is impossible to rely solely on hippocampal and adjacent temporal lobe sections for the diagnosis of AD. Within the neocortical mantle, neurofibrillary tangles are found widely distributed in the cortex, though as with senile plaques, there is a marked tendency to spare the primary cortical areas.

One important practical point in the microscopic examination of the brain in AD is that visualization of neurofibrillary pathology requires the use of special stains which may be one of a number of silver stains,

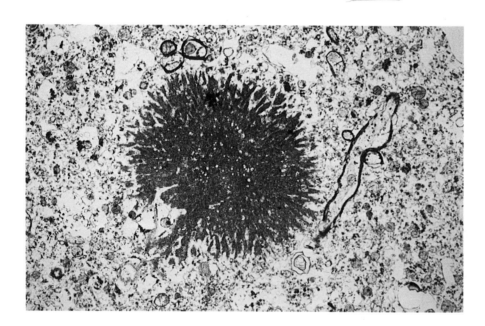

Fig. 4a.10. Electron micrograph of a mature plaque core showing the characteristic fibrillar organization of amyloid (Uranyl acetate/lead citrate ×2500)

immunocytochemical techniques for amyloid or neurofibrillary epitopes, or thioflavine A. It is effectively
impossible accurately to estimate the degree of neurofibrillary pathology with haematoxylin and eosin or other
routine histological stains. Although individual tangles
may be quite easy to identify in the hippocampal
pyramidal cell layer using H&E, it is much more difficult

to see them in the neocortex. A feature that can be
evaluated with H&E is the degree of attenuation of the
neuropil that occurs as a result of neuronal loss in AD
(Fig. 4a–13). The attenuation is most conspicuous in
layers one and two of the cortex and usually most severe
in the temporal lobe. This can range from a change in the
density of the neuropil that just allows the individual

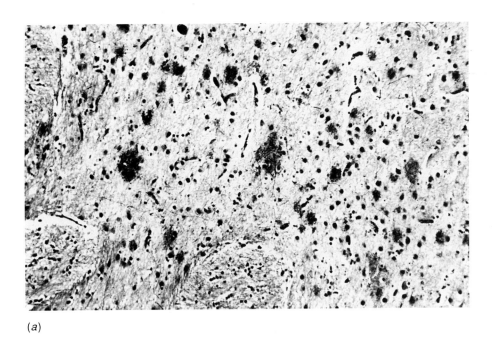

(a)

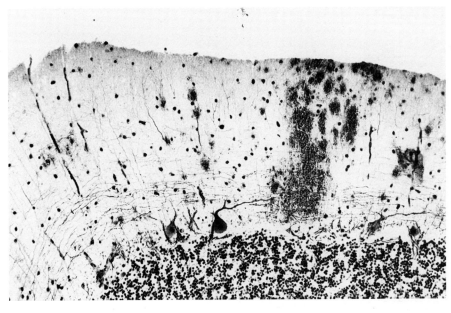

(b)

Fig. 4a.11. (a) Diffuse plaques in the
putamen. (Bielschowsky × 125) (b)
Diffuse plaques in the molecular
layer of the cerebellum.
(Bielschowsky × 125)

processes to begin to be distinguished to a severe microvacuolation and collapse of the upper cortical layers (Brun & Englund, 1981). This vacuolation has sometimes been confused with the vacuolar change that occurs in Creutzfeldt–Jakob disease, although its location in the upper layers of the cortex is uncharacteristic for this disease. Smith *et al.* (1987) showed that to some degree this vacuolar change could be found in the temporal lobe in a majority of cases of AD (Fig. 4a.14).

The conformation of neurofibrillary tangles is very dependent on the neuron in which they accumulate so that the archetypal 'flame-shaped' tangle is found in large pyramidal neurones such as those in the hippocampal pyramidal cell layer, while globose tangles

are more typically seen in neurones such as those in the basal nucleus of Meynert and the locus ceruleus (Fig. 4a.15). Ultrastructurally, neurofibrillary tangles are composed of swaths of intracytoplasmic paired helical filaments (phf) with a diameter of about 20 nm. and a periodicity of 80 nm. (Fig. 4a.16) which displace the cytoplasmic contents and the nucleus (Fig. 4a.17). The paired helical filaments of the neurofibrillary tangle are very insoluble, so insoluble, in fact, that they remain within the neuropil as 'ghost' or 'tombstone' tangles after the death and degeneration of the cell in which they developed. In this condition they can still be stained by silver stains such as Bielschowsky and can be easily differentiated from intracellular tangles by

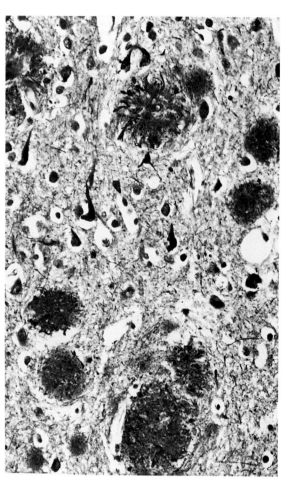

Fig. 4a.12. Typical appearance at medium power of cortex in Alzheimer's disease showing the combination of mature plaques with prominent neuritic reaction, neurofibrillary tangles and neuropil threads scattered in the intervening neuropil. (Bielschowsky ×125)

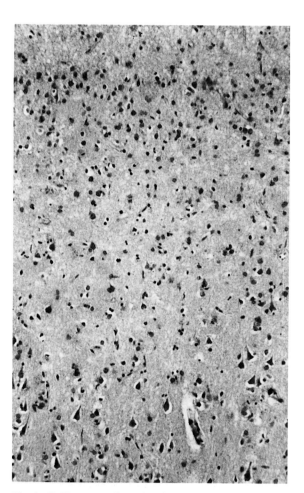

Fig. 4a.13. Haematoxylin and eosin stain of the upper layers of parietal cortex in severe Alzheimer's disease showing marked neuronal loss and neuropil pruning. The faint nodularity seen in this photograph is a reflection of the presence of numerous neuritic plaques. (H&E ×50)

their different staining intensity (Figs. 4a.18). Free in the neuropil the tangles become coated with other molecules and develop different immunochemical reactivity, for example to antibodies directed against glial fibrillary acidic protein (GFAP), ubiquitin and apolipoprotein E (Yamaguchi *et al.*, 1994). A small fraction are also immunoreactive to the amyloid β/A4 protein (Tabaton *et al.*, 1991 Yamaguchi *et al.*, 1991). This process is reflected ultrastructurally, in that 'ghost tangles' lose the characteristic paired helical conformation of the intracellular tangle and become thicker straight filaments (Figs. 4a.19, 4a.20).

As described in the section on plaques, the development of dystrophic neurites, which is associated with the coalescence of dispersed β/A4 protein into focal deposits of fibrillary β/A4 protein amyloid, is one of the stages in the evolution of the mature plaque. The third expression of neuritic pathology, the neuropil threads (Braak *et al.*, 1986) are found between the plaques and tangles in the neocortex, entorhinal cortex and amygdala (Fig. 4a.12) and also in subcortical areas such as the periaqueductal grey. As with the dystrophic neurites, their staining and immunochemical characteristics resemble neurofibrillary tangles, and ultrastructurally they contain paired helical filaments. Their presence is thought to reflect dendritic sprouting by neurons affected by tangle formation and they are a manifestation of neuritic pathology (Braak & Braak, 1988; Ihara, 1988).

Subcortical pathology in AD

The cortical pathology in AD is so dramatic that it tends to overwhelm the considerable subcortical changes that are also found. In terms of senile plaque distribution, as well as the cortex, neuritic plaques can easily be found in the hypothalamus and mamilliary bodies, the olfactory bulbs (Esiri & Wilcock, 1984) and the midbrain tegmentum. Smaller numbers may also be found in the region of the basal forebrain and floor of the fourth ventricle.

The subcortical neuritic pathology is also conspicuous. The nucleus basalis of Meynert in the basal forebrain is a conspicuous site of neurofibrillary tangle formation (Whitehouse *et al.*, 1981, 1982; Rogers, Brogan & Mirra, 1985) and has been the subject of a large number of studies (Tomlinson, 1992). The importance of this region is that the large neurons of the nucleus basalis of Meynert are the source of cholinergic input to the cortex and loss of cholinergic supply and choline acetyl transferase in the cerebral cortex is perhaps the most well-established neurochemical change in AD (Davies & Maloney 1976). The consensus of the numerous studies of the nucleus basalis is that there is loss of between 40 and 70% of the neurons in this nucleus in AD (Arendt *et al.*, 1993; Wilcock *et al.*, 1988) and a generally good correlation with the neurochemical change in the cortex, the severity of the dementia and the degree of Alzheimer change seen histologically (Wilcock *et al.*, 1982). There is some evidence that there is a greater degree of nucleus basalis neuron loss in younger patients (Tagliavini & Pilleri, 1983; Whitehouse *et al.*, 1983). It is also reported that the part of the

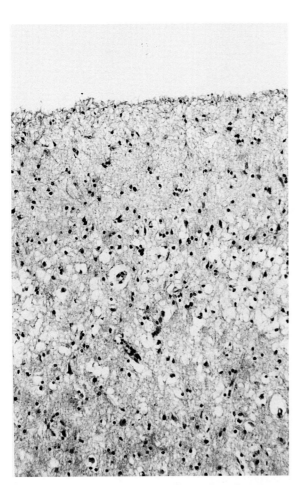

Fig. 4a.14. Haematoxylin and eosin-stained section showing the 'spongy' vacuolation of the upper layers of the cortex seen in some cases of Alzheimer's disease. This change resembles that seen in the fronto-temporal dementias. In Creutzfeldt–Jakob disease changes are more pronounced in the lower layers of the cortex. (H&E × 125)

nucleus that supplies the temporal lobe is more severely affected (Wilcock *et al.*, 1988).

The other major sites of subcortical tangle formation and neuronal loss are the periaqueductal grey matter and the dorsal raphe which are the source of serotonergic supply to the cortex (Tomlinson, 1989) and the locus ceruleus (Mann *et al.*, 1980) which is the main source of noradrenergic supply. In all these regions there is a tendency for a degree of neuronal loss to occur with age and in the raphe, this age related neuronal loss is often accompanied by a degree of tangle formation. The age related changes in these regions are, however, almost always considerably less than that seen in patients with AD. In line with the reduction in noradrenergic and serotonergic neurons, there are also changes in cortical transmitter content and associated metabolites and marker enzymes, although the correlations among neuronal loss, tangle formation, neurochemistry and clinical symptomatology are less straightforward then for the cholinergic system.

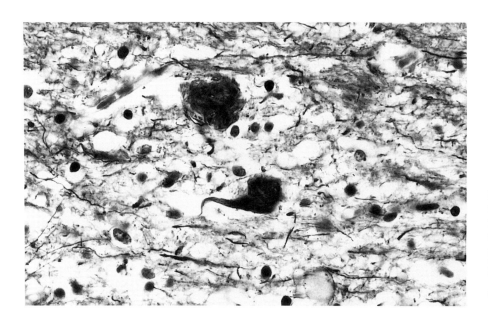

Fig. 4a.15. The general shape of the neuron defines the configuration of tangles that form within the cell. In this illustration of two neurofibrillary tangles from the basal nucleus of Meynert, one has a 'pyramidal' configuration while the other is 'globose'. (Bielschowsky × 250)

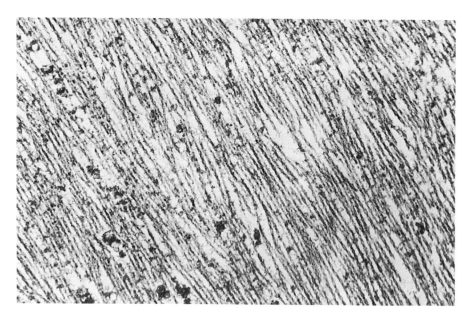

Fig. 4a.16. High power illustration of the characteristic paired helical filaments that are the major constituent of neurofibrillary tangles (Uranyl acetate/lead citrate × 60 000)

Congophilic angiopathy

Amyloid deposition (congophilic angiopathy) in the cerebral arteries has been recognized since the beginning of this century and its association with Alzheimer's disease was also recognized early in the study of the disease (Vintners, 1987). Amyloid can be formed by molecules that have the capacity to aggregate in a conformation called a β pleated sheet so that amyloid is derived from a number of different sources. Most of the systemic causes of amyloid deposition are not associated with any amyloid deposition in the cerebral vasculature. Cerebral vascular amyloid deposition, although particularly associated with Alzheimer's disease, also occurs in a number of other disease states including prion disease, where the amyloid is derived from the prion protein, and in the Icelandic form of hereditary cerebral haemorrhage with amyloidosis (HCHWA) where the genetic defect is located in the gene for cystatin C (Cohen et al., 1983, Jensson et al., 1987). Focal vascular amyloid deposition has also been described in vascular malformations (Hart

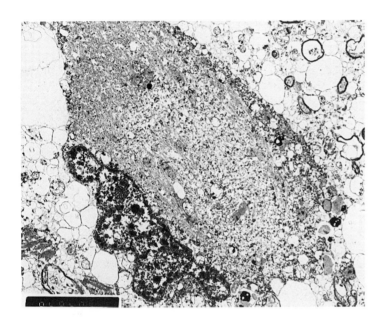

Fig. 4a.17. Low power electron micrograph of an intracellular neurofibrillary tangle. (Uranyl acetate/lead citrate × 3000)

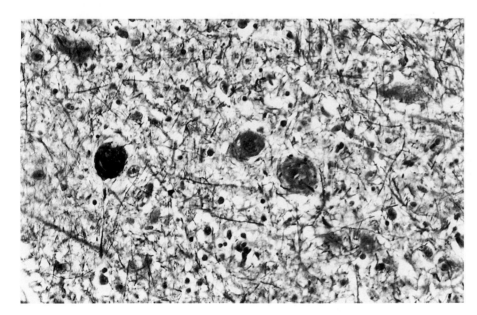

Fig. 4a.18. Intracellular and extracellular 'ghost' or 'tombstone' globose tangles in the basal nucleus of Meynert. The extracellular tangles are significantly less intensely stained in the Bielschowsky stain. (Bielschowsky × 250)

et al., 1988) and after radiation therapy (Mandybur & Gore, 1969). In some respects, the amyloid hypothesis of AD started with congophilic angiopathy when Glenner and Wong (1984) first sequenced the cerebrovascular amyloid and showed that it was a previously undescribed amino acid sequence. Using protein chemical and immunocytochemical methods, this protein subunit was subsequently shown to be shared between cerebrovascular amyloid and diffuse and neuritic plaques, although the latter appear to contain a slightly shortened form of

the protein with 40 amino acids ($A\beta1$–40) rather than the $A\beta1$–42 (43) form that appears to predominate in diffuse plaques (Iwatsubo *et al.*, 1994). Both forms of the $\beta/A4$ polypeptide are present in cerebrovascular amyloid (Joachim *et al.*, 1988; Roher *et al.*, 1993).

Congophilic angiopathy is an almost invariable finding in AD, the frequency being to some extent dependent on how hard it is looked for, (Mandybur, 1975; Joachim *et al.*, 1988), but is also common in elderly patients without AD (Vintners & Gilbert, 1983; Esiri & Wilcock,

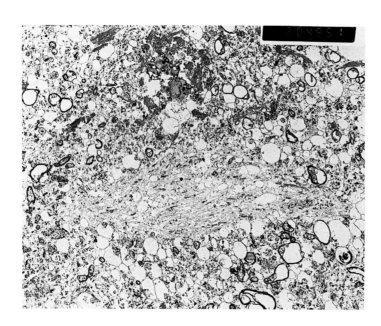

Fig. 4a.19. Low power electron micrograph of an extracellular, 'ghost' or 'tombstone' tangle. No cell membrane or nucleus is present, and degenerate organelles are present forming vacuoles between the tangle material. (Uranyl acetate/lead citrate × 2500)

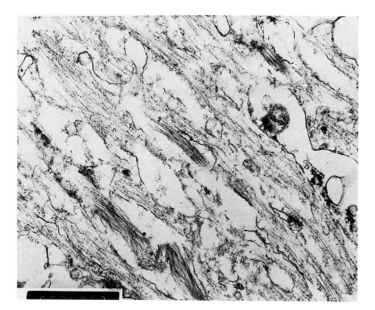

Fig. 4a.20. Higher power view of the fibrils shows that the paired helical configuration has been lost and replaced by straight filaments. The degenerate organelles between the fibrils are clearly seen at this power. (Uranyl acetate/lead citrate × 30 000)

1986). As with AD, the incidence rises with increasing age. The distribution and severity of amyloid angiopathy is unconnected to the severity of the Alzheimer changes or the duration of the disease and as such is of no diagnostic value, although it is reported to be related to the apolipoprotein E genotype (see below).

Congophilic (amyloid) angiopathy characteristically affects the smaller branches of the sulcal arteries and the penetrating arteries in the cerebral cortex. Within the cerebral cortex (Figs. 4a.21, 3.16). Both the long and short penetrating arteries are affected, but, with the long penetrating arteries that supply the white matter, amyloid is found only in the section of the artery passing through the cortex. When the artery enters the subcortical white matter, the amyloid deposition stops, although there may be other vascular wall changes. In general, when there is significant amyloid angiopathy the deposition tends to be most pronounced in the occipital lobe, and least conspicuous in the temporal lobe (Tomonaga, 1981; Vintners & Gilbert, 1983). The other major site at which amyloid angiopathy is found is in the cerebellum, where most of the deposition is in the small subarachnoid arteries. Some regions of the cerebral hemisphere, specifically the white matter, the basal ganglia, most of the thalamus and often the hippocampus are notably spared amyloid deposition, although the amygdala is often affected and the dorso-medial nucleus of the thamalus may also show pericapillary vascular amyloid deposition.

Microscopically, the amyloid is deposited in the walls of the smaller arteries, first tending to surround the smooth muscle cells that comprise the muscular wall of the vessel and eventually replacing them (Figs. 4a.22, 23 and 24). This process can be followed ultrastructurally, with smooth muscle cells becoming progressively surrounded by a thickening band of amyloid fibrils. At a later stage the smooth muscle cells undergo degeneration and at the final stage the entire wall of the vessel is composed of a dense meshwork of amyloid fibrils with no surviving cellular components except for the endothelial cells lining the lumen of the artery (Fig. 4a.25). At the intermediate stage, where the smooth muscle cells are surrounded, but have not yet degenerated, the amyloid can be seen in light microscopy as congophilic rings in the wall of the vessel. A recognized complication of amyloid angiopathy is an increased incidence of lobar haemorrhage, which can be recurrent. Curiously, the haemorrhages are typically subcortical rather than intracortical and so occur from vessels that are not themselves affected by amyloid deposition. A further peculiarity of these haemorrhages is that they tend to occur in the frontal lobes, and not in the parietooccipital lobes where the angiopathy is most severe (Gilbert & Vintners, 1983). Single lobar haemorrhages are usually associated with a focal neurological syndrome, but if they are multiple, they can cause, or contribute to cognitive decline. Since many of the patients have concomitant AD it can be hard to assess the significance of amyloid associated haemorrhages to cognitive decline, but cases of recurrent haemorrhage

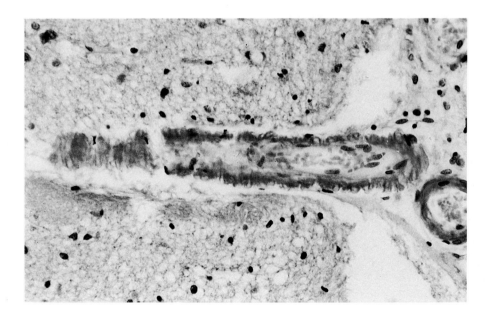

Fig. 4a.21. Congo red stain of amyloid angiopathy in a small artery entering the cortex from the subarachnoid space. Amyloid can be seen surrounding the smooth muscle cells in the wall of the artery. Amyloid deposits are also present in the parenchyma adjacent to the artery but separated from it by the Virchow–Robin space. (Congo red × 125)

with progressive dementia in the absence of marked plaque and tangle formation have been described (Okazaki, Reagan & Campbell 1979; Griffiths *et al.*, 1982).

It is not known whether there is a close relationship between the mechanisms of amyloid formation and deposition in blood vessel walls and the amyloid deposition that occurs in plaques and plaque cores. The disconnection between the severity of amyloid angiopathy and the severity of Alzheimer change in the parenchyma suggests that different cell biological mechanisms may govern the formation of amyloid in the two circumstances. Conceivably, for example, there could be a different pathway leading to the formation of the amyloid β protein, and certainly, if tissue factors play a significant part in the conversion of the β/A4 protein from the soluble form to the fibrillar form of amyloid β/A4 pleated sheets they can be expected to be different in the cerebral parenchyma and in the wall of a blood vessel. However, there are clearly some common factors

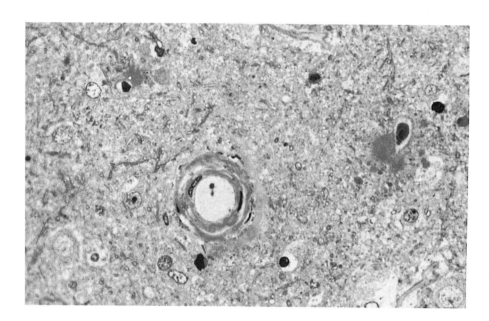

Fig. 4a.22. Semi-thin resin embedded section of cerebral cortex with amyloid angiopathy affecting a small arteriole and two capillaries with amyloid deposition. (Toluidine blue × 250)

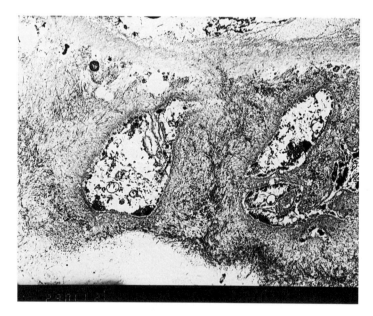

Fig. 4a.23. Electron micrograph of a relatively early stage of amyloid deposition with amyloid fibril deposition in the spaces between the smooth muscle cells. (Uranyl acetate/lead citrate × 7000)

in the increased production of β/A4 protein amyloid as there are examples of early Alzheimer changes in Down's syndrome that are accompanied by congophilic angiopathy. This finding indicates that the additional chromosome 21, perhaps merely by increasing the production of the β/A4 protein, is affecting the formation and deposition of amyloid in both the cerebral parenchyma and the cerebral vessels.

One interesting microscopic feature that demonstrates the significance of amyloid deposition in the generation of plaque neuritic reactions is the phenomenon of perivascular plaque formation (Fig. 4a.26). Perivascular plaques are often present in cases with severe amyloid angiopathy and the wall of an intracortical vessel is completely replaced by amyloid. When this occurs, there can be extension of amyloid deposition across the Virchow–Robin space and into the adjacent cerebral parenchyma. It should be noted that perivascular plaques are only seen when there is massive deposition of amyloid in the vessel so that it is reasonable to conclude that the amyloid being deposited is arising from the blood vessel, rather than arising in the parenchyma and being deposited secondarily in the blood vessel. Ultrastructurally, this deposition very much resembles that seen in ordinary plaque cores with 'fingers' of amyloid fibrils extending into the tissue. This may be

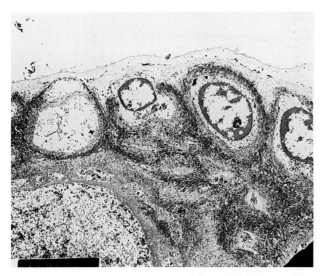

Fig. 4a.24. Electron micrograph of a later stage of amyloid deposition where the smooth muscle cells are more closely invested by amyloid. In some cases the smooth muscle cells are entirely surrounded by amyloid fibrils. This is analogous to the situation seen in the light micrography Fig. 4.21. (Uranyl acetate/lead citrate × 5000)

accompanied by a marked neuritic reaction associated with this amyloid. It is not credible to assume that there is any particular tissue selectivity about the location of this extension of amyloid into the cortex. This suggests that it is some aspect of the presence of the amyloid that generates the neuritic reaction in otherwise unaffected neuropil. On the subject of vascular deposition of amyloid, there are occasional cases where there is very marked pericapillary deposition of amyloid. This almost always occurs in the context of AD, although there are occasional cases of marked pericapillary amyloid deposition with very little in the way of plaque and tangle formation (Figs 4a.27, 28). A further feature sometimes seen in cases with severe disease is the subpial deposition of amyloid (Fig. 4a.29).

White matter changes in Alzheimer's disease

The development of CT and subsequently MRI opened new horizons in the examination of the brain in life and, not surprisingly, revealed some unexpected aspects of disease. A striking finding is that many older people have periventricular and diffuse white matter regions of low density, a group of changes that have been called leukoaraiosis (Hachinski, Potter & Merskey, 1987). In general, MRI is more sensitive than CT in detecting this type of change which can be seen in patients with cerebrovascular disease (Erkinjuntti et al., 1987; Aharon-Peretz, Cummings & Hill, 1988) but also in asymptomatic patients and in patients with AD (Awad et al., 1986, Erkinjuntti et al., 1987, 1989; George et al., 1986a, b; Mirsen et al., 1991). Most studies suggest that the strongest correlates of the more severe grades of radiological change are advancing age and cerebrovascular disease (Awad et al., 1986; Brilliant et al., 1995). In terms of cognitive function, results have been ambiguous, but it is probably fair to conclude that there is no clear and consistent relationship between the severity of leukoaraiosis and any degree of cognitive decline (Brilliant 1995).

Pathological studies of the white matter in AD (Brun & Englund, 1986) have shown some degree of white matter change in approximately 60% of patients, with severe changes being present in about 20% of patients. The pathological change consists of a diffuse incomplete demyelination with some associated loss of axons and a mild reactive astrocytosis. Occasional macrophages are also found. The blood vessels show a variable hyaline thickening. These changes are similar to those described in Binswanger's disease, but lack the cavitating and frankly necrotic lesions that are usually present in this disease (Caplan & Schoene, 1978; De Reuck *et al.*, 1980). The severity of the white matter changes was unrelated to either the distribution or the severity of the Alzheimer process in the grey matter, so that the changes were not likely to be the result of wallerian degeneration of white matter axons secondary to cortical neuronal loss (Brun & Englund, 1986; Englund, Brun & Alling, 1988, Brilliant *et al.*, 1995). The absence of any degree of change in

45% of patients with AD also supports this conclusion. There is also no correlation with distribution or severity of amyloid angiopathy (Englund *et al.*, 1988; Janota *et al.*, 1989). The absence of significant associations with the severity of AD or AD associated structural changes in blood vessels suggest that, although a frequent finding in AD, the white matter lesion is not specifically related to the Alzheimer process.

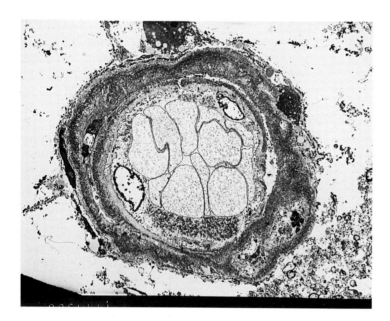

Fig. 4a.25. In the most advanced stage of amyloid deposition, the smooth muscle cells, as in this example, degenerate and the wall of the vessel is composed almost entirely of amyloid. Even at this stage the endothelial cells remain intact. (Uranyl acetate/lead citrate ×1500)

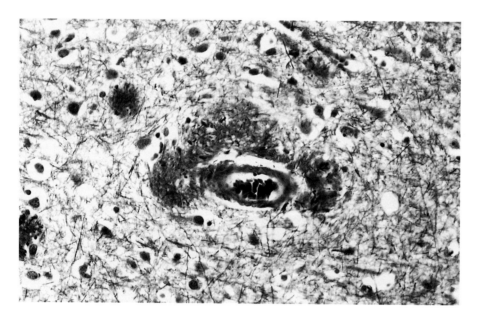

Fig. 4a.26. Bielschowsky silver stain of a perivascular plaque showing amyloid and neuritic reaction in the parenchyma around a small arteriole with amyloid angiopathy. (Bielschowsky ×250)

PATTERN OF DEVELOPMENT OF AD CHANGES AND THEIR RELATION TO THE SYMPTOMS OF DEMENTIA

This discussion can be broken into three areas of interest:

1. Spatial and temporal distribution of AD changes (see Chapter 1)
2. Clinical correlates of regional and laminar specific pathology (see Chapter 1)
3. Significance of plaques and tangles in the symptoms of dementia

As has been described in Chapter 1 there have been a number of correlative studies of the overall severity of the dementia of AD with a morphological indicator of the overall burden of disease. The balance of scientific opinion is that, in terms of Alzheimer pathology, neurofibrillary tangle numbers or some other reflection of neurofibrillary pathology are the best pre-

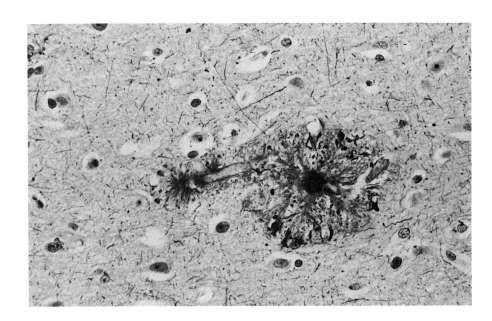

Fig. 4a.27. Pericapillary plaque formation with marked neuritic reaction around a pericapillary amyloid deposit. A further smaller reaction is also present further along the same capillary. (Bielschowsky × 250)

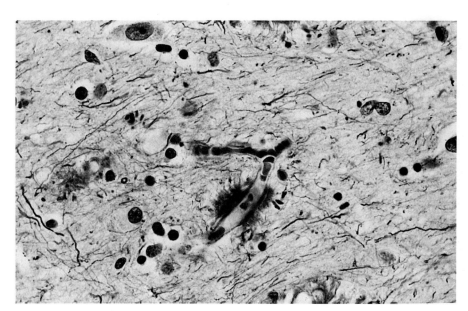

Fig. 4a.28. Pericapillary amyloid showing the very characteristic fibrillar appearance of amyloid deposits. (Bielschowsky × 250)

dictor of overall cognitive decline (Wilcock & Esiri, 1982; Neary *et al.*, 1986; Terry *et al.*, 1991; McKee, Kosik & Kowall, 1991; Morris *et al.*, 1991, Arriagada *et al.*, 1992; Crystal *et al.*, 1988; Berg *et al.*, 1993). A concept that is at variance with these studies is that of 'plaque only' AD (Terry *et al.*, 1987) where it was proposed that in the elderly population (over 80 years) there was a group of demented patients with AD where the only pathological manifestation was the presence of senile plaques. Closer examination of this group of patients suggests that almost all cases of 'plaque only' AD are cases where there is mixed disease and, in particular, a high prevalence of cortical Lewy bodies. The dementia in these patients is then a reflection of the effects of the early stage of two dementing diseases with additive effects. Thus, in cases of suspected AD, when only plaques are found, a search should be made for another disease, very often Parkinson's disease or cerebrovascular disease, that might be contributing to the symptoms of dementia.

Progressing from this correlation between the symptoms of dementia and the overall burden of neuritic pathology, recent studies have begun to look more closely at the different regions of the cortex and have found that dementia scores are correlated most closely with the burden of neurofibrillary pathology in the frontal and parietal lobes (Nagy *et al.*, 1995). In a further refinement, some investigators have looked beyond plaques and tangles to parameters such as neuronal loss and reductions in synaptic density as more

direct reflections of functional impairment of the different regions of the brain. Current studies suggest that the strongest correlate with pre-mortem dementia is neocortical synapse density in the mid-frontal lobe (Terry *et al.*, 1991; Masliah *et al.*, 1991, De Kosky *et al.*, 1990).

In a parallel development, there has also been increasing attention paid to different aspects of cognitive decline so that, for example, in a recent study, Samuel *et al.* (1994) using a combination of neuropsychological tests have found that changes in higher cortical functions such as conceptualization, attention and initiation were most strongly correlated with alterations in midfrontal synapse density while, for the more memory-orientated tests, the strongest predictor was neurofibrillary tangle formation in the nucleus basalis of Meynert. In another study (Nagy *et al.*, 1995) memory deficits correlated closely with the severity of hippocampal neurofibrillary tangle formation.

This chapter has, as its major focus, the dementia associated with AD, and most published work has been directed towards correlating pathological and neurochemical features of the disease with quantitative measures of cognitive decline. However, many of the most distressing features of the disease, particularly for family members and other carers, are actually the behavioural changes such as incessant wandering, aggression, paranoia, sexual disinhibition and depression that often accompany the dementia and are most frequently the symptoms that precipitate the need for

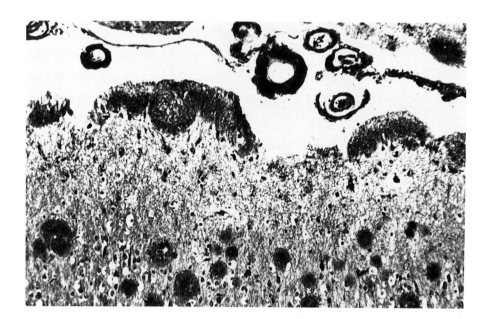

Fig. 4a.29. Subpial deposition of amyloid in a case with numerous amyloid plaques and severe amyloid angiopathy. (Bielschowsky × 125)

institutional care (Wilcock & Jacoby, 1991), Psychiatric symptoms may also be among the earliest presenting symptoms of AD (Becker *et al.*, 1994) and there is a recent study that shows that their presence can be a predictor of a faster cognitive decline (Chui *et al.*, 1994). In this important field there has been much less systematic work than in relation to the dementia of AD but it is an area that is beginning to generate significant interest. There are some studies which suggest, for example, that the depression is associated with neuronal loss in the locus ceruleus and reduced levels of noradrenaline in the cortex (Hope & Fairburn 1992; Zubenko, Moossy & Kopp, 1990; Zweig *et al.*, 1988), although there is not a good correlation between the severity of the neuronal loss and the severity of the depressive symptoms. Similarly, other studies have suggested that aggressive behaviour is correlated with evidence of diminished 5HT function in frontal cortex (Chan-Palay & Assan, 1989; Palmer *et al.*, 1988). However, in what may become a recurring theme of clinico-pathological correlative studies of psychiatric features, Chen *et al.* (1992, personal communication) have shown that, although there is 40% loss of 5HT neurons in the dorsal raphe nucleus in AD cases with aggressive behaviour compared to controls, there is no correlation between the severity of neuronal loss in this region and the severity of cognitive or behavioural changes during life. Attention is now being turned to investigations of possible changes in cortical 5HT innervation and metabolism. This whole area of neurochemical and receptor changes in the behavioural changes in AD is only at the beginning of investigation and the correlations, given the complexity introduced by the existence of multiple different receptor types for transmitters such as 5HT and dopamine, are likely to be complex and interdependent.

What may be a harbinger of the conceptual problems that are likely to result from this complexity is the current difficulty in clarifying the relationship between dopamine deficiencies, a possible cholinergic–monoaminergic imbalance, and the presence of hallucinations (Perry *et al.*, 1990a, 1991) in patients with dementia. At a morphological level, this debate takes the form of whether a clinical history of hallucinations is associated with the finding of Lewy bodies in the cerebral cortex and substantia nigra (Perry *et al.*, 1990a) and to what extent the concomitant presence of AD changes, particularly the presence of senile plaques, is a necessary accompaniment of cortical

Lewy bodies or a coincidental finding. The suggested association between cortical Lewy bodies and senile plaques raises the question of a more than incidental relationship between AD, Parkinson's disease and what has come variously to be called diffuse Lewy body disease (Yoshimura, 1983; Kosaka *et al.*, 1984, Gibb, Esiri & Lees, 1985; Burkhardt *et al.*, 1988; Dickson *et al.*, 1989; Lennox *et al.* 1989, Kosaka, 1990; Crystal *et al.*, 1990; Sugiyama, 1994), senile dementia of the Lewy body type (Perry *et al.*, 1990b) and the Lewy body variant of Alzheimer's disease (Hansen *et al.*, 1990). This whole rather convoluted and controversial topic is considered in more detail in Chapter 6.

Another aspect of the clinical presentation of AD that has begun to be addressed is possible differences arising from the genetic heterogeneity of AD. Although the different genetic subtypes and sporadic late onset disease seem to have a very similar pattern of progressive cognitive decline, Haltia *et al.* (1994), in a study of Finnish chromosome 14 encoded AD suggests that this group of patients has a high frequency of myoclonus and epilepsy. This is a combination of symptoms and signs that is otherwise very rare in AD, and has led many of these patients to be considered to have prion disease prior to definitive diagnosis. Another difference in this group is the generally earlier age of onset of symptoms which is usually before the age of 50 years, in contrast to the families with genetic abnormalities in the amyloid precursor protein where onset tends to be between the ages of 50 and 60 years.

DIAGNOSTIC CRITERIA

One of the most vexed questions in the pathological study of Alzheimer's disease is that of the criteria that should be used for the diagnosis. In their seminal studies of the disease, Tomlinson and colleagues found what they construed to be a relationship between the number of senile plaques and the severity of cognitive decline. For a long time this formulation was considered to be acceptable and found its most concrete expression in Khatchaturian's article (1985) reporting the results of a workshop sponsored by the National Institute of Aging (NIA), the American Association of Retired Persons (AARP), the National Institute of Neurological and Communicative Disorders and Stroke (NINCDS) and the National Institute of Mental Health (NIMH).

The consensus of the neuropathological panel at this workshop was that the diagnosis could be made based on the mean number of senile plaques in three regions of neocortex taken from the temporal, frontal and parietal lobes (areas not specified) and graduated for age, so that, with increasing age, a greater number of plaques was necessary for the diagnosis to be considered secure. The panel considered that tangles would often be present, but that the diagnosis was not conditional on their presence. The insecurity of the criteria adopted was highlighted by a later paragraph of the report suggesting that a reduction (possibly of up to 50%) in the number of plaques required for the diagnosis would be acceptable in patients with a clinical history of dementia. The Khatchaturian criteria specifically enshrined the possibility of making the diagnosis of AD in the absence of a history of dementia and without the necessity of being able to find neurofibrillary tangles, particularly in patients over the age of 75 years.

This concentration on senile plaques as a diagnostic indicator was also adopted by the consortium to establish a registry for Alzheimer's disease (CERAD), but with a number of very significant differences. First, they introduced the formulation of possible, probable and definite AD on the basis of age-related numbers of plaques estimated in a semi-quantitative way and the presence or absence of a clinical history of dementia. Using CERAD criteria, in the absence of a clinical history of dementia, no matter how severe the Alzheimer changes only a diagnosis of possible AD can be made, so that this constitutes acceptance of the proposition that there are no absolute morphologic criteria for the diagnosis of AD. Secondly, the CERAD criteria, as revised, require the semi-quantitation of neuritic plaques and ignore diffuse ones altogether.

Tierney *et al.* (1988) applied a range of diagnostic criteria for AD but included the presence of neurofibrillary tangles in the requirement for diagnosis and by varying the criteria obtained clinico-pathologic agreement ranging from 64 to 86%.

The three sets of major diagnostic criteria for AD are summarized below:

Khatchaturian

Technique
Not stated.

Sample
1. Three regions of neocortex (frontal, temporal parietal)
2. Hippocampus
3. Amygdala
4. Basal ganglia

5. Substantia nigra
6. Cerebellar cortex
7. Spinal cord

Histological criteria (per × 200 field)
< 50yrs: > 2–5 neuritic plaques and tangles
50–65   :8 or more senile plaques (tangle +)
66–75   :10 or more senile plaques (tangle +)
> 75   :15 or more senile plaques (tangle + / −)

Plaque numbers reduced by up to 50% with + history of dementia

Comments
In use, there are practical problems particularly in relation to achieving a 'mean' involvement with only 3 areas, and the nature of the plaques that count, the age effect and the 'possible' allowance for the presence of clinical dementia. A problem with these criteria is their dependence on uncharacterized plaque counts. There has always been a contrary position that has emphasized the importance of neuritic pathology in relation to the presence of dementia. This position has been reinforced over the years by reports of individuals or small series of unequivocally non-demented patients who were well examined in life, but who, on post-mortem examination were found to fulfil Khatchaturian criteria for Alzheimer's disease in terms of plaque counts (Crystal *et al.*, 1988).

CERAD

Technique
Bielschowsky recommended, but alternatives acceptable.

Sample
1. Middle frontal gyrus
2. Superior and middle temporal gyrus
3. Inferior parietal lobule
4. Anterior cingulate gyrus
5. Hippocampus
6. Entorhinal cortex and amygdala
7. Midbrain including substantia nigra.

Additional sections possible

Histological criteria
1. Neuritic plaque assessment
2. Semi-quantitative assessment of area of maximum

involvement matching this with illustrations of neuritic plaque densities representing each of three scores

3. In frontal, temporal or parietal cortex
4. Age-related plaque score.

Ranks
Possible, probable or definite
Requires history of dementia

Comments
CERAD have just issued their most recent update. It includes some refinement of the definitions of possible AD and Parkinson's disease and makes some specific suggestions about sections to take for the diagnosis of cerebrovascular dementia.

Tierney

Technique
Bielschowsky

Sample
1. Frontal ($\times$ 5), temporal ($\times$ 5), parietal ($\times$ 3), occipital ($\times$ 1)
2. Allocortex (inc. hippocampus) ($\times$ 3)
3. Amygdala
4. Basal ganglia, thalamus, basal nucleus
5. Mesencephalon, pons medulla (all $\times$ 3)
6. Cerebellum

Histologic criteria
A1 one or more NFT and one or more neuritic plaque per $\times$ 25 field in hippocampus (neocortical findings ignored)
A2 one or more NFT and one or more neuritic plaque per $\times$ 25 field in both neocortex and hippocampus.
A3 one or more NFT and one or more neuritic plaque per $\times$ 25 field in neocortex (hippocampal findings ignored) ($+$ vascular exclusion criteria).

Comments
A strictly numerical system. Our experience with Tierney A3 (Nagy et al., 1995) is that it is rather too strict and leads to the exclusion of cases that have significant disease burden and cognitive decline and that the A1 and A2 criteria are too heavily biased to hippocampal neuritic change to be really useful.

STAGING THE SEVERITY OF AD PATHOLOGY
A set of criteria has been advanced by Braak and Braak (1991) as a means of semi-quantitatively staging the severity of Alzheimer pathological change. The stages that are defined by this system span the pre-clinical and symptomatic phases of what is presumed to be the progressive accumulation of plaques and tangles over time and their progressively wider dissemination through the brain.

Braak

Technique
100 μm sections/Gallyas

Samples
Anterior hippocampus
Posterior hippocampus
Occipital

Histological criteria
Semi-quantitative ($+$ / $+$ $+$ $+$) of NFT and neuropil threads

Comments
The use of this system has a significant technical problem in that the nature of the section preparation (100 μm) and staining protocols are probably too difficult and restrictive to be used on a routine basis. It will be important to establish whether this system can be adapted for routine use.

Choice of histopathological criteria
There are a number of issues that are relevant to the choice of histopathological criteria for the diagnosis of AD (Mirra, Hart & Terry, 1993). An important initial point is that the selection of diagnostic criteria is influenced by their intended use. For example, criteria for general use of multi-centre brain banking might be different from those adopted in an individual laboratory for a specific research purpose. In this chapter we are concerned with diagnostic criteria for general rather than research use. Starting from the first principles, whatever diagnostic criteria are advocated they should meet four practical tests. These are that the criteria should be:

1. *Simple*: Since whatever is suggested must be capable of being performed in a variety of

laboratories and used by a wide range of people trained to different standards, it must be very straightforward. In practice, this means that it should not require either elaborate sampling or complex staining.

2. *Transferable*: Any set of criteria intended for general use should be able to be applied in different centres and give the same result.

3. *Validated*: What is adopted should, if possible, already have wide international experience of use. It would not be sensible to propose an entirely novel protocol for the diagnosis of AD.

4. *Versatile*: The practical reality of the neuropathological examination of patients with dementia is that some of the cases that get submitted with a clinical diagnosis of Alzheimer's disease will have some other dementing disease. This means that, in selecting a diagnostic protocol for general use, the diagnosis of Alzheimer's disease should not be considered in isolation from that of other dementing diseases that will be encountered by any laboratory that accepts cases with a clinical diagnosis of Alzheimer's disease.

Some assessment of the merits of the available diagnostic criteria for AD can be gained by examining them in using the criteria described above.

1. Simple

In technical terms Khatchaturian, CERAD and Tierney are all within the compass of standard neuropathological techniques. Braak staging is more difficult to accommodate within the standard laboratory procedures.

In procedural terms, in the assessment of severity of disease, there is a practical difference between the measurement of mean or maximum involvement. For example, Khatchaturian requires mean counts, although we have found in practice that the three-field requirement is really not sufficient to obtain a mean value as the variation in cortical involvement is considerable. CERAD, on the other hand, calls for assessment of maximum involvement. Our experience has been that it is quite easy in practice to go to the area of maximum involvement. This is a significant practical advantage in using a system, such as CERAD, that requires assessment of the maximum extent of disease. One of the practical problems in using CERAD is in the definition of a neuritic plaque, about which there is an inevitable imprecision that sometimes causes prob-

lems of interpretation and assessment of severity of disease.

2. Transferable

This is a very important requirement, particularly since the diagnosis of AD rests on a form of quantitative estimation of the amount of pathological change. In relation to this, a European multi-centre study supported by EURAGE was published by Duyckaerts *et al.* (1990) which showed that there was marked variation in absolute numerical values in plaque and tangle counts from different centres, although there was much better agreement among the different centres about the ranking of the cases submitted. More recently, similar results have been obtained by Dr Mirra and her collaborators in CERAD (Mirra *et al.* 1994). In a study of differences among laboratories using the same staining techniques as in the EURAGE study, although the specific numbers were very variable among the different centres, when a semi-quantitative rather than a quantitative method was used (i.e. the methodology suggested by CERAD) the different laboratories were very close in the order in which they ranked the cases for severity. These findings demonstrate that numerical methods can not at present be recommended for use as the basis of a diagnostic standard where different laboratories will be using a common assessment methodology. In individual laboratories, where there is a specific research purpose and a much more detailed methodology, strictly quantitative methods are more appropriate.

3. Validated

As has been described, the major currently existing diagnostic standards for AD are those of Khatchaturian, CERAD, and Tierney. Both Khatchaturian and CERAD have had very wide exposure. In relation to the various diagnostic criteria for AD, we in Oxford have been collecting prospectively assessed cases for the last few years in the OPTIMA (Oxford Project to Investigate Memory and Ageing) project and have performed a comparative assessment of the Khatchaturian, CERAD and Tierney A3 staging in relation to the cognitive status prior to death (Nagy *et al.*, 1995). Overall, CERAD offers the best correlation. This is true even though the best correlation in terms of individual microscopic findings is with tangle numbers in the frontal and parietal lobes. As already mentioned, this reflects the fact that CERAD requires the age-adjusted semi-quantitative assessment of neuritic plaques and not just total plaques and is therefore really more a measure of neuritic pathology than plaque number. Validation requires that known non demented as well as demented cases are analysed to discover the 'false positive' rate that a given set of criteria may produce. This has unfortunately not been carried out for any of the above criteria as yet.

4. Versatile

In this area CERAD stands alone since, of the currently available diagnostic criteria, it is the only one that explicitly envisages the possibility of diagnoses other than AD.

Overall, this review of the currently available diagnostic criteria for AD clearly brings us to the conclusion that CERAD (or a modification) should be recommended as the standard diagnostic tool for AD. No single diagnostic protocol is likely to be completely satisfactory for all purposes, but in our view CERAD has the merits of being:

a.   Relatively simple
b.   Has been successfully applied in a number of different centres.
c.   Has obtained wide national and international recognition and is regularly updated.
d.   A diagnostic protocol that is able to be used for most if not all cases that are submitted as dementia (a significant fraction of which will not be AD).

Beyond the selection of suitable diagnostic criteria there are two other practical aspects to the diagnosis of AD.

The use of clinical information in the diagnosis of AD

This is not really considered in most of the pathological diagnostic criteria for AD, except to the extent that 'dementia' may or may not be present clinically, although both Khatchaturian and CERAD require some clinical information to complete the assessment. Any discussion of the role of clinical information raises the question of whether the diagnosis of AD can be made in a patient with no history of dementia because the patient has never been examined – Khatchaturian and CERAD both have (albeit rather different) answers to this particular conundrum. Using the Khatchaturian criteria, a history of dementia allows the possible reduction in the amount of pathological change required for the diagnosis and specifically admits the possibility of making the diagnosis of AD in the absence of any clinical history of dementia. By contrast, CERAD allows only the diagnosis of possible AD in the absence of a history of dementia, no matter how severe the pathological changes.

A related question is what sort of clinical information is desirable in the study of patients with AD. At a recent MRC sponsored conference on brain banking in dementia it was suggested that minimum clinical information in dementia should consist of:

a.   A clinical vignette
b.   A clinical diagnosis made on operation criteria (DSM III)
c.   A standardized rating of mental function (eg. MMSE)
d.   A dementia severity rating
e.   Preferably recurrent testing at 6-month intervals if possible.

Differential diagnosis

There are three aspects to this question. The first is that of the differential diagnosis of patients with dementia who are submitted for neuropathological examination with a clinical diagnosis of 'Alzheimer's disease'. This is adequately covered in the requirement for versatility in the diagnostic protocol.

The second is the rather shorter list of conditions that could be mistaken histopathologically for AD. About the only disease that could be seriously confused with AD would be Gerstmann–Sträussler syndrome where, as is not infrequent, the neocortical amyloid deposits are accompanied by marked tangle formation. While this can certainly occur and make the neocortical appearance possible to confuse with AD, the microscopic appearance of the cerebellum is usually quite characteristic in GSS and markedly different from AD. If there is any doubt, immunocytochemistry could be used to define the prion origin for the amyloid deposits in GSS. A second differential involves cortical Lewy body disease in which plaques occur in cortex more abundantly than might be expected by chance. Most cases of cortical Lewy body disease have almost exclusively non-neuritic plaques in cortex but some cases also have neuritic plaques. Thus, it is necessary to examine all cases of suspected AD for the possible presence of cortical Lewy bodies. Such a search is indicated if there are Lewy bodies in the substantia nigra (see further discussion in Chapter 6). A third differential that may be mentioned is progressive supranuclear palsy in which quite extensive neurofibrillary pathology may be present in the cortex. However, in this condition there is usually macroscopic dilatation of the fourth ventricle, not seen in AD, and abundant microscopic subcortical pathology, as described in Chapter 10, also not seen in AD. Even in the cortex, neurofibrillary pathology shows a subtly different distribution in progressive supranuclear palsy than in AD with, for example, neurofibrillary tangles in the dentate gyrus of the hippocampus.

The third aspect in the differential diagnosis of AD is the question of how to classify the non-demented aged with some Alzheimer changes. This is where, as a practical matter, we need to distinguish between a staging system such as the Braak classification and diagnostic criteria for AD. The question that is being asked here is what can and can not be included in the diagnosis of AD, and is there such a thing as 'pre-Alzheimer's disease' (i.e. patients that are going to go on to develop dementia) that can be identified neuropathologically before the patient has any symptoms of dementia? What view is taken on this depends very much on how the pathophysiology of AD is envisaged. If β/A4 protein amyloid deposition is considered to be an essential and early stage in the process that leads to the development of neuritic pathology in AD, then restricted neurofibrillary change or amyloid deposition without cortical neuritic pathology might represent a presymptomatic stage of Alzheimer's disease. This is a point made by Braak in his stages 1–4 where tangles are confined to the hippocampus and entorhinal cortex.

Our view on this is that, although it is in fact a very important practical issue, there is currently insufficient information to offer useful guidance. We regard this very much as an area for active research that will require the examination of a large number of non-demented prospectively assessed controls to be able to formulate an answer to this question.

A minimalist approach to the pathological diagnosis of AD

The pathological scenario that we have been discussing in the last few paragraphs, and which reflects the whole thrust of this volume, has been geared towards the needs of those with a specific interest in dementia in general and AD in particular. Somewhat reluctantly, we are forced to acknowledge that there is also another world where a more ruthlessly pragmatic approach to diagnosis is frequently taken. The needs of the pathologist working in this milieu can be encapsulated in the question 'what is the minimum sampling and staining required to make the diagnosis of AD?'

While we have had to suppress all our neuro-

pathological instincts to write this, we have concluded that the short answer is two sections, each of which can be accommodated on a standard slide. Our recommended sections are:

1. Frontal or parietal convexity.
2. Lateral temporal lobe, which should include the middle temporal gyrus.

The sections should be stained with H&E and a silver stain, preferably one that shows both plaques and tangles. It is perhaps worth mentioning that, in a minimalist approach, we specifically do not recommend sampling the hippocampus. Ball and colleagues (1977) have shown that the appearance of the hippocampus in AD is unreliable from a diagnostic standpoint. In this situation the appearance of the hippocampus can be quite misleading since there are frequently moderate and even large numbers of neurofibrillary tangles present in aged people with no significant cognitive decline. Conversely, in AD the severity of the neuronal loss can sometimes produce the appearance of very little neuritic pathology.

In the frontal or parietal lobe section, the presence of significant numbers of tangles, which will invariably be accompanied by neuritic plaques, will be sufficient to make the diagnosis of AD. The rationale for also taking a section of temporal lobe is that, particularly in very old patients, it is our judgement that AD can be present with significant lateral temporal lobe tangle formation but relatively few, if any, tangles being found in the frontal or parietal lobes. It is possible, however, that many of these patients may have other processes such as diffuse Lewy body formation that might be contributing to their dementia.

The reason for not relying only on a temporal lobe section is that in younger patients with only moderate temporal lobe Alzheimer pathology, the absence of frontal or parietal lobe involvement would dissuade us from making the diagnosis of AD.

As might be expected, the minimalist approach comes with the neuropathological equivalent of a government health warning to the effect that, although these two sections will allow the diagnosis of AD to be made, they are not adequate for the diagnosis of almost all other causes of dementia. Hence, dementia as a result of another process will not be diagnosable, and, further, other processes contributing to the dementia will also probably be missed.

PATHOGENESIS OF ALZHEIMER'S DISEASE

Particularly in the past decade there has been an enormous expansion in the volume of published work on AD. This reflects both the wide recognition of the social and financial impact of AD in an ageing population and the major advances that have occurred in our understanding of the pathogenesis of the Alzheimer process over the last decade. What follows is the briefest of surveys, that covers only the major highlights of the story as it is currently understood and refers directly to only a small fraction of the published literature. As with all fields of scientific endeavour, one of the features of the progress of ideas is unpredictability. What seems like an obvious line of advance can be diverted into quite another channel by an unexpected finding. At the time of writing, what might best be called the 'amyloid hypothesis' of AD pathogenesis probably commands the widest general support with the AD research community, but there is no security of tenure in science and it should certainly not be regarded as received and immutable wisdom.

To maintain some sort of organization it has been divided into sections on molecular genetics, neuritic pathology and amyloid. There is necessarily considerable overlap among these areas and this inevitably generates some repetition, for which reader toleration is requested. For those wishing to delve further into the labyrinth of AD pathogenesis, there are a number of excellent recent introductory reviews by recognized experts in their field that provide an initial guide down the various avenues of current AD research. For the molecular genetics and familial AD these include: Clark and Goate (1993); St George-Hyslop (1993); Mullen & Crawford (1993); Rossor (1992); Van Broeckhoven (1995). Tau protein and neurofibrillary pathology: Kosik (1992), Goedert (1993). β/A4-amyloid protection and its metabolism: Joachim & Selkoe (1992); Selkoe (1993), Mattson et al. (1993), Smith and Anderton (1994). Two of the major players in the ApoE and amyloid stories have recently summarized their positions in adjacent articles (Selkoe, 1994; Roses, 1994) with Hyman and Terry (1994) acting as referee in an accompanying editorial. However, AD research is so fast-moving that, by the time any review, and certainly any book, is printed, there will have already been some significant recent results that will modify, though hopefully not completely overturn, our current concepts of pathogenesis in AD.

Molecular genetics

As has been described, epidemiological studies of AD looking for risk factors for the development of the disease have consistently shown the importance of the presence of a positive family history for the disease. Although most cases of AD are not clearly familial, there are a minority of families, most with early onset disease, in which AD appears to be inherited in the manner of an autosomal dominant gene. In those families without a clear inheritance pattern, although first-degree relatives are at increased risk of developing the disease, there is wide divergence of opinion as to the extent of the risk (Huff et al., 1988; Breitner et al., 1988; Van Duijn et al., 1991; Heyman et al., 1984; Rocca et al., 1986).

The study of the molecular genetics of AD is relatively young, but its earliest results (St. George-Hyslop et al., 1990) confirmed earlier suggestions (Mayeux, Stern & Spanton, 1985) that what we call AD is aetiologically heterogeneous, and later findings unambiguously have confirmed this supposition (Hyman & Tanzi, 1995). In overall terms, what has been shown is that, in early onset AD, there are familial cases that are inherited in a mendelian pattern that have been linked to mutations of genes on chromosomes 1, 14 and 21 and that, together, they probably account for almost all these inherited cases. In addition to these cases inherited as a result of a genetic defect, the allelic inheritance of the apolipoprotein gene on chromosome 19 has a large influence on the susceptibility to the development of AD in older age groups. It is also the case that there are large numbers of late onset cases that are familial, but that in these cases no clear inheritance pattern is evident suggesting that, although there is a major genetic component, it is polygenic.

Early onset familial AD

Chromosome 21

Molecular genetic interest initially focussed on chromosome 21 because of the long recognized association between Down's syndrome (trisomy 21) and Alzheimer change in that virtually all Down's syndrome patients who survive into their fourth decade develop the pathological features of AD (Heston & Mastri, 1977). The attraction of chromosome 21 was significantly increased when it was recognized that the gene for the β/A4-amyloid precursor protein, which is the source of the specific β/A4 protein that forms the amyloid deposits at the centre of the plaques in AD, and is also deposited in the cerebral vessels, was located on the long arm of this chromosome close to the Down's syndrome critical region. Not surprisingly, attention was concentrated on the β/A4 amyloid precursor protein (βAPP) gene, as the potential source of the genetic defect responsible for familial AD (St George-Hyslop et al., 1987). Although the search for a specific linkage with the APP gene was initially unsuccessful (Schellenberg et al., 1988; Tanzi et al., 1987; van Broechhaven et al., 1987), Goate et al. (1991) found evidence of linkage of AD to chromosome 21 in a single family. Subsequently this was shown to be the result of a valine-to-isoleucine substitution at codon 717 of the APP770 which is in the transmembrane portion of the βAPP and just outside the β/A4 region of the protein. By late 1993 a total of 11 families had been identified with this mutation that segregates with AD (Naruse et al., 1991; Yoshioka et al., 1991, Karlinsky et al., 1992; Fidani et al., 1992; Sorbi et al., 1993). Conversely, the mutation has not been found to be present in normal individuals or in a large number of other families who do not have early onset AD. As has been indicated above, this sort of mutation is associated with early onset disease, and in the affected families, mean age of onset has been in the fifth and sixth decades (Hardy et al., 1991).

A number of other mutations have been described in the APP gene on chromosome 21. Two are at the same location as that described by Goate et al. (1991) (APP717) but substitute glycine and phenylalanine for the valine normally present at this location (Chartier-Harlin et al., 1991a,b; Murrell et al., 1991; Kennedy et al., 1993; Farlow et al., 1994). A double point mutation has also been described at APP670/671 in a Swedish familial AD kindred (Mullen et al., 1992a).

All the families with mutations in these two locations show early onset AD, but there are other mutations in the APP gene that manifest not as a progressive dementia, but as hereditary cerebral haemorrhage with amyloidosis. In the affected families there is large-scale deposition of amyloid in cerebral vessels and the formation of numerous diffuse plaques in the cerebral parenchyma. Affected individuals tend to suffer from recurrent cerebral haemorrhages starting in their 40s. The first family with this disease was found to have a mutation at APP693 that results in the substitution of glutamine for glutamic acid (Levy et al., 1990) although in a subsequent family with a similar phenotype, the affected individuals have an amino acid substitution at codon 692 (Hendriks et al., 1992). This second family is particularly interesting in that the family members with the gene defect may present either with cerebral haemorrhages or with dementia although it is not known what factors influence the mode of presentation.

In addition to these symptomatic gene defects, genetic study of the APP gene has revealed a small number of other point mutations that have no clear association with AD either because they were found in normal individuals or in single patients where there was no evidence of segregation with disease (Clark & Goate, 1993).

Although the findings on chromosome 21 are very interesting and indicate that there are circumstances where modification of the APP gene can lead to the development of AD, it must also be remembered that linkage to genetic abnormalities on chromosome 21 is present in only a very small fraction (probably only 2–3%) of the early onset familial cases of AD (van Broeckhoven et al., 1987; Chartier-Harlan et al., 1991b). The recognition of this resulted in the search for linkage to early onset familial disease on other chromosomes.

Chromosome 14

At least four studies of familial groups have indicated linkage of early onset familial AD to a locus on the long arm of chromosome 14 (Schellenberg et al., 1992b; van Broeckhoven et al., 1992; St. George-Hyslop et al., 1992; Mullan et al., 1992a; Haltia et al., 1994). In contrast to the rather small fraction of early onset familial AD cases linked to abnormalities on chromosome 21, as many as 70% of cases of early onset familial AD may link to the locus on chromosome 14. Many of these cases also have an unusually early onset (approximately a decade earlier than those with chromosome 21 mutations) suggesting that the defect has a fundamental effect on the processes leading to the development of AD.

In initial studies of this chromosome the region flanking the disease locus was first narrowed to a 8.9 megabase region at 14q24.3. Candidate genes for the AD disease locus included promising contenders such as HSPA-2, a 70 kD heat shock protein, the proto-oncogene c-Fos, which is a DNA binding regulatory protein and α-1-antichymotrypsin. However, science advances in mysterious ways and these seemingly promising contenders appear all to have been eliminated by Sherrington et al. (1995) who have cloned a gene that they have designated S182 from six linked pedigrees where there are five different missense mutations found only in family members with AD. Not a great deal is currently known about this 467 amino acid protein but it has a very characteristic structure with seven linked transmembrane regions, with regions 6 and 7 being linked by a longer sequence than the others. The molecular configuration is indicative of an integral membrane protein that might be a receptor or a channel component. A protein with known homology appears to be a constituent of Golgi derived membranes in the sperm of *Caenorhabditis elegans* and immunocytochemical studies of A182 suggest an intracellular location in both Golgi and endoplasmic reticulum. Several defects have already been located in S182, most of which seem to be concentrated in the second and third transmembrane regions and in the connecting sequence between transmembrane regions 6 and 7. The nature of the metabolic disturbance introduced by the genetic defects is not clearly established as yet although there are some suggestions that cells from patients with defects in the S182 gene make increased amounts of β-amyloid. However, as noted by Selkoe (1995) in his commentary on the findings of Sherrington *et al.*, 'speculating about the malfunction of a newly discovered gene whose product has not even been seen, let alone characterised, is risky!'

Chromosome 1

Chromosomes 21 and 14 do not exhaust the possible locations for genetic abnormalities associated with early onset familial AD. In the course of their studies of genetically related Volga German families, Schellenberg *et al.*, (1992*b*), have demonstrated that the disease in these families with early onset disease is not linked to abnormalities on either chromosome 14 or 21. The genetic defect in this group has recently been identified in a gene at chromosome 1q31–42 as a molecule with a very high degree of structural and amino acid sequence homology to the S182 protein coded for on chromosome 14, including the characteristic 7 transmembrane regions (Levy-Lahad *et al.*, 1995*a*, *b*). Because of the structural homology, the gene product has been initially referred to as STM 2 (standing for second seven transmembrane gene associated with AD but is now more frequently called presenilin 2). Within the transmembrane regions of the molecule 84% of the amino acid sequence is identical in S182 and STM2. This high degree of homology was in fact a significant element in the identification of this particular gene as the most probable candidate gene for the cause of AD in the Volga German families. Another source of similarity between STM2 and S182 is that the genetic defect in the Volga German families on STM2 has been located close to the beginning of one of the transmembrane regions, as also are several of the reported mutations in the S182 gene. It seems very likely that mutations of the gene on chromosome 1 will have generally similar metabolic

effects to the S182 gene on chromosome 14, and will also prove to be the cause of AD in other families with AD that have genetic defects that are as yet unidentified.

The mechanisms by which these mutations in the APP gene, on chromosome 14 and chromosome 1 produce AD are not addressed by molecular genetic techniques. However, in relation to APP gene defects on chromosome 21, one highly suggestive finding is that cells *in vitro* transfected with APP containing the 670/671 mutation have been found to have a 5–8 fold increase in β/A4 production (Cai, Golde & Younkin, 1993). Increased β/A4 production could plausibly be associated with an increased likelihood of amyloid deposition, thereby initiating the pathophysiologic cascade leading to the development of AD. The consequences to APP metabolism of the other mutations of the APP gene have not yet been established. Effects on β/A4 production and metabolism clearly need to be looked for in mutations of chromosomes 1 and 14 as well as chromosome 21. However, the possibility that some of the effects of chromosome mutations, especially those that do not directly affect the APP gene, operate remotely or on selected cell populations such as for example, microglial cells, may make them difficult to investigate in *in vitro* systems.

Late-onset AD

Most of the genetic linkage and molecular studies have concentrated on families with early disease, and there has been relatively little work on the genetics of late onset disease. This is largely because of the inherent and ineradicable difficulties of working with older age groups. However, AD has frequently been observed to cluster in families with late onset although, because the disease is so common in the elderly population, some degree of familial clustering can be expected for non-genetic reasons.

Chromosome 19

The prevailing view is that most of the late onset forms of AD are multifactorial in origin with contributions from genetic and environmental influences. In this group the predominant genetic influences are presumed to be polygenic and large scale segregation analyses in this group of patients has suggested that a major gene effect was responsible for only about 4% of the variance (Farrar *et al.*, 1991). However, linkage analysis in families with late onset AD suggested an association with markers on the proximal part of the long arm of chromosome 19 at position q13.2 (Pericak-Vance *et al.*, 1991).

Alzheimer's disease and the apolipoproteins

Two genes that map to the appropriate region on chromosome 19q13.2 are those for apolipoprotein CII and apolipoprotein E and association studies have been carried out for both of these genes. Apolipoprotein C2 (ApoC2) was found to be significantly increased in affected family members in 23 families (Schellenberg *et al.*, 1987, 1992*a*). Perhaps more significantly, in the initial report, the frequency of the ε4 allele of Apolipoprotein E was increased from 13% to 48% in a group of 30 AD patients from different families (Strittmatter *et al.*, 1993). These results effectively were duplicated in numerous subsequent studies of familial and sporadic late onset cases which show a significantly increased frequency of the ε4 allele compared to age and gender matched controls (Corder *et al.*, 1993; Chartier-Harlin *et al.*, 1994; Saunders *et al.*, 1993; Mayeux *et al.*, 1993; Noguchi, Murakami & Yamada, 1993; Payami *et al.*, 1993).

The, already considerable, interest in the apolipoprotein gene was greatly augmented when it was shown by the Duke University group that while the possession of the ε4 allele is associated with an increase in the frequency of AD, the frequency of the ε2 allele in patients with AD is markedly lower than in the normal population (Corder *et al.*, 1994). Possession of the ε2 allele therefore confers protection against the development of Alzheimer's disease. This result has been strengthened by studies in our own OPTIMA population of prospectively assessed post-mortem confirmed cases of AD (Smith *et al.*, 1994). Interestingly, ApoE genes do not seem to have any effect on the incidence of either Parkinson's disease or diffuse Lewy body disease (Benjamin *et al.*, 1994*b*), and it has been recently reported that there is no association between apolipoprotein ε4 and AD in Nigerians (Osuntokun *et al.*, 1995), although interestingly there is a reported association in African Americans (Hendrie *et al.*, 1995). It has also been shown that possession of the ε2 allele also protects against heart disease and leads to an increase in the frequency of the ε2 allele in centenarians compared to younger age groups (Menzel *et al.*, 1983). This finding demonstrates that the protective effect cannot be an artefact of early death from other causes of patients with the ε2 allele who, had they survived, would subsequently have gone on to develop AD.

It is not at all clear how the known functions of these proteins could be relevant to the development of AD. It is possible to envisage ways that they might influence the processing of βAPP and apoE has been detected in amyloid deposits (of both Alzheimer and non-Alzheimer type), neurofibrillary tangles and congophilic angiopathy (Namba *et al.*, 1991). There are also some indications that the different isoforms of apoE bind amyloid to different degrees, with the ε4 isoform having a more rapid binding (Strittmatter *et al.*, 1993). This has led to the suggestion that apoE might, in some way, enhance the sequestration of soluble β/A4 into plaques and thus hasten the development of one of the significant morphologic manifestations of AD. It has been reported that patients with the ε4 allele have significantly greater vascular and plaque β/A4 deposition in the cerebral cortex (Schmechel *et al.*, 1993). At the molecular level there has been great interest in the interaction between the different apolipoprotein alleles and β/A4. Ma *et al.* (1994) have shown that Apo ε4 produces a greater acceleration in amyloid fibril formation than either apo ε2 or apo ε3. In an interesting correlation with the recent evidence that the predominant β/A4 species in plaques is Aβ1–42(43) it was also shown that the effect of apo ε4 was significantly more pronounced on Aβ1–42(43) than on Aβ1–40. While not conclusive these recent results tend to suggest that the presence of the apo ε4 allele might be expected to enhance any tendency to fibrillar amyloid deposition and plaque formation and might therefore be expected to favour the development of AD (Younkin, 1995). A recent study from Finland (Polvikoski *et al.*, 1995) has shown that there is a correlation between apoliprotein E genotype and the presence of dementia, the frequency and degree of cortical amyloid deposition, and the number of neurofibrillary tangles in a community study of patients over the age of 85 years. These features were all found to the greatest degree in patients with the ε4/ε4 or ε4/ε3 genotype, and to a progressively lesser degree in patients with the ε3/ε3 and ε3/ε2 genotypes. In terms of the dementia, 28 of 33 patients carrying the ε4 allele were demented, although the presence of 5 patients carrying the ε4 allele who were not demented shows that other factors must be involved in the development of dementia and confirms the status of the apoliprotein status as a major risk factor for the development of dementia.

A rather more heterodox view of the significance of the ε4 isoform in AD that has recently been put forward by Rose and Strittmatter is that the association might take the form of preferential protection of patients with the apo ε2 genes making such patients less likely to develop AD. Their suggestion is that this might occur by differences in the binding to tau protein which would prevent, or at least influence, the abnormal phosphorylation of tau that occurs in the formation of neurofibrillary pathology (Roses, 1994). There have been a number of detailed objections raised to this suggestion, not least the way in which it bypasses the role of β/A4 protein amyloid (Selkoe, 1994; Strittmatter *et al.*, 1994), and it remains highly speculative. In one significant respect the debate about the significance of the apolipoproteins coded for on chromosome 19 differs from the other genetic associations of AD in that there is no suggestion of a genetic defect on chromosome 19, but rather that the different normal apolipoprotein alleles confer a different predisposition to develop AD. The apolipoproteins are more properly considered as normally occurring genetically determined risk factors for AD not genetic defects that initiate or accelerate the pathophysiology of the Alzheimer process.

By introducing the topic of the amyloid precursor protein the discussion of the molecular biology of AD, has to a degree anticipated the examination of the cellular pathophysiology. The two major neuropathological features of Alzheimer's disease are senile plaques and neurofibrillary pathology. There is, as indicated, clear evidence to suggest that the development of neuritic pathology in the form of neurofibrillary tangles and other neuritic components is the key determinant of the development of the dementia seen in AD. Neuritic pathology however, is not unique to Alzheimer's disease, occurring for example in other degenerative diseases such as progressive Supranuclear Palsy, ALS/Parkinsonism/Dementia of Guam, and Gerstmann–Sträussler–Scheinker syndrome.

Amyloid in Alzheimer's disease

Unlike neurofibrillary pathology, which occurs in a number of quite disparate pathological processes, the amyloid that is deposited in AD is rather more specific. To claim that it is deposited in AD is rather more specific. To claim that it is unique to AD would not be quite correct, since amyloid angiopathy is quite frequently seen in the brains of older people who do not have AD. As mentioned above in the discussion of the molecular biology of chromosome 21, there is a hereditary disease characterized by deposition of vascular amyloid that results in recurrent cerebral haemorrhage without the necessary presence of dementia or other features of AD. However, the existence of some families with early onset AD associated with a genetic abnormality in the APP gene establishes amyloid deposition as one of the central processes in the development of AD. Hence, an understanding of the pathophysiology and consequences of amyloid production and deposition are

central to an understanding of the pathophysiology of AD itself, and over the past decade an enormous volume of published work has focused on the process of amyloid production and deposition in aged brains and AD.

Metabolism of APP and production of β/A4

As has already been mentioned, the amyloid in AD is produced from the β amyloid precursor protein (βAPP) located on chromosome 21. This protein is actually a small family of transmembrane glycoproteins that exists in at least four forms, that arise as a result of variable exon splicing of a single gene. Two forms, βAPP^{751} and βAPP^{770} contain a Kunitz-type protease inhibitor (KPI) domain, while the other two, βAPP^{695} and βAPP^{714} do not (Neve, Finch & Dawes, 1988). The function of the molecule is not known, although its primary structure with an intracellular C-terminus, a transmembrane region and an extracellular N-terminus have led to the suggestion that it may function as a cell surface receptor (Kang *et al.*, 1987).

βAPP is expressed in almost all mammalian cells and shows a high degree of evolutionary conservation. Although the function of βAPP is not known, there are several circumstances that alter its cellular expression. These include metabolic insults such as ischaemia and head trauma, and also exposure to excitotoxins, all of which upregulate expression of βAPP. βAPP levels also vary during development and in response to neurotrophic factors and cytokines. None of these influences gives any very specific indication of βAPP function, but have suggested that it might have a role in neuronal plasticity and the responses of the brain to trauma or other damage. In AD there is deposition of what is called β/A4-amyloid that is derived from a fragment of this molecule. Conceptually, the process of amyloid formation could be a result of excess production of amyloid β as a result of overexpression of the βAPP gene, the production of an abnormal gene product or altered processing of normally derived β-amyloid fragment. The heterogeneity that we have already seen in the genetic influences on the development of AD make it probable that all three of these mechanisms operate in the pathogenesis of AD.

The β/A4-amyloid protein (β/A4) deposited in AD is composed of a hydrophobic peptide derived from the βAPP that is 40–42 amino acids long derived from a part of the βAPP molecule 12–14 of which are intramembranous with a 28 amino acid extracellular segment (Kang *et al.*, 1987). There is now a considerable body of literature on the possible mechanisms of production of $\beta/A4$ from the APP. At least three different cellular mechanisms of APP processing have been discovered. One mechanism is the action of the so-called α-secretase which cleaves intact *in situ* APP just outside the transmembrane region. This mode of processing precludes $\beta/A4$ protein production because the cleavage site is within the $\beta/A4$ protein region. The action of this enzyme releases a soluble product (APP$_s$) into the medium (Esch *et al.*, 1990). However, studies have shown that this mechanism probably accounts for a minority fraction of cellular APP processing and this finding, together with the obvious fact of $\beta/A4$ deposition in many aged brains, prompted the search for alternative methods of APP processing that would release the $\beta/A4$ fragment and permit the deposition of $\beta/A4$ amyloid.

This search rapidly led to the discovery of a lysosomal pathway processing APP, which is capable of producing Aβ. Protein chemical studies demonstrating the accumulation of $\beta/A4$-containing fragments in cells in which lysosomal function has been inhibited have been supported by the direct immunocytochemical demonstration of $\beta/A4$ epitopes in lysosomes (Golde *et al.*, 1992). Further evidence for the existence of a lysosomal pathway was the demonstration that APP labelled with antibodies or biotin is incorporated into lysosomes (Benowitz *et al.*, 1989; Hass *et al.*, 1992*a*).

To these two pathways, a third has recently been added with the discovery that $\beta/A4$ is normally secreted as a soluble peptide into biological media (Hass *et al.*, 1992*b*; Seubert *et al.*, 1992; Shoji *et al.*, 1992). This process seems to occur in the absence of any membrane injury and to be a normal part of the metabolism of the cell, and its occurrence suggests that $\beta/A4$ production is not necessarily a manifestation of aberrant intermediary metabolism in a damaged or defective cell. The $\beta/A4$ so produced has been detected using $\beta/A4$ antibodies to immunoprecipitate the conditioned media. Sequencing of the immunoprecipitated material shows it to be $\beta/A4^{32-34}$. This form of $\beta/A4$ secretion has been found in a variety of cells types in culture including human neurons, astrocytes and endothelial cells, but, in these experiments, is not detectable in lysosomes. The site of production of the $\beta/A4$ in this processing pathway is not certain, although the Golgi apparatus has been suggested as one possibility. One possibility that is raised by the finding of $\beta/A4$ secretion as a result of normal intermediary metabolism is that it might have a normal physiological function.

Currently, this is a speculative suggestion, that is made at least credible by its action to produce trophic effects on neurones when added to culture medium and the recent demonstration of its ability to interact with extracellular matrix components to promote neurite outgrowth (Selkoe, 1994).

Neurotoxicity of amyloid

A more conventional role for $\beta/A4$ is that of a neurotoxin, this being a more obvious way in which the deposition of amyloid could be a harbinger for the subsequent development of neuritic pathology. One of the difficulties in accepting a simple model of $\beta/A4$ as a significant neurotoxin is the existence of the diffuse plaque. As described earlier, diffuse plaques are 'amorphous' deposits of $\beta/A4$ that occur in grey matter and that are not apparently associated with any disturbance in the tissue. There is no detectable sign of damage to neurons or glia in association with these deposits, a finding that indicates that the mere presence of $\beta/A4$ alone does not produce detectable parenchymal damage. This has been seen by some as a major objection to the 'amyloid hypothesis' of AD, but the deposition of $\beta/A4$ and its evolution into $\beta/A4$ protein amyloid is a multistage process of which the deposition of $\beta/A4$ in the tissue is only the first. The evolution of the mature plaque, from the initial deposition of $\beta/A4$ to a senile plaque with a central core of fibrillar $\beta/A4$ protein amyloid surrounded by a halo of distorted phf containing neurites, is a process that offers several possible avenues that could lead to local cell damage (for ref. see Smith & Anderton, 1994).

In diffuse plaques, although $\beta/A4$ is present, ultrastructural examination shows few or none of the fibrils characteristic of the amyloid seen in mature plaque cores and amyloid angiopathy. The development of the more conventional plaque core involves a molecular conformational change of the $\beta/A4$ peptide to a β-pleated sheet and the aggregation of these changed molecules into fibrils. This change in physico-chemical state of $\beta/A4$ could, of itself, substantially alter its local effects. In support of this suggestion there is some experimental evidence that the use of '*in vitro* aged' Aβ, where prolonged incubation of synthetic peptides in buffer leads to conformational change and aggregation, can increase the toxicity of $\beta/A4$ for cultured neurones. This conformational change in $\beta/A4$ is a key step in the pathophysiology of AD, since it converts $\beta/A4$ into a form that is associated with the onset of a cascade of tissue damage that leads to the neuritic change that correlates with the dementia of AD. The mechanisms that bring about the conformational change in the brain during life are not known, but tissue factors must play a role, since, as noted earlier, while there is progressive accumulation of neuritic plaques in cerebral cortex, this does not occur in the basal ganglia or the cerebellum. In these two areas of the brain, β/A4 remains in diffuse unaggregated form and stimulates little or no neuritic reaction, even when there is prominent neuritic pathology elsewhere in the brain. One natural mechanism that could have a role in the conversion of β/A4 from a non-aggregating to an aggregating form is the action of free radicals. Dyrks et al. (1993) have shown that β/A4 expressed in an *in vitro* system did not spontaneously aggregate, but could be converted into an aggregating form of similar pattern to that of β/A4 isolated from brain by exposure to free radical generating systems. They also showed that the conversion process was inhibited by the addition of free radical scavengers such as ascorbic acid. Conformational change and fibril aggregation is not the only change affecting β/A4 during the formation of a mature plaque. The deposition of amyloid fibrils in the tissue is also associated with the progressive accumulation of a number of other amyloid associated proteins such as components of the complement pathway, apolipoprotein E, α_1-antichymotrypsin and heparan sulphate proteoglycans. These are all potentially active locally although the sum of their actions is hard to predict.

Neurofibrillary pathology

Although the role of β/A4 amyloid protein in the pathogenesis of AD has attracted a great deal of attention, the mere deposition of the β/A4 protein in the tissues is insufficient to produce cognitive decline in the patients. There are a number of good studies of β/A4 protein amyloid deposition and non-neuritic senile plaques that show significant overlap between normals and patients with symptomatic AD (Crystal et al., 1988, 1993; Davies et al., 1988). The best correlations of morphological change with cognitive decline are with the formation of neuritic pathology. As has been described earlier, neuritic pathology occurs in three basic forms; neurofibrillary tangles that develop in the cell bodies and apical dendrites of neurones, the so-called neuropil threads which form in distal dendrites and the abnormal dilated tortuous neurites seen in association with some amyloid deposits (neuritic plaques) (See Chapter 1). All these structures have in common the presence of paired helical filaments (phf) as their major

component and a smaller component of straight filaments. PHF are relatively insoluble so that the degeneration of the nerve cell does not result in the immediate dissolution of the phf which remain as extracellular 'ghost' tangles that can be seen in the neuropil. Ghost tangles are most prominent in the entorhinal cortex and the hippocampus where they may be present in large numbers, but can usually be seen in other areas such as the nucleus basalis of Meynert, the periaqueductal grey and the raphe and the locus ceruleus. Curiously, they are rarely conspicuous in the neocortex, even when there are large numbers of intracellular tangles.

Although characteristic of AD, it is very important to recognize that, unlike the β-amyloid protein, neurofibrillary tangles are not specific to the Alzheimer process. They are found in a number of different disorders, notably progressive supranuclear palsy and subacute sclerosing panencephalitis where there is no amyloid deposition, and also in Gerstmann–Sträussler syndrome where there is amyloid deposition, but in this disease the amyloid is composed of a completely different protein, prion protein. Tangles should therefore be seen, at least to some extent, as a final common path of different pathophysiological processes of neuronal damage. The challenge in each of the diseases where tangles are formed is to elucidate the cell biology that leads to their formation.

Composition of tangles

There has been a large amount of work relating to the molecular biology and chemistry of neurofibrillary pathology and tau and other proteins and recent reviews include those of Kosik (1992), Goedert (1993) and Smith and Anderton (1994). phf are composed almost entirely of an abnormally phosphorylated variant of a normally occurring cellular protein associated with microtubules called tau. When combined into tangles, phf are extremely insoluble and correspondingly hard to study, but there is a phase where phf have formed within the cytoplasm but not yet aggregated into tangles and in this dispersed form phf are much more soluble. Work on tau and neurofibrillary pathology has been greatly aided by the discovery in 1991 of extraction techniques for the dispersed phf. In the normal adult cell tau is produced in six isoforms ranging in size from 352 to 441 amino acids with three or four sets of tandem repeats and lettered A–F in order of increasing size (Goedert et al., 1989; Himmler, 1989). Foetal cells produce only isoform A. Much of the work done on the function of this protein has been done *in vitro*, but it is almost certain that the normal function of this protein is to promote the formation and increase the stability of the cytoplasmic microtubules. Experiments in which anti-sense oligonucleotides to block the function of tau have been inserted in developing neurones show that this prevents differentiation of neurites into the axon and suggest that tau is important in the development of axonal morphology. This is reflected in the presence of microtubules within the normal axon and it is reasonable to suppose that any process that seriously disrupts the formation and stability of microtubules would have a significant effect on axonal morphology and functions such as rapid axonal transport in which microtubules play a critical role.

Phosphorylation of tau and the formation of phf

Normal adult tau has a number of phosphorylation sites that play a key role in its normal physiological function. Increasing the phosphorylation state reduces the degree of binding of tau to microtubules (Bramblett *et al.*, 1993) and regulation of the processes of phosphorylation and dephosphorylation of tau is probably critical to its normal function. In tau isolated from material obtained at post-mortem, a major difference between normal functioning tau and the tau protein found in neurofibrillary tangles and phf is that the tau in phf is much more heavily phosphorylated (Lee *et al.*, 1991; Hasagawa *et al.*, 1992). Curiously, as was suggested by the fact that antibodies to foetal tau label neurofibrillary tangles while antibodies to normal adult tau do not, foetal tau is much more heavily phosphorylated than the normal adult isoforms isolated from post-mortem brain. In this respect it more closely resembles the degree of phosphorylation seen in phf tau. These results tended to suggest that abnormal hyperphosphorylation was an essential feature of the conversion of normal tau into phf tau (Trojanowski *et al.*, 1993a, b; Goedert, 1993). However, an aspect of the difficulties in working with human disease for which there is not a good animal model is illustrated by the recent finding that soluble tau isolated from brain biopsies where there is no post-mortem delay has a similar degree of phosphorylation to phf tau (Matsuo *et al.*, 1994). The difference between the phosphorylation state of post-mortem and biopsy-derived tau is attributed to the continuing action of dephosphorylating enzymes in the post-mortem interval. This suggests that the phosphorylation of tau seen in phf is not simply the result of excessive phosphorylation, but rather a result of either a change in the balance of phosphorylating and dephosphorylating enzymes in the

AD brain or an increase in the stability of the phosphorylation state of tau in AD. Studies on tau extracted from phf have demonstrated that the phosphorylation is not specific to any of the particular isoforms of the protein since all the six adult isoforms are present in the phf in the same proportions as in normal brain (Goedert *et al.*, 1992). As would be expected, the major consequence of this change in phosphorylation state is that phosphorylated tau has a much lower affinity for microtubules than normal tau. That this loss of affinity is a result of the phosphorylation can be shown by the fact that tau extracted from dispersed phf and subsequently dephosphorylated has a normal affinity for microtubules. As with the formation of β/A4-protein amyloid from non-fibrillar β/A4, the steps in the assembly of dispersed phf from phosphorylated tau and their subsequent aggregation into neurofibrillary tangles are not clearly defined, but it has been shown that phf-like filaments can self-assemble *in vitro* from bacterially expressed fragments of tau. A difference between the tau in dispersed phf and the phf aggregated into neurofibrillary tangles is that in dispersed phf the whole tau molecule is present, while in the tangle fragments only the carboxy terminus half of the tau molecule is present and the protein is also ubiquitinated.

From these studies of the biochemistry of tau it is clear that regulation of the phosphorylation state of the tau protein is a key event in the process of the formation of phf and neurofibrillary pathology from tau protein. Attention is now shifting to looking for the candidate enzymes that could perform the phosphorylation and dephosphorylation and the events that could control or modify their activity. Examination of the sequence of phf tau has shown that there are between six and eight sites on the molecule that are phosphorylated in phf tau, and most of them are next to a proline residue. Hence, the most obvious candidates for the enzymes that perform the phosphorylation are what are called proline directed kinases. If the abnormal phosphorylation of tau seen in phf is a consequence of hyperactivity of the normal mechanism of phosphorylation, there are a number of candidate proline directed enzymes that are capable of phosphorylating tau such as microtubule associated protein (MAP) kinases, glycogen synthase kinase (GSK) 3 and other proline directed kinases. Protein phosphatases 2A (PP2A) and 2B (PP2B) (for references see Matsuo *et al.*, 1994) have been identified as being able to dephosphorylate tau. The abnormal phosphorylation of tau that occurs in AD implies that the normal regulatory mechanism that controls the phosphorylation state of tau has broken down but currently it is not known where the regulatory defect, or defects, are located.

The precise effects of the reduction in binding of tau to microtubules on the formation, stability and function of the microtubular apparatus of the cell are not known, but in the presence of a significant accumulation of phf there is a reduction in the normal cytoskeletal content of microtubules and neurofilaments. Given the wide distribution of phf in cell bodies and neuropil threads, it is not difficult to surmise that the extensive cytoskeletal disruption that this implies would be associated with a severe disruption of axonal transport and cell metabolism and could ultimately produce an accelerated cell death (Lee & Trojanowski, 1992; Trojanowski *et al.*, 1993*a*, *b*). Another possible mechanism of cell damage is that the hyperphosphorylation of tau is a reflection of a more generalized activation of kinases in the affected neurons that might be a manifestation of disordered regulation of intracellular calcium. There is certainly evidence of abnormalities of calcium regulating proteins including protein kinases that are altered in AD and a suggestion of increased protease activity including calcium activated proteases. It is at this level that a possible connection between tissue deposition of β/A4 and neurofibrillary pathology is beginning to emerge (Mattson *et al.*, 1993). Whatever the precise mechanism, as an empirical observation, it is abundantly clear from the presence within tissue of 'ghost' extracellular tangles that the presence of tangles within cells is associated with cell death and that the development of neurofibrillary pathology is seriously detrimental to cell health.

Regulation of tau and its association with amyloid

The amyloid hypothesis depends on the demonstration that there is a causative relation between the production and/or deposition of extracellular β/A4 and the later development of pathological changes among which are intracellular neurofibrillary pathology, loss of synapses and neuronal death. However, the study of the toxic effects of β/A4 has been complicated by inconsistent results with β/A4 being reported to have both neurotrophic and neurotoxic effects on neurons in culture. There is now increasing evidence that for the β/A4 molecule to be neurotoxic it has to be aggregated into fibrils. What is not clear is the mechanism of this toxic effect, although a number of possibilities have been advanced, and whether β/A4 acts alone or in concert with other influences such as excitotoxins, free radicals, ischaemia or hormonal effects. A possible direct connection between amyloid, and hyperphosphorylated tau,

and therefore with neurofibrillary pathology comes from reports that β/A4 can induce the formation of calcium channels in artificial membranes (Arispe *et al.*, 1993), and can amplify Ca^{2+} signalling in neurons (Hartman *et al.*, 1993). At least in principle this could prove a mechanism to permit increased or unregulated entry of Ca^{2+} into affected cells leading to inappropriate activation of calcium activated kinases, including those that could hyperphosphorylate the tau protein. It is exceedingly unlikely that amyloid cytotoxicity will be shown to be as simple as this mechanism suggests. This is particularly the case bearing in mind the slowness of the process of development of neurofibrillary pathology and, as indicated from the study of patients with Down's syndrome, the number of years that elapse from the first deposition of non-fibrillary β/A4 to the final flowering (if that is the appropriate word) of Alzheimer pathology that follows over the following two decades. This very tardiness argues for a small, but perhaps persistent, perturbation in neuronal metabolism, that results in the slow but relentless accumulation of damage that is eventually sufficient to cause neuronal death, having first progressively compromised neuronal function.

Although not universally accepted, there is a considerable body of scientific opinion that regards amyloid production and deposition as the starting point of a pathophysiologic process that ultimately leads to the development of the neuritic changes that are closely correlated with the dementia of AD. If what might be called the 'amyloid hypothesis' is to be accepted, there are a number of general questions that can be posed. Some questions, such as the protein chemical nature of the amyloid and the identity of the APP have already been answered. Others, such as the metabolic pathways by which β/A4 (the polypeptide that forms the amyloid) are derived from the APP, are in the process of solution while there remain still further major questions to be answered. At the time of writing these include:

1. The role of the gene defects on chromosomes 1 and 14 that is associated with early onset familial AD

The nature of these defects will be an important test of the 'amyloid hypothesis'. If they are shown to be associated with significant and appropriate changes in the metabolism of βAPP and/or the formation of the β/A4 polypeptide or its aggregation into an amyloid they will give a powerful boost to the hypothesis. If not, a rethink will almost certainly be required, which will direct AD research along what might be quite another avenue.

2. The identification of the cellular source or sources of the APP from which the β/A4 is derived

The importance of this question relates in part to possible therapeutic avenues, since a significant non-CNS source for either βAPP or β/A4 may exist. In some cases with AD, there is a very prominent vascular and perivascular component to the deposition of amyloid, and a marked perivascular neuritic response. This is shown in two ways; sometimes pericapillary amyloid deposition is very marked (Figs. 4a.28 and 4a.29), and usually this is most easily seen when there is not a marked neuritic reaction to the deposition of the amyloid. In other cases, deposition of amyloid in the penetrating arteries of the cortex is associated with a prominent neuritic reaction in the surrounding neuropil. Ultrastructurally this is seen when amyloid deposition extends across the perivascular space into the perivascular parenchyma. Such prominent vascular and perivascular deposition raises the possibility of a vascular source for the β/A4 and therefore the possibility that the circulation could be the source of either the βAPP or the β/A4.

3. What factors govern the conversion of soluble Aβ into insoluble amyloid fibrils?

In this area the interaction between the various forms of β/A4, but principally Aβ1–42(43), and other amyloid associated molecules such as α1-antichymotrypsin, the alleles of apolipoprotein E, and other factors such as complement factors will certainly be areas of interest. The identification of the (probably) intrinsic tissue factors that seem to maintain plaques in the diffuse form in the basal ganglia and the cerebellum may also provide some interesting insights into the mechanisms of the changes that occur between early diffuse and mature neuritic plaques.

4. What determines the location of the amyloid deposits?

One of the striking features of amyloid deposition in AD is its focal nature. This is true of cerebrovascular and parenchymal amyloid. In the parenchyma, there appears to be a maximum diameter for senile plaques of any age and configuration. In the vascular system, systemic vessels are unaffected and amyloid deposition is often notably focal with a segment of a cerebral vessel with considerable amyloid deposition in the wall being adjacent to a region with no discernible amyloid deposition. It is possible that, once amyloid begins to be deposited, its presence acts as a catalyst for further amyloid deposition. The mechanism for this could be that amyloid associated proteins were involved in the conversion of β/A4 from the non-fibrillar to the fibrillar form and there is, as has been described some evidence to support this suggestion.

5. What is the precise cell biological connection between the extracellular deposition of amyloid and the intracellular development of neuritic pathology?

As has been indicated, the outline of possible connections is beginning to be discerned in the association between amyloid and cellular damage and the possible interactions between calcium influx, protease activation and hyperphosphorylation of tau.

For the clinical scientist who interacts with patients, perhaps the most attractive feature of the 'amyloid hypothesis' is that, if it turns out to be substantially correct, it will almost certainly open up a number of potential therapeutic options. With this hypothesis, any method of retarding the deposition of 'neurotoxic' forms of β/A4 opens up the possibility that the sequence of events that results in the development of dementia in the patient could be retarded, or even arrested. The most immediately obvious are ways in which the production of β/A4 and the aggregation and deposition of amyloid fibrils, could be influenced. The fact that the deposition of amyloid significantly antedates the development of neuritic pathology, only increases the attraction of the hypothesis. It offers the possibility that interfering with the production of β/A4 or its conversion into fibrous amyloid would be interrupting the Alzheimer process at the earliest possible stage. This would be the greatest benefit to the very large numbers of people who, if the process cannot be arrested, will face the certain prospect of a progressive and irreversible dementia with all the personal, family and social consequences that this implies.

REFERENCES

Alzheimer A (1907) Über eine eigenartige Erkrankung der Hirnrinde. *Allg Zeitsch Psychiat* 64: 146–8.

Amaducci LA, Rocca, WA, Schoenberg BS (1986) Origin of the distinction between Alzheimer's disease and senile dementia. *Neurology* 36: 1497–9.

Aharon-Peretz J, Cummings JL, Hill MA (1988) Vascular dementia and dementia of Alzheimer type: cognition, ventricular size and leukoaraiosis. *Arch Neurol* 45: 719–21.

Arendt T, Bigl, V, Arendt A, Tennstedt A (1983) Loss of neurons in the nucleus basalis of Meynert in Alzheimer's disease, paralysis agitans and Korsakoff's disease. *Acta Neuropath* 61: 101–8.

Arispe N, Pollard HB, Rojas E (1993) Giant multilevel cation channels formed by Alzheimer disease β Protein [AβP-(1–40)] in bilayer membranes. *Proc Nat Acad Sci USA* 90: 10573–7.

Aronson MK, Ooi WL, Morgenstern H *et al* (1990) Women, myocardial infarction, and dementia in the very old. *Neurology* 40: 1102–6.

Arriagada PW, Growdon JH, Hedley-Whyte ET, Hyman BT (1992) Neurofibrillary tangles not senile plaques parallel duration and severity of Alzheimer's disease. *Neurology* 42: 631–9.

Awad, IA, Spetzler RE, Hodak JA, Awad CA, Carey R (1986) Incidental subcortical lesions identified on magnetic resonance imaging in the elderly. I. Correlation with age and cerebrovascular risk factors. *Stroke* 17: 1084–9.

Azzarelli B, Muller J, Ghetti B, Dykan M, Conneally PM (1985) Cerebellar plaques in familial Alzheimer's disease (Gerstmann–Sträussler–Scheinker variant?). *Acta Neuropath Berl* 65: 235–46.

Bachman DL, Wolf PA, Linn R (1992) Prevalence of dementia and probable senile dementia of the Alzheimer type in the Framingham study. *Neurology* 42: 115–19.

Ball MJ (1977) Neuronal loss, neurofibrillary tangles and granulovacuolar degeneration in the hippocampus with aging and dementia. *Acta Neuropath* 37: 111–18.

Bancher C, Braak H, Fischer P, Jellinger KA (1993) Neuropathological staging of Alzheimer lesions and intellectual status in Alzheimer's and Parkinson's disease patients. *Neurosci Lett* 162: 179–82.

Beard CM, Kokman E, Offord K, Kurland LT (1992) Lack of association between Alzheimer's disease and education, occupation, marital status, or living arrangement. *Neurology* 42: 2063–8.

Becker JT, Boller F, Lopez OL, Saxton J, McGonigle KL (1994) The natural history of Alzheimer's Disease. *Arch Neurol* 51: 585–94.

Benjamin R, Leake A, McArthur FK *et al* (1994a) Protective effect of apoE ε2 in Alzheimer's disease. *Lancet* 344: 473.

Benjamin R, Leake A, Edwardson JA *et al* (1994b) Apolipoprotein E genes in Lewy body and Parkinson's disease. *Lancet* 343: 1565.

Benowitz LI, Rodriguez W, Paskevich P, Muson EJ, Schenk D, Neve RL (1989) The amyloid precursor protein is concentrated in neuronal lyosomes in normal and Alzheimer disease subjects. *Exp Neurol* 106: 237–50.

Berg L, McKeel DW Jr, Miller JP, Baly J, Morris JC (1993) Neuropathological indexes of Alzheimer's disease in demented and nondemented persons aged 80 years and older. *Arch Neurol* 50: 349–58.

Berthier ML, Leiguarda R, Starkstein SE, Seviever G, Taratuto AL (1991) Alzheimer's disease in a patient with posterior cortical atrophy. J. Neurol. *Neurosurg Psychiat* 54: 1110–11.

Bird TD, Lampe TH, Nemens EJ *et al* (1987) Familial Alzheimer's disease in American descendents of the volga Germans: probable founder effect. *Ann Neurol* 23: 25–31.

Blessed, G, Tomlinson BE, Roth M (1968) The association between quantitative measures of dementia and of senile changes in the cerebral grey matter of elderly subjects. *Br J Psychiat* 114: 797–811.

Blocq P, Marinesco G (1892) Sur les lésions et la pathogénie de l'épilepsie dit essentiel. *Sem Med* 12: 445–6.

Bonaiuto S, Rocca WA, Lippi A *et al* (1990) Impact of education and occupation on prevalence of Alzheimer's disease (AD) and multi-infarct dementia (MID) in Appignano, Macerata Province, Italy [abstract] *Neurology* 40 (suppl 1): 346.

Braak H, Braak E (1988) Neuropil threads occur in dendrites of tangle bearing nerve cells. *Neuropathol Appl Neurobiol* 14: 39–44.

Braak H, Braak E (1991) Neuropathological staging of Alzheimer-related changes. *Acta Neuropath Berl* 82: 239–59.

Braak H, Braak E, Grunde-Iqbal I, Iqbal K (1986) Occurrence of neuropil threads in the senile human brain and in Alzheimer's disease: a third location of paired helical filaments outside of neurofibrillary tangles and neuritic plaques. *Neurosci Lett* 65: 351–5.

Bramblett GT, Goedert M, Jakes R, Merrick SE, Trojanowski JQ, Lee VM-Y (1993) Abnormal tau phosphorylation at Ser^{396} in Alzheimer's disease recapitulates development and contributes to reduced microtubule binding. *Neuron* 10: 1089–99.

Brashear HR, Godec MS, Carlsen J (1988) The distribution of neuritic plaques and acetylcholinesterase staining in the amygdala in Alzheimer's disease. *Neurology* 38: 1694–9.

Brayne C (1993) Clinico-pathological studies of the dementia from an epidemiological point of view. *Br J Psychiat* 162: 439–46.

Breitner JC, Silverman JM, Mohs RC, Davis KL (1988) Familial aggregation in Alzheimer disease: comparison of risk among relatives of early- and late-onset cases, and among male and female relatives in successive generations. *Neurology* 38: 207–12.

Brenner DE, Kukull WA, van Belle G *et al* (1993) Relationship between cigarette smoking and Alzheimer's disease in a population-based case-control study. *Neurology* 43: 293–300.

Brilliant M, Hughes, L, Anderson D, Ghobrial M, Elble R (1995) Rarified white matter in patients with Alzheimer's disease. *Alzheimer Dis Assoc Discord* 9: 39–46.

Brün A, Englund E (1981) Regional pattern of degeneration in Alzheimer's disease: neuronal loss and histopathological grading. *Histopathology* 5: 549–64.

Brün A, Englund E (1986) A white matter disorder in dementia of the Alzheimer type: a pathoanatomical study. *Ann Neurol* 19: 253–62.

Burkhardt CR, Filley CM, Kleinschmidt-DeMasters BK *et al* (1988) Diffuse Lewy body disease and progressive dementia. *Neurology* 38: 1520–8.

Burns A, Luthert P, Levy R *et al* (1990) Accuracy of clinical diagnosis of Alzheimer's disease. *Br Med J* 301: 48.

Burns A, Levy R, Jacoby R (1991) Diagnosis of Alzheimer's disease *Br Med J* 302: 48.

Byrne EJ (1991) Diagnosis of Alzheimer's disease. *Br Med J* 1991: 302: 48.

Cai ZD, Golde TE, Younkin SG (1993) Release of excess amyloid β-protein from a mutant amyloid β protein precursor. *Science* 259: 514–16.

Caplan LR, Schoene WC (1978) Clinical features of subcortical arteriosclerotic encephalopathy (Binswanger's disease) *Neurology* 28: 1206–15.

Chan-Palay V, Assan E (1989) Alterations in catecholamine neurones of the locus caeruleus in senile dementia of the Alzheimer type and in Parkinson's disease with and without dementia and depression. *J Comp Neurol* 287: 373–92.

Chartier-Harlin MC, Parfitt M, Legrain S *et al* (1994) Apolipoprotein E, epsilon 4 allele as a major risk factor for sporadic early and late-onset forms of Alzheimer's disease: analysis of the 19q13.2 chromosomal region. *Hum Mol Genet* 3: 569–74.

Chartier-Harlin MC, Crawford F, Houlden H *et al* (1991*a*) Early-onset Alzheimer's disease caused by mutation at codon 717 of the β-amyloid precursor protein gene. *Nature* 353: 844–6.

Chartier-Harlin MC, Crawford F, Hamandi K *et al* (1991*b*) Screening for the beta amyloid precursor protein mutation (APP717 Val-Ile) in extended pedigrees with early-onset Alzheimer's disease. *Neurosci Lett* 129: 134–5.

Chui HC, Lyness SA, Sobel E, Schneider LS (1994) Extrapyramidal signs and psychiatric symptoms predict faster cognitive decline in Alzheimer's disease. *Arch Neurol* 51: 676–81.

Clark, RF, Goate AM (1993) Molecular genetics of Alzheimer's disease. *Arch Neurol* 50: 1164–72.

Claus JJ, van Harskamp F, Breteler MMB, Krenning EP, de Koning I, van der Kammen TJM, Hofman A, Hasan D (1994) The diagnostic value of SPECT with Tc 99m HMPAO in Alzheimer's disease: a population study. *Neurology* 44: 454–61.

Cohen DH, Feiner H, Jensson O, Frangione B (1983) Amyloid fibril in hereditary cerebral haermorrhage with amyloidosis (HCHWA) is related to the gastroenteropancreatic neuroendocrine protein gamma trace. *J Exp Med* 158: 623–8.

Cook RH, Schenk SA, Clark DB (1981) Twins with Alzheimer's disease. *Arch Neurol* 38: 300–1.

Corder EH, Saunders A, Strittmatter WJ *et al* (1993) Gene dosage of apolipoprotein E type 4 allele and the risk for Alzheimer's disease in late onset families. *Science* 261: 921–3.

Corder EH, Saunders AM, Risch NJ *et al* (1994) Protective effect of apolipoprotein E type 2 allele for late onset Alzheimer disease. *Nature Genet* 7: 180–4.

Corsellis JAN (1962) *Mental Illness and the Aging Brain.* Oxford University Press.

Corsellis JAN (1976) Aging and the Dementias. In Blackwood W, Corsellis JAN, (eds) *Greenfield's Neuropathology.* Edward Arnold London. pp. 796–848.

Corsellis JAN, Bruton CJ, Freeman-Browne D (1973) The aftermath of boxing. *Psychol Med* 3: 270–3.

Crystal H, Dickson D, Fuld P *et al* (1988) Clinico-pathological studies in dementia: Non-demented subjects with pathologically confirmed Alzheimer's disease. *Neurology* 38: 1682–7.

Crystal HW, Dickson DW, Lizardi JE *et al* (1990) Antemortem diagnosis of Diffuse Lewy body disease. *Neurology* 40: 1523–8.

Crystal HA, Dickson DW, Sliwinski MJ *et al* (1993) Pathological markers associated with normal aging and dementia in the elderly. *Ann Neurol* 34: 566–73.

Dale GE, Leigh PN, Luthert P, Anderton BH, Roberts GW (1991) Neurofibrillary tangles in dementia pugilistica are ubiquitinated. *J Neurol Neurosurg Psychiat* 54: 116–18.

Dartigues JF, Gagnon M, Michel P *et al* (1991) Le programme de recherche Paquid sur l'epidemiologie de la demence: methods et resultats initiaux. *Rev Neurol Paris* 147: 225–30.

Davies L, Wolska B, Hilbich C *et al* (1988) A4 amyloid protein deposition and the diagnosis of Alzheimer's disease: prevalence in aged brains determined by immunocytochemistry compared with conventional neuropathological techniques. *Neurology* 38: 1688–93.

Davies P, Maloney AJF (1976) Selective loss of central cholinergic neurons in Alzheimer's disease *Lancet* ii: 1403.

Davis PC, Gray L, Albert M *et al* (1992) The Consortium to Establish a Registry for Alzheimer's Disease (CERAD). Part III. Reliability of a standardised MRI evaluation of Alzheimer's disease. *Neurology* 42: 1676–80.

De Kosky ST, Scheff SW (1990) Synapse loss in frontal cortex biopsies in Alzheimer's disease: correlation with cognitive severity. *Ann Neurol* 27: 457–64.

De Leon MJ, George AE, Stylopoulos LA, Smith G, Miller DC (1989) Early marker for Alzheimer's disease: the atrophic hippocampus. *Lancet* ii: 672–3.

De Reuck J, Crevits L, De Coster W, Sieben G, van der Eecken H (1980) Pathogenesis of Binswanger chronic progressive subcortical encephalopathy. *Neurology* 30: 920–8.

Dickson DW, Crystal H, Mattiace LA *et al* (1989) Diffuse Lewy body disease: light and electron microscopic immunocytochemistry of senile plaques. *Acta Neuropath* 78: 572–84.

Duyckaerts C, Delaere P, Hauw JJ *et al* (1990) Rating of the lesions in senile dementia of the Alzheimer type: concordance between laboratories. A European multi-centre study under the auspices of EURAGE. *J Neurol Sci* 97: 295–326.

Dyrks T, Dyrks E, Hartmann T, Masters CL, Beyreuter K (1993) Radicals as mediators for the amyloidognic transformation of βA4-bearing APP fragments. In Corain B, Iqbal K, Nicolini M, Windblad B, Wisniewski H (eds) *Alzheimer's Disease: Advances in Clinical and Basic Research*. John Wiley & Sons, pp. 497–505.

Englund E, Brun A, Alling C (1988) White matter changes in dementia of Alzheimer's type: biochemical and neuropathological correlates. *Brain* 111: 1425–39.

Erkinjuntti T, Ketonen L, Sulkava R, Sipponen J, Vuoriahlo M, Iivanainen M (1987) Do white matter changes on MRI and CT differentiate vascular dementia from Alzheimer's disease? *J Neurol Neurosurg Psychiat* 50: 37–42.

Erkinjuntti T, Sulkava R, Palo J, Ketonen L (1989) White matter low attenuation on CT in Alzheimer's disease. *Arch Gerontol Geriatr* 8: 95–104.

Erkinjuntti T, Lee DH, Gao F *et al* (1993) Temporal lobe atrophy on magnetic resonance imaging in the diagnosis of early Alzheimer's disease. *Arch Neurol* 50: 305–10.

Esch FS, Keim PS, Beattie EC *et al* (1990) Cleavage of amyloid β-peptide during constitutive processing of its precursor. *Science* 248: 1122–4.

Esiri MM, Wilcock GK (1984) The olfactory bulbs in Alzheimer's disease. *J Neurol Neurosurg Psychiat* 47: 56–60.

Esiri MM, Wilcock GK (1986) Cerebral amyloid angiopathy in dementia and old age. *J Neurol Neurosurg Psychiat* 49: 1221–6.

Esiri MM, Pearson RCA, Powell TPS (1986) The cortex of the primary auditory area in Alzheimer's disease. *Brain Res* 366: 385–7.

Evans DA, Funkenstein HH, Albert MS *et al* (1989) Prevalence of Alzheimer's disease in a community population of older persons. *JAMA* 262: 2551–6.

Farlow M, Murrell J, Ghetti B, Unverzagt F, Zeldenrust S, Benson M (1994) Clinical characteristics in a kindred with early onset Alzheimer's disease and their linkage to a G-T change at position 2149 of the amyloid precursor protein gene. *Neurology* 44: 105–11.

Farrar LA, Myers RH, Connor L *et al* (1991) Segregation analysis reveals evidence for a major gene for Alzheimer's disease. *Am J Hum Genet* 48: 1026–33.

Fidani L, Rooke K, Chartier-Harlin MC *et al* (1992) Screening for mutations in the open reading frame and promoter of the β-amyloid precursor protein gene in familial Alzheimer's disease: identification of a further family with APP717Val → Ile. *Hum Mol Genet* 1: 165–8.

Fillit H, Weinreb H, Cholst I *et al* (1986) Observations in a preliminary open trial of estradiol therapy for senile dementia Psychoneuroendocrinology 11: 337–45.

Fischer O (1907) Miliare Nekrosen mit drusigen Wucherungen der Neurofibrillen, eine regelmässige Veränderung der Hirnrinde bei seniler Demenz. *Monatssch Psychiat Neurol* 22: 361–72.

Frataglioni L, Grut M, Forsell Y, Viitanen M, Graftström M, Holmén K, Ericsson K, Bäckman L, Ahlbom A, Winblad B (1991) Prevalence of Alzheimer's disease and other dementias in an elderly urban population; relationship with age, sex and education. *Neurology* 41: 1886–92.

Friedland RP (1993) Epidemiology, education, and the ecology of Alzheimer's disease. *Neurology* 43: 246–9.

Galasko D, Hansen LA, Katzman R, Wiederholt W, Masliah E, Terry R, Hill R, Lessin P, Thal LJ (1994) Clinical-Neuropathological correlations in Alzheimer's disease and related dementias. *Arch Neurol* 51: 888–95.

Gearing M, Mirra SS, Hedgreen JC, Sumi SM, Hansen LA, Heyman A (1995) The Consortium to Establish a Registry for Alzheimer's Disease (CERAD). Part X. Neuropathology confirmation of the clinical diagnosis of Alzheimer's disease. *Neurology* 45: 461–6.

Gentleman SM, Roberts GW (1991) Risk factors in Alzheimer's disease. *Br Med J* 304: 118–19.

George AE, deLeon MJ, Gentes CI *et al* (1986*a*) Leukoencephalopathy in normal and pathologic aging I. CT of brain lucencies. AJNR 7: 561–6.

George AE, deLeon MJ, Kalnin A, Rosner L, Goodgold A, Chase N (1986*b*) Leukoencephalopathy in normal and pathologic aging. II. MRI of brain lucencies. AJNR 8: 567–70.

George AE, de Leon MJ, Stylopoulos LA *et al* (1990) CT diagnostic features of Alzheimer's disease: importance of the choroidal/hippocampal fissure complex. *Am J Neuroradiol* 11: 101–7.

Ghetti B, Tagliavini F, Masters CL *et al* (1989) Gerstmann –Sträussler–Scheinker disease. II Neurofibrillary tangles and plaques with PrP amyloid coexist in an affected family. *Neurology* 39: 1453–61.

Gibb WRG, Esiri MM, Lees AJ (1985) Clinical and pathological features of diffuse cortical Lewy body disease (Lewy body dementia) *Brain* 110: 1131–53.

Gilbert JJ, Vintners HV (1983) Cerebral amyloid angiopathy: incidence and complications in the aging brain I. Cerebral haemorrhage. *Stroke* 14: 915–23.

Gilleard CJ, Kellett JM, Coles JA, Millard, PH, Honavar M, Lantos PL (1992) The St. George's dementia bed investigation study: a comparison of clinical and pathological diagnosis. *Acta Psychiatr Scand* 85: 264–9.

Glenner GG, Wong, CW (1984) Alzheimer's disease: initial report of the purification and characterisation of novel cerebrovascular amyloid protein. *Biochem Biophys Res Comm* 120: 885–90.

Goate A, Chartier-Harlin MC, Mullen M *et al* (1991) Segregation of a missense mutation in the amyloid precursor protein gene with familial Alzheimer's disease, *Nature* 349: 704–6.

Goedert M (1993) Tau protein and the neurofibrillary pathology of Alzheimer's disease. *Trends Neurosci* 16: 460–5.

Goedert M, Spillantini MG, Cairns NG, Crowther RA (1992) Tau protein of Alzheimer's paired helical filaments: abnormal phosphorylation of all six brain isoforms. *Neuron* 8: 159–68.

Goedert M, Spillantini MG, Jakes R, Rutherford D, Crowther

RA (1989) Multiple isoforms of human microtubule associated protein tau: sequences and localisation in neurofibrillary tangles of Alzheimer's disease. *Neuron* 3: 519–26.

Golde TE, Estus S, Younkin LH, Selkoe DJ, Younkin SG (1992) Processing of the amyloid protein precursor to potentially amyloidogenic carboxyl-terminal derivatives. *Science* 255: 728–30.

Gorelick PB, Freels S, Harris Y, Dollear BS, Billingsley M, Brown N (1994) Epidemiology of vascular and Alzheimer's dementia among African Americans in Chicago, Ill. Baseline frequency and comparison of risk factors. *Neurology* 44: 1391–6.

Graves, AB, van Duijn CM, Chandra V *et al* (1991) Alcohol and tobacco consumption as risk factors for Alzheimer's disease. *Int J Epidemiol* 20 (suppl 2): S48–57.

Griffiths RA, Mortimer TF, Oppenheimer DR, Spalding, JMK (1982) Congophilic angiopathy of the brain: a clinical and pathological report on two siblings. *J Neurol Neurosurg Psychiat* 45: 396–408.

Hachinski VV, Iliff LD, Zihkla *et al* (1975) Cerebral blood flow in dementia. *Arch Neurol* 32: 632–7.

Hachinski VC, Potter P, Merskey H (1987) Leuko-araiosis *Arch Neurol* 44: 21–3.

Hagnell O, Öjesö L, Rorsman B (1992) Incidence of dementia in the Lundby study. *Neuroepidemiology* 11 (suppl 1): 61–6.

Haltia M, Viitanan M, Sulkava R *et al* (1994) Chromosome 14 encoded Alzheimer's disease: genetic and clinicopathological description. *Ann Neurol* 36: 362–7.

Hamos, JE, DeGennaro LJ, Drachman, DA (1989) Synaptic loss in Alzheimer's disease and other dementias. *Neurology* 39: 355–61.

Hansen L, Salmon D, Galasko D, Masliah E, Katzman R, DeTeresa R, Thal L, Pay MM, Hofstetter R, Klauber M, Rice V, Butters N, Alford M (1990) The Lewy body variant of Alzheimer's disease: a clinical and pathologic entity. *Neurology* 40: 1–8.

Hardy J, Mullan M, Chartier-Harlan MC, Brown J, Goate A, Rossor M *et al* (1991) Molecular classification of Alzheimer's disease. *Lancet* 337: 1342–3.

Hart MN, Merz, P, Bennett-Gray J, Menezes AH, Goeken JA, Schelper RL, Wisniewski HM (1988) β-amyloid protein of Alzheimer's disease is found in cerebral and spinal cord malformations. *Am J Path* 132: 167–72.

Hartmann H, Eckert A, Müller WE (1993) β-amyloid protein amplifies calcium signalling in central neurons from the adult mouse. *Biochem. Biophys. Res. Commun.* 194: 1216–20.

Hasagawa M, Morishima-Kawashima M, Takio K, Suzuki M, Litani K, Ihara Y (1992) Protein sequence and mass spectrometric analyses of tau in the Alzheimer's disease brain. *J Biol Chem* 267: 17047–54.

Hass C, Koo EH, Mellon A, Hung AY, Selkoe DJ (1992*a*) Targetting of cell surface β-amyloid precursor to lysosomes: Alternative processing into amyloid bearing fragments. *Nature* 357: 500–3.

Hass C, Schlossmacher MG, Hung AY *et al* (1992*b*) Amyloid β-peptide is produced by cultured cells during normal metabolism. *Nature* 359: 322–5.

Henderson AS (1986) The epidemiology of Alzheimer's disease. *Br Med Bull* 42: 3–10.

Henderson VW, Buckwalter JG (1994) Cognitive deficits in men and women with Alzheimer's disease. *Neurology* 44: 90–6.

Henderson VW, Paganini-Hill A, Emanual CK, Dunn ME, Buckwalter JG (1994) Estrogen replacement therapy in older women. Comparisons between Alzheimer's disease cases and non-demented control subjects. *Arch Neurol* 51: 896–900.

Hendrie HC, Hall KS, Hui S *et al* (1995) Apolipoprotein E genotypes and Alzheimer's disease in a community study of elderly African Americans. *Ann Neurol* 37: 118–20.

Hendriks L, Van Duijn CM, Cras P *et al* (1992) Presenile dementia and cerebral haemorrhage linked to a mutation at codon 692 of the β-amyloid precursor protein gene. *Nature Genet* 1: 218–21.

Heston L, Mastri A (1977) The genetics of Alzheimer's disease: associations with haematologic malignancy and Down's syndrome. *Arch Gen Psychiat* 34: 976–81.

Heyman A, Wilkinson WE, Stafford JA (1984) Alzheimer's disease: a study of epidemiological aspects. *Ann Neurol* 15: 335–41.

Heyman A, Fillenbaum G, Prosnitz B *et al* (1991) Estimated prevalence of dementia among elderly black and white community-residents. *Arch Neurol* 48: 594–8.

Hill LR, Klauber MR, Salmon DP *et al* (1993) Function status, education and the diagnosis of dementia in the Shanghai survey. *Neurology* 43: 138–45.

Himmler A (1989) Structure of the bovine tau gene: alternatively spliced transcripts generate a protein family. *Mol Cell Biol* 9: 1389–95.

Hofman A, Rocca WA, Brayne C *et al* (1991) The prevalence of dementia in Europe: a collaborative study of 1980–1990 findings. *Int J Epidemiol* 20: 736–48.

Homer A, Honavar M, Lantos P, Hastie I, Kellet J, Millard P (1988) Diagnosing dementia: do we get it right? *Br Med J* 297: 894–6.

Honjo H, Ogino Y, Naitoh K *et al* (1989) *In vivo* effects by oestrone sulphate on the central nervous system – senile dementia (Alzheimer type) *J Steroid Biochem* 34: 521–5.

Hope T, Fairburn CG (1992) The present behavioural examination (PBE): the development of an interview to measure current behavioural abnormalities. *Psychol Med* 22: 223–30.

Hubbard BM, Anderson JM (1981*a*) Age, senile dementia and ventricular enlargement. *J Neurol Neurosurg Psychiat* 44: 631–5.

Hubbard BM, Anderson JM (1981*b*) A quantitative study of cerebral atrophy in old age and senile dementia. *J Neurol Sci* 50: 135–45.

Huff J, Auerbach J, Chackravarti A, Boller F (1988) Risk of dementia in relatives of patients with Alzheimer's disease. *Neurology* 38: 786–90.

Hyman BT, Terry RD (1994) Apolipoprotein E, Aβ, and Alzheimer disease. An editorial comment. *J Neuropath Exp Neurol* 53: 427–8.

Hyman BT, Tanzi R (1995) Molecular epidemiology of Alzheimer's disease. *N Engl J Med* 333: 1283–4.

Ihara Y (1988) Massive somatodendritic sprouting of cortical neurons of Alzheimer's disease. *Brain Res* 459: 138–44.

Iwatsubo T, Odaka A, Suzuki N, Mizusawa H, Nukina N, Ihara Y (1994) Visualization of Aβ42(43) and Aβ40 in senile plaques with endspecific Aβ monoclonals: Evidence that initially deposited species is Aβ42(43). *Neuron* 13: 45–53.

Iwatsubo T, Mann DMA, Odaka A, Suzuki N, Ihara Y (1995) Amyloid β protein (Aβ) deposition: Aβ42(43) precedes Aβ40 in Down syndrome. *Ann Neurol* 37: 294–9.

Jack CR, Petersen RC, Obrien PC et al (1992) MR based hippocampal volumetry in the diagnosis of Alzheimer's disease. *Neurology* 42: 183–8.

Janota I, Mirsen TR, Hachinski VC, Lee DH, Merskey H (1989) Neuropathological correlates of leuko-araiosis. *Arch Neurol* 46: 1124–8.

Jarvik LF, Ruth V, Matsuyama SS (1980) Organic brain syndrome and aging. A six year follow-up of surviving twins. *Arch Gen Psychiat* 37: 280–6.

Jellinger K (1976) Neuropathological aspects of dementias resulting from abnormal blood and cerebrospinal fluid dynamics. *Acta Neurol Belg* 76: 83–102.

Jellinger K, Danielczyk W, Fischer P, Gabriel E (1990) Clinicopathological analysis of dementia disorders in the elderly. *J Neurol Sci* 95: 239–58.

Jensson O, Gudmundsson G, Arnason A et al (1987) Hereditary cystatin C (γ-trace) amyloid angiopathy of the CNS causing cerebral haemorrhage. *Acta Neurol Scand* 76: 102–14.

Joachim CL, Morris JH, Schoene WC (1986) Neuropathological findings in six cases of dementia with severe focal atrophy. *J Neuropath Exp Neurol* 49: 275(abst).

Joachim CL, Morris, JH, Selkoe DJ (1988) Clinically diagnosed Alzheimer's disease: autopsy results in 150 cases. *Ann Neurol* 24: 50–6.

Joachim CL, Duffy LK, Morris JH, Selkoe DJ (1984) Protein-chemical and immunocytochemical studies of meningovascular β-amyloid protein in Alzheimer's disease and normal aging. *Brain Res* 474: 100–11.

Joachim CL, Morris DJ, Selkoe DJ (1989) Diffuse senile plaques occur commonly in the cerebellum in Alzheimer's disease. *Am J Path* 135: 309–19.

Joachim CL, Selkoe DJ (1992) The seminal role of β-amyloid in the pathogenesis of Alzheimer's disease. *Alzheimer Dis Assoc Disord* 6: 7–34.

Jobst KA, Smith AD, Barker CS et al (1992) Association of atrophy of the medial temporal lobe with reduced blood flow in the posterior parieto-temporal cortex in patients with a clinical and pathological diagnosis of Alzheimer's disease. *J Neurol Neurosurg Psychiat* 55: 190–4.

Jobst KA, Smith AD, Szatmari M et al. (1991) Detection in life of confirmed Alzheimer's disease using a simple measurement of medial temporal lobe atrophy by computed tomography. *Lancet* 340: 1179–83.

Jobst KA, Smith AD, Szatmari M et al. (1994a) Rapidly progressing atrophy of medial temporal lobe in Alzheimer's disease. *Lancet* 343: 829–31.

Jobst KA, Hindley NJ, King E, Smith AD (1994b) The diagnosis of Alzheimer's disease: a question of image? *J Clin Psychiat* 55: [11 suppl.]: 22–31.

Jorm, AF, Korten AE, Henderson AS (1987) The prevalence of dementia: a quantitative integration of the literature. *Acta Psychiatr Scand* 76: 465–79.

Kang J, Lemaire H, Unterbeck A, Salbaum JM, Masters CL, Grzeschik et al (1987) The precursor of Alzheimer's disease amyloid A4 protein resembles a cell surface receptor. *Nature* 325: 733–6.

Karlinsky H, Vaula G, Haines JL et al (1992) Molecular and prospective phenotypic characterisation of a pedigree with familial Alzheimer disease and a missense mutation in codon 717 of the β-amyloid precursor protein (APP) gene. *Neurology* 42: 1445–53.

Katzman R, Aronson M, Fuld P et al (1989) Development of dementing illnesses in an 80 year old cohort. *Ann Neurol* 25: 317–24.

Katzman R (1993a) Clinical and epidemiological aspects of Alzheimer's disease. *Clin Neurosci* 1: 165–70.

Katzman R (1993b) Education and the prevalence of dementia and Alzheimer's disease. *Neurology* 43: 13–20.

Katzman R, Terry RD, deTeresa R et al (1988) Clinical, pathologic and neurochemical changes in dementia: a subgroup with preserved mental status and numerous neocortical plaques. *Ann Neurol* 23: 138–44.

Kellett JM, Gilleard C, Homer A, Millard P (1991) Diagnosis of Alzheimer's disease. *Br Med J* 302: 47.

Kennedy AM, Newman S, McCaddon A et al (1993) Familial Alzheimer's disease: a pedigree with a mis-sense mutation in the amyloid precursor protein (amyloid precursor protein 717 valine-glycine) *Brain* 116: 309–24.

Kesslak JP, Nalcioglu O, Cotman CW (1991) Quantification of magnetic resonance scans for hippocampal and parahippocampal atrophy in Alzheimer's disease. *Neurology* 41: 51–4.

Khatchaturian ZS (1985) Diagnosis of Alzheimer's disease. *Arch Neurol* 42: 1097–105.

Kido DK, Caine ED, LeMay M et al (1989) Temporal lobe atrophy in patients with Alzheimer's disease: a CT study. *Am J Neuroradiol* 10: 551–5.

Kokmen E, Beard CM, Offord KP, Kurland LT (1989) Prevalence of medically defined dementia in a defined United States population. *Neurology* 39: 773–6.

Korczyn AD, Kahana E, Galper Y (1991) Epidemiology of dementia in Ashkelon, Israel. *Neuroepidemiology* 10: 100.

Kornfield M (1984) Gerstmann–Sträussler syndrome with features of Alzheimer's disease: two entities or one? *Neuropathol Exp Neurol* 43: 321.

Kosaka K (1990) Diffuse Lewy body disease in Japan. *J Neurol* 237: 197–204.

Kosaka K, Yoshimura M, Ikaeda K, Budka H (1984) Diffuse type of Lewy body disease: progressive dementia with abundant cortical Lewy bodies and senile changes of varying degree – a new disease? *Clin Neuropath* 3: 185–92.

Kosik K (1992) Alzheimer's disease: a cell biological perspective. *Science* 256: 780–3.

Kukull WA, Larson EB, Reifler BV, Lampe TH, Yearby MS, Hughes JP (1990) The validity of three clinical diagnostic criteria for Alzheimer's disease. *Neurology* 40: 1364–9.

Kumar A, Schapiro MB, Grady CL *et al* (1991) Anatomic, metabolic, neuropsychological and molecular genetic studies on three pairs of identical twins discordant for dementia of the Alzheimer type. *Arch Neurol* 48: 160–8.

Lee VM-Y, Balin BJ, Otvos L Jr, Trojanowski JQ (1991) A68: a major subunit of paired helical filaments and derivatived forms of normal tau. *Science* 251: 675–8.

Lee VM-Y, Trojanowski JQ (1992) The disordered neuronal cytoskeleton in Alzheimer's disease. *Curr Opin Neurobiol* 2: 653–6.

Lennox, G, Lowe J, Landon M *et al* (1989) Diffuse Lewy body disease: correlative neuropathology using anti-ubiquitin immunocytochemistry. *J Neurol Neurosurg Psychiat* 52: 1236–47.

Levine DN, Lee JM, Fisher CM (1993) The visual variant of Alzheimer's disease: a clinicopathological case study. *Neurology* 43: 305–13.

Levy E, Carman, MD, Fernandez-Madrid IJ *et al* (1990) Mutation of the Alzheimer's disease amyloid gene in hereditary cerebral haermorrhage, Dutch type. *Science* 248: 1124–6.

Levy-Lahad E, Wijsman E, Nemens E *et al* (1995a) A familial Alzheimer's disease locus on chromosome 1. *Science* 269: 970–3.

Levy-Lahad E, Wasco W, Poorkaj P *et al* (1995b) Candidate gene for the chromosome 1 familial Alzheimer's disease locus. *Science* 269: 973–7.

Lindley RI, Dennis MS (1991) Diagnosis of Alzheimer's disease. *Br Med J* 302: 47.

Lopez OL, Swihart AA, Becker JT, Reinmuth OM, Reynolds CF, Rezek DL, Daly FL III (1990) Reliability of NINCDS-ADRDA clinical criteria for the diagnosis of Alzheimer's disease. *Neurology* 40: 1517–22.

Ma J, Yee A Jr, Brewer HB *et al* (1994) Amyloid associated proteins α1-antichymotrypsin and apolipoprotein E promote assembly of Alzheimer β protein into filaments. *Nature* 372: 92–4.

Mandybur TI, Gore I (1969) Amyloid in late post-irradiation necrosis of the brain. *Neurology* 19: 983–92.

Mandybur TI (1975) The incidence of cerebral amyloid angiopathy in Alzheimer's disease. *Neurology* 25: 120–6.

Mann DMA, Lincoln J, Yates PO, Stamp JE, Toper S (1980) Changes in the monoamine-containing neurons of the human central nervous system in senile dementia. *Br J Psychiat* 136: 533–41.

Manning FC (1991) Diagnosis of Alzheimer's disease. *Br Med J* 302: 47–8.

Martin EM, Wilson RS, Penn RD *et al* (1987) Cortical biopsy results in Alzheimer's disease: correlation with cortical deficits. *Neurology* 37: 1201–4.

Martin RL, Gerteis G, Gabrielli WJF (1988) A family-genetic study of dementia of Alzheimer type. *Arch Gen Psychiat* 45: 894–900.

Martins JJ, Gheuens J, Bruyland MD *et al* (1991) Early-onset Alzheimer's disease in 2 large Belgian families. *Neurology* 41: 62–8.

Masliah E, Terry RD, DeTeresa R, Hansen LA (1989) Immunohistochemical quantitation of the synapse related protein synaptophysin in Alzheimer's disease. *Neurosci Lett* 103: 234–8.

Masliah E, Terry RD, Alford M, DeTeresa RM, Hansen LA (1991) Cortical and subcortical patterns of synaptophysin-like immunoreactivity in Alzheimer's disease. *Am J Pathol* 138: 235–46.

Matsuo ES, Shin R-W, Billingsley ML, Van deVoorde A, O'Connor M, Trojanowski JQ, Lee VM-Y (1994) Biopsy-derived adult human brain tau is phosphorylated at many of the same sites as an Alzheimer's disease paired helical filament tau. *Neuron* 13: 989–1002.

Mattson MP, Barger, SW, Cheng B *et al* (1993) β-amyloid precursor protein metabolites and loss of neuronal Ca²⁺ homeostatis in Alzheimer's disease. *Trends Neurosci* 16: 409–14.

Mayeux R, Stern Y, Ottman R *et al* (1993) The apolipoprotein ε4 allele in patients with Alzheimer's disease. *Ann Neurol* 34: 752–4.

Mayeux R, Stern Y, Spanton S (1985) Heterogeneity in dementia of the Alzheimer type. *Neurology* 35: 453–61.

McKee AC, Kosik KS, Kowall NW (1991) Neuritic pathology and dementia in Alzheimer's disease. *Ann Neurol* 30: 156–65.

McKhann G, Drachamnn D, Folstein M *et al* (1984) Clinical diagnosis of Alzheimer's disease: Report of the NINCDS-ADRDA workgroup under the auspices of the Department of Health and Human Services task force on Alzheimer's disease. *Neurology* 34: 939–44.

McMenemey WH (1958) The dementias and progressive disease of the basal ganglia. In Greenfield JG, Blackwood W, McMenemey WH, Meyer A, Norman RM (eds.) *Neuropathology* Edward Arnold, London. pp. 475–528.

McMenemey WH (1963) The dementias and progressive disease of the basal ganglia. In Blackwood W, McMenemey WH, Meyer A, Norman RM, Russel DS (eds.) *Greenfield's Neuropathology* Edward Arnold, London. pp. 520–81.

Mendez MF, Zander BA (1991) Dementia presenting with aphasia: clinical characteristics. *J Neurol Neurosurg Psychiat* 54: 542–5.

Mendez MF, Mastri AR, Sung, JH, Frey WH (1992) Clinically diagnosed Alzheimer disease: neuropathologic findings in 650 cases. *Alzheimer Dis Assoc Disord* 6: 35–43.

Menzel H-J, Kladetzky RG, Assmann G (1983) Apolipoprotein E polymorphisms and coronary artery disease. *Arteriosclerosis* 3: 310–15.

Miller FD, Hicks SP, D'Amato CJ, Landis JR (1984) A descriptive study of neuritic plaques and neurofibrillary tangles in an autopsy population. *Am J Epidemiol* 120: 331–41.

Mirra SS, Heyman A, McKeel D, Sumi SM, Crain BJ, Brownlee LM, Vogel FS, Hughes JP, van Belle G, Berg L (1991) The Consortium to Establish a Registry for Alzheimer's Disease (CERAD). Part II Standardization of the neuropathologic assessment of Alzheimer's disease. *Neurology* 41: 479–86.

Mirra SS, Hart MN, Terry RD (1993) Making the diagnosis of Alzheimer's disease. A primer for practising pathologists. *Arch Pathol Lab Med* 117: 132–44.

Mirra SS, Gearing M, McKeel DW, Crain BJ, Hughes JP, van Belle G, Heyman A (1994) Interlaboratory comparison of neuropathology assessments in Alzheimer's disease: a study of the consortium to establish a registry of Alzheimer's disease (CERAD) *J Neuropath Exp Neurol* 53: 303–15.

Mirsen TR, Lee DH, Wong CJ *et al* (1991) Clinical correlates of white matter changes on magnetic resonance imaging scans of the brain. *Arch Neurol* 48: 1015–21.

Mölsä PK, Martiilla RJ, Rinne UK (1982) Epidemiology of dementia in a Finnish population. *Acta Neurol Scand* 65: 541–52.

Mölsä PK, Sako E, Paljarvi L, Rinne JO, Rinne UK (1987) Alzheimer's disease: neuropathological correlates of cognitive and motor disorders. *Acta Neurol Scand* 75: 376–84.

de la Monte SM (1989) Quantitation of cerebral atrophy in preclinical and end stage Alzheimer's disease. Ann Neurol 25: 450–9.

Morris JC, Heyman A, Mohs RC *et al* (1989) The Consortium to Establish a Registry for Alzheimer's Disease (CERAD). Part I Clinical and neuropsychological assessment of Alzheimer's disease. *Neurology* 39: 1159–65.

Morris JC, McKeel DW, Storandt M *et al* (1991) Very mild Alzheimer's disease: informant-based clinical, psychometric, and pathologic distinction from normal aging. *Neurology* 41: 469–78.

Morris JC (1994) Differential diagnosis of Alzheimer's disease. *Clin Geriat Med* 10: 257–76.

Mortimer JA, van Duijn CM, Chandra V *et al* (1991) Head trauma as a risk factor for Alzheimer's disease: a collaborative reanalysis of case control studies. *Int J Epidemiol* 20 (suppl 2): S28–35.

Mullen M, Crawford F, Axelman K *et al* (1992a) A new

mutation in APP demonstrates that pathogenic mutations for probable Alzheimer's disease frame the β-amyloid sequence. *Nature Genet* 1: 345–7.

Mullen M, Houlden H, Windelspecht M *et al* (1992b) A locus for familial early-onset Alzheimer's disease on the long arm of chromosome 14, proximal to the α-1 antichymotripsin gene. *Nature Genet* 2: 340–2.

Mullen M, Crawford F (1993) Genetic and molecular advances in Alzheimer's disease. *Trends Neurosci* 16: 398–403.

Murphy GM, Forno LS, Scardina JM, Eng LF, Cordell B (1994) Development of a monoclonal antibody specific for the COOH terminal of β-amyloid 1042 and its immunohistochemical reactivity in Alzheimer's disease and related disorders. *Am J Path* 144: 1082–8.

Murrel J, Farlow M, Ghetti B, Benson MD (1991) A mutation in the amyloid precursor protein associated with hereditary Alzheimer's disease. *Science* 254: 97–9.

Murrel J, Crawford F, Axelman K *et al* (1992) A pathogenic mutation for probable Alzheimer's disease in the APP gene at the *N*-terminus of β-amyloid. *Nature Genet* 1: 345–7.

Nagy Z, Esiri MM, Jobst, KA *et al.* (1995) Relative roles of plaques and tangles in the dementia of Alzheimer's disease. *Dementia* 6: 21–31.

Namba Y, Tomonage M, Kawasaki H *et al* (1991) Apolipoprotein E immunoreactivity in cerebral amyloid deposits and neurofibrillary tangles in Alzheimer's disease and Kuru plaque amyloid in Creutzfeldt–Jakob disease. *Brain Res* 541: 163–6.

Naruse S, Igarashi S, Kobayashi H *et al* (1991) Mis-sense mutation Val–Ile in exon 17 of amyloid precursor protein in Japanese familial Alzheimer's disease. *Lancet* 337: 978–9.

Neary D, Snowden JS, Mann DMA, Bowen DM, Sims NR, Northern B, Yeats PO, Davison Am (1986) Alzheimer's disease – a correlative study. *J Neurol Neurosurg Psychiat* 49–229.

Neve RL, Finch EA, Dawes LR (1988) Expression of the Alzheimer amyloid precursor gene transcripts in the human brain *Neuron* 1: 669–77.

Nochlin D, Sumi SM, Bird TD *et al* (1989) Familial dementia with PrP positive amyloid plaques: a variant of Gerstmann-Sträussler syndrome. *Neurology* 39: 910–18.

Noguchi S, Murakami N, Yamada N (1993) Apolipoprotein E genotype and Alzheimer's disease. *Lancet* 342: 737.

O'Connor DW, Pollit PA, Treasure FP (1991) The influence of education and social class on the diagnosis of dementia in a community population. *Psychol Med* 21: 219–34.

Ogomori K, Kitamato T, Tateishi J *et al* (1988) β-Protein amyloid is widely distributed in the central nervous system of patients with Alzheimer's disease. *Am J Path* 134: 243–51.

Ogunniyi AO, Osuntokun BO, Ledwauwa UG, Falope ZF (1992) Rarity of dementia (by DSM IIIR) in an urban community in Nigeria. *East Afr Med J* 69: 10–14.

Okazaki H, Reagan TJ, Campbell RJ (1979) Clinicopathologic

studies of primary cerebral amyloid angiopathy. *Mayo Clin Proc* 54: 22–31.

Osuntokun BO, Ogunniyi AO, Akang EEU *et al* (1994) βA4-amyloid in the brains of non-demented Nigerian Africans. *Lancet* 343: 56.

Osuntokun BO, Ogunniyi AO, Ledwauwa UG (1992) Alzheimer's disease in Nigerians? *Afr J Med Sci* 21: 71–7.

Osuntokun BO, Sahota A, Ogunniyi AO *et al* (1995) Lack of association between Apolipoprotein Eε4 and Alzheimer's disease in elderly Nigerians. *Ann Neurol* 38: 463–5.

Palmer AM, Stratmann GC, Procter AW, Bowen DM (1988) Possible neurotransmitter basis of behavioural changes in Alzheimer's disease. *Ann Neurol* 23: 616–20.

Pasquier F, Bail L, Lebert F *et al* (1994) Determination of medial temporal lobe atrophy in early Alzheimer's disease with computed tomography. *Lancet* 343: 861 (letter).

Payami H, Kaye J, Heston L *et al* (1993) Apolipoprotein E genotypes and Alzheimer's disease. *Lancet* 342: 738.

Pericak-Vance MA, Bedout JL, Gaskell PC *et al* (1991) Linkage studies in familial Alzheimer's disease – evidence for chromosome 19 linkage. *Am J Hum Genet* 48: 1034–40.

Perry EK, Tomlinson BE, Blessed G *et al* (1978) Correlation of cholinergic abnormalities with senile plaques and mental test scores in senile dementia. *Br Med J* 1457–9.

Perry EK, Marshall E, Kerwin J, Smith CJ, Jabeen S, Cheng AV, Perry RH (1990a) Evidence of a monoaminergic cholinergic imbalance related to visual hallucinations in Lewy body dementia. *J Neurochem* 55: 1454–6.

Perry EK, McKeith I, Thompson P *et al.* (1991) Topography, extent and clinical relevance of neurochemical deficits in dementia of Lewy body type, Parkinson's disease and Alzheimer's disease. *Ann NY Acad Sci* 197–202.

Perry RH, Irving D, Blessed G, Fairburn A, Perry EK (1990b) Senile dementia of Lewy body type – Lewy body dementia: a clinically and neuropathologically distinct form of Lewy body dementia in the elderly. *J Neurol Sci* 95: 119–35.

Podlisny MB, Lee G, Selkoe DJ (1987) Gene dosage of the amyloid β precursor protein in Alzheimer's disease. *Science* 238: 669–71.

Polvikoski T, Sulkava R, Haltia M *et al* (1995) Apolipoprotein E, dementia and cortical deposition of β-amyloid protein. *N Engl J Med* 333: 1242–7.

Prince M, Cullen M, Mann A (1994) Risk factors for Alzheimer's disease and dementia: a case control study based on the MRC elderly hypertension trial. *Neurology* 44: 97–104.

Ragers J, Cooper NR, Webster S *et al* (1992) Complement activation by β-amyloid in Alzheimer disease. *Proc Natl Acad Sci USA* 89: 10016–20.

Raghaven R, Khin-Nu C, Brown AG (1994) Gender differences in the phenotypic expression of Alzheimer's disease in Down's syndrome (Trisomy 21) *Neuroreport* 5: 1393–6.

Rapoport SI, Pettigrew KD, Schapiro MB (1991) Discordance and concordance of dementia of the Alzheimer type (DAT) in monozygotic twins indicate heritable and sporadic forms of Alzheimer's disease. *Neurology* 41: 1549–53.

Risse SC, Raskind MA, Nochlin D *et al* (1990) Neuropathological findings in patients with clinical diagnoses of probable Alzheimer's disease. *Am J Psychiat* 147: 168–72.

Roberts GW, Allsop D, Bruton CJ (1990) The occult aftermath of boxing. *J Neurol Neurosurg Psychiat* 53: 373–8.

Roberts GW, Gentleman SM, Lynch A, Murray L, Landon M, Graham DI (1994) β Amyloid protein in the brain after severe head injury: implications for the pathogenesis of Alzheimer's disease. *J Neurol Neurosurg Psychiat* 57: 419–25.

Rocca WA, Amaducci LA, Schoenberg BS (1986) Epidemiology of clinically diagnosed Alzheimer's disease. *Ann Neurol* 19: 415–24.

Rocca WA, Baniauto S, Lippi A *et al* (1990) Prevalence of clinically diagnosed Alzheimer's disease and other dementing disorders: a door-to-door survey in Appignano, Macerata Province, Italy. *Neurology* 40: 626–31.

Rocca WA, Hofman A, Brayne C *et al* (1991) Frequency and distribution of Alzheimer's disease in Europe: a collaborative study of 1980–1990 prevalence findings. *Ann Neurol* 30: 381–90.

Rogers JD, Brogan D, Mirra S (1985) The nucleus basalis of Meynert in Neurological disease: a quantitative morphological study. *Ann Neurol* 17: 163–70.

Roher AE, Lowenson JD, Clark S, Woods AS, Cotter RJ, Gowing E, Ball MJ (1993) β-amyloid (1–42) is a major component of cerebrovascular amyloid deposits: implications for the pathology of Alzheimer disease. *Proc Natl Acad Sci USA* 90: 10836–40.

Roses AD, Pericak-Vance MA, Saunders, AM *et al* (1994) Complex genetic disease: can genetic strategies in Alzheimer's disease and new genetic mechanisms be applied to epilepsy. *Epilepsia* 35 Suppl 1: 520–8.

Roses AD (1994) Apolipoprotein E affects the rate of Alzheimer disease expression: β-amyloid burden is a secondary consequence dependent on APOE genotype and duration of disease. *J Neuropath Exp Neurol* 53: 429–37.

Rossor MN (1992) Familial Alzheimer's disease. In *Clinical Neurology* 1. Ballière-Tindall, pp. 517–534.

Roth M, Tomlinson BE, Blessed G (1966) Correlation between scores for dementia and counts of 'senile plaques' in cerebral grey matter of elderly subjects. *Nature* 209: 109–10.

Samuel W, Terry RD, DeTeresa R, Butters N, Masliah E (1994) Clinical correlates of cortical and nucleus basalis pathology in Alzheimer dementia. *Arch Neurol* 51: 772–8.

Saunders A, Strittmatter WJ, Schmechel D *et al* (1993) Association of apolipoprotein E allele ε4 with the late onset familial and sporadic Alzheimer's disease. *Neurology* 43: 1467–72.

Schellenberg GD, Deeb SS, Boehnke M *et al* (1987) Association of apolipoprotein CII allele with familial dementia of the Alzheimer type. *J. Neurogenet* 4: 97–108.

Schellenberg GD, Boehnke M, Wijsman EM *et al* (1992a)

Genetic association and linkage analysis of the ApoCII locus and familial Alzheimer disease. *Ann Neurol* 31: 223–7.

Schellenberg GD, Bird TD, Wijsman EM *et al* (1992b) Genetic linkage evidence for a familial Alzheimer's disease locus on chr 14. *Science* 258: 868–71.

Schellenberg GD, Bird TD, Wijsman EM *et al* (1988) Absence of linkage of chromosome 21q21 markers to familial Alzheimer's disease. *Science* 241: 1507–10.

Schmechel WJ, Saunders A, Strittmatter D *et al* (1993) Increased amyloid β-peptide deposition in cerebral cortex as a consequence of apolipoproein E genotype in late-onset Alzheimer disease. *Proc Natl Acad Sci USA* 90: 9649–53.

Schoenberg BS, Anderson DW, Haerer AF (1985) Severe dementia: prevalence and clinical features in a bi-racial US population. *Arch Neurol* 42: 740–3.

Schoenberg BS, Kokmen E, Okazaki H (1987) Alzheimer's disease and other dementing illnesses in a defined United States population: incidence rates and clinical features. *Ann Neurol* 22: 724–9.

Seab JP, Jagust WJ, Wong ST *et al* (1988) Quantitative NMR measurements of hippocampal atrophy in Alzheimer's disease. *Magn Reson Med* 8: 200–8.

Selkoe DJ (1993) Physiological production of the β-Amyloid protein and the mechanism of Alzheimer's disease. *Trends Neurosci* 16: 403–9.

Selkoe DJ (1994) Alzheimer's Disease: a central role for amyloid. *J Neuropath Exp Neurol* 53: 438–47.

Selkoe DJ (1995) Missense on the membrane. *Nature* 375: 734.

Seubert P, Vigo-Pelfrey C, Esch F *et al* (1992) Isolation and quantitation of soluble Alzheimer's β-peptide from biological fluids. *Nature* 359: 325–7.

Sherrington R, Rogaev EI, Liang Y *et al* (1995) Cloning of a gene bearing missense mutations in early-onset familial Alzheimer's disease. *Nature* 375: 754–60.

Shoji M, Golde TE, Ghiso J *et al* (1992) Production of the Alzheimer amyloid β protein by normal protolytic processing. *Science* 258: 126–9.

Skoog I, Nilsson L, Palmertz B *et al* (1993) A population based study of dementia in 85-year-olds. *N Engl J Med* 328: 153–8.

Smith AD, Johnson C, Sim E *et al* (1994) Protective effect of ApoE ε2 in Alzheimer's disease. *Lancet* 344: 473–4.

Smith C, Anderton BH (1994) The molecular pathology of Alzheimer's disease: are we any closer to understanding the neurodegenerative process? *Neuropath Appl Neurobiol* 20: 322–38.

Smith TW, Anwer U, De Girolami U, Drachman DA (1987) Vacuolar change in Alzheimer's disease. *Arch Neurol* 44: 1225–8.

Snowden DA, Ostwald SK, Kane RL (1989) Education, survival and independence in elderly Catholic sisters, 1936–1988. *Am J Epidemol* 130: 999–1012.

Sorbi S, Nacmias B, Forlio P, Placentini S, Amaducci L (1993) APP717 and Alzheimer's disease in Italy. *Nature Genet* 4: 10.

Sparks DL, Hunsaker JC, Scheff SW *et al* (1990) Cortical senile plaques in coronary artery disease, aging and Alzheimer's disease. *Neurobiol Aging* 11: 601–8.

St George-Hyslop PH (1993) Recent advances in the molecular genetics of Alzheimer's disease. *Clin Neurosci* 1: 171–5.

St George-Hyslop P, Haines J, Rogaeva EA *et al* (1992) Genetic evidence for a novel familial Alzheimer disease gene on chromosome 14. *Nature Genet* 2: 331–4.

St George-Hyslop PH, Haines JL, Farrar LA *et al* (1990) Genetic linkage studies suggest that Alzheimer's disease is not a single homogeneous disorder. *Nature* 347: 194–7.

St George-Hyslop PH, Tanzi RE, Podlisky RJ *et al* (1987) The genetic defect causing familial Alzheimer's disease maps on chromosome 21. *Science* 235: 885–90.

Strittmatter WJ, Saunders A, Schmechel D *et al* (1993) Apolipoprotein E: high affinity binding to β/A4 amyloid and increased frequency of type 4 allele in familial Alzheimer's disease. *Proc Natl Acad Sci USA* 90: 1977–81.

Strittmatter WJ, Weisgraber KH, Goedert M *et al* (1994) Hypothesis: microtubule instability and paired helical filament formation in the Alzheimer's disease brain are related to apo E genotype. *Exp Neurol* 125: 163–71.

Sugiyama H, Hainfellner JA, Yoshimura M, Budka H (1994) Neocortical changes in Parkinson's disease revisited. *Clin Neuropathol* 13: 55–9.

Sulkava R, Haltia M, Paetau A *et al* (1983) Accuracy of clinical diagnosis in primary degenerative dementia: correlation with neuropathological findings. *J Neurol Neurosurg Psychiat* 46: 9–13.

Sulkava R, Wikström J, Aromaa A *et al* (1985) Prevalence of severe dementia in Finland. *Neurology* 35: 1025–9.

Tabaton M, Cammarata S, Manetto V *et al* (1991) Ultrastructural localisation of β-amyloid, τ, and ubiquitin epitopes in extracellular neurofibrillary tangles. *Proc Natl Acad Sci USA* 88: 2098–102.

Tagliavini F, Pilleri G (1983) Neuronal counts in basal nucleus of Meynert in Alzheimer's disease and simple senile dementia. *Lancet* 1: 469–70.

Tanzi R, Bird ED, Latt SA, Neve RL (1987) The amyloid β-protein gene is not duplicated in brains from patients with Alzheimer's disease. *Science* 238: 666–9.

Terry RD, Hansen LA, DeTeresa R *et al* (1987) Senile dementia of the Alzheimer type without neocortical neurofibrillary tangles. *J Neuropath Exp Neurol* 46: 262–8.

Terry RD, Peck A, DeTeresa R, Schecter R, Hourupian DS (1981) Some morphometric aspects of the brain in senile dementia of the Alzheimer type. *Ann Neurol* 10: 184–92.

Terry RD, Masliah E, Salmon DP, Butters N, DeTeresa R, Hill R, Hansen LA, Katzman R (1991) Physical bases of cognitive alteration in Alzheimer's disease: synaptic loss is the major correlate of cognitive impairment. *Ann Neurol* 30: 572–80.

Tierney MC, Fisher RH, Lewis AJ *et al* (1988) The NINCDS-ADRDA work group criteria for the clinical diagnosis of probable Alzheimer's disease: a clinicopathologic study of 57 cases. *Neurology* 38: 359–64.

Tomlinson BE (1989) The neuropathology of Alzheimer's disease – issues in need of resolution. (second Dorothy S. Russell memorial lecture) *Neuropathol Appl Neurobiol* 15: 491–512.

Tomlinson BE (1992) Aging and the dementias. In Adams JH, Duchen LW (eds) *Greenfield's Neuropathology*. 5th edn, Oxford University Press, New York, pp. 1284–410.

Tomlinson BE, Blessed G, Roth M (1968) Observations on the brains of non-demented old people. *J Neurol Sci* 7: 331–56.

Tomlinson BE, Blessed G, Roth M (1970) Observations on the brains of demented old people. *J Neurol Sci* 11: 205–42.

Tomonaga M (1981) Cerebral amyloid angiopathy in the elderly. *J Am Geriatr Soc* 29: 151–7.

Toran-Allerand CD, Miranda RC, Bentham WDL *et al* (1992) Estrogen receptors colocalise with low affinity nerve growth receptor in cholinergic neurons of the basal forebrain. *Proc Natl Acad Sci USA* 89: 4668–72.

Tozer R (1991) Diagnosis of Alzheimer's disease. *Br Med J* 302: 48.

Trojanowski JQ, Schmidt ML, Shin R-W, Bramblett GT, Rao D, Lee VM-Y (1993a) Altered tau and neurofilament proteins in neurodegenerative diseases: Diagnostic implications for Alzheimer's disease and Lewy body dementias. *Brain Pathol* 3: 445–64.

Trojanowski JQ, Schmidt ML, Shin R-W, Bramblett GT, Rao D, Lee VM-Y (1993b) PHFτ(A68): from pathological marker to potential mediator of neuronal dysfunction and neuronal degeneration in Alzheimer's disease. *Clin Neurosci* 1: 184–91.

Tsuda T, Lopez Rogaeva EA *et al* (1994) Are the associations between Alzheimer's disease and polymorphisms in the Apolipoprotein E and the apolipoprotein CII genes due to linkage dysequilibrium? *Ann Neurol* 36: 97–100.

Van Broeckhoven C (1995) Molecular genetics of Alzheimer's disease: Identifications of genes and gene mutations. *Eur Neurol* 35: 8–19.

Van Broeckhoven C, Backhovens H, Cruts M *et al* (1992) Mapping of a gene predisposing to early-onset Alzheimer's disease to chromosome 14q24.3. *Nature Genet* 2: 335–9.

Van Broeckhoven C, Genthe AM, Vandenberghe A *et al* (1987) Failure of familial Alzheimer's disease to segregate with the A4 amyloid gene in several European families. *Nature* 329: 153–5.

van Duijn CM, Clayton D, Chandra CM *et al* (1991) Familial aggregation of Alzheimer's disease and related disorders: a collaborative reanalysis of case-control studies. *Int J Epidemiol* 20(suppl 2): S13–20.

Victoroff J, Ross W, Benson DF, Verity A, Vinters HV (1994) Posterior cortical atrophy: Neuropathologic correlations. *Arch Neurol* 51: 269–74.

Vinters HV, Gilbert JJ (1983) Cerebral amyloid angiopathy: Incidence and complications in the aging brain II The distribution of amyloid vascular changes. *Stroke* 14: 924–8.

Vinters HV (1987) Cerebral amyloid angiopathy: a critical review. *Stroke* 18: 311–24.

Wade JPH, Mirsen TR, Hachinski VC *et al* (1987) The clinical diagnosis of Alzheimer's disease. *Arch Neurol* 44: 24–9.

Wernicke TF, Reischies FM (1994) Prevalence of dementia in old age: clinical diagnoses in subjects aged 95 and older. *Neurology* 44: 250–3.

Whitehouse PJ, Price DL, Clark AW, Coyle JT, DeLong MR (1981) Alzheimer disease: evidence for selective loss of cholinergic neurons in the nucleus basalis. *Ann Neurol* 10: 122–6.

Whitehouse PJ, Price DL, Struble RG, Clark AW, Coyle JT, DeLong MR (1982) Alzheimer's disease and senile dementia: loss of neurons in the basal forebrain. *Science* 215: 1237–9.

Whitehouse PJ, Hedreen JC, White CL III, Clark AW, Price DL (1983) Neuronal loss in the basal forebrain cholinergic system is more marked in Alzheimer's disease than in senile dementia of the Alzheimer type. *Ann Neurol* 13: 243–8.

Wilcock GK, Esiri MM (1982) Plaques, tangles and dementia. A quantitative study. *J Neurol Sci* 56: 434–56.

Wilcock GK, Esiri MM, Bowen, DM Smith CCT (1982) Alzheimer's disease. Correlation of cortical choline acetyl transferase activity with the severity of dementia and histological abnormalities. *J Neurol Sci* 57: 407–17.

Wilcock GK, Esiri MM, Bowen DM, Hughes AO (1988) The differential involvement of subcortical nuclei in senile dementia of the Alzheimer type. *J Neurol Neurosurg Psychiat* 51: 842–9.

Wilcock GK, Jacoby R (1991) In Jacoby R, Oppenheimer C (eds) *Psychiatry in the Elderly*. Oxford University Press, pp. 586–605.

Yamaguchi H, Nakazato Y, Hirai S, Shiji M, Harigaya Y (1989) Electron micrograph of diffuse plaques: initial stage of senile plaque formation in the Alzheimer brain. *Am J Path* 135: 593–7.

Yamaguchi H, Nakazato Y, Shiji M *et al* (1991) Secondary deposition of β amyloid within extracellular neurofibrillary tangles in Alzheimer-type dementia. *Am J Pathol* 138: 699–705.

Yamaguchi H, Koji I, Sugihara S *et al* (1994) Presence of apolipoprotein E on extracellular neurofibrillary tangles and on meningeal blood vessels precedes the Alzheimer β-amyloid deposition. *Acta Neuropathol* 88: 413–19.

Yoshimura M (1983) Cortical changes in the parkinsonian brain: a contribution to the delineation of 'diffuse Lewy body disease'. *J Neurol* 229: 17–32.

Yoshioka K, Miki T, Katsuya Ogihara T, Sakaki Y (1991) The 717 Val–Ile substitution in amyloid precursor protein is associated with familial Alzheimer's disease regardless of ethnic groups. *Biochem Biophys Res Commun* 178: 1141–6.

Younkin SG (1995) Evidence that Aβ42 is the real culprit in Alzheimer's disease. *Ann Neurol* 37: 287–8.

Zhang, M, Katzman R, Jin H *et al* (1990) The prevalence of dementia and Alzheimer's disease in Shanghai, China.

Impact of age, gender and education. *Ann Neurol* 27: 428–37.

Zubenko GS, Moossy J, Kopp U (1990) Neurochemical correlates of major depression in primary dementia. *Arch Neurol* 47: 209–14.

Zweig RM, Ross CA, Hendreen JC, Steele C, Cardillo JE, Whitehouse PJ, Folstein MF, Price DL (1988) The neuropathology of aminergic nuclei in Alzheimer's disease. *Ann Neurol* 24: 233–42.

Neuropathological changes of Alzheimer's disease in persons with Down's syndrome

D. M. A. Mann

Introduction
Gross changes in the brain in Down's syndrome
Neuronal fallout in Down's syndrome
Neurochemical changes in elderly persons with Down's syndrome
The prevalence and distribution of senile plaques and neurofibrillary tangles in the brain in Down's syndrome
The morphological and immunohistochemical appearance of SP and NFT in Down's syndrome
Conclusion
Chronological studies of the time course of pathological events

INTRODUCTION

Down's syndrome (DS) is the most common clinical syndrome associated with mental handicap, occurring in about 1/1000 live births (Adams *et al.*, 1981) and accounting for about 17% of the total mentally handicapped population (Heller, 1969). While an association between DS and dementia was noted over a century ago by Fraser & Mitchell (1876), who wrote 'in not a few instances, however, death was attributed to nothing more than a general decay – a sort of precipitated senility', it was not until much later (Struwe, 1929; Jervis, 1948) that the linkage between this 'senile decay' and the presence within the brain of the pathological lesions of Alzheimer's disease (AD), namely senile plaques (SP) and neurofibrillary tangles (NFT), was noted. Over the past 20 years, it has now become apparent that nearly all persons with DS who live beyond 40 years of age show SP and NFT within their brains that seemingly mimic those of AD itself.

The more vigorous and successful treatment of cardiac and infective disease during infancy in DS has much increased life expectancy, from around 9 years early this century, to a level whereby as many as 70% of persons can now expect to live beyond 50 years of age (Dupont, Vaeth & Videbech, 1986; Baird & Sadovnick, 1987), particularly if cardiac abnormalities are not present. This increased longevity has latterly given rise to a substantial population of elderly people with DS and with this the problems of 'precocious ageing' and dementia have gained prominence. Moreover, the apparent predictability of the pathology of AD in such persons, should they live long enough, has provided a unique opportunity in humans to detect the early changes of this destructive process and to follow them through in time to that end-point characteristically seen at autopsy in persons in the general population dying with AD itself.

In this review, the pathological features of AD in individuals with DS will be described and how the evolution of such changes helps in understanding the pathogenesis of AD will be discussed.

GROSS CHANGES IN THE BRAIN IN DOWN'S SYNDROME

Although the presence of Alzheimer-type pathology in the brains of elderly DS individuals is well recognized (see later), it is equally well known that the brains of children and young adults with DS, but without SP and NFT, are defective, showing distinctive gross neuropathological changes as well as specific abnormalities of nerve cell number and neuronal connectivity; changes presumably responsible in some way for dictating the basic mental handicap. Hence, alterations in brain size and structure in older DS individuals have to be set in context of those fundamental alterations occurring in earlier life; direct comparisons between elderly DS patients and non-demented persons of the same age in the general population may not be strictly tenable.

In gross terms, the weight of the brain in younger individuals with DS is usually low for age. For example, in the combined studies of Benda (1960), Solitaire & Lamarche (1967), Whalley (1982), Wisniewski et al. (1985a) and Mann & Esiri (1989), out of 106 patients, over 8 but under 50 years of age, the brain weight exceeded 1200 g in only 21 (20%) and fell below 1000 g in 16 (15%) patients; few mentally able persons of that age-range would have a brain weight under 1200 g and certainly none under 1000 g. In morphology, the brain in DS is 'rounded' and usually shows a foreshortening in the anterior–posterior dimension (Davidoff, 1928; Crome & Stern, 1972) due particularly to the relative smallness of the frontal lobes (Crome & Stern, 1972; Wisniewski et al., 1985a). The cerebellum may also be small (Crome & Stern, 1972), as is the hippocampus (Sylvester, 1983; Wisniewski et al., 1985a). The frontal gyri and those of the temporal lobe, especially the superior temporal gyrus, may show an incomplete eversion (Davidoff, 1928). These changes might account for the low (for age) brain weight commonplace in such DS individuals. The incompletely developed DS brain also shows structural abnormalities with a low (for age) number of nerve cells in regions such as the temporal (Ross, Galaburda & Kemper, 1984; Mann et al., 1987a; Mann, 1988b) and other areas of cortex (Colon, 1972; Ross et al., 1984; Wisniewski, Laure-Kamionowska & Wisniewski, 1984; Wisniewski et al., 1986), the hippocampus (Ball & Nuttall, 1980) and the subcortex and brainstem (Gandolfi, Horoupian & De Teresa, 1981; McGeer et al., 1985; Casanova et al., 1985; Mann et al., 1987a; Mann, 1988b). Abnormalities in dendritic spines (Marin-Padilla, 1976; Suetsuga & Mehraein, 1980; Takashima et al., 1981; Becker, Armstrong & Chan, 1986; Ferrer & Gullotta, 1990), an arrested synaptogenesis (Wisniewski et al., 1984, 1986) and a delayed post-natal myelination (Wisniewski & Schmidt-Sidor, 1986) have also been reported.

After the age of 50 years, however, the weight of the brain in DS does fall when compared to younger DS individuals (see Wisniewski et al., 1985a). Hence, in the combined studies of Solitaire & Lamarche (1967), Whalley (1982), Wisniewski et al. (1985a) and Mann (1988b), out of a total of 75 patients over 50 years of age, only 7 (9%) still had a brain weight over 1200 g but 39 (52%) now had a brain weight below 1000 g. Morphometric analysis (De La Monte & Hedley-White, 1990) shows

that, when the basic underdevelopment of the frontal and anterior temporal lobes in younger DS individuals is taken into account, the additional decrease in brain size (and presumably weight also) that occurs in DS in later life is brought about, as in AD (De La Monte, 1989; Mann, 1991), by a loss of tissue, both grey and white, especially from posterior parts of the brain. Such changes (presumably) relate to the onset and progression of Alzheimer-type pathology in such regions; a finding underscored by the similar reductions in brain weight (in percentage terms) occurring in elderly, as compared to younger, DS individuals and in patients with AD, when related to non-demented persons in the general population (Mann, Royston & Ravindra. 1990b).

Serial CT scanning (Schapiro et al., 1989) shows that, while healthy young persons with DS have smaller brains than persons of that age within the general population (see above), older DS subjects have a reduced brain size when compared to such younger DS individuals, and that this declines further with age and upon onset of dementia. Hence, although their brains are smaller than usual, younger DS patients still have a normal (proportionately to size) cerebral regional glucose utilization (Schapiro et al., 1990) and blood flow (Risberg, 1980; Schapiro et al., 1988) whereas in elderly patients, as in AD, both of these parameters are reduced, particularly in the temporal and posterior parietal cortex, both in relationship to younger DS individuals (Schapiro et al., 1987) or to normal, non-Down's, persons of that age (Melamed et al., 1987).

NEURONAL FALLOUT IN DOWN'S SYNDROME

The cerebral atrophy of AD is brought about by a shrinkage and loss of neurones within particular cortical and subcortical structures and by the loss of pathways connecting such areas (see previously and Mann, 1985, 1988a for reviews). Most severely affected cells are the large pyramidal cells of the layers III and V of the cerebral cortex and those of the hippocampus; the cholinergic cells of the basal forebrain system, the noradrenergic cells of the locus caeruleus and the serotonergic cells in the dorsal raphe also undergo (often severe) neuronal fallout with atrophy of survivors.

In elderly patients with DS (as in AD, when compared to similarly aged persons in the general population) there is a low number (for age) of pyramidal (Mann, Yates & Marcyniuk, 1985a) and non-pyramidal (Kobayashi et al., 1990) nerve cells in areas of the temporal cortex, hippocampus (Ball & Nuttall, 1980) and entorhinal cortex (Hyman & Mann, 1991). The nucleus basalis (Mann, Yates & Marcyniuk, 1984; Mann *et al.*, 1985*b*; Price *et al.*, 1982; Casanova *et al.*, 1985), locus caeruleus (Mann *et al.*, 1984, 1985*b*; Marcyniuk, Mann & Yates, 1988; German *et al.*, 1992), dorsal raphe (Mann *et al.*, 1984, 1985*b*) and ventral tegmentum (Mann, Yates & Marcyniuk, 1987*b*; Gibb *et al.*, 1989) are also grossly depleted of nerve cells. Considerable atrophy of surviving nerve cells of these types also takes place as is witnessed by the low values for nucleolar size (an index of ribosomal RNA synthesis and cellular protein synthetic activity) in remaining cells (Mann *et al.*, 1984, 1985*a*, *b*, 1987*a*).

However, bearing in mind what has been said previously, it cannot be assumed, *prima facie*, that these low values for cell number and nucleolar volume represent the 'actual' level of change in such elderly DS subjects associated with the development of Alzheimer-type pathology, since it is clear (see earlier) that younger individuals with DS may not start out with the same complement of nerve cells (and perhaps nucleolar size also) as their non-DS counterparts in the general population. When this is taken into account (by making comparisons with young DS individuals rather than with young adults in the general population) (Mann *et al.*, 1987*a*, 1990*b*), it is apparent that an actual loss and atrophy of nerve cells in all of these regions does indeed occur. While the extent of the reduction in cell number seems broadly similar in DS to that in AD (Mann *et al.*, 1987*a*) for many brain areas (e.g. hippocampus, nucleus basalis, locus caeruleus and dorsal raphe), in other regions (e.g. temporal cortex) it is significantly less than in AD. Likewise the extent of cellular atrophy (i.e. the reduction in nucleolar size) does not parallel that in AD (Mann *et al.*, 1987*a*, 1990*b*), being less in DS in all these aforementioned areas. These differences may be of importance (see later) in connection with the failure of some elderly persons with DS to develop dementia despite the presence of abundant Alzheimer-type changes in their brains.

NEUROCHEMICAL CHANGES IN ELDERLY PERSONS WITH DOWN'S SYNDROME

In AD, nerve cell loss and atrophy leads to associated reductions in neurochemical markers (i.e. transmitter levels, enzyme activities or receptor densities) in regions of brain containing the cell bodies or nerve terminals comprising such affected systems (see previously and

Mann & Yates, 1986 for review). In elderly individuals with DS, low levels of choline acetyl transferase (ChAT) within the cerebral cortex and other brain regions has been reported (Yates *et al.*, 1980, 1983; Godridge *et al.*, 1987). Noradrenaline (Yates *et al.*, 1981, 1983; Reynolds & Godridge, 1985; Godridge *et al.*, 1987) and 5-hydroxytryptamine (Yates, Simpson & Gordon, 1986; Godridge *et al.*, 1987) levels are reduced in cortex and other areas. Losses of glutamate (Reynolds & Warner, 1988) and GABA (Reynolds & Warner, 1988) in cerebral cortex have been reported, as have reductions in D-^{3}H aspartate binding (Simpson *et al.*, 1989). Dopamine levels appear to be unaltered (Yates *et al.*, 1983; Godridge *et al.*, 1987). The amount of somatostatin also appears to be low in elderly DS brains (Pierotti *et al.*, 1986). Although it should be kept in mind that the whole of these neurochemical studies in DS has been based on a very small number of cases (some 10–20 in total) together with an absence or a paucity of relevant control data taken from younger DS individuals *without* Alzheimer-type changes (about 6 in total), the findings are still consistent with the view that, as in AD, such low values do indicate an actual transmitter loss and likewise reflect the atrophy and fall-out of parental neurones.

THE PREVALENCE AND DISTRIBUTION OF SENILE PLAQUES AND NEUROFIBRILLARY TANGLES IN THE BRAIN IN DOWN'S SYNDROME

The occurrence of SP or NFT or both within one or more brain regions in persons with DS at different times of life has been the subject of numerous case reports and some more extensive surveys (e.g. Struwe, 1929; Bertrand & Koffas, 1946; Jervis, 1948; Solitaire & Lamarche, 1966; Neumann, 1967; Haberland, 1969; Olson & Shaw, 1969; Malamud, 1972; O'Hara, 1972; Burger & Vogel, 1973; Schochet, Lampert & McCormick, 1973; Ellis, McCulloch & Corley, 1974; Reid & Maloney, 1974; Crapper *et al.*, 1975; Rees, 1977; Murdoch & Adams, 1977; Wisniewski *et al.*, 1979, 1985*a*, *b*; Ball & Nuttall, 1980; Ropper & Williams, 1980; Blumbergs, Beran & Hicks, 1981; Pogacar & Rubio, 1982; Whalley, 1982; Yates *et al.*, 1983; Sylvester, 1983; Ross *et al.*, 1984; Mann *et al.*, 1984, 1985*a*, 1986, 1987*a*, 1990*a*, *b*; Mann & Esiri, 1989; Belza & Urich, 1986; Motte & Williams, 1989; Giaccone *et al.*, 1989; De La Monte & Hedley-White, 1990; Ferrer & Gullotta, 1990). These 39 studies encompass some 434 patients, aged from under 10 years to over 70 years. When classic silver (e.g. Bodian, Palmgren, Bielschowsky) staining methods

Table 4b-1. *Prevalence of senile plaques and neurofibrillary tangles in the brains of patients with Down's syndrome: reviewed data analysed by age*

Age range (years)	Total number of patients	Number showing plaques and tangles	Percentage of patients affected
0–9	38	0	0
10–19	81	6	7.4
20–29	59	10	16.9
30–39	45	36	80.0
All < 39	223	52	23.3
40–49	62	61	98.4
50–59	98	96	98.0
60–69	48	48	100.0
70–79	3	3	100.0
All > 40	211	208	98.6
All patients 0–79	434	260	59.9

were employed, the presence of (any) SP or NFT or both, was noted in 260 (59.9%) of these patients (Table 4b-1). When analysed by decade, typical SP (see later) together with, or without, NFT first appeared, infrequently, during the second decade of life and increased rapidly through the third and fourth decades such that nearly 100% prevalence was reported in patients aged 40–60 years and exactly 100% in those over 60 years of age. In summary, of those 211 patients *over* 40 years of age surveyed here, 208 (98.6%) showed SP *and* NFT whereas only 52 of 223 patients (23.3%) *under* 40 years showed *either* SP or NFT or *both* changes. It seems therefore that in DS there is a transitional period, usually between 20 and 40 years of age, during which the absence of SP and NFT in any part of the brain changes into a widespread presence throughout the brain and that this change occurs in virtually all patients. So far, only three persons over the age of 40 years with the DS phenotype have been claimed not to show any SP or NFT at all within their brains (see Murdoch & Adams, 1977; Whalley, 1982). In one of these persons, a 55 year-old woman, the karyotype was that of a chromosomal mosaic (Whalley, 1982), whereas in another, a 49 year-old woman (Whalley, 1982) the karyotype was that of a full trisomy 21. However, in this patient the brain weight was a most unusual 1520 g and the histological examinations were insufficiently extensive to definitely exclude the presence

of SP and NFT *anywhere* in the brain. The third such potential patient was briefly referred to in a letter by Murdoch & Adams (1977) in which they reported on a 56 year-old man whose brain was said not to contain either SP or NFT. How extensive the pathological investigations had been in this case is not clear, nor were any details of karyotype presented. Therefore, from these limited data, it is still uncertain as to whether any exceptions from the usual association between DS and the presence of SP and NFT in later life do indeed exist.

This present survey also shows that, while in most, if not all, patients over 50 years of age SP and NFT *always* occur together and in high numbers, in those patients under this age a more variable picture is seen. For example, within those studies (Struwe, 1929; Jervis, 1948; Olson & Shaw, 1969; Burger & Vogel, 1973; Schochet *et al.*, 1973; Wisniewski *et al.*, 1979, 1985a; Ball & Nuttall, 1980; Ropper & Williams, 1980; Yates *et al.*, 1983; Sylvester, 1983; Ross *et al.*, 1984; Mann *et al.*, 1986; Mann & Esiri, 1989; Motte & Williams, 1989; Giaccone *et al.*, 1989) in which patients aged between 6 and 50 years were represented and in which the presence of SP and NFT in different brain regions was investigated separately (giving a total of 94 brains), 43 patients showed neither SP nor NFT in any area examined, 41 showed SP and NFT *together* in all areas examined or in the hippocampus alone, but at least 10 patients in 5 studies (see Struwe, 1929; Jervis, 1948; Burger & Vogel, 1973; Motte & Williams, 1989; Giaccone *et al.*, 1989) seemed to show *only SP* alone in one or more regions. However, because in most instances, surveys were limited either to frontal cortex or hippocampus, or both, it is possible that some NFT might have occurred in other areas not investigated. *In no patient however did NFT occur in the absence of SP.*

In all studies reported so far (Solitaire & Lamarche, 1966; Olson & Shaw, 1969; Burger & Vogel, 1973; Reid & Maloney, 1974; Crapper *et al.*, 1975; Rees, 1977; Wisniewski *et al.*, 1985b; Motte & Williams, 1989; Rafalowska *et al.*, 1988), including our own (Mann *et al.*, 1984, 1985a, 1986, 1987a, 1990b), the *pattern of involvement* of brain structures by SP and NFT, in persons with DS who live beyond 50 years of age, seems to closely follow that typically seen in AD (for review, see Mann, 1985, 1988a). For example, in such elderly and established cases of DS the amygdala, hippocampus and association areas of frontal, temporal and parietal cortex and especially the outer laminae (Rafalowska *et al.*, 1988) are all strongly favoured by SP formation, whereas the visual, motor and somatosensory cortex are less affected (Mann *et al.*, 1986; Motte & Williams, 1989). Nerve cells in the olfactory nuclei and tracts are also affected by NFT (Mann *et al.*, 1986; Mann, Tucker & Yates, 1988*a*) and sometimes also by SP. Typical SP are not seen in the cerebellar cortex (see later) nor are NFT present in Purkinje cells though occasionally nerve cells of the dentate nucleus contain NFT (Mann *et al.*, 1990*a*). The nucleus basalis, locus caeruleus and raphe are all severely affected by NFT (Mann *et al.*, 1984, 1985*b*, 1986). Whether the *density* of SP and NFT within affected brain regions is also similar in middle-aged persons with DS to that seen in patients with AD is not clear. Ball & Nuttall (1980) estimated that NFT density in the hippocampus of two patients with DS fell within that range encountered in eight patients with AD; SP were not quantified. Ropper & Williams (1980) estimated SP and NFT densities in the hippocampus of 8 persons over 50 years of age with DS and, although no data was presented, these were said to be comparable with levels in 'demented old people'. More recently, work by us (Mann, 1988*b*) suggests differences might occur; for example, in 15 persons with DS over 50 years of age the mean SP density in the temporal cortex was less than that in ten patients of that age with AD whereas NFT densities were equivalent in both groups. However, in the hippocampus, in DS, both SP and NFT densities far exceeded those usually seen in AD.

THE MORPHOLOGICAL AND IMMUNOHISTOCHEMICAL APPEARANCE OF SP AND NFT IN DOWN'S SYNDROME

Plaques
The similarities in appearance between SP and NFT of patients with DS and those typically seen in AD (see earlier and Wisniewski & Terry (1973) for light and electron microscope appearances of SP and NFT in AD), have been emphasized at both light (Struwe, 1929; Jervis, 1948; Solitaire & Lamarche, 1966; Olson & Shaw, 1969; Burger & Vogel, 1973) and electron (O'Hara, 1972; Schochet *et al.*, 1973; Ellis *et al.*, 1974) microscope levels. However, a high proportion of amorphous plaque cores dissimilar to those of AD, being larger and having the amyloid fibrils less compact and lacking, under Congo red birefringence, the well-defined typical polarization cross has been reported (Masters *et al.*, 1985; Allsop *et al.*, 1986). Although these observations were made on biochemically isolated plaque cores rather than on SP *in situ* we too have observed these amorphous SP to be more common in DS after 50 years of age, and especially

so within the amygdala and entorhinal cortex (Mann *et al.*, 1986). Assuming that, in DS, patients start to form and accumulate SP (and NFT) at 30–40 years of age, then the pathological picture seen at death may have been evolving in many patients for at least 20 years. In AD, the usual duration of illness is about 5 to 10 years, only occasionally exceeding 15 years. Differences in SP morphology between DS and AD may thus only represent variations in the 'stages' of their natural history consequent upon this longer pathological course.

The proteinaceous, β-pleated, congophilic material (amyloid) that comprises much of the 'core' of typical SP in AD (and DS), consists of a polypeptide of 39–42 amino acids (Masters *et al.*, 1985) now termed β/A4 peptide (according to molecular weight, 4.2 kD, and ability to polymerize spontaneously into a β-pleated configuration). β/A4 is formed through an alternative cleavage of a larger precursor molecule, amyloid precursor protein, APP (Esch *et al.*, 1990; Sisodia *et al.*, 1990) which spans the nerve cell membrane, having a small intracellular domain and a much larger extracellular domain (Kang *et al.*, 1987). APP is coded by a gene located on the long arm of chromosome 21 and may function as a cell surface receptor or have secretory or cell adhesion properties (Kang *et al.*, 1987). This same, or at least a very similar, β/A4 molecule is also present within the walls of arteries that in AD display 'congophilic angiopathy' (Glenner & Wong, 1984*a*: Joachim *et al.*, 1988). Glenner & Wong (1984*b*) have shown that the β/4 molecule of AD is also present in arterial walls in DS and Masters *et al.* (1985) report that the β/A4 of plaque cores in DS, is identical to that of plaque cores in AD. Microchemical analysis of the non-proteinaceous residue of plaque cores in both AD and DS (Masters *et al.*, 1985; Edwardson *et al.*, 1986; Edwardson & Candy, 1989) reveals much aluminium and silicon, possibly co-localized in the form of an aluminosilicate.

Surrounding the amyloid core are various cellular and non-cellular (more β/A4) elements. Unusual accumulation of glycoproteins, probably as oligosaccharides, are present in the plaque periphery (Szumanska *et al.*, 1987; Mann *et al.*, 1988*b*, 1989*a*) though the precise molecular nature of these, as well as the cellular elements within which they are contained, remain to be characterized. Heparan sulphate proteoglycan (HSPG) is also accumulated within SP, both in AD and DS (Snow *et al.*, 1990). Glial cells are usually present within SP, both in AD and DS; microglia are often intimately associated with the amyloid cores (Wegiel & Wisniewski, 1990; Mann, Younis & Jones, 1992*c*) whereas astrocytes and their processes are more abundant in the periphery though these can often extend throughout the plaque region (Murphy *et al.*, 1990; Mann *et al.*, 1992*c*).

Recently, immunohistochemistry, using antibodies directed against β/A4 has revealed that, in the cortex in AD, besides the typical cored SP there are (often many more) 'diffuse' types of deposits (see previously and Ogomori *et al.*, 1989; Ikeda, Allsop & Glenner, 1989*a*; Tagliavini *et al.*, 1988; Yamaguchi *et al.*, 1988; Wisniewski *et al.*, 1989; Mann *et al.*, 1990*a*). Similar deposits are widely seen in the cortex, hippocampus and amygdala in DS (Mann *et al.*, 1989*a*, 1990*a*: Mann & Esiri, 1989; Allsop *et al.*, 1989; Ikeda *et al.*, 1989*b*; Giaccone *et al.*, 1989; Rumble *et al.*, 1989; Murphy *et al.*, 1990; Snow *et al.*, 1990; Spargo *et al.*, 1990). These, in both conditions, do not seem to be associated with a neuritic component nor do they usually display much (if any) astrocytic reaction (Murphy *et al.*, 1990; Mann *et al.*, 1992*c*), though they do contain microglia (Mann *et al.*, 1992*c*) and often show much accumulation of oligosaccharide (Mann *et al.*, 1989*a*). Importantly, β immunostaining has also shown that, in both AD and DS, non-cortical areas such as the cerebellum (Ogomori *et al.*, 1989; Ikeda *et al.*, 1989*a*; Joachim, Morris & Selkoe, 1989; Yamaguchi *et al.*, 1989; Wisniewski *et al.*, 1989; Mann *et al.*, 1990*a*) and striatum (Ogomori *et al.*, 1989; Suenaga *et al.*, 1990) contain many similarly diffuse, β/A4 deposits. These also contain microglial cells but, in contrast to the cerebral cortical deposits, do not show much (if any) accumulation of oligosaccharide (Mann *et al.*, 1992*c*); they are never associated with a neuritic element and astrocytes are only infrequently present (Mann *et al.*, 1992*c*).

Tangles

Immunohistochemistry indicates that the microtubule-associated protein, tau, is most probably the major antigenic determinant of the paired helical filaments (PHF) of the NFT in AD (see earlier and Wood *et al.*, 1986; Kosik, Joachim & Selkoe, 1986; Ihara *et al.*, 1986; Delacourte & Defossez, 1986). The presence of tau within PHF has been confirmed by direct protein analysis (Goedert *et al.*, 1988; Wischik *et al.*, 1988; Kondo *et al.*, 1988) which in conjunction with other immunohistochemical studies (e.g. Kosik *et al.*, 1988) implies that the *whole* of the tau molecule is incorporated into PHF via its microtubule binding region and exists in an abnormally phosphorylated state (Wood *et al.*, 1986). Immunostaining (Perry *et al.*, 1987; Lowe *et al.*, 1988; Lennox *et al.*, 1988) and direct protein analysis (Mori, Kondo & Ihara, 1987) have shown another protein, ubiquitin, also to form an important part of the

NFT. Lectin histochemistry (Szumanska *et al.*, 1987; Mann *et al.*, 1988*b*; Sparkman *et al.*, 1990) has revealed the NFT to contain, or at least to be associated with, certain saccharide sequences.

These properties of the NFT in AD seem to hold in DS. Cross-reactivity between the NFT of AD and DS occurred with an antibody to neurofilament protein (Anderton *et al.*, 1982). The NFT of DS is similarly immunoreactive to tau and ubiquitin as that of AD (Mann *et al.*, 1989*b*; Murphy *et al.*, 1990). Immunoblotting (Flament, Delacourte & Mann, 1990; Hanger *et al.*, 1991) shows similar mobility profiles for tau proteins in elderly DS brains as in AD. However, in DS, NFT do not seem to interact with lectins (Mann *et al.*, unpublished data).

Other pathological similarities

Granulovacuolar degeneration of neurones in the hippocampus and particularly in area CA1 is, as in AD, a feature of DS at middle age (Solitaire & Lamarche, 1966; Olson & Shaw, 1969; Burger & Vogel, 1973; Ellis *et al.*, 1974; Ball & Nuttall, 1980). Like AD, Hirano bodies are commonly present in this same part of the hippocampus in such older persons with DS (Burger & Vogel, 1973; Ellis *et al.*, 1974). Calcification of the walls of the larger arteries of the globus pallidus, and a deposition of calcified deposits (calcospherites) around capillaries in this same brain region, is often seen in AD, particularly in late onset cases (Mann, 1988*c*). Elderly patients with DS often show an excessive (for age) calcification of this part of the basal ganglia (Wisniewski *et al.*, 1982; Takashima & Becker, 1986; Mann, 1988*c*), though it is not clear whether this change is related to ageing alone or whether the additional burden of AD has a bearing on its frequent occurrence. Again, as in younger patients with AD uncomplicated by single or multiple lacunar or embolic infarcts, atherosclerosis of the major vessels at the base of the brain is a conspicuously negative finding in (elderly) patients with DS (Olson & Shaw, 1969; Burger & Vogel, 1973, Murdoch *et al.*, 1977; Mann, 1988*b*). However, a severe deposition of β/A4 protein within the walls of large meningeal arteries, especially those supplying the posterior hemispheres and cerebellum and within the walls of some intraparenchymal arteries, is a feature of most middle aged patients with DS (Mann *et al.*, 1990*a*), as well as in many of those with AD. Such a vascular amyloidosis is also associated with a deposition of HSPG (Snow *et al.*, 1990). Other changes, involving a deposition of glycoproteins within the endothelium or basement membrane and detectable by lectin histochemistry, occur after the age of 50 years in the small arteries of the cortex and hippocampus (Mann *et al.*, 1992*d*). Similar changes are present in AD, but in both instances seem unrelated to the deposition in vessels of β/A4 protein; their pathological significance remains uncertain though they may result in, or stem from a compromise in the blood–brain barrier that might have a bearing on the neuronal loss and atrophy taking place at that time of life.

CONCLUSION

Hence, in general, it seems that differences in SP and NFT structure or chemistry between AD and DS are slight; patterns of neuronal damage and loss of transmitters also appear similar. Any variations that may possibly occur might reflect differences in patient life history (e.g. community versus institutional life) or the differing time courses of evolution of pathology and not necessarily be of major aetiological or pathogenetic significance. Moreover, the changes of AD in elderly patients with DS are not due to mental handicap, *per se*, since Malamud (1972) found that, while such changes were present in all patients with DS over 40 years of age, SP and NFT occurred in only 31 of 225 (14%) other (non-DS) mentally handicapped persons, of that age; a prevalence rate probably similar to that of the elderly in the general population.

Therefore, it seems safe to conclude that the pathological changes which develop in the brain in DS during late adult life are indeed those of AD. Although the development of changes in DS is undoubtedly related to the chromosomal alterations that characterize and underpin the disorder, it is not yet certain to what extent a triplication of chromosome 21 is necessary for both expression of Alzheimer-type pathology as well as the typical DS phenotype. Since most cases of DS are those of a full trisomy 21 (Hook, 1981; Gilbert & Opitz, 1982) all will have, as such, a complete genomic triplication and all might be expected to show Alzheimer-type pathology, as indeed they probably do (see earlier). However, some 4–6% of persons with phenotypical DS are 'translocational' (Hook, 1981; Gilbert & Opitz, 1982) with only a partial triplication of chromosome 21 (usually the most distal part of the long arm, a portion obligatory for expression of the DS phenotype). Whether, and to what extent, these translocational patients also show Alzheimer-type changes is not known; in some patients genes dictating SP and NFT formation could be inherited independently (in normal amounts) from those (in triplicate) which determine the DS phenotype. Such patients could thus greatly help to resolve which genes on chromosome 21 are mandatory

to the expression of AD, not only in DS but in the general population as well.

Dementia in Down's syndrome

The question as to whether all patients with DS who live beyond 40 years of age, and whose brains show SP and NFT in quantities sufficient to signal AD in the general population, do indeed also become demented is still unresolved. Most clinically based studies (Owens, Dawson & Losin, 1971; Dalton, Crapper & Schlotterer, 1974; Wisniewski *et al.*, 1978, 1985*b*, 1986; Lott & Lai, 1982; Miniszek, 1983; Thase *et al.*, 1984; Dalton & Crapper, 1984, 1986; Hewitt, Carter & Jancar, 1985; Schapiro *et al.*, 1986; Fenner, Hewitt & Torpy, 1987; Zigman *et al.*, 1987; Silverstein, Herbs & Miller, 1988; Lai & Williams, 1989; Evenhuis, 1990) show that many, and sometimes all, patients beyond this age display signs of mental deterioration or behavioural regression though few(er) present an overt clinical deterioration that can be convincingly defined as dementia. Arguments concerning the acquisition of relevant data that reflect the burden of an additional deficit upon a basic mental retardation and the difficulties in extracting meaningful clinical data from retrospective records not specifically kept for the purpose of charting changes in cognitive function are no doubt applicable and may go a long way towards explaining these apparent inconsistencies. Furthermore, the changes in visual memory in later life, used to mark onset of dementia in several studies, could represent the effects of early deficiencies in the visual cortex (Wisniewski *et al.*, 1984) aggravated by ageing instead of those of AD; to what extent therefore simply 'growing older' precipitates (many of) the mental and behavioural changes of later life is not known. Hence, because there is no established method for the diagnosis of dementia in DS in particular, or in the mentally handicapped in general, it is hardly surprising that such wide variations in the assessed prevalence rate of dementia in elderly DS persons exist.

Nonetheless, despite the difficulties in assessing dementia in DS, a number of studies have identified persons with numerous SP and NFT in their brains (and who, had they not had DS would have been said to have had AD) who have failed even with careful scrutiny to undergo any apparent change in mental state or behaviour in later life (Wisniewski & Rabe, 1986; Wisniewski *et al.*, 1987; Mann *et al.*, 1990*b*, Evenhuis, 1990).

In order to explain this paradox, Wisniewski has argued (Wiesniewski & Rabe, 1986; Wisniewski *et al.*, 1987) that a threshold effect might operate, dictating that a certain level of pathology must accrue before clinical dementia becomes apparent. This threshold level might be higher in the 'cognitively blunted' DS brain, though it is also possible that being 'less sensitive' functionally the DS brain can tolerate a greater level of pathology. Earlier, it was suggested that non-demented elderly DS persons, while still showing above 'threshold' numbers of SP and NFT might not have lost as many nerve cells as their demented counterparts. We have recently examined this possibility (Mann *et al.*, 1990*b*) but find that the two non-demented elderly DS persons identified in this study in fact showed just as great a loss of nerve cells as the eight demented persons of that age. However, like Wisniewski (Wisniewski & Rabe, 1986; Wisniewski *et al.*, 1987), we found such non-demented patients to have fewer neocortical SP and NFT than their demented counterparts though the significance of this finding in functional terms is unclear.

There is clearly therefore a great need to produce diagnostic criteria that differentiate clinically the 'malignant' changes of AD from those insidious ones of ageing, *per se*, within DS individuals. These, together with longitudinal studies in which properly selected (according to karyotype) persons are appropriately and regularly tested and whose brains are thoroughly examined at postmortem, should enable the onset and clinical progression of Alzheimer-related degenerative changes to be accurately recorded. Only then may this apparent discrepancy become reconcilable.

CHRONOLOGICAL STUDIES OF THE TIME COURSE OF PATHOLOGICAL EVENTS IN DS

The structural and biochemical changes present in children with DS, while of potential importance to the understanding of the pathophysiology conferring the basic mental handicap, offer no immediate clues as to why (perhaps all) such persons also ultimately develop AD. However, because of the transitional period of 20–30 years in DS, during which the absence of Alzheimer-type changes develops into a (virtually) predictable presence, it is possible to reconstruct a chronological course of pathological events by pooling cross-sectional data from individuals with DS dying before, during and after this transitional period. It is not practical to carry out this kind of study on patients with AD itself, since, in these, tissues are only usually available at postmortem and then mostly from clinical and pathological 'end-stage' cases in whom the early changes of the disease will either no longer be present or will not be easily identifiable. Moreover, it is not possible with any degree of certainty to differentiate those (non-

demented) persons showing early pathological stages of AD from other patients also showing such minimal changes but who may not necessarily have developed the full-blown pathological picture of AD, and become demented, had they lived longer.

We have studied in recent years (Mann *et al.*, 1989*a, b*, 1990*b*, 1992*c*; Mann & Esiri, 1989) the brains from (currently) 43 individuals with DS, ranging from 13 to 71 years of age and have employed a variety of histological probes designed to detect the presence of many of the molecular and cellular elements within SP and NFT that have been described earlier. Using markers for β/A4, tau, ubiquitin, PHF, oligosaccharides or glial cells we were unable to detect any changes at all in our youngest patient, aged 13 years. However, between this and 50 years of age we observed (see Mann *et al.*, 1989*a, b*, 1992*c*; Mann & Esiri, 1989) a sequence of changes (Fig. 4b.1) within the cerebral cortex and hippocampus that were initiated by the deposition of β/A4 protein, in the form of diffuse plaques (see Fig. 4b.1). Soon *afterwards* activated microglial cells became present within these amyloid deposits and at this same site accumulations of glycoconjugates, and other granular material detectable by anti-ubiquitin appeared. Later, 'cored' amyloid deposits containing many more activated microglia, much ubiquitinated material and larger quantities of oligosaccharide were seen. These cored deposits were reactive with anti-tau and anti-GFAP and contained filamentous structures (PHF), immunoreactive with anti-ubiquitin. At this stage, NFT were only occasionally present in the cerebral cortex but were numerous in the hippocampus, especially in areas CAI and subiculum, entorhinal cortex and amygdala. After 50 years of age a pathological picture indistinguishable from that of AD was seen in all DS patients. Loss of neurones from cortical areas rich in NFT then occurred (Mann *et al.*, 1990*b*) and in most patients (see previously) there was a progressive deterioration in behaviour and personality (Mann *et al.*, 1990*b*). Deposition of β/A4 within the cerebellar cortex occurred about 5 years *after* that in the cerebral cortex and, although the prevalence of this increased with age, such deposits never became associated with a neuritic change nor did NFT become present in Purkinje or other cerebellar cortical cells (Mann *et al.*, 1990*a*).

Therefore, using this particular range of molecular markers, it seems that the onset and progression of the pathological cascade of AD in patients with DS is triggered by events that lead to a deposition of β/A4 protein within the cerebral cortex (Fig. 4b-1). Other less extensive studies on similarly younger persons with DS

(Allsop et al., 1989; Ikeda et al., 1989b; Giaccone et al., 1989; Rumble et al., 1989; Murphy et al., 1990) also point towards this conclusion and the work of Snow et al. (1990) accords with our own observations of an early accumulation of glycoconjugates within such cortical deposits. As mentioned earlier, β/A4 is produced from APP via an alternative breakdown mechanism (Esch et al., 1990; Sisodia et al., 1990). APP seems to be over-expressed in DS (Rumble et al., 1989), and it is therefore possible that imbalances in the handling of an over-production of APP on the one hand, and a relative insufficiency of normal processing factors on the other, might lead to a progressive β/A4 deposition through a 'feeding' of alternative (secondary) catabolic mechanisms (Fig. 4b-2). Experimental work, using transgenic mice that over-express APP_{751} in relationship to APP_{695} (Quon et al., 1991), shows that an over-expression of APP can indeed lead to diffuse β/A4 deposition, though whether the other changes of AD (i.e. the neuritic plaques, NFT and nerve cell loss) can be ultimately induced in this way remains to be demonstrated.

In AD itself, however, it is well known that the APP gene does not exist in triplicate nor is APP over-expressed. Some cases of AD can be inherited at an early age in an apparently autosomally dominant fashion. While in most such families both the APP gene and its products appear normal, it has recently been discovered in a number of European (Goate et al., 1991; Chartier-Harlin et al., 1991), American (Murrell et al., 1991), and Japanese (Naruse et al., 1991) families that there are point mutations at codon 717 of the APP gene

that lead to (three different) single amino acid substitutions in the APP molecule. All three mutations seem to be associated with a typical AD pathology (Murrell et al., 1991; Naruse et al., 1991; Mann et al., 1992a) though variations (e.g. presence of Lewy bodies in brain stem neurones) have been observed in one instance (Lantos et al., 1992). The implication of these latter studies is that mutations within codon 717 of the APP molecule are also pathogenic (Fig. 4b-2) and in some way, per-haps again involving an abnormal processing of APP, lead to the pathological outcome of AD. As in DS, it is not clear how such a mutation might dictate the time of onset (usually at around 40–50 years of age) in these patients.

Whether β/A4 protein is itself neurotoxic and thereby responsible, per se, for the generation of all subsequent pathological events is still far from clear; it might simply represent a relatively innocuous marker of a wider ranging process that carries in its wake other changes certain of which might lead to the 'malignant' neurofib-rillary alterations and eventual cell death. In humans, deposition of β/A4 can, and frequently does, occur in the absence of any neuritic changes and NFT formation. This is particularly so, in both AD and DS, in areas such as the striatum (Suenaga et al., 1990) and cerebellum (Joachim et al., 1989; Mann et al., 1990a), but it can even occur within the cerebral cortex and hippocampus in conditions other than AD (and DS) (Mann & Jones, 1990; Mann et al., 1992b). Hence, in AD and DS, PHF formation may proceed in parallel to, but not necessarily as a direct consequence of, β/A4 formation. It is possible

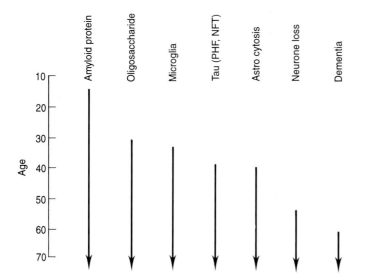

Fig. 4b.1. Time course of pathological events in Down's syndrome patients of different ages.

that a further fragment of the APP molecule, released during cleavage, could be responsible for, or modulate, PHF formation. What that factor might be is not known though it seems clear that it is an entity that must be specific for AD and perhaps more importantly one that is specifically produced by the cerebral cortex in AD (if it is produced in other regions (e.g. cerebellum) in AD it does not affect local neurones in the same way. The fact that the APP molecule is glycosylated (Kang *et al.*, 1987) and the observations that unusual and excessive accumulations of glycoproteins and proteoglycans occur within the cerebral cortical (Szumanska *et al.*, 1987; Mann *et al.*, 1988*b*, 1989*a*; Snow *et al.*, 1990), but not the cerebellar cortical (Mann *et al.*, 1990*a*; Snow *et al.*, 1990) amyloid deposits, in both AD and DS, suggests that oligosaccharides, possibly derived from APP, could be factors that mediate such neuritic changes.

Therefore, at present, it seems that, although DS and AS appear largely homogenous in pathological terms, the mechanisms driving the destructive process(es) behind each are different and diverse. In DS, because of the triplication of chromosome 21, there is over-expression and mismetabolism of APP, though this is perhaps only one of the (many) potential ways by which a common pathological end-point can be brought about. Other factors, some genetic, some possibly non-genetic, clearly exist and interplay within other persons in the general population (Fig. 4b-2) but none the less are ultimately responsible for producing the same disease phenotype that we presently call 'Alzheimer's disease'.

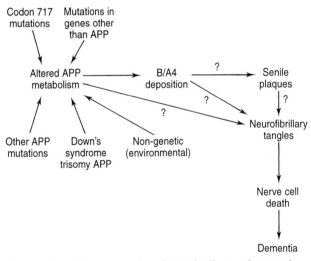

Fig. 4b.2. Possible pathogenetic pathways leading to plaque and tangle formation, nerve cell death and dementia in Down's syndrome and Alzheimer's disease.

REFERENCES

Adams MM, Erickson, JD, Layde PM, Oakley GP (1981) Down's syndrome. Recent trends in the United States. *J Am Med Ass* 246: 758–60.

Allsop D, Kidd M, Landon M, Tomlinson A (1986) Isolated senile plaque cores in Alzheimer's disease and Down's syndrome show differences in morphology. *J Neurol Neurosurg Psychiat* 49: 886–92.

Allsop D, Haga, S-I, Haga C, Ikeda S-I, Mann DMA, Ishii T. (1989) Early senile plaques in Down's syndrome brains show a close relationship with cell bodies of neurones. *Neuropath Appl Neurobiol* 15: 531–42.

Anderton BH, Breinburg D, Downes MJ, Green PJ, Tomlinson BE, Ulrich J, Wood JN, Kahn J. (1982) Monoclonal antibodies show that neurofibrillary tangles and neurofilaments share antigenic determinants. *Nature* 298: 87–96.

Baird PA, Sadovnick AD (1987) Life expectancy in Down's syndrome. *J Paediat* 110: 849–54.

Ball MJ, Nuttall K (1980) Neurofibrillary tangles and granulovacuolar degeneration and neurone loss in Down's syndrome: quantitative comparison with Alzheimer's dementia. *Ann Neurol* 7: 462–5.

Becker LA, Armstrong DL, Chan F (1986) Dendritic atrophy in children with Down's syndrome. *Ann Neurol* 20: 520–6.

Belza MG, Urich H (1986) Cerebral amyloid angiopathy in Down's syndrome. *Clin Neuropathol* 6: 257–60.

Benda CE (1960) *The Child with Mongolism (Congenital Acromicria)*. Grune & Stratton, New York.

Bertrand I, Koffas D (1946) Cas d' idiotie mongolienne adult avec nombreuses plaques seniles et concretions calcaires pallidales. *Rev Neurol (Paris)* 78: 338–45.

Blumbergs P, Beran R, Hicks P (1981) Myoclonus in Down's syndrome. Association with Alzheimer's disease. *Arch Neurol* 38: 453–4.

Burger PC, Vogel FS (1973) The development of the pathological changes of Alzheimer's disease and senile dementia in patients with Down's syndrome. *Am J Path* 73: 457–76.

Casanova MF, Walker LC, Whitehouse PJ, Price DL (1985) Abnormalities of the nucleus basalis in Down's syndrome. *Ann Neurol* 18: 310–13.

Chartier-Harlin MC, Crawford F, Houlden H, Warren A, Hughes D, Fidani L, Goate A, Rossor M, Roques P, Hardy J, Mullan M (1991) Mutations at codon 717 of the β amyloid precursor protein gene cause Alzheimer's disease. *Nature* 353: 84–6.

Colon EJ (1972) The structure of the cerebral cortex in Down's syndrome. *Neuropaediatrics* 3: 362–76.

Crapper DR, Dalton AJ, Skopitz M, Scott JW, Hachinski VC (1975) Alzheimer degeneration in Down's syndrome. *Arch Neurol* 32: 618–23.

Crome L, Stern J (1972) *Pathology of Mental Retardation*, 2nd edn., Williams & Wilkins, Baltimore.

Dalton AJ, Crapper DR, Schlotterer CR (1974) Alzheimer's disease in Down's syndrome: visual retention deficits. *Cortex* 10: 366–77.

Dalton AJ, Crapper DR (1984) Incidence of memory deterioration in ageing persons with Down's syndrome. In Berg JM (ed.) *Perspectives and Progress in Mental Retardation*, Vol. 2, University Park Press, Baltimore, pp 55–62.

Dalton AJ, Crapper DR (1986) Clinical expression of Alzheimer's disease in Down's syndrome. *Psychiat Clin N Am* 4: 659–70.

Davidoff LM (1928) The brain in mongolian idiocy. *Arch Neurol Psychiat* 20: 1229–57.

Delacourte A, Defossez A (1986) Alzheimer's disease tau proteins, the promoting factors of microtubule assembly, are major components of paired helical filaments. *J Neurol Sci* 76: 173–86.

De la Monte S (1989) Quantitation of cerebral atrophy in preclinical and end-stage Alzheimer's disease. *Ann Neurol* 25: 450–9.

De la Monte SM, Hedley-White ET (1990) Small cerebral hemispheres in adults with Down's syndrome. Contributions of developmental arrest and lesions of Alzheimer's disease. *J Neuropath Exp Neurol* 49: 509–20.

Dupont A, Vaeth M, Videbech P (1986) Mortality and life expectancy of Down's syndrome in Denmark. *J Ment Defic Res* 30: 111–20.

Edwardson JA, Candy JM (1989) Aluminium and the pathogenesis of senile plaques in Alzheimer's disease, Down's syndrome and chronic renal dialysis. *Ann Med* 21: 95–7.

Edwardson JA, Klinowsky J, Oakley AE, Perry RH, Candy JM (1986) In Evered D, O'Connor M (eds), *Silicon Biochemistry* Ciba Foundation Symposium No. 121, Wiley & Sons, Chichester, UK, pp 160–79.

Ellis WG, McCulloch JR, Corley CL (1974) Presenile dementia in Down's syndrome. Ultrastructural identity with Alzheimer's disease. *Neurology* 24: 101–6.

Esch ES, Kelm P, Beattie EC, Blancher RW, Cowell AR, Olstersdorf T, McClure D, Ward IJ (1990) Cleavage of amyloid β peptide during constitutive processing of its precursor. *Science* 248: 1122–4.

Evenhuis HM (1990) The natural history of dementia in Down's syndrome. *Arch Neurol* 47: 263–7.

Fenner ME, Hewitt KE, Torpy DM (1987) Down's syndrome: intellectual and behavioural functioning during adulthood. *J Ment Defic Res* 31: 241–9.

Ferrer I, Gullotta F (1990) Down's syndrome and Alzheimer's disease: dendritic spine counts in the hippocampus. *Acta Neuropathol* 79: 680–5.

Flament S, Delacourte A, Mann DMA (1990) Phosphorylation of tau proteins: a major event during the process of neurofibrillary degeneration. Comparisons between Alzheimer's disease and Down's syndrome. *Brain Res* 516: 15–19.

Fraser J, Mitchell A (1876) Kalmuc idiocy: report of a case with autopsy with notes on 62 cases. *J Ment Sci* 22: 161–9.

Gandolfi A, Horoupian DS, DeTeresa, RM (1981) Pathology of the auditory system in trisomies with morphometric and quantitative study of the ventral cochlear nucleus. *J Neurol Sci* 51: 43–50.

German DC, Manaye KF, White CL, Woodward DJ, McIntire DD, Smith WK, Kalaria RN, Mann DMA (1992) Disease specific patterns of locus caeruleus cell loss: Parkinson's disease, Alzheimer's disease and Down's syndrome. *Ann Neurol* 32: 667–76.

Giaccone G, Tagliavini F, Linoli G, Bouras C, Frigero L, Frangione B, Bugiani O (1989) Down patients: extracellular preamyloid deposits precede neuritic degeneration and senile plaques. *Neurosci Lett* 97: 232–8.

Gibb WRG, Mountjoy CQ, Mann DMA, Lees AJ (1989) The substantia nigra and ventral tegmental area in Alzheimer's disease and Down's syndrome. *J Neurol Neurosurg Psychiat* 52: 193–200.

Gilbert EF, Opitz JM (1982) Developmental and other pathological changes in syndromes caused by chromosomal abnormalities. *Perspect Paediat Path* 7: 1–63.

Glenner GG, Wong CW (1984a) Alzheimer's disease: initial report of the purification and characterization of a novel cerebrovascular amyloid protein. *Biochem Biophys Res Commun* 120: 885–90.

Glenner GG, Wong CW (1984b) Alzheimer's disease and Down's syndrome: sharing a unique cerebrovascular amyloid fibril. *Biochem Biophys Res Commun* 122: 1131–5.

Goate A, Chartier-Harlin MC, Mullan M, Brown, J, Crawford F, Fidani L, Gioffra L, Haynes A, Irving N, James L, Mant R, Newton P, Rooke K, Roques P, Talbot C, Pericak-Vance M, Roses AD, Williamson R, Rossor M, Owen M, Hardy JA (1991). Segregation of a missense mutation in the amyloid precursor gene with familial Alzheimer's disease. *Nature* 349: 704–6.

Godridge H, Reynolds GP, Czudek C, Calcutt NA, Benton M (1987) Alzheimer-like neurotransmitter deficits in adult Down's syndrome brain tissue. *J Neurol Neurosurg Psychiat* 50: 775–8.

Goedert M, Wischik C, Crowther RA, Walker JE, Klug A (1988) Cloning and sequencing of the cDNA encoding a core protein of the paired helical filament of Alzheimer's disease: identification as the microtubule associated protein, tau. *Proc Nat Acad Sci USA*, 85: 4051–5.

Haberland C (1969) Alzheimer's disease in Down's syndrome: clinical and neuropathological observations. *Acta Neurol Belg* 69: 369–80.

Hanger DP, Brion, J-P, Gallo J-M, Cairns NJ, Luthert PJ, Anderton BH (1991) Tau in Alzheimer's disease and Down's syndrome is insoluble and abnormally phosphorylated. *Biochem J* 275: 99–104.

Heller JH (1969) Human chromosome abnormalities as related to physical and mental dysfunction. *J Hered* 60: 239–52.

Hewitt KE, Carter G, Jancar J (1985) Ageing in Down's syndrome. *Br J Psychiat* 147: 58–62.

Hook EB (1981). Down's syndrome: its frequency in human populations and some factors pertinent to variations in rates. In de la Cruz FF, Gerald PS (eds) *Trisomy 21 (Down's Syndrome): Research Perspectives*, University Park Press, Baltimore USA, pp 3–68.

Hyman BT, Mann DMA (1991) Alzheimer-type pathological changes in Down's individuals of various ages. In Iqbal K, McLachlan DRC, Winblad B, Wisniewski H M (eds), *Alzheimer's disease: Basic Mechanisms, Diagnosis and Therapeutic Strategies*. Wiley, New York, pp 105–13.

Ihara Y, Nukina N, Miura R, Ogawara M (1986) Phosphorylated tau protein is integrated into paired helical filaments in Alzheimer's disease. *J Biochem (Jpn)* 99: 1807–10.

Ikeda S-I, Allsop D, Glenner GG (1989a) The morphology and distribution of plaque and related deposits in the brains of Alzheimer's disease and control cases: an immunohistochemical study using amyloid β protein antibody. *Lab Invest* 60: 113–22.

Ikeda S-I, Yanagisawa N, Allsop D, Glenner GG (1989b) Evidence of amyloid β protein immunoreactive early plaque lesions in Down's syndrome brains. *Lab Invest* 61: 133–7.

Jervis GA (1948) Early senile dementia and mongoloid idiocy. *Am J Psychiat* 105: 102–6.

Joachim CL, Duffy LK, Morris JH, Selkoe DJ (1988) Protein chemical and immunocytochemical studies of meningovascular β amyloid protein in Alzheimer's disease and normal ageing. *Brain Res* 474: 100–11.

Joachim CL, Morris JH, Selkoe DJ (1989) Diffuse amyloid plaques occur commonly in the cerebellum in Alzheimer's disease. *Am J Path* 135: 309–19.

Kang J, Lemaire H-G, Unterbeck A, Salbaum JM, Masters CL, Grzeschik K-H, Multhaup G, Beyreuther K, Muller-Hill B (1987) The precursor of Alzheimer's disease amyloid A4 protein resembles a cell surface receptor. *Nature* 325: 733–6.

Kobayashi K, Emson PC, Mountjoy CQ, Thornton SN, Lawson DEM, Mann DMA (1990) Cerebral cortical calbindin D_{28k} and parvalbumin neurones in Down's syndrome. *Neurosci Lett* 113: 17–22.

Kondo J, Honda T, Mori H, Hamada Y, Miura R, Ogawara M, Ihara Y (1988) The carboxyl third of tau is tightly bound to paired helical filaments. *Neuron* 1: 827–34.

Kosik KS, Joachim CL, Selkoe DJ (1986) Microtubule associated protein tau is a major antigenic component of paired helical filaments in Alzheimer's disease. *Proc Nat Acad Sci USA* 83: 4044–8.

Kosik KS, Orecchio LD, Binder LI, Trojanowski JQ, Lee V M-Y, Lee G (1988) Epitopes that span the tau molecule are shared with PHF. *Neuron* 1: 817–25.

Lai F, Williams RA (1989) Alzheimer's disease in Down's syndrome. *Neurology* 37: 332–9.

Lantos P, Luthert PJ, Hanger D, Anderton BH, Mullan M, Rossor M (1992) Familial Alzheimer's disease with the amyloid precursor protein position 717 mutation and sporadic Alzheimer's disease have the same cytoskeletal pathology. *Neurosci Lett* 137: 220–4.

Lennox G, Lowe JS, Morrell K, Landon M, Mayer RJ (1988) Ubiquitin is a component of neurofibrillary tangles in a variety of neurodegenerative disorders. *Neurosci Lett* 94: 211–17.

Lott IT, Lai F (1982) Dementia in Down's syndrome; observations from a neurology clinic. *Appl Res Ment Retard* 3: 233–9.

Lowe J, Blanchard A, Morrell K, Lennox G, Reynolds L, Billett M, Landon M, Mayer RJ (1988) Ubiquitin is a common factor in intermediate filament inclusion bodies of diverse type in man including those of Parkinson's disease, Pick's disease and Alzheimer's disease, as well as Rosenthal fibres in cerebellar astrocytomas, cytoplasmic bodies in muscle and Mallory bodies in alcoholic liver disease. *J Path* 155: 9–15.

Malamud N (1972) Neuropathology of organic brain syndromes associated with ageing. In Gaitz CM (ed), *Ageing and the Brain: Advances in Behavioral Biology vol* 3, Plenum Press, New York, pp 63–87.

Mann DMA (1985) The neuropathology of Alzheimer's disease: a review with pathogenetic, aetiological and therapeutic considerations. *Mech Ageing Dev* 31: 213–55.

Mann DMA (1988a) Neuropathological and neurochemical aspects of Alzheimer's disease. In Iversen LL, Iversen SD, Snyder S (eds), *Handbook of Psychopharmacology*, vol 20. Plenum Press, New York, pp 1–67.

Mann DMA (1988b). The pathological association between Down's syndrome and Alzheimer's disease. *Mech Ageing Dev* 43, 99–136.

Mann DMA (1988c) Calcification of the basal ganglia in Down's syndrome and Alzheimer's disease. *Acta Neuropathol* 76: 595–8.

Mann DMA (1991) The topographic distribution of brain atrophy in Alzheimer's disease. *Acta Neuropathol* 83: 81–6.

Mann DMA, Esiri MM (1989) Regional acquisition of plaques and tangles in Down's syndrome patients under 50 years of age. *J Neurol Sci* 89: 169–79.

Mann DMA, Jones D (1990) Amyloid (A4) protein deposition in the brains of persons with dementing disorders other than Alzheimer's disease and Down's syndrome. *Neurosci Lett* 109: 68–75.

Mann DMA, Yates PO (1986) Neurotransmitter deficits in Alzheimer's disease and in other dementing disorders. *Hum Neurobiol* 5: 147–58.

Mann DMA, Yates, PO, Marcyniuk B (1984) Alzheimer's presenile dementia, senile dementia of Alzheimer type and Down's syndrome in middle age form an age-related continuum of pathological changes. *Neuropath Appl Neurobiol* 10: 185–207.

Mann DMA, Yates, PO, Marcyniuk B (1985a) Some morphometric observations on the cerebral cortex and hippocampus in presenile Alzheimer's disease, senile dementia of Alzheimer type and Down's syndrome in middle age. *J Neurol Sci* 69: 139–59.

Mann DMA, Yates, PO, Marcyniuk B, Ravindra CR (1985*b*) Pathological evidence for neurotransmitter deficits in Down's syndrome of middle age. *J Ment Defic Res* 29: 125–35.

Mann DMA, Yates, PO, Marcyniuk B, Ravindra CR (1986) The topography of plaques and tangles in Down's syndrome patients of different ages. *Neuropath Appl Neurobiol* 12: 447–57.

Mann DMA, Yates PO, Marcyniuk B, Ravindra CR (1987*a*) Loss of nerve cells from cortical and subcortical areas in Down's syndrome patients at middle age: quantitative comparisons with younger Down's patients and patients with Alzheimer's disease. *J Neurol Sci* 80: 79–89.

Mann DMA, Yates PO, Marcyniuk B (1987*b*) Dopaminergic neurotransmitter systems in Alzheimer's disease and in Down's syndrome at middle age. *J Neurol Neurosurg Psychiat* 50: 341–4.

Mann DMA, Tucker CM, Yates PO (1988*a*) Alzheimer's disease: an olfactory connection? *Mech Ageing Dev* 42: 1–15.

Mann DMA, Bonshek RE, Marcyniuk B, Stoddart RW, Torgerson E (1988*b*) Saccharides of senile plaques and neurofibrillary tangles in Alzheimer's disease. *Neurosci Lett* 85: 277–82.

Mann DMA, Brown AMT, Prinja D, Davies CA, Beyreuther K, Masters CL, Landon M (1989*a*) An analysis of the morphology of senile plaques in Down's syndrome patients of different ages using immunocytochemical and lectin histochemical methods. *Neuropath Appl Neurobiol* 15: 317–29.

Mann DMA, Prinja D, Davies CA, Ihara Y, Delacourte A, Defossez A, Mayer RJ, Landon M (1989*b*) Immunocytochemical profile of neurofibrillary tangles in Down's syndrome patients of different ages. *J Neurol Sci* 92: 247–60.

Mann DMA, Jones D, Prinja D, Purkiss MS (1990*a*) The prevalence of amyloid (A4) protein deposits within the cerebral and cerebellar cortex in Alzheimer's disease and Down's syndrome. *Acta Neuropathol* 80: 318–27.

Mann DMA, Royston MC, Ravindra CR (1990*b*) Some morphometric observations on the brains of patients with Down's syndrome: their relationship to age and dementia. *J Neurol Sci* 99: 153–64.

Mann DMA, Jones D, Snowden JS, Neary D, Hardy J (1992*a*) Pathological changes in the brain of a patient with familial Alzheimer's disease having a missense mutation at codon 717 in the amyloid precursor protein gene. *Neurosci Lett* 137: 225–8.

Mann DMA, Jones D, South PW, Snowden JS, Neary D (1992*b*) Deposition of amyloid β protein in non-Alzheimer dementias; evidence for a neuronal origin of parenchymal deposits of β protein in neurodegenerative disease. *Acta Neuropathol* 83: 415–19.

Mann DMA, Younis N, Stoddart RW, Jones D (1992*c*) The time course of pathological events concerned with plaque formation in Down's syndrome with particular reference to the involvement of microglial cells. *Neurodegeneration* 1: 201–15.

Mann DMA, Purkiss MS, Bonshek RE, Jones D, Brown AMT, Stoddart RW (1992*d*) Lectin histochemistry of cerebral microvessels in ageing, Alzheimer's disease and Down's syndrome. *Neurobiol Ageing*, 13: 137–43.

Marcyniuk B, Mann DMA, Yates PO (1988) Topography of nerve cell loss from the locus caeruleus in middle aged persons with Down's syndrome. *J Neurol Sci* 83: 15–24.

Marin-Padilla M (1976) Pyramidal cell abnormalities in the motor cortex of a child with Down's syndrome. A Golgi study. *J Comp Neurol* 167: 63–82.

Masters CL, Simms G, Weinmann NA, Multhaup G, McDonald BL, Beyreuther K (1985) Amyloid plaque core protein in Alzheimer's disease and Down's syndrome. *Proc Nat Acad Sci USA* 82: 4245–9.

McGeer EG, Norman M, Boyes B, O'Kosky J, Suzuki J, McGeer PL (1985) Acetylcholine and aromatic amine systems in post mortem brain of an infant with Down's syndrome. *Exp Neurol* 87: 557–60.

Melamed E, Mildworf B, Sharav T, Benlenky L, Wertman E (1987) Regional cerebral blood flow in Down's syndrome. *Ann Neurol* 22: 275–8.

Miniszek NA (1983) Development of Alzheimer's disease in Down's syndrome individuals. *Am J Ment Defic* 87: 377–85.

Mori H, Kondo J, Ihara Y (1987) Ubiquitin is a component of paired helical filament in Alzheimer's disease. *Science* 235: 1641–4.

Motte J, Williams RS (1989) Age-related changes in the density and morphology of plaques and neurofibrillary tangles in Down's syndrome brains. *Acta Neuropathol* 77: 535–46.

Murdoch JC, Adams H (1977) Reply to W. Hughes. *Br Med J* 2: 702.

Murdoch JC, Rodger JC, Rao SS, Fletcher CD, Donnigan MG (1977) Down's syndrome: an atheroma-free model. *Br Med J* 2: 226–8.

Murphy GM, Eng LF, Ellis WG, Perry G, Meissner LC, Tinklenberg JR (1990) Antigenic profile of plaques and neurofibrillary tangles in the amygdala in Down's syndrome: a comparison with Alzheimer's disease. *Brain Res* 537: 102–8.

Murrell J, Farlow M, Ghetti B, Benson MD (1991) A mutation in the amyloid precursor protein associated with hereditary Alzheimer's disease. *Science* 254: 97–9.

Naruse S, Igarashi S, Aoki K, Kaneko K, Iihara K, Miyatake T, Kobayashi H, Inuzuka T, Shimizu T, Kojima T, Tsuji S (1991) Mis-sense mutation val → ile in exon 17 of amyloid precursor protein gene in Japanese familial Alzheimer's disease. *Lancet* 337: 978–9.

Neumann NA (1967) Langdon Down syndrome and Alzheimer's disease. *J Neuropath Exp Neurol* 26: 149–50.

Ogomori K, Kitamoto T, Tateishi J, Sato Y, Suetsugu M, Abe

M (1989) β protein amyloid is widely distributed in the central nervous system of patients with Alzheimer's disease. *Am J Path* 134: 243–51.

O'Hara PT (1972) Electronmicroscopical study of the brain in Down's syndrome. *Brain* 95: 681–4.

Olson MI, Shaw CM (1969) Presenile dementia and Alzheimer's disease in mongolism. *Brain* 92: 147–56.

Owens D, Dawson JC, Losin S (1971) Alzheimer's disease in Down's syndrome. *Am J Ment Defic* 75: 606–12.

Perry G, Friedman R, Shaw G, Chau V (1987) Ubiquitin is detected in neurofibrillary tangles and senile plaque neurites of Alzheimer's disease brains. *Proc Nat Acad Sci*, USA 84: 3033–6.

Pierotti AR, Harmar AJ, Simpson J, Yates CM (1986) High molecular weight forms of somatostatin are reduced in Alzheimer's disease and Down's syndrome. *Neurosci Lett* 63: 141–6.

Pogacar S, Rubio A (1982) Morphological features of Pick's and atypical Alzheimer's disease in Down's syndrome. *Acta Neuropathol* 58: 249–54.

Price DL, Whitehouse PJ, Struble RG, Coyle JT, Clark AW, DeLong MR, Cork LC, Hedreen JC (1982) Alzheimer's disease and Down's syndrome. *Ann NY Acad Sci* 396: 145–64.

Quon D, Wang Y, Catalano R, Scardina JM, Murakami K, Cordell B (1991) Formation of β amyloid protein in brains of transgenic mice. *Nature* 352: 239–41.

Rafalowska J, Barcikowska M, Wen GY, Wisniewski HM (1988) Laminar distribution of neuritic plaques in normal ageing, Alzheimer's disease and Down's syndrome. *Acta Neuropathol* 77: 21–5.

Rees S (1977) The incidence of ultrastructural abnormalities in the cortex of two retarded human brains (Down's syndrome). *Acta Neuropathol* 37: 65–8.

Reid AH, Maloney AFJ (1974) Giant cell arteritis and arteriolitis associated with amyloid angiopathy in an elderly mongol. *Acta Neuropathol* 27: 131–7.

Reynolds GP, Godridge H (1985) Alzheimer-like monoamine deficits in adults with Down's syndrome. *Lancet* ii: 1368–9.

Reynolds GP, Warner CEJ (1988) Amino acid transmitter deficits in adult Down's syndrome brain tissue. *Neurosci Lett* 94: 224–7.

Risberg J (1980) Regional cerebral blood flow measurements by 133 Xe inhalation: methodology and application in neuropathology and psychiatry. *Brain Lang* 9: 9–34.

Ropper AH, Williams RS (1980) Relationship between plaques and tangles and dementia in Down's syndrome. *Neurology*, 30: 639–44.

Ross MH, Galaburda AM, Kemper TL (1984) Down's syndrome: is there a decreased population of neurones? *Neurology* 34: 909–16.

Rumble B, Retallack R, Hilbich C, Simms G, Multhaup G, Martins R, Masters CL, Beyreuther K (1989) Amyloid (A4) protein and its precursor in Down's syndrome and Alzheimer's disease. *New Engl J Med* 320: 1446–52.

Schapiro MB, Haxby JV, Grady CL, Rapoport SI (1986) Cerebral glucose utilization, quantitative tomography and cognitive function in adult Down's syndrome. In Epstein CJ (ed), *Neurobiology of Down's Syndrome*, Raven Press, New York, pp 89–108.

Schapiro MB, Haxby JV, Grady CL, Duara R, Schlageter NL, White B, Moore A, Sundaram M, Larson SM, Rapoport SI (1987) Decline in cerebral glucose utilization and cognitive function with ageing in Down's syndrome. *J Neurol Neurosurg Psychiat* 50: 766–74.

Schapiro MB, Berman KF, Friedland RP, Weinberger DR, Rapoport SI (1988) Regional blood flow is not reduced in young adult Down's syndrome. *Ann Neurol* 24: 310.

Schapiro MB, Luxenberg JS, Kaye JA, Haxby JV, Friedland RP, Rapoport SI (1989) Serial quantitative CT analysis of brain morphometrics in adult Down's syndrome at different ages. *Neurology* 39: 1349–53.

Schapiro MB, Grady CL, Kumar A, Herscovitch P, Haxy JV, Moore A, White P, Friedland RP, Rapoport SI (1990) Regional cerebral glucose metabolism is normal in young adults with Down's syndrome. *J Cereb Blood Flow Metab* 10: 199–206.

Schochet SS, Lampert PW, McCormick WF (1973) Neurofibrillary tangles in patients with Down's syndrome: a light and electron microscope study. *Acta Neuropathol* 23: 342–6.

Silverstein AB, Herbs D, Miller TJ (1988) Effects of age on the adaptive behaviour of institutionalized and non-institutionalized individuals with Down's syndrome. *Am J Ment Retard* 92: 455–60.

Simpson MD, Slater P, Cross AJ, Mann DMA, Royston MC, Deakin JFW, Reynolds GP (1989) Reduced D-[³H] aspartate binding in Down's syndrome brains. *Brain Res* 484: 273–8.

Sisodia SS, Koo EH, Beyreuther K, Unterbeck A, Price DL (1990) Evidence that β amyloid protein in Alzheimer's disease is not derived by normal processing. *Science* 248: 492–5.

Snow AD, Mar H, Nochlin D, Sekiguchi RT, Kimata K, Koike Y, Wight TN (1990) Early accumulation of heparan sulphate in neurones and in the beta-amyloid protein containing lesions of Alzheimer's disease and Down's syndrome. *Am J Path* 137: 1253–70.

Solitaire GB, Lamarche JB (1966) Alzheimer's disease and senile dementia as seen in mongoloids: neuropathological observations. *Am J Ment Defic* 70: 840–8.

Solitaire GB, Lamarche JB (1967) Brain weight in the adult mongol. *J Ment Defic Res* 11: 79–84.

Spargo E, Luthert PJ, Anderton BH, Bruce M, Smith D, Lantos PL (1990) Antibodies raised against different portions of A4 protein identity a subset of plaques in Down's syndrome. *Neurosci Lett* 115: 345–50.

Sparkman DR, Hill SJ, White CL (1990) Paired helical filaments are not major binding sites for WGA and DBA agglutinins in neurofibrillary tangles of Alzheimer's disease. *Acta Neuropathol* 79: 640–6.

Struwe F (1929) Histopathologische Untersuchungen uber Enstehung und Wesen der senilen plaques. *Zeitsch Neurol Psychol* 122: 291–307.

Suenaga T, Hirano A, Llena JF, Yen S-H, Dickson DW (1990) Modified Bielschowsky staining and immunohistochemical studies on striatal plaques in Alzheimer's disease. *Acta Neuropathol* 80: 280–6.

Suetsuga M, Mehraein P (1980) Spine distribution along the apical dendrite of the pyramidal neurones in Down's syndrome. A quantitative Golgi study. *Acta Neuropathol* 50: 207–10.

Sylvester PE (1983) The hippocampus in Down's syndrome. *J Ment Defic Res* 27: 227–36.

Szumanska G, Vorbrodt AW, Mandybur TI, Wisniewski HM (1987) Lectin histochemistry of plaques and tangles in Alzheimer's disease. *Acta Neuropathol* 73: 1–11.

Tagliavini F, Giaccone G, Frangione B, Bugiani O (1988) Preamyloid deposits in the cerebral cortex of patients with Alzheimer's disease and non-demented individuals. *Neurosci Lett* 93: 191–6.

Takashima S, Becker LE (1985) Basal ganglia calcification in Down's syndrome. *J Neurol, Neurosurg Psychiat* 48: 61–4.

Takashima S, Becker LE, Armstrong DL, Chan FW (1981) Abnormal neuronal development in the visual cortex of the human fetus and infant with Down's syndrome. *Brain Res* 225: 1–21.

Thase ME, Tigner R, Smeltzer D, Liss L (1984) Age-related neuropsychological deficits in Down's syndrome. *Biol Psychiat* 19: 571–85.

Wegiel J, Wisniewski HM (1990) The complex of microglial cells and amyloid star in 3-dimensional reconstruction. *Acta Neuropath* 81: 116–24.

Whalley LJ (1982) The dementia of Down's syndrome and its relevance to aetiological studies of Alzheimer's disease. *Ann N Y Acad Sci* 396: 39–53.

Wischik C, Novak M, Thagersen HC, Edwards PC, Runswick MJ, Jakes R, Klug A (1988) Isolation of a fragment of tau derived from the core of the paired helical filament of Alzheimer's disease. *Proc Nat Acad Sci, USA*, 85: 4506–10.

Wisniewski HM, Terry RD (1973) Re-examination of the pathogenesis of the senile plaque. In Zimmerman HM (ed), *Progress in Neuropathology vol 2*. Grune and Stratton, New York, pp 1–26.

Wisniewski HM, Rabe A (1986) Discrepancy between Alzheimer-type neuropathology and dementia in persons with Down's syndrome. *Ann N Y Acad Sci* 477: 247–60.

Wisniewski HM, Rabe A, Wisniewski KE (1987) Neuropathology and dementia in people with Down's syndrome. *Banbury Report 27: Molecular Neuropathology of Ageing*, pp 399–413.

Wisniewski HM, Bancher C, Barcikowska M, Wen GY, Currie J (1989) Spectrum of morphological appearance of amyloid deposits in Alzheimer's disease. *Acta Neuropathol* 78: 337–47.

Wisniewski KE, Schmidt-Sidor B (1986) Myelination in Down's syndrome brains (pre- and post-natal maturation) and some clinical-pathological correlations. *Ann Neurol* 20: 429–30.

Wisniewski KE, Howe J, Gwyn-Williams D, Wisniewski HM (1978) Precocious ageing and dementia in patients with Down's syndrome. *Biol Psychiat* 13: 619–27.

Wisniewski KE, Jervis GA, Moretz RC, Wisniewski HM (1979) Alzheimer neurofibrillary tangles in diseases other than senile and presenile dementia. *Ann Neurol* 7: 462–5.

Wisniewski KE, Frenchy JH, Rosen JF, Kozlowski PB, Tenner M, Wisniewski HM (1982) Basal ganglia calcification (BGC) in Down's syndrome (DS) – another manifestation of premature ageing. *Ann N Y Acad Sci* 396: 179–89.

Wisniewski KE, Laure-Kamionowska M, Wisniewski HM (1984) Evidence of arrest of neurogenesis and synaptogenesis in brains of patients with Down's syndrome. *New Engl J Med* 311: 1187–8.

Wisniewski KE, Wisniewski HM, Wen GY (1985a) Occurrence of neuropathological changes and dementia of Alzheimer's disease in Down's syndrome. *Ann Neurol* 17: 278–82.

Wisniewski KE, Dalton AJ, Crapper-McLachlan DR, Wen GY, Wisniewski HM (1985b) Alzheimer's disease in Down's syndrome. Clinicopathologic studies. *Neurology* 35: 957–61.

Wisniewski KE, Laure-Kamionowska M, Connell F, Wen GY (1986) Neuronal density and synpatogenesis in the postnatal stage of brain maturation in Down's syndrome. In Epstein CJ (ed), *The Neurobiology of Down's syndrome*, Raven Press, New York, pp 29–44.

Wood, JG, Mirra SS, Pollock NJ, Binder LI (1986) Neurofibrillary tangles of Alzheimer's disease share antigenic determinants with the axonal microtubule associated protein tau. *Proc Nat Acad Sci, USA* 83: 4040–3.

Yamaguchi H, Hirai S, Morimatsu M, Shoji M, Harigaya Y (1988) Diffuse type of senile plaque in the brains of Alzheimer type dementia. *Acta Neuropath* 76: 541–9.

Yamaguchi H, Hirai S, Morimatsu M, Shoji M, Nakazato Y (1989) Diffuse type of senile plaque in the cerebellum of Alzheimer type dementia as detected by β-protein immunostaining. *Acta Neuropath* 77: 314–19.

Yates, CM, Simpson J, Maloney AFJ, Gordon A, Reid AH (1980) Alzheimer-like cholinergic deficiency in Down's syndrome. *Lancet* ii: 979.

Yates CM, Ritchie IM, Simpson J, Maloney AFJ, Gordon A (1981) Noradrenaline in Alzheimer type dementia and Down's syndrome. *Lancet* ii: 39–40.

Yates CM, Simpson A, Gordon A, Maloney AFJ, Allison Y, Ritchie IM, Urquhart A (1983) Catecholamines and cholinergic enzymes in presenile and senile Alzheimer-type dementia and Down's syndrome. *Brain Res* 280: 119–26.

Yates CM, Simpson J, Gordon A (1986) Regional brain 5-hydroxytryptamine levels are reduced in senile Down's syndrome as in Alzheimer's disease. *Neurosci Lett* 65: 189–92.

Zigman WB, Schopf N, Lubin RA, Silverman WP (1987) Premature regression of adults with Down's syndrome. *Am J Ment Defic* 92: 161–8.

CHAPTER FIVE

Vascular dementia

J. H. Morris

Introduction
How frequent is vascular dementia?
How does cerebrovascular disease produce dementia?
Aetiology of vascular dementia
Neuropathological criteria for vascular dementia

INTRODUCTION

One of the most controversial and difficult areas in the pathology of dementia is the role of cerbrovascular disease in dementia. That cerebrovascular disease can cause dementia is not in doubt, it is the frequency with which this occurs and the way that the dementia is produced that are contentious (Brust, 1983, 1988, O'Brien, 1988). Most of the main problems in assessing the significance and pathophysiology of cerebrovascular disease in the aetiology of dementia can be discussed under one of the following three questions:

1. What is the frequency of dementia in association with cerebrovascular disease?
2. What effects does vascular disease have on the nervous system and how does it produce dementia?
3. What are the neuropathological criteria for the diagnosis of dementia caused by cerebrovascular disease?

However, even before embarking on the discussion of the big questions we should address one of the small, but surprisingly intractable, questions in cerebrovascular disease which is 'what should we call the cognitive decline associated with cerebrovascular disease?' A variety of terms have been used for the presumed causal association between cerebrovascular disease and cognitive decline, but there is no entirely satisfactory term. The originally favoured term of atherosclerotic dementia has largely been replaced by multi-infarct dementia (MID) (Hachinski et al., 1974, 1975)

which has an appealing resonance but is unsatisfactory. A fundamental problem with MID as a general term is that it is misleading because it implies a degree of pathological precision that is, unfortunately, belied by the variation and complexity of cerebrovascular disease associated with cognitive decline. It is misleading, not because there is no such entity as multi-infarct dementia, but because its use implies that there is a single aetiology for the dementia of cerebrovascular disease.

There are several features of cerebrovascular disease that are not easily reconciled with MID as a generally applicable concept (Parnetti et al. 1990). First, one of the most striking features of cerebrovascular disease is its variability, a fact that accounts for a considerable part of the difficulties in describing it and ascribing clinical significance to its presence. A second, and more important, objection is that a significant feature of the brains from patients with dementia associated with cerebrovascular disease is that they almost all have, in addition to any focal infarcts, widespread diffuse cerebrovascular disease. While it is certainly true that focal infarction alone, without diffuse vascular disease, can produce defects in cognitive function, the cognitive defects such isolated infarcts produce tend to be rather specific types of loss of function. An example is the amnestic state secondary to bilateral hippocampal damage that can follow bilateral posterior cerebral artery infarctions. These cases, although very striking when encountered, are the exception rather than the rule.

The more usual finding in dementia associated with cerebral infarcts is the presence of a number of separ-

Table 5.1.

	Sample size	Vascular dementia	Mixed dementia	Total (%) vasc. Dis.
Corsellis (1962)	89	42(47%)	17(19%)	66
Tomlinson *et al.* (1970)	50	9(17%)	9(18%)	35
Sourander & Sjogren (1970)	258	72(28%)	—	28
Malamud (1972)	1255	356(29%)	283(23%)	52
Todorov *et al.* (1975)	675	123(18%)	241(36%)	54
Jellinger (1977)	1009	225(22%)	136(14%)	36
Loeb & Gandolfo (1983)	101	(29%)		29
Mölsä *et al.* (1985)	58	11(19%)	6(10%)	29
Barclay *et al.* (1985)	311	69(22%)	43(14%)	36
Esiri & Wilcock (1986)	86	18(21%)	11(13%)	34
Ulrich *et al.* (1986)	54	9/11(17–20%)	6/10(11–19%)	28/39
Boller *et al.* (1989)	54	4(7%)	3(6%)	13
Jellinger *et al.* (1990)	675	106(16%)	53(8%)	24

ate infarcts, the accumulated burden of which could reasonably be expected to produce significant impairment of function of the brain, an impairment that would include a degree of cognitive decline. However, the presence of multiple infarctions, whether thrombotic or embolic in origin, almost invariably carries with it the implication of a considerable degree of diffuse cerebrovascular disease in addition to that which is manifested as focal infarctions. At the other end of the neuropathological spectrum of cerebrovascular disease are the patients who have only diffuse cerebrovascular disease with few or no actual discrete cerebral infarcts. In contrast to the patients with infarcts who usually manifest quite prominent focal neurological signs, these patients may present with a dementia that can be very difficult to distinguish from a degenerative disease such as Alzheimer's disease. The existence of these patients with predominantly, or exclusively, diffuse small vessel cerebrovascular disease, and the presence of some degree of diffuse cerebrovascular disease in almost all patients with focal cerebrovascular disease makes multi-infarct dementia unsatisfactory as a general term. Although, as a debating point, this smacks a little of pedantry, the continuing use of such an unsatisfactory general term should be avoided if a better alternative could be offered. To evade the charge of misrepresentation, authors can be forced into all sorts of circumlocutions such as *dementia associated with cerebrovascular disease*, which is probably the most correct general term but is far too cumbersome. The shortest and probably most convenient term is *vascular dementia* which, although los-

ing something in precision, is sufficiently general and is the term that will be used in this chapter.

HOW FREQUENT IS VASCULAR DEMENTIA?

Historical overview

Over the last 30 years there have been a number of clinical and pathological studies of patients with dementia which have considered the frequency of vascular dementia and dementia in which vascular disease was considered to play a significant role in the cognitive decline. Some of the major studies are listed in Table 5.1.

Although not the first, among the most influential publications on the subject of vascular dementia are those of Tomlinson and colleagues (1970). In brief, they compared the brains of 50 demented old people with those of undemented controls and found that 17% had definite or probable 'arteriosclerotic dementia' and a similar fraction a combination of 'arteriosclerotic dementia' and Alzheimer's disease. Thus in approximately one-third of the patients studied, cerebrovascular disease was adjudged to play a major part in the causation of the dementia and in one-sixth it was the sole cause.

Their observations of vascular disease were predominantly focused on the presence of infarctions, and they concluded that only when there was a large volume of infarction (usually more than 100 ml) was there a significant association with the presence of dementia. One of the interesting aspects of this study, which illustrates the continuing difficulties in this field, is that in their analysis of the infarcts they did not consider 'the possibility of ischaemic lesions affecting areas of brain likely to be particularly important in relation to producing features of dementia'. Completely to ignore the significance of location seems to conflict with the generally held view of the localization of function within the nervous system, and the frequent observation that patients with damage to specific regions of the brain can have significant problems with cognitive function. The converse is also true; large infarcts with prominent focal signs can occur without producing a dementia.

Without going into a detailed exegesis of each of the studies listed in Table 5.1 they demonstrate what, at first sight, is a very wide spread in their estimates of 'significant' cerebrovascular disease in dementia that ranges between 75% and 13%, with pure 'vascular dementia' rates between 7% and 29%. Looking at this Table it is noteworthy both that the highest rates of vascular disease and the greatest variation in the rates of 'significant' cerebrovascular disease is greatest in the studies performed in the 1960s and 1970s. There are a number of possible explanations for this. One is that, in line with the secular reduction in cardiovascular disease, there has been a reduction in the effects on the nervous system. Another possibility is that one of the contributors to this variation is that these studies were performed in the period before the widespread availability of modern neuroimaging. In this context it is perhaps significant that all the studies in the decade of the 1980s have produced much more consistent results, with rates of 'significant' vascular disease in the 29–39% range. It seems from these studies that it would be reasonable to consider cerebrovascular disease to be the principal aetiological factor in approximately one-fifth of the cases of dementia and a significant contributor in a further eighth of the cases.

The problem with many of these studies is that, in most cases, the nature of the cognitive decline was not extensively investigated. Thus, for example, in Corsellis's (1962) paper the patients were classified only into 'organic psychosis'. These studies, which seem to indicate a substantial element of vascular disease in the causation of dementia have been performed on a largely uncharacterized population. Many of the problems of interpretation of these studies are bedevilled by what might be called the three 'Ds' of the dementia of cerebrovascular disease: Derivation, Definition, Degree.

Derivation

As demonstrated in Table 5.1, pathological surveys of dementia have yielded variations in estimates of the prevalence of vascular dementia ranging from 30% to 70%. In general, the estimated prevalence of vascular dementia has, if anything, been declining. This could be a real decline, paralleling the decline in the incidence of stroke and cerebral haemorrhage that has been attributed to the improvements in the management of hypertension, but part of the variation in frequency is undoubtedly influenced by the source from which the study patients are derived.

All the studies of the relative frequency of vascular dementia have been beset by the problems of case selection. In any given study the nature of the patient population surveyed is markedly influenced by the nature of the institutions surveyed and the interests and training of the referring clinicians. Studies such as that of Joachim, Morris and Selkoe (1988), for example, where the selection criterion was clinical diagnosis of a degenerative dementia, are by definition biased towards the degenerative dementias. In this sort of study patients with evident focal signs produced by stroke are very likely to be excluded. Similarly, where the majority of the patient population has been referred to a neurologist for investigation, the presence of prominent focal neurological signs and imaging evidence of cerebral infarction will tend to result in these patients being classified as having particular stroke syndromes, rather than a vascular dementia. Conversely, patients who present with mood alterations are much more likely to be referred to psychiatric hospitals and from community hospitals the focus might, in a similar group of patients, tend to be on the cognitive decline rather than on the focal neurology and result in their being classified as demented rather than having a specific stroke syndrome. Differences in national patterns of health care also have significant influences on the pattern of patient referral. In the USA, for example, the number of neurologists per head of population is about six times that in the UK. Consequently, patients with cognitive decline in the USA have a much greater likelihood of being referred to a neurologist with consequent differences in their pattern of investigation and classification. Even in studies aimed at clinico-pathological correlation, the nature of the institution or institutions surveyed will have an effect on patient selection.

A community-based study of cognitive decline with adequate pathological follow-up of the patients who die would provide the best indication of the extent of dementia associated with cerebrovascular disease. However, these are very large and complex studies, and even a purely clinical study, such as the East Boston study

(Evans *et al.*, 1989), is a major and expensive undertaking. At the time of writing, no such large-scale study has been published. Even this ideal is not without problems of bias given that temporally limited studies will tend to be biassed towards patients with more serious disease who die relatively quickly. There is also the likelihood of geographical variation in the amount of vascular disease between urban and rural areas and the known, and very substantial, variation in degree of vascular disease among different populations. All these confounding factors mean that there is no straightforward or simple answer to the question 'How important is cerebrovascular disease in the causation of dementia?'

Definition

A significant part of the problem of determining the prevalence and significance of vascular causes of dementia lies in the definition that is adopted for the clinical syndrome of dementia. The combination of this difficulty and the relatively uncertain correlation between clinical and pathological diagnosis means that, unlike Alzheimer's disease, there is no good age-related prevalence data for vascular dementia (Rocca *et al.*, 1991). In the most generally accepted sense of the term, dementia can be considered to be a syndrome characterized by the presence of a generalized decline in the 'higher mental functions'. We tend to think of dementia in terms of the archetypal patient with advanced Alzheimer's disease and the genuinely global decline in higher mental function suffered by these patients to be the quintessential 'real dementia'; the gold standard against which other types of cognitive decline are tested to see whether they can meet the standard. What this formulation ignores is that, in its early stages, Alzheimer's disease can present with a variety of rather focal defects of function such as mood alteration, memory problems and language difficulties. Thus, at the time of the initial presentation, the decline in higher mental function in Alzheimer's disease is not necessarily global, at least as far as clinical testing is concerned. The generalized decline in higher mental functions may be only a later stage of the clinical evolution of the disease. Parenthetically, from a practical diagnostic standpoint, it is the early stages where firm diagnostic criteria would be most valuable. By the time the patient is globally demented, the diagnostic position, although not certain, is usually much clearer.

Applied rigorously, a requirement for truly generalized intellectual deterioration would exclude many cases of cognitive decline secondary to cerebrovascular disease. Whether a single stroke, or focal cerebrovascular disease, can be said to cause a dementia depends largely on how strictly the requirement is for a generalized deterioration in mental function. A requirement for generalized cognitive impairment along the lines of that seen in Alzheimer's disease would certainly exclude amnestic states such as those resulting from bilateral posterior cerebral infarctions that produce bilateral hippocampal damage, or anterior thalamic infarctions, which are the usual cause of the so-called 'thalamic dementias'. This point is often side-stepped by using the term 'cognitive impairment' rather than dementia. Although convenient, this manoeuvre has contributed to the continuing confusion in this field by using terminology that is not clearly defined.

One factor in the debate over definition is the method used to assess cognitive function. There has been considerable difficulty in defining the most appropriate criteria for dementia in vascular dementia (Tatemichi *et al.*, 1992; Chui *et al.*, 1992, Román *et al.*, 1993). In many, if not most, cases, the mental function of the patient will have been assessed by one or more of a number of cognitive function rating scales, and a phenomenological label based on the score using such scales. It is not within the terms of reference of this volume (and certainly beyond the competence of this author) to evaluate the various dementia rating scales. However, it is appropriate to point out that the degree to which their questions reflect different brain functions (and therefore different brain regions) will be biased to disease affecting those regions. As a straightforward example of the effect, as noted by Liu *et al.* (1992), many questions in dementia rating scales are concerned with language, and patients with language disorders will score particularly poorly in such scales. Other areas, such as, for example, right parietal function, may be relatively less emphasized and, using such a rating scale, patients may score well even with severe right parietal dysfunction. When groups of patients are being surveyed for the presence of defects in higher mental function, the limitations of the way that the cognitive decline was defined and measured, must be borne in mind. This caveat applies *a fortiori* in cases where cognitive decline is assessed without specific neuropsychological assessment of cognitive function.

Terminology should be a servant not a master, and it is important not to get bogged down trying to decide whether the patient does or does not have a dementia *sensu strictu*. It is worth emphasizing that the term dementia, like stroke, is one of those old-fashioned medical terms that is clinically very useful but pathologically imprecise. It embraces a loosely defined and variable set of neurological and neuropsychological phenomena. When the term dementia was coined, the state of neurological knowledge was such that it was the end point of the investigative process. Over the years, the advances in the understanding of the causes of cognitive decline mean that dementia has become a phenomenological description, not a diagnosis, and describing a patient as sufferig from dementia is now the first stage of the diagnostic process rather than the last. The purpose of the diagnostic process is to reach a conclusion about the pathophysiology of the cognitive decline, not to split hairs about the name to be applied to the clinical phenomenology. However, while advances in neuropathological knowledge mean that the diagnostic candidates in cognitive decline and dementia are now mostly defined fairly well pathologically, clinical investigative methods in most cases are unable to provide a definitive diagnosis. Although considerable progress has been made, particularly through refinements in neuroimaging, the final diagnosis, in most cases of dementia, can currently only be made by neuropathological examination of the brain.

Not unnaturally, this fact has blunted the enthusiasm of some clinicians to explore the possibilities of clinical diagnosis in cases of cognitive decline. However, while certainty is not yet attainable, detailed clinico-pathological studies of prospectively assessed patients is producing some refinement in the ability of *in vivo* methods to arrive at a probable pathological diagnosis. Practically, what is needed is to move away from the use of global terms such as dementia to a more refined clinical analysis of the cognitive decline which may be more revealing of the site, distribution and character of the pathological process. It is likely that this more refined analysis will be in terms of neurological and neuropsychological phenomenology, and also make use of the ever-expanding range and sophistication of neuroimaging techniques such as CT, MRI and SPECT (Fisher *et al.*, 1992).

Degree
Cerebrovascular disease is common, and increases in prevalence in older age-groups and a majority of persons dying in their 60s and 70s have some evidence of cerebrovascular disease. Numerous patients have some degree of focal or diffuse vascular disease, either in the form of small, or even quite large, infarcts, or lacunes, or arteriolar sclerosis of the white matter, and are apparently unscathed from the standpoint of their cognitive function. Most of these people have no evidence of any degree of cognitive decline, let alone a decline severe enough to label as dementia. Clearly, it is possible, and indeed common, to have a degree of cerebrovascular disease and be asymptomatic. Unfortunately for the pathologist, there is no signpost to mark the passage of the Rubicon after which the amount of vascular disease is symptomatic.

With focal disease, Tomlinson, Blessed and Roth (1968, 1970) adopted an essentially arbitrary standard of volume of infarction that was necessary to produce dementia that took no account of location of the infarction within the brain. Given the distributed function of the brain, it seems unlikely that there is no spatial significance in the distribution of infarcts in dementia associated with cerebrovascular disease. This has been confirmed by a recent quantitative MRI study of vascular dementia which has indicated, not surprisingly, that left hemisphere infarction has a more significant association with dementia than right hemisphere infarction (Liu *et al.*, 1992). With modern neuroimaging, which can generate volumetric indices and define the location of the infarcted tissue precisely, there seems no reason why the associations of focal vascular disease, i.e. multiple infarcts, with dementia cannot be greatly refined.

The situation for diffuse cerebrovascular disease is nothing like as rosy, principally because the pathological changes represent a continuum that progresses through arteriolar sclerosis and perivascular gliosis to a much more diffuse loss of white matter with no easily definable steps along the way to mark the points of 'significant' diffuse vascular disease. As will be discussed in the section on 'Binswanger's disease', this area also seems much less amenable to investigation because of the lack of good clinico-pathological correlation between the imaging studies (CT and MRI) and both the clinical symptoms and pathological findings.

The influence of neuroimaging
The key event that altered the investigation of cognitive decline was the advent of modern neuroimaging, initially computed tomography and subsequently, magnetic resonance imaging. The fact that many of the larger-scale studies occurred before this era makes them very difficult to interpret in modern terms, when the availability of neuroimaging would completely change the pattern of investigation of many of these patients. This aspect is discussed in more detail in the subsequent section on clinical criteria for vascular dementia.

In the last 20 years there have been enormous advances in neuroimaging principally in the form of computed tomography (CT) and magnetic resonance imaging (MRI). The major influence of the increasing availability of modern neuroimaging from the early to mid-1970s has been its effect in extending the clinical diagnostic spectrum. The (relative) ease with which images of the brain could be generated by, initially, CT, produced a revolution in the investigation of cognitive decline. Prior to the advent of CT the information about, for example, ventricular size, could be obtained only indirectly and at some risk to the patient. It also required both a considerable degree of patient co-operation and the expenditure of considerable inpatient and professional time. The difficulties inherent in the investigations were sufficiently great that they were undertaken in comparatively few patients, and specific diagnoses were correspondingly rare. The availability and use of CT both widened the range and increased the precision of the diagnostic spectrum of cognitive decline to the extent that 'organic brain disease' has ceased to be, to most modern eyes, a diagnostically respectable term. Subsequent advances in neuroimaging have produced further changes in the assessment of cerebrovascular disease and, characteristically it might be thought, both simplified and complicated the assessment.

During what might be called the halcyon days of neuroimaging, just after the advent of the CT scan, the task of the physician in trying to decide whether or not the patient had had a 'stroke' was considerably eased. This encouraged the classification of a great many patients with cognitive decline into the group of 'vascular dementias' on the grounds that they had unequivocal evidence of cerebro-vascular disease. Demonstrating the presence of cerebrovascular disease is not, however, the same as being able reasonably to conclude that the vascular disease is actually responsible for the cognitive decline. As has been noted, a problem with the diagnosis of vascular dementia is that both cerebrovascular disease and dementia are common and many patients have both.

The imaging of focal infarction has made the investigation of patients with focal signs much easier and provided reliable differentiation among infarcts, haemorrhages and other types of disease presenting as 'strokes'. A more controversial area of CT imaging is the pathological significance and clinico-pathological correlations of the white matter low density and periventricular low density seen in a number of patients with cognitive decline. The arrival of MRI scanning has further refined the imaging of focal infarction and added several new twists to the problem of generalized and focal white matter damage in the form of 'unidentified bright objects' (UBOs) and other more diffuse changes in white matter signal visible principally on T2 imaging. The problems of the interpretation of white matter changes on CT and MRI is discussed at greater length in the section on Binswanger's disease.

As might be surmised, if the clinical phenomenology of cognitive decline can be ambiguous, the same is true for the investigations. Neuroimagings by CT and MR have made enormous strides, and new MR techniques (Fisher et al., 1992) in combination with more arcane investigations such as SPECT (Tohgi et al., 1991), PET (Mielke et al., 1992) and MRS (Petroff et al., 1992) can be expected to provide further advances. However, even with the best imaging, there currently remains a substantial residuum of cases where the pathological diagnosis is not clear, even after all investigations.

Clinical criteria for vascular dementia

The lack of clarity in definition and neuroimaging has been complemented by an equal difficulty in establishing clear clinical diagnostic criteria for the diagnosis of vascular dementia. Although this is not primarily a clinical treatise, some indication of the evolution of clinical criteria is appropriate.

In 1974 and subsequently Hachinski and his colleagues (1974, 1975) developed an 'ischaemic score' using a number of clinical features (13 in all) such as an abrupt onset, stepwise deterioration and the presence of focal symptoms and signs as indicators of vascular aetiology in patients with cognitive decline. Subsequent evaluation of the use of the ischaemic score has indicated that it attaches undue weight to the presence of focal signs. This had the effect of widening the clinical definition of vascular dementia to the point where significant evidence of cerebrovascular disease in a patient with cognitive impairment will tend to classify the patient as having vascular dementia. However, as Tomlinson and colleagues pointed out in 1976, '...experience also shows that one must never assume that, because multiple infarcts are present, this is the sole cause or contributing factor of the dementia...'. Studies of neuropathological validation of the Hachinski ischaemic score indicate that its strict application tends to overestimate the contribution of vascular disease to dementia largely drawn from the patients with mixed pathology where cerebrovascular disease co-exists with another, and often more significant, cause of dementia

(Rosen *et al.*, 1980, Fischer *et al.*, 1991; Mölsä *et al.*, 1985). This has led to suggested revisions (Loeb & Gandolfo, 1983) and some questioning of its utility (Liston & La Rue, 1983).

A more recent international attempt to establish diagnostic criteria for vascular dementia was reported by Román and colleagues (1993) in the report of the NINDS-AIREN International workshop in 1991. The aim of the workshop was to define diagnostic criteria for research studies. In this, they establish a series of sets of criteria for probable and possible vascular dementia that include features of the history, clinical examination and radiologic imaging studies. They also included a series of features that they considered made the diagnosis of vascular dementia uncertain or unlikely, again including lack of evidence of vascular disease on neuroimaging.

Accuracy of the clinical diagnosis of vascular dementia
There have been few specific attempts to define the accuracy of clinical diagnosis of vascular dementia by pathological confirmation, and available estimates have produced a wide variation in diagnostic accuracy (Todorov *et al.*, 1975; Mölsä *et al.*, 1985). This is, in part, a reflection of the methodological problems arising from the uncertainty over the best criteria for both the clinical and pathological diagnosis of vascular dementia. The lack of clear information is expressed by the contrasting views of Brust (1988) and O'Brien (1988) in adjacent articles who aver that vascular dementia is over- and under- diagnosed, respectively. One recent specific study of the accuracy of clinical diagnosis of vascular dementia is that of Erkinjuntti *et al.* (1988) who reported a diagnostic accuracy of 85% in pathological study of 27 patients with a clinical diagnosis of vascular dementia. This degree of accuracy is similar to that achieved with Alzheimer's disease and is considerably higher than most previous studies of vascular dementia. However, the patients in this study had been subject to an extensive clinical investigation including neuropsychological and neuroradiological studies, and it seems likely that this study is close to the best practically achievable result using clinical methods.

As examplified by the pathological studies referred to earlier, most workers have tended to concentrate on studies of the frequency and nature of cerebrovascular disease in cases of dementia. As we have seen, this results in estimates of vascular dementia in the range of 20%, with cerebrovascular disease making a significant contribution to the symptoms in a further 10–15% of patients.

However, this question can be approached in terms of the frequency of the development of dementia in a population with a history of stroke. This type of study has tended to be purely clinical and thus to suffer from the major disadvantage of such studies which is the lack of pathological verification of the clinical diagnoses. This is particularly important in dementia related to vascular disease where small-scale studies have shown that, while the presence of vascular disease is reliably detected, there is poor discrimination between cognitive decline as a result of vascular disease alone and cognitive decline that is the result of the combination of vascular disease and a degenerative disease. Hence, in studies of this type there is a tendency to over-estimate the contribution of vascular disease to dementia.

The authors of such studies are, of course, perfectly aware of the limitations of clinical methods in this respect and attempt to compensate for them. In the most ambitious recent study of dementia in patients with stroke Tatemichi *et al.* (1992) studied 251 patients aged ≥ 60 years with ischaemic strokes. In this study the cognitive function of the patients was assessed 3 months after the stroke, and dementia was found in just over 26% of the patients, compared to 3.2% in an age-matched control sample drawn from the community. This frequency of dementia in stroke patients is in general agreement with a number of other smaller studies.

Tatemichi *et al.* went on to a further refinement of this prevalence by distinguishing between dementia secondary to preexisting degenerative disease (assumed to be AD), vascular dementia (either directly related to the region of the stroke or unrelated), and other causes of dementia. Based principally on a temporal association of the onset of the cognitive decline with the stroke, vascular disease was considered to be the cause in approximately two-thirds of the cases of dementia. Overall, they concluded that the prevalence of dementia directly attributable to stroke was approximately 15% in the cohort surveyed. Of the group of patients with dementia associated with vascular disease, they considered that in approximately 40% of the cases the location of the stroke or strokes accounted for the dementia, while in the other 60% they considered that the location of the vascular disease did not explain the dementia syndrome (using, 'traditional concepts of functional neuroanatomy'). They also found that age and level of education were independent contributors to the incidence of dementia in the population surveyed.

Can cerebrovascular disease produce a progressive dementing syndrome?

From a practical standpoint it would be helpful to have some indication of whether and how often cerebrovascular disease alone can produce a progressive generalized dementing syndrome that clinically resembles that produced by a 'degenerative' disease such as Alzheimer's disease (Tatemichi, 1990). Perhaps the best empirical information about this comes from selected series such as that of Boller, Lopez and Moossy (1989) in which patients with an obvious vascular aetiology were excluded and Joachim et al. (1988) where patients were referred to an Alzheimer's disease research group from a large variety of community sources with a clinical diagnosis of presumed Alzheimer's disease. In Boller's series only 4 out of 54 cases were considered to have multi-infarct dementia while in Joachim's group, out of 150 cases only 3 (2%) were considered to be demented on the basis of cerebrovascular disease alone and, in a further 11 cases, strokes were thought to have contributed to the dementia. These findings suggest that vascular disease may occasionally produce a dementia clinically resembling that of Alzheimer's disease, but that it is not a common event.

Another group of vascular disease patients that might be expected to produce a progressive dementing disease most resembling that of a degenerative dementia would be those with diffuse non-occlusive cerebrovascular disease of the 'Binswanger' type. This produces a diffuse loss of white matter that is considered to lead to progressive disconnection of the cerebral cortex from the deeper structures. Clinical studies have shown that 'Binswanger's disease' does produce a progressive dementing syndrome that, however, does not particularly resemble the dementia of Alzheimer's disease. Some authorities, notably Caplan and Schoene (1978), consider that 'Binswanger's disease' has a characteristic clinical picture, although this is not universally accepted (Babikian & Ropper, 1987).

HOW DOES CEREBROVASCULAR DISEASE PRODUCE DEMENTIA?

Before discussing the ways that vascular disease can produce dementia, it is appropriate to review briefly the types of brain damage that are produced by vascular disease. Vascular disease has a wide range of effects on the nervous system, and affects the performance of the brain in a number of different ways. Probably the most relevant way to start to systematize its effects is to begin by dividing them into focal and diffuse.

Focal cerebrovascular disease consists, for the most part, of the various types of infarct that occur in the brain as a result of thrombotic or embolic vascular occlusions. At least in principle, it is possible to describe, with a reasonable degree of precision, the location and extent of focal cerebrovascular disease. With a fair degree of labour, or with more computing and memory power and better software, the infarcts can be defined in terms of the volume and regions of the brain that are damaged. Furthermore, using modern neuroimaging, this may be done in life. With focal cerebrovascular disease there is not usually any difficulty in deciding whether or not there is a lesion present and cerebrovascular disease is at least potentially amenable to analysis by what are fundamentally conventional methods.

Diffuse cerebrovascular disease is rather different and the problems of description and analysis are very much more intractable. The major aetiological factor in the development of diffuse disease is hypertension, although, as a result of the well known association of hypertension with the development of atherosclerosis there is also an established connection with focal cerebrovascular disease and in many patients both focal and diffuse disease are present.

Many of the diffuse effects of hypertension are manifested through changes in the structure and function of the relatively small arteries in the brain, though they tend to affect different regions in different ways and to different degrees. As far as the production of cognitive decline is concerned, the major regions of interest are the white matter of the cerebral hemispheres and the deep grey nuclei, particularly the thalamus. Although diffuse vascular disease is very important in the causation of cognitive decline, no entirely satisfactory or easy way to describe it has yet been devised. The principal reason for this is that the diffuse changes are expressed as a pathological continuum. This brings two major problems, the first being that such processes are not easy to describe with any precision in terms of either their severity or their distribution. The second problem is that many of the diffuse vascular and parenchymal changes that are found in patients with cognitive decline can also be seen in patients with no known history of cognitive failure, or even in patients who have been shown to have normal cognitive function. It is also very probable that some of the clinically apparent effects of vascular disease on the nervous system are dynamic and relate to blood flow and vessel wall metabolic function. These functions are reflected only very indirectly in morphological changes in blood vessels and the brain.

Although for convenience of description, the focal and diffuse effects of cerebrovascular disease will be treated as if they were separate, it is important to recognize that they frequently co-exist. It is quite possible to conceive that a moderate degree of diffuse disease that was insufficient to produce cognitive decline might, with the addition of some focal disease, become symptomatic. As if the problems of description were not sufficient, the complexity of mixed disease within a single aetiological category has to be added to the difficulties of interpretation of cerebrovascular disease!

MECHANISMS OF VASCULAR DEMENTIA

In the past few years there have been several thoughtful examinations of the ways in which cerebral vascular disease produces dementia (Scheinberg, 1988; Tatemichi, 1990; Loeb, 1990; Garcia & Brown, 1992). Most of the authors of these separate studies were participants in the NINDS-AIRED International workshop entitled Vascular Dementia: diagnostic criteria for research studies (Román *et al.*, 1993), which suggested six general ways that cerebrovascular disease could produce dementia. The three major categories of vascular disease that they identified are:

1. *Multi-infarct dementia*
2. *Strategic single infarct dementia*
3. *Small vessel disease*

While this formulation is very helpful in that it indicates the three major types of vascular disease that are encountered, it needs to be recognized as a considerable simplification, notably in the frequent presence of a degree of small vessel disease in many of the cases of so-called 'multi-infarct dementia' and 'strategic single infarct dementia'. Nevertheless it fulfils a need for a framework into which to fit a description of the range of vascular disease that is encountered in patients with cognitive decline.

Multi-infarct dementia

This is the classical concept where the combined effect of a number of different infarcts has a cumulative effect on cognitive function sufficient to produce a dementia. The common expression of this type of cerebrovascular disease is illustrated in Fig. 5.1, but occasionally the multiple infarcts can be very large numbers of microinfarcts (Fig. 5.2). There are many variations in this particular theme, but most cases will be found to have bilateral infarcts affecting parts of the middle cerebral

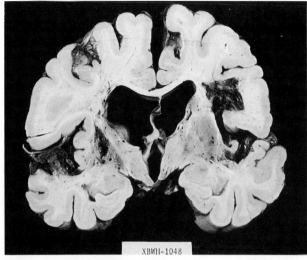

(a)

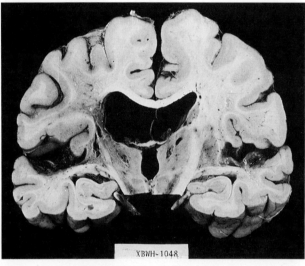

(b)

Fig. 5.1. Multi-infarct dementia: two adjacent brain slices from a patient with multi-infarct dementia showing the variety and severity of tissue destruction commonly seen in these patients.

(a) In the more anterior slice there is infarction in the territories of the inferior division of both middle cerebral arteries, part of the superior division of the right middle cerebral artery and in the left caudate and putamen involving the intervening internal capsule. This damage has resulted in significant enlargement of the right lateral ventricle and third ventricle and gross enlargement of the left lateral ventricle.

(b) In the posterior slice, there are still infarctions in both inferior divisions of the middle cerebral arteries, the left putamen and an additional extensive area of damage in the white matter of the left centrum semiovale. There are also at least three identifiable lacunes in the thalami.

artery territories of both hemispheres, often with additional damage in the basal ganglia and thalamus.

Strategic single infarct dementia

The striking feature of individual cerebral infarctions is how few of them cause mental dysfunction resembling a dementia. Major left hemisphere infarcts with significant hemiparesis and language disorder may not produce gross cognitive decline. A caveat here is that it is very difficult to evaluate the cognitive function of patients with severe aphasia. However, there are a number of areas in the brain where a single infarct can produce a restricted but significant impairment in cognitive function. As has been discussed, if the dementia associated with advanced neurodegenerative disease is used as the necessary standard, many of these cases are not *sensu stricti* examples of dementia because the cognitive decline associated with these infarcts cannot be said to be generalized.

As listed by NINDS-AIREN, the major examples of

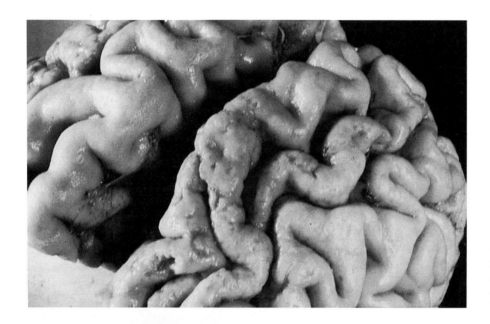

Fig. 5.2. Multi-infarct dementia: the pattern and severity of granular atrophy of the cortex seen in patients who have large numbers of microemboli. In this brain it is conspicuous that the most severe damage is seen in the parasagittal boundary zone regions.

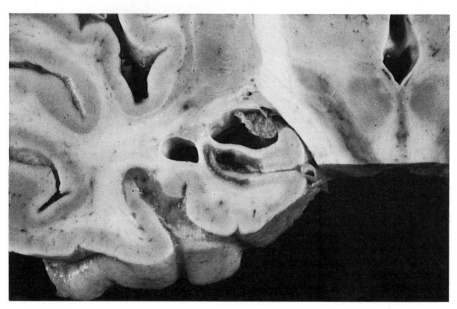

Fig. 5.3. Infarction of the hippocampus and part of the parahippocampal gyrus as a result of occlusion of the posterior cerebral artery. Bilateral occlusion of the posterior cerebral artery can result in bilateral hippocampal infarction with severe effects on memory.

vascular territories infarction of which is associated with changes in cognitive function are:

Angular gyrus infarction: Cognitive function abnormalities are a fluent aphasia, alexia with agraphia, memory disturbance, spatial disorientation and constructional disturbances.

Bilateral posterior cerebral infarction (Fig. 5.3): This will produce bitemporal and occipital infarctions. The bilateral hippocampal infarction produces an amnestic state. This may be accompanied by psychomotor agitation, confusion, and visual impairment and hallucinations. Very occasionally, a rather similar amnestic state can occur when bilateral convexity subdural haematomas produce chronic distortion and compression of the temporal lobes that results in temporal lobe atrophy. This situation would probably be included in the category of 'haemorrhagic dementia' in the NINDS-AIREN classification (see below).

Anterior cerebral artery infarcts: These are associated with abulia, transcortical motor aphasia, memory impairment and dyspraxia.

Right middle cerebral artery infarcts: This may be associated with confusional episodes and psychosis.

Parietal lobe infarcts: There are cognitive and behavioural abnormalities in addition to the spatial perceptive disorder.

Thalamic infarctions (Fig. 5.4): These are particularly of the anterior and intralaminar nuclei. Infarctions in this region produce predominantly a profound memory disturbance similar to that seen in Korsakoff's psychosis and what is termed an amnestic dementia.

Basal forebrain lesions: There are amnesia and behavioural changes.

Small vessel disease

This heading embraces a wide range of morphological changes in the brain. At its extremes of pathological expression, it includes two major patterns of vascular diseases, Binswanger's disease, first described in 1894,

and the état lacunaire described by Pierre Marie in 1901, both which have a long provenance in neurological literature that, to some degree reflects the controversy over their significance.

Diffuse vascular disease is hard to characterize because, while its effects may be most obvious in one particular region, small vessels throughout the brain are affected and the pathological changes are manifested as a continuum of progressively more severe damage. It also needs to be emphasized here that the two different pathological expressions of small vessel disease, small vessel occlusions that produce lacunes, and more diffuse damage, often co-exist. This is not surprising since they are different expressions of small vessel disease resulting from hypertension. Thus, for example, the presence of occasional lacunes is frequent in cases of subcortical leukoencephalopathy and, conversely, there is often evidence of some degree of diffuse damage in cases of lacunar disease.

All regions of the brain are exposed to some extent to the effects of diffuse cerebrovascular disease but the brunt of the damage is borne by the white matter and the deep grey nuclei. Despite the fact that the cerebral cortex is notably sensitive to ischaemia, and that it is most severely affected in the focal vascular disease exemplified by cerebral infarction, it shows little if any damage in diffuse cerebrovascular disease when examined with the normal neuropathological techniques. By contrast, the white matter and the deep grey nuclei show what appear to be a hierarchy of progressively more severe damage and it is therefore in the white matter and deep grey nuclei that the morphological effects of diffuse cerebrovascular disease are most appropriately sought.

The major morphological changes in diffuse cerebrovascular disease can be described under four headings:

a. Arterial wall changes
b. Expansion of the Virchow–Robin spaces,
c. Perivascular parenchymal rarefaction and gliosis
d. Diffuse white matter disease (Binswanger change/subcortical leukoencephalopathy).

In general, these changes can be thought of as sequential and additive, so that, for example, the arterial wall changes can be seen in the absence of any of the other morphological features, but if there is perivascular parenchymal rarefaction and gliosis, there will also be expansion of the Virchow–Robin spaces and arterial wall changes.

Arterial wall changes
In diffuse cerebrovascular disease the blood vessels of interest are the smaller arteries and arterioles. Large vessel cerebral atherosclerosis, although very relevant to

the development of focal infarcts in the deep grey nuclei, has no specific relationship to diffuse vascular disease of the white matter.

The small vessels particularly affected are the long penetrating arteries that supply the hemispheric white matter and the penetrating arteries supplying the deep grey nuclei (basal ganglia and thalamus) and their

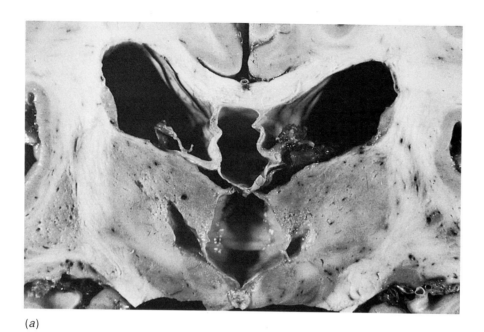

(a)

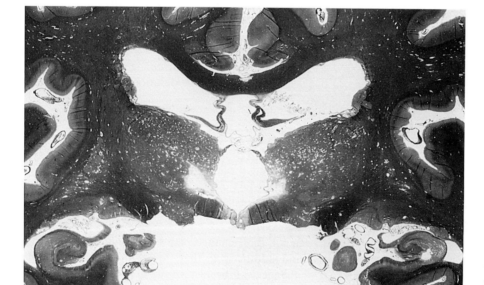

(b)

Fig. 5.4 (a). Cognitive decline as a result of strategic specific infarctions: the macroscopic appearance of the thalamus in a patient with mesencephalic artery syndrome that has produced bilateral thalamic damage with cognitive impairment. Some indication of the degree of tissue loss from the thalamus is provided by the degree of dilatation of the third ventricle.

(b). This photograph of a large microscopic section of the case illustrated in Fig. 5.4(a) shows that remaining relatively intact thalamic tissue has a markedly vacuolated appearance. This indicates that, as is so frequently the case in cerebrovascular disease, in addition to the infarctions that can be seen with the naked eye, there is significant coexisting small vessel disease that adds to the effect of the large vessel disease.

branches. In the white matter, the characteristic change is a hyaline thickening of the walls of the long penetrating arteries, with loss of the normal smooth muscle cell population of the vessel wall (Fig. 5.5). The thickening can be very marked and the wall thickness can come to comprise 75% of the total diameter of the arteriole. It can be seen in the absence of any other change and is probably one of the least specific pathological reactions to systemic hypertension. It can certainly be seen in patients with a history of hypertension and no evidence of cognitive decline.

In the basal ganglia, because the arteries are larger in diameter, changes are generally similar to those that are seen in large diameter arteries with medial fibrosis,

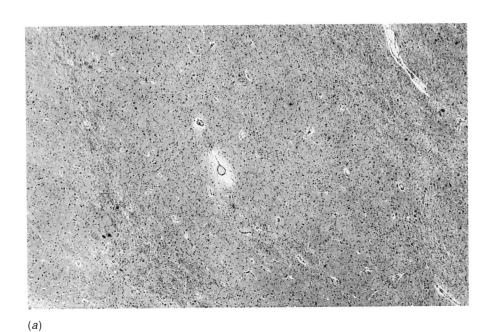

(a)

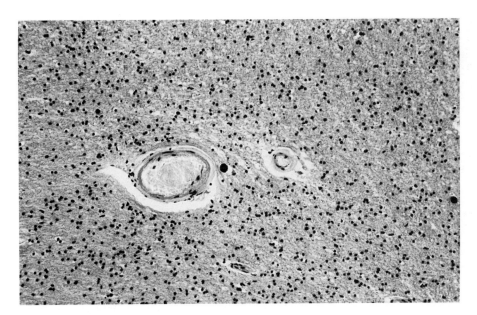

(b)

Fig. 5.5 (a). Mild non-occlusive small vessel disease in the thalamus. There is thickening of the walls of small arterioles and some expansion of the Virchow–Robin spaces. H&E × 50. (b) The white matter in these cases often shows arteriolar sclerosis without expansion of the Virchow–Robin spaces. (H&E × 125)

intimal thickening and, sometimes, focal atherosclerotic changes.

Expansion of the Virchow–Robin spaces (L'État Criblé)

The expansion of the Virchow–Robin space that occurs in hypertensive cerebrovascular disease is multifactorial and reflects both changes in the arteries and volume losses in the parenchyma. Although expansion of the Virchow–Robin spaces can be seen in the white matter, it is most conspicuous in the deep grey nuclei. This is probably a reflection of the fact that the arteries in the deep grey nuclei are larger in diameter than the long penetrating arteries of the white matter and therefore

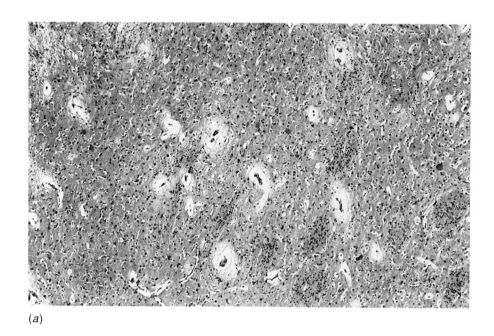

(a)

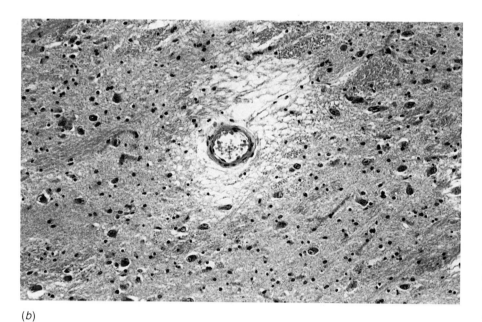

(b)

Fig. 5.6. (a). Low power view of moderate small vessel disease with expansion of the Virchow–Robin spaces and loosening and gliosis in the perivascular neuropil. (H&E × 50) (b). At higher magnification, it can be seen that the neuropil beyond the region of neuropil loosening and attentuation is well preserved. H&E × 125. (c) The same degree of damage in white matter with marked expansion of the Virchow–Robin spaces but rather less conspicuous loosening of the neuropil. (H&E × 125)

have a more conspicuous Virchow–Robin space. In these arteries, the putative pathophysiological mechanism of expansion of the Virchow–Robin spaces is the spiralling of the artery that occurs in hypertension. This converts the ordinarily straight course of the artery into a corkscrew-like spiral, and the process of formation of this spiral configuration will naturally tend to produce enlargement of the Virchow–Robin space. In accordance with this hypothesis, the artery is most often seen to one side of the enlarged Virchow–Robin space (Fig. 5.6c).

The expansion of the Virchow–Robin spaces around the lenticulo-striate arteries can be very marked close to their origin and large enough to be easily visualized by imaging studies of the brain. The expansion can be mistaken for a lacune by the inexperienced neuroradiologist. Unfortunately, the terminology is very imprecise, and some authorities are prepared to designate this widespread expansion of the Virchow–Robin spaces in the deep grey nuclei as a variant of the so-called 'état lacunaire'. Others prefer to reserve the term lacune for small focal necrotic lesions. In our opinion the use of the term lacune for an expansion of the Virchow–Robin space runs the risk of confusing two processes that would be better kept separate.

In the white matter, this change is most usually seen in association with parenchymal changes described below and in this region the expansion more reflects tissue damage and consequent reduction in parenchymal volume.

Perivascular parenchymal rarefaction and gliosis

This change affects both white and grey matter, although it tends to be most noticeable in the deep grey nuclei. It consists of a loosening, vacuolation and gliosis of the neuropil surrounding the small arteries and arterioles that permeate the deep grey nuclei and the white matter. Neurons do not appear to be particularly susceptible to this process, and may still be present in affected regions (Fig. 5.6).

When this change is present, it tends to affect all the deep grey nuclei but to rather different degrees. In a given case the globus pallidus usually shows the most severe changes, with marked vacuolation, while the thalamus shows less severe changes and the caudate/putamen is the least dramatically affected. Within the thalamus there is also some tendency for the different subnuclei to show different degrees of perivascular loosening. This difference in apparent susceptibility probably reflects the different structure of the neuropil in the various nuclei which render them more or less likely to show this change. There are considerable variations in severity, with some cases showing severe damage and considerable neuronal loss (Fig. 5.7).

In the white matter, a morphologically similar type of

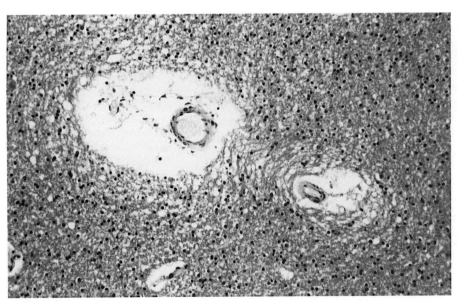

(c)

change is usually present. It tends to be particularly conspicuous around arterioles showing the most marked hyaline thickening.

Diffuse white matter rarefaction (Binswanger change/subcortical leukoencephalopathy)

The gross features of what has come to be called Binswanger change were first described by the eponymous Otto in a paper presented at the annual meeting of the Society of German Alienists in Dresden in 1894 (Blass, Hoyer & Nitsch, 1991). They consist of a marked atrophy of white matter and gross ventricular dilatation with notable sparing of the cortex. These findings occurred in a patient who had undergone a progressive

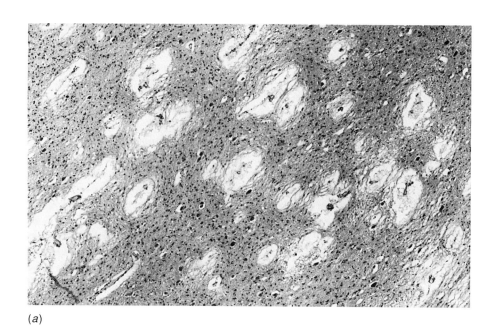

(a)

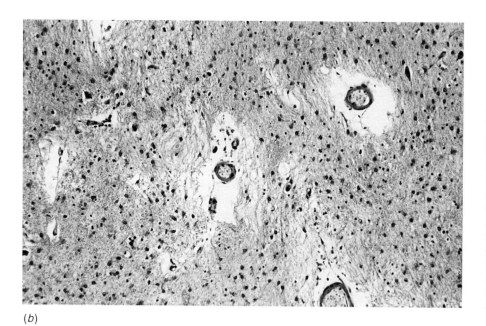

(b)

Fig. 5.7. (a). Severe small vessel disease with gross expansion of the Virchow–Robin spaces. This is the sort of microscopic appearance that is seen in cases such as that illustrated in Fig. 5.4. (H&E ×50) (b). Higher magnification of this case shows that beyond the region of obviously attenuated neuropil surrounding the vessels, there is severe neuronal loss and gliosis (H&E ×125) (c) Severe non-occlusive small vessel disease is often coupled with small focal infarctions and perivascular collections of macrophages as seen in this illustration. (H&E ×50)

mental deterioration, culminating in severe dementia over a course of about 10 years. Alzheimer (1902) expanded Binswanger's gross description, adding that the shrunken white matter was firm and mottled. He also described the microscopic finding of extensive loss of myelin with relative sparing of the subcortical U-fibres and convolutional white matter. Also noted was the presence of expansion of the Virchow–Robin spaces (état criblé), numerous small areas of infarction in the affected white matter and lacunes in the deep grey nuclei and brainstem.

There have been a number of clinical and pathological studies with and without attempted clinico-pathological correlation. Over the past two decades, reports have included those from Burger, Burch and Kunze (1976), Caplan and Schoene (1978), Rosenberg *et al.* (1979), Goto, Ishii and Fukasawa (1981), Janota (1981), Tomonaga *et al.* (1982), Loizou *et al.* (1982) and Dubas *et al.* (1985). Recent reviews of the topic include contributions by Babikian and Ropper (1987) and a particularly illuminating account by C. Miller Fisher (1989). All these studies have amplified descriptions of the changes by Binswanger and Alzheimer but have not, in any essentials, altered the pathological and clinical archetype which is that of a widespread disease of the white matter of the cerebral hemispheres with relative sparing of the cortical ribbon in a patient with a progressive dementia.

The external appearance of the brain in cases of Binswanger's disease is not usually at all impressive. The brain weight tends to be well maintained, and there is no marked gyral atrophy. There is also no particular tendency for large vessel atherosclerosis to occur in Binswanger's disease. Miller Fisher (1989), in his analysis, published case notes that large vessel atherosclerosis was absent or virtually absent in 22% of the cases. On brain slices, the most marked feature is usually dilatation of the lateral and third ventricles which were reported to be moderately or greatly enlarged in 81% of cases (Fig. 5.8).

Although the gross appearance of the brain in Binswanger's encephalopathy indicates considerable tissue loss, the real extent of the damage to the deep, hemispheric white matter is revealed only by study of microscope slides, and is one of the situations in which whole mount slides of hemispheres are most useful (Fig. 5.9). Gross examination of such a section stained for myelin shows, as described by Alzheimer, marked pallor that usually affects both hemispheres to a similar degree. The pallor is not homogeneous, but variable in degree, sometimes with perivascular accentuation and may be patchy or confluent and show small foci of actual tissue lysis; the term 'moth eaten' is almost irresistible. Usually, the pallor is most severe in the deeper regions of the white matter and periventricularly. More peripherally, the pallor becomes less intense and more focal, with only foci of perivascular myelin loss. In regions of more

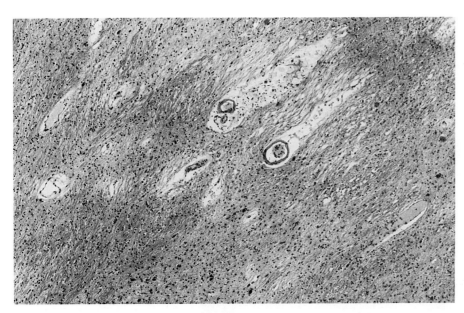

(*c*)

compacted myelin, the internal capsule tends to be spared, and the corpus callosum, although often markedly reduced in thickness, does not show the severity of pallor displayed by the periventicular white matter. These changes may be seen at any section of the hemisphere, but are often prominent in frontal and parietal planes. Curiously, although there is severe and widespread damage to the white matter of the cerebral hemispheres, the white matter of the cerebellar hemispheres is relatively spared.

Microscopic examination of the affected white matter shows widespread but variable pruning of the parenchymal elements of the white matter with loss of both axons and myelin from the white matter, that in some places is almost total (Fig. 5.10). The loss of myelin is rather greater than the axonal pruning. Within the variable picture, in the most severely affected areas, there are foci of frank tissue destruction with the formation of lacunes, and, at the other end of the pathological spectrum, only a mild general attenuation of myelin staining, with the individual myelinated axons being more distinguishable than is normal within white matter. C. Miller Fisher rightly describes the appearance as being that of 'diffuse incomplete demyelination'. In most of the affected areas there is a reduction in the number of oligodendrocytes and an accompanying but variable reactive astrocytosis. Surprisingly, in view of the degree of tissue loss, macrophages are often not very conspicuous, a fact that probably reflects the slow pathological evolution of the white matter damage and therefore the prolonged clinical course. In the regions of frank tissue destruction, foamy macrophages are present if the damage is relatively recent, and within the more diffusely damaged areas, scattered macrophages may also be found, often in fields, as though a particular area has undergone damage over a relatively similar time course while a neighbouring region has not. Occasional macrophages are also present in the Virchow–Robin spaces around the blood vessels in the affected areas. As can be seen on gross examination, the subcortical U-fibres tend to be spared and the damage, when it is present, tends to be most conspicuous in the fronto-parietal white matter, although some authorities report that the most severe microscopic changes are to be found in the occipital lobes. The blood vessel changes are very much those previously described above with marked hyaline thickening of the long penetrating arteries. In keeping with the severe loss of parenchyma, there is conspicuous enlargement of the perivascular Virchow–Robin spaces.

Clinical features

The clinical features of Binswanger's encephalopathy have been well described in a number of places, but good summaries are provided by both Babikian and Ropper and Miller Fisher. Specific diagnostic criteria were advanced by Bennet et al. (1990) that incorporate both clinical and radiological findings.

Hypertension is an almost invariable feature of patients with Binswanger's disease (98% (40 of 41) in Babikian and Ropper's review). The age of onset is

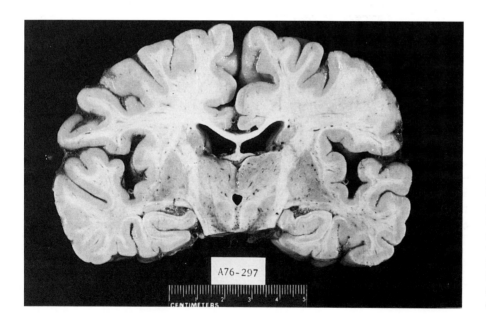

A76-297

Fig. 5.8. Binswanger's disease (sub-cortical leukoencephalopathy): Macroscopic picture of a case of Binswanger's disease. There is remarkably little obvious parenchymal change or ventricular dilatation. Other than the expansion of the Sylvian fissures, the most conspicuous change is attenuation of the corpus callosum.

variable, but more than 80% of cases occur in the sixth and seventh decades, and approximately equal numbers of males and females are affected.

The details of the clinical phenomenology are very variable, but Miller Fisher, after reviewing 50 pathologically confirmed cases in the literature, has suggested the following four basic patterns of clinical presentation and evolution.

a. Slowly progressive dementia with repeated strokes and/or transient ischaemic attacks (TIAs)

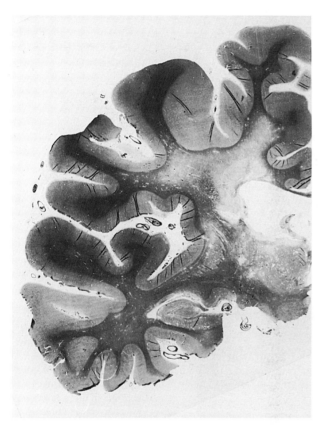

Fig. 5.9. Binswanger's Disease (sub-cortical leukoencephalopathy): Photograph of a luxol fast blue stained giant section of cerebral hemisphere of the case illustrated in Fig. 5.10. Despite the inconspicuous findings on macroscopic examination there is severe attenuation of stainable myelin in the hemispheric white matter of the fronto-parietal lobe. The overlying cortex is well preserved and there are no focal infarcts. The severe attenuation of the corpus callosum is noteworthy and reflects the degree of axonal damage that has occurred. Damage of this severity could be expected to produce significant disconnection between the deep grey nuclei and the cortex. In the plane of section stained, the thalamus also shows some small vessel disease.

or subacutely evolving neurological deficits.

b. Slowly progressive dementia with subacute evolving neurological deficits but without recognizable strokes or TIAs.

c. Dementia which evolves late after strokes, TIAs or subacute evolving neurological deficits.

d. Dementia without stroke, TIA or other abrupt event but with accruing neurological signs of unrecognized time of onset and unobtrusive evolution.

In almost all cases, an intellectual deficit is apparent early in the course of the disease and a memory disorder is often described as one of the early symptoms. The patients are frequently described as confused, inattentive and vague. Mood changes are frequent and, as the disease advances, the familiar changes of a widespread decline in higher mental function become apparent with a general slowness of function merging into a global dementia. In addition to the general failure of higher mental function, a very large number of different focal neurologic deficits have been described, accompanying the progressive intellectual decline of Binswanger's disease. Prominent among these are difficulties with walking and balance, and small strokes giving pure motor pareses.

Correlations with neuroimaging
Binswanger's disease is an area where the correlation of imaging and pathology is of some importance.

CT findings: The CT findings in Binswanger's disease consist of a non-contrast enhancing low density that is most prominent close to the ventricles and diminishes in severity as it extends into the hemispheric white matter. The most frequently used term for this CT finding has been periventricular low density, often abbreviated to PVLD. It has been repeatedly confirmed by clinico-pathologic studies that PVLD in demented patients clinically thought to have Binswanger's disease is well correlated with the presence of the white matter lesions characteristic of Binswanger's disease. In his 1989 review, Miller Fisher noted some 22 cases of pathologically confirmed Binswanger's disease that had been studied by CT, all of which supported this conclusion. This conclusion now seems sufficiently soundly based that it would be difficult to accept the diagnosis of Binswanger's disease in a patient with a normal appearing CT scan.

Thus far, all is plain sailing; the problem with the interpretation of PVLD comes from studies of non-demented patients and patients with other forms of dementia. When patients with PVLD are studied (rather than patients with dementia), it emerges that up to 60% of them do not have dementia (Goto *et al.*, 1981; George *et al.*, 1986). Pathological studies of brains showing

PVLD appear to show that the neuroradiological finding is reliable in the sense that there is a good correlation between the presence of the pathological substrate of Binswanger change (arteriolar sclerosis, diffuse loss of myelin and axons) and the presence of PVLD, but a poor correlation with the presence of dementia (Lotz, Ballinger & Quisling, 1986). There is also the suggestion that

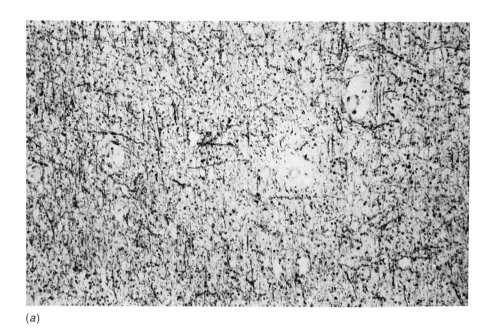

(a)

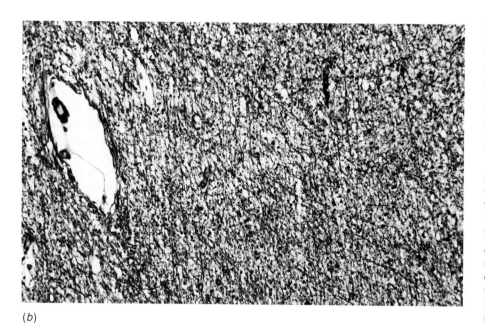

(b)

Fig. 5.10. (*a*). When examined microscopically, a luxol fast blue stain of the white matter from a case of Binswanger's disease shows only scattered preserved myelinated axons. Although the axonal loss is most severe around the blood vessel in the centre of the picture there is also widespread diffuse reduction in the density of myelinated fibres in the affected white matter. (H&E × 50) (*b*). A similarly stained section from a patient with mild small vessel disease of the white matter. There is marked dilatation of the Virchow–Robin space around the blood vessel but no clear attenuation of the perivascular neuropil. The difference in the density of myelinated fibres between this illustration and the case of Binswanger's disease in Fig. 5.10(*a*) is very striking. (H&E × 50)

minor degrees of Binswanger change can be found in the absence of CT abnormalities.

MRI findings: The principal MRI findings fall into two classes, diffuse changes seen on both T1 and T2 sequences, and, in T2 images, the 'unidentified bright objects' (UBOs) also known as white matter hyperintense foci. In general terms the diffuse MRI changes are equivalent to the PVLD seen on CT scanning, but as visualized by the T2 sequence, MRI is generally considered to be somewhat more sensitive than CT while the T1 images tend to be inferior to CT scanning. For the diffuse lesions, the equivalence between MRI and CT means that the same general correlations between imaging and pathology and imaging and clinical expression are valid. Broadly speaking, in cases of Binswanger's disease, diffuse white matter lesions are invariably present on MRI and there is a good correlation between the MRI signal changes and the distribution and type of pathological change (Révész *et al.*, 1989). However, as with CT there are numerous false positives where MRI changes are not accompanied by any clinical symptoms or signs. Since MRI tends to be more sensitive than CT to diffuse changes, the pathological changes seen with the lesser degrees of MRI signal change are quite inconspicuous, and it is not surprising that patients with these lesser degrees of abnormality were asymptomatic.

This is not the place for a detailed examination of correlative studies of the UBOs but in a careful study by Awad *et al.* (1986) of post-mortem scanned brains they showed that UBOs were associated with the presence of several types of abnormality ranging from dilatation of the Virchow–Robin space (état criblé) to parenchymal changes of focal gliosis and axonal loss.

PATHOGENESIS

The pathophysiology of the white matter damage in Binswanger's disease is not clearly understood, but whatever explanation is to be evolved it must take account of the importance of hypertension in the development of Binswanger change. All clinical studies of patients with Binswanger's disease have shown a prevalence of hypertension in more than 90% of the patients. From another standpoint, studies of patients with the CT and MRI findings of PVLD or PVH on MRI have shown that the overwhelming majority of patients with these imaging findings also have hypertension. Supporting evidence for the importance of the association with hypertension comes from the presence of lacunes in more than 85% of cases of Binswanger's

disease. The doyen of lacunar disease, C. Miller Fisher, is on record that the presence of lacunar disease is related to hypertension in more than 90% of cases. The combination of both a history of hypertension and the almost invariable presence of some degree of lacunar disease in Binswanger's disease is strong evidence for the importance of hypertension in its pathophysiology.

Beyond this testimony to the importance of hypertension, there is little agreement as to the specifics of the pathophysiology of the white matter damage. One of the reasons for the difficulty in arriving at a more precise concept of the pathogenesis of Binswanger change is that the processes of damage are relatively slow and progressive and that dynamic factors interacting with structural changes almost certainly play a major role in the evolution of the degeneration of the axons and myelin. The most obvious dynamic factors that could be involved are variations in blood pressure and cerebral perfusion pressures, changes in the permeability of the blood–brain barrier in respect of both electrolytes and proteins, and changes in CSF pressures. All these can be affected by the presence of hypertension and can also undergo changes over a variety of time courses, some of which may be quite prolonged by the normal standards of physiologic measurement. Thus, even if they could be measured at a single point in time, the value measured might not reflect a significant alteration in a pattern of variation. It may also be that treatment of established hypertension could even have an adverse effect. It has been suggested that compensatory mechanisms evolved to protect the tissue from the effects of hypertension could result in relative tissue ischaemia when the blood pressure was returned to a more normal range by antihypertensive medication.

The most straightforward suggestions of aetiology are those that involve tissue ischaemia in the distal fields of supply of the thickened penetrating arteries which are almost all end arteries. If the cause is simple ischaemia, it is not likely that the ischaemia is a result of vascular occlusion, as this is notably rare in examination of the long penetrating arteries in Binswanger's disease, although Okeda (1973) has stated that vascular occlusion is more common in Binswanger's disease than in hypertension alone. Even if this is accepted, the type of damage seen in Binswanger's disease is not what is usually found in vascular occlusions, since occlusions of long penetrating arteries that supply the deep white matter produce focal infarctions that are linear and follow the course of the occluded artery, not the diffuse changes actually seen in Binswanger's disease. Most of the suggestions related to ischaemia are that there is generally reduced flow through the thickened long penetrating arteries. The reduced flow is thought to result in relative tissue ischaemia, perhaps occurring on an intermittent basis during periods of actual or 'relative' hypotension when the usually elevated blood pressure is within the normal range. The ischaemia would be expected to be most severe in the 'border zone' of the deep white matter between the penetrating arteries supplying the white matter and the blood supply of the deep grey nuclei which is the zone principally affected in Binswanger change (De Reuck et al., 1980). There have been a number of refinements of this view, such as that of Okeda (1973) who suggested that autoregulatory activity in the short, penetrating arteries supplying the cortext could result in a relative 'shunting' of flow to the arteries supplying the deep, white matter which results in inappropriate thickening of these arteries and an impaired microcirculation.

The view that the damage is all a result of simple ischaemia as a result of the changes in the arteries has an engaging simplicity and immediate plausibility, but is not without its detractors. One problem is the suggestion from three sources that the vascular changes can occur independently of hypertension. There are certainly a few cases of Binswanger's disease where there is no history of hypertension (Loizou et al., 1982; Caplan & Schoene, 1978; Goto et al., 1981). A possibility in these rare cases of Binswanger's disease without a history of hypertension is that they represent unrecognized examples of hereditary liability to vascular dementia where the findings are similar to Binswanger's disease but hypertension is characteristically absent (see below). Hypertension is also absent in the white matter disease associated with congophilic angiopathy and Alzheimer's disease where there is both pruning of axons and myelin in the deep white matter and hyaline thickening of the arteries of the white matter. Brun and Englund (1986) sought to distinguish the vascular changes seen in Alzheimer's disease from those seen in Binswanger's disease. They drew attention to the lack of any history of hypertension in the patients with Alzheimer's disease and, morphologically, to the absence of vascular hypertensive changes and, in the parenchyma, regions of complete infarction and lacunar disease in these patients.

There is also evidence from radiological studies that white matter changes are more severe in patients with vascular dementia than in Alzheimer's disease (Aharon-Peretz, Cummings & Hill, 1988). Perfusion studies have also shown lower blood flow in subcortical structures in vascular dementia compared to Alzheimer's disease and

suggest a different aetiology for the white matter disease in vascular dementia (Kawamura et al., 1993). Studies of brain oedema (Feigin & Popoff, 1963) have also suggested that the vascular changes can occur as a result of the oedema rather than being its cause. The most direct test of the significance of ischaemia would be repeatedly to measure the degree of oxygen extraction from the circulation in the deep white matter, an experiment that has yet to be performed. It is technically difficult to get accurate measurements of blood flow and oxygen extraction in the periventricular white matter but what data there is from older subjects have not indicated an increase in the oxygen extraction fraction in either grey or white matter. SPECT (Tohgi et al., 1991) and PET (Yao et al., 1990) studies, however, lend some credence to the ischaemic hypothesis in that they have suggested that there is a reduction in cerebral perfusion and white matter oxygenation in cerebrovascular dementia of the Binswanger type that occurs early in the course of the disease. It is also reported that the severity of the changes in perfusion and oxygenation is correlated with the severity of the dementia. The perfusion reduction is predominantly in the frontal lobes which parallels the neuroimaging studies (though not the rather fewer cases studied pathologically), suggesting that the white matter disease tends to start in the frontal lobes and remains most prominent in this region of the brain.

At present, no coherent pathophysiological mechanism can be advanced to explain the findings in Binswanger's disease; it can be accepted that the condition is usually a consequence of hypertension, but the precise mechanism or mechanisms by which it acts to produce both the vascular changes and the diffuse incomplete demyelination remain(s) to be elucidated.

White matter small vessel disease and amyloid angiopathy

Studies on cases of presumed Alzheimer's disease have shown an incidence of some degree of PVLD in up to 30% of cases of AD, but with a poor correlation with the severity of the dementia. The presence of white matter changes in Alzheimer's disease is well established. In their pathoanatomical study, Brun and Englund (1986) found some degree of diffuse white matter disease in more than 60% of the cases, and severe changes in about 20% of the total sample. As already mentioned, the pathological findings had some similarities to those in Binswanger's disease with diffuse incomplete loss of myelin and axons combined with a hyaline thickening of the small arteries supplying the white matter. In this study there was no correlation between either the distribution or the severity of the Alzheimer cortical changes and the severity and distribution of the diffuse white matter loss, nor did the white matter loss appear to be correlated with the presence or severity of congophilic angiopathy. However, a correlation between white matter loss and congophilic angiopathy has been reported by Dubas et al. (1985) and Gray et al. (1985), but in at least some of the cases studied, the interpretation, both in terms of imaging and pathology, is complicated by the presence of focal haemorrhage.

Lacunar disease

All the deep grey nuclei have a similar pattern of blood supply, being fed by small arteries that are direct branches of large arteries, there being no progressive arterial arborization to smaller and smaller diameters. This is the case both for the lenticulo-striate branches of the middle cerebral artery that supplies the basal ganglia, and the branches from the initial segment of the posterior cerebral artery that enter through the posterior perforated substance to supply the thalamus. Although this pattern of blood supply is quite different from that of white matter, it also confers on these nuclei a peculiar vulnerability to vascular disease. Where the white matter is vulnerable because the long penetrating arteries are at the distal end of a very long arterial arborization, the deep grey nuclei are vulnerable because their blood supply lacks the protection of an arborization. Being direct branches of large arteries, the arterial supply of the deep grey nuclei is immediately exposed to the effects of hypertension. In this context, it is probably significant that all three regions of the brain supplied in this manner, the basal ganglia, thalamus and pons (supplied by branches from the basilar artery) are sites of predilection for hypertensive haemorrhages and lacunar disease.

By comparison with the tortuosities of Binswanger's disease, lacunar disease is relatively straightforward. Lacunes themselves are small cavitary lesions found within the brain parenchyma that are the result of occlusions of small penetrating branches of the large diameter arteries of the brain. They range in size between 2 mm and 2 cm. In old lesions the gliotic reaction in the wall gives it a fibrillary and sometimes trabeculated appearance. They tend to occur in patients with a history of hypertension and almost certainly have multiple aetiologies. Some will certainly be the consequence of small emboli, probably atherosclerotic, but in others there are marked changes in the vascular wall, a change descriptively called 'lipohyalinosis' by Fisher (1969), in which the vessel is occluded and the arterial wall is

grossly disrupted and generate. Lacunes are not distributed randomly in the brain. Because of their tendency to occur in the penetrating branches of large diameter arteries, they are most typically found in the deep grey nuclei, internal capsule and the basis pontis, although the deep hemispheric white matter can also be affected through occlusions of the long penetrating arteries.

Individual lacunes are certainly easy to identify and, as single entities, tend to be either asymptomatic or, if located in a clinically eloquent area of the brain such as the internal capsule or the basis pontis, produce sharply defined focal neurological symptoms and signs. Clinically, a large number of individual neurologic syndromes have been described in association with single lacunes (Fisher, 1982). Examples include pure sensory strokes, pure motor hemipareses or monopareses. Equally important is that dementia is one the syndromes not associated with individual lacunes, although a single example of memory loss as a result of bilateral infarction of the pillars of the fornix has been described. In C. Miller Fisher's memorable paraphrase, 'lacunes lick the psyche and bite the soma, just the opposite to senile dementia' (Fisher, 1968). However, although ordinarily not associated with dementia, they are clearly associated with cognitive decline when they present in large numbers (del Ser et al., 1990). Lacunes, when numerous, are an indicator of the presence of widespread severe small vessel disease, and this has been called the lacunar state or, more evocatively for Anglo-Saxons, l'état lacunaire.

L'État Lacunaire (lacunar state)

L'état lacunaire was first described by Pierre Marie (1901). In the original description it was associated with chronic progressive neurological decline including dysarthria, incontinence, imbalance, pseudobulbar palsy and some degree of dementia. Modern experience is that such patients are considerably less frequently encountered than in earlier epochs and it has been suggested by Fisher (1982) that a number of the early cases may have been undiagnosed cases of normal pressure hydrocephalus. The impression of a reduction in frequency of the lacunar state has found some confirmation in two studies between 1950–54 (Fisher, 1965) and 1975–76 by C. Miller Fisher (1982) who found a decrease in both the number of brains with lacunes (from 11% to 8%) and the average number of lacunes per case (from 3.3 to 2.5). In the 1950–54 study more than 10 lacunes were found in some of the cases, while in the later study no case contained more than seven lesions. He attributed this decline in both incidence and severity to the more effective treatment of hypertension which has made a rarity of the florid lacunar states previously seen. It would seem therefore that the dementia associated with l'état lacunaire should be regarded as a rather rare bird. However, although rare, the lacunar state is not entirely extinct since occasional cases with numerous lacunes still occur. Those where there is a significant degree of cognitive decline tend to have many lesions in the deep grey nuclei and particularly the thalamus (Fig. 5.11). The widespread nature of the small vessel disease in this condition is reflected by the fact that microscopic examination of the affected regions usually reveals many other non-cavitary ischaemic lesions in addition to the lacunes seen on gross examination of the brain (Fig. 5.12).

While the above mechanisms undoubtedly account for the vast majority of cases of vascular dementia, the authors of the NINDS-AIRED workshop also suggested three other mechanisms by which vascular disease could cause dementia, none of which are common causes of dementia. These are:

4. *Hypoperfusion* where dementia followed an episode of cerebral ischaemia following cardiac arrest or hypotension.
5. *Haemorrhagic dementia* which included dementia as a result of chronic subdural haematoma, subarachnoid haemorrhage or intracerebral haematoma.
6. *Other mechanisms* which included combinations of the five preceding causes and other, as yet unknown, mechanisms.

AETIOLOGY OF VASCULAR DEMENTIA

As has been clear from the discussion thus far, the aetiology of vascular dementia is associated overwhelmingly with the interacting pathophysiological processes of hypertension and atherosclerosis each of which reinforce the effect of the other. As risk factors for the development of atherosclerosis, hyperlipidaemia, smoking and diabetes all tend to raise the chance of developing vascular dementia in individual patients (del Ser *et al.*, 1990; Gorelick *et al.*, 1993). Similarly, the largely unknown forces that affect the prevalence of primary hypertension and its various secondary causes are factors in the incidence and prevalence of vascular dementia. The dominant role of hypertension and atherosclerosis in vascular dementia of necessity also places these patients in a significantly higher risk category for cardiovascular death.

Hypertension and atherosclerosis

The direct effects of hypertension are of necessity diffuse in that, when it is present, all vessels are exposed to hypertension. However, although all vessels are exposed to hypertension, the effects are not the same. This is made most obvious by considering the effects of hypertension on the short penetrating arteries that supply the cerebral cortex and the long, penetrating arteries that pass through the cortex to supply the white matter. While the arterioles in the white matter can become markedly thickened and hyalinized and the white matter diffusely attenuated, the short penetrating arteries and

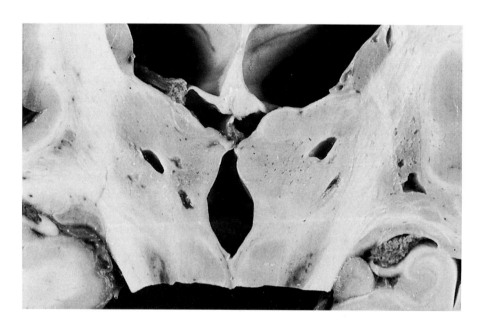

Fig. 5.11. Lacunar state: in this patient who suffered from a stepwise cognitive decline there are at least seven lacunes of varying size in this plane of section of the thalamus and posterior putamen. Other planes of section in this case showed additional lacunes with very little focal vascular disease elsewhere in the brain.

the overlying cortex rarely show any changes. As has been described, small vessel changes are also prominent in the deep grey nuclei of the basal ganglia and thalamus.

By contrast to the diffuse and widespread effects of hypertension, atherosclerosis is almost always focal and exerts its influence locally either through stenosis, thrombosis or embolism. Probably the commonest site of vascular thrombosis secondary to atherosclerosis is the internal carotid artery at the bifurcation, and it is good practice always to examine the carotid bifurcations in patients who come to post-mortem examination. Thrombosis of the intracranial arteries is distinctly rarer, with the basilar artery being the most commonly affected.

Embolic disease
Although atheroemboli are very important and probably the commonest type of embolus encountered in vascular dementia, the existence of cognitive decline secondary to strategic single infarcts means that other sources of emboli can certainly be associated with cognitive decline and that cognitive decline does not invariably occur in the context of widespread cerebrovascular disease.

The twin aetiologies of hypertension and atherosclerosis account for almost all cases of vascular dementia, but there are a small number of other conditions that affect blood vessels and can produce dementia.

Hereditary liability to stroke
There are a large number of rare but well-established conditions that confer a hereditary liability to recurrent cerebral infarcts and are therefore potential causes of vascular dementia (Natowicz & Kelly, 1987). They include conditions such as homocysteinuria, varieties of the dyslipoproteinaemias, and Fabry's disease among many others.

Two groups merit specific mention, the first being the hereditary cerebral amyloidoses that are described in Chapter 12. The second is a condition that is now becoming best known by its acronym, CADASIL.

Cerebral autosomal dominant arteriopathy with subcortical infarcts and leukoencephalopathy (CADASIL)
Over the years there have been a number of reports of a familial syndrome characterized by subcortical ischaemic strokes with dementia and a leukoencephalopathy that resembles Binswanger's disease (Davous & Fallet-Bianco, 1991; Sourander & Wallinder, 1977;

Stevens, Hewlett & Brownall, 1977; Sonninen & Savontaus, 1987; Tournier-Lasserve et al., 1991; Mas, Dilouya & Recondo, 1992). Although there are some differences among the families reported in these studies, the overall similarity in genetic transmission as an autosomal dominant and the parallels of clinical and pathological expression of disease suggest that they all belong in a similar category now often called CADASIL.

Clinically, these cases present with recurrent episodes of focal cerebral dysfunction that affect mostly subcortical structures. The onset of the disease tends to be in the 30s and 40s with a duration of between 10 and 15 years. The clinical syndrome is rather similar to that reported in Binswanger's disease (Caplan & Schoene, 1978; Babikian & Ropper, 1987) but with the notable exception that these patients have no history of findings of hypertension and no other identifiable risk factors for cerebrovascular disease. A number of patients also report migraine-like headaches. In accordance with the predominantly subcortical nature of the clinical symptoms, imaging studies show predominantly white matter abnormalities (leukoaraiosis) on CT and T_2-weighted MRI scans that again resemble Binswanger's disease (Tourneir-Lasserve et al., 1991; Mas et al., 1992). Lacunar infarcts and other infarcts in the deep grey nuclei are also frequently seen on imaging studies of these patients. Changes can be seen in symptomatic patients and also in some asymptomatic family members.

Pathologically, the changes in the white matter are very similar to those seen in Binswanger's disease with diffuse and focal myelin loss and pallor with sparing of subcortical U-fibres. As indicated by neuroradiological studies, basal ganglia and thalamic infarcts are seen. In the vascular system the changes are seen predominantly in smaller arteries in the white matter and deep grey nuclei, but changes can also be seen in the small arteries in the subarachnoid space and these have been used for diagnostic purposes (Lammie et al., 1995). The changes consist of degeneration of the media with thickening and hyalinization of the arterial wall, marked splitting and reduplication of the elastic lamina and intimal thickening, all leading to marked narrowing or occlusion of the vessel lumen. In one report (Sourander & Willander, 1977), a scant perivascular infiltration with mononuclear inflammatory cells was recorded, but there are no other indications to suggest that this is an inflammatory vasculopathy. No amyloid deposition is present. Periodic acid-Schiff stains of affected vessels show positive staining granular material in the muscle cells of small parenchymal and subarachnoid arteries (Baudrimont et *al.*, 1993) and electron microscopy shows collections of granular electron dense material that is considered to be diagnostic of the condition (Baudrimont *et al.*, 1993; Gray *et al.*, 1994). The vascular changes are not restricted to brain and similar ultrastructural findings have been recorded in sural nerve and skin biopsies that can be used to confirm a clinical diagnosis (Schröder *et al.*, 1995; Ruchoux *et al.* 1994; Lechner-Scott *et al.*, 1996). The genetic locus of this hereditary syndrome is reported to be chromosome 19q12 (Tournier-Lasserve *et al.*, 1993; Jung *et al.*, 1995), but the affected gene has not been established. In view of the report of migraine-like headaches in some of the patients, it might be significant that this genetic locus is also linked to familial hemiplegic migraine. The pathophysiology of the vascular changes is likewise unclear, but if it could be discovered it might cast considerable light on the process leading to vascular and parenchymal damage in hypertension.

Vasculitis

Vasculitis occurs in a number of clinical forms which have varying effects on the nervous system (Moore & Cupps, 1983). The principal clinically defined varieties of vasculitis are the polyarteritis nodosa group, hypersensitivity angiitis, Wegener's granulomatosis (Nishino *et al.*, 1993), isolated angiitis of the nervous system, giant cell arteritis, and Behcet's disease. These different entities affect the nervous system to different degrees and in different ways, but problems with higher nervous system function and cognitive decline are one of the ways that

vasculitis affecting the nervous system can become manifest.

With the possible exception of hypersensitivity angiitis, it is probably true to say that any of the major groups of arteritis characterized above can present with generalized encephalopathy, memory loss and behavioural changes that could fall within the category of dementia. It is certainly reasonable to add that such general features are frequently accompanied by other focal symptoms and signs such as cranial neuropathies and focal cerebral defects that suggest a multifocal process. Since they are also systemic diseases, effects on other organ systems are usually present and may dominate the clinical picture. Further, to distinguish these conditions from atherosclerotic vascular disease, the time-scale of the process is almost invariably compressed and is spread over weeks to months rather than the months to years that elapse in atherosclerotic disease.

Isolated angiitis of the nervous system

The most challenging situation is perhaps that which occurs in isolated angiitis of the nervous system when systemic effects are not present (Kolodney *et al.*, 1968; Calabrese & Malleck, 1987; Cupps, Moore & Fauci, 1983). In this condition there is focal inflammation and necrosis in the walls of leptomeningeal and parenchymal arteries. The inflammation is typically lymphoplasmacytic with macrophages and, in most cases, also giant cells and formation of granulomas; hence the alternative name of granulomatous angiitis of the CNS. The condi-

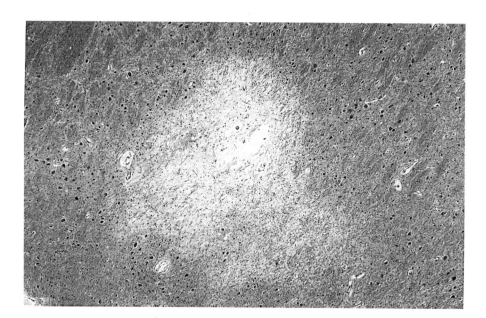

Fig. 5.12. Microscopic examination of the same case as Fig. 5.11 showed, in addition to the lacunes, scattered areas of non-cavitated focal ischaemic damage. As can be seen from this illustration, the neuropil between the focal lesions is well preserved. (H&E ×50)

tion may present with confusion and intellectual deterioration, although this is nearly always accompanied by headache. Although sometimes absent early in the course, focal neurological signs usually occur at some time. In most cases granulomatous angiitis is subacutely progressive over weeks to months but has been recorded to 'grumble' on for years. The pathologist becomes involved in these cases because they usually produce considerable diagnostic uncertainty and, even when angiography demonstrates segmental narrowing and beading of affecting arteries, there is sometimes a need to confirm this pathologically. There have also been cases where angiography has been normal but biopsy has shown the presence of arteritis in the smaller vessels not visualized by radiographic techniques (Moore, 1989). In such cases a leptomeningeal and parenchymal biopsy has sometimes proved positive (Hughes & Brownell, 1966; Harrison, 1976; Jellinger, 1977).

Giant cell (temporal) arteritis

This affects arteries in the distribution of the carotid and, less frequently, vertebral arteries (Wilkinson & Russell, 1972). Visual involvement is the most common manifestation, and CNS abnormalities are relatively uncommon. Bilateral carotid involvement has been reported to produce global mental deterioration (Howard *et al.*, 1984).

Buerger's disease

Another condition within the spectrum of vasculitis that can present with dementia is the cerebral form of thromboangiitis obliterans (Buerger's disease) (Lie, 1988). This condition, as is widely recognized, is almost invariably associated with a history of cigarette smoking, but the precise nature of the aetiological connection between the two remains elusive. Although rare in Europe and North America, thromboangiitis obliterans is common in other parts of the world, notably Japan, India and Israel. In most cases, the disease is generalized and thus occasionally affects the brain, but Lindenberg and Spatz (1940) described a cerebral form of the disease that they divided into types I and II which tended to affect large basal arteries (type I) or distal branches (type II). Both these variants were associated with the presence of vascular dementia, although it was reported to be more common in the type II disease. In a recent report of what has been called Spatz-Lindenberg disease (SLD), Zhan, Beyreuther & Schmitt (1993) attempted to compare synaptophysin loss in SLD with that in Alzheimer's disease and showed similar degrees of loss, although the significance and interpretation of this finding was not clear.

Collagen vascular disease

Systemic lupus erythematosis (SLE)

SLE is the collagen vascular disease with the most frequent involvement of the central nervous system. Although neurological disease is rarely a presenting sign, there is a high frequency of involvement at some-

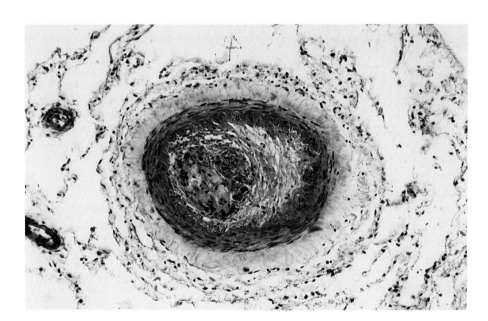

Fig. 5.13. Systemic lupus erythematosus (SLE). The vascular changes in the vasculopathy of SLE are concentrated in the intima, with, as in this illustration, relative sparing of the media. In arteritides such as polyarteritis nodosa, the principal focus of the inflammatory infiltrate and tissue damage is in the muscular media of the artery. (H&E × 125)

time during the course of the disease, estimates varying between 10 and 75% of patients in different series (Lim *et al.*, 1988; Bluestein, 1987), with neurological symptoms being more frequent in the later and more severe stages (Johnson & Richardson, 1968). SLE has a range of effects on the nervous system, some of which, such as the cranial neuropathies, cerebrovascular accidents and chorea, reflect focal disease. Given the role of single strategic infarction in vascular dementia, even focal disease can produce cognitive decline, although this is not common (Mitsias & Levine, 1994). Diffuse effects such as confusional states, and acute delirium, delusions and other more generalized disturbances of cerebral function are quite common, and dementia has also been described.

Although vasculitis has always been regarded as one of the major pathological mechanisms in SLE, the extent of the identifiable vasculitic changes in the brain have always been much less than would be expected from the severity of the symptoms and signs (Johnson & Richardson, 1968). Occasional examples of a conventional acute vasculitis, with an acute inflammatory reaction within the arterial wall, sometimes with a giant cell reaction, and necrosis of the vessel wall, are seen in SLE, but this is quite a rare finding. The more frequent observation is a 'vasculopathy' with hyaline thickening of the wall of the blood vessel, fibrinoid degeneration and endothelial proliferation (Ellis & Verity, 1979; Ellison *et al.*, 1993) (Fig. 5.13). The aetiology of this vascular lesion is not clear but Ellison *et al.* have shown the presence of platelet-derived material within the thickened wall of these abnormal vessels. The disparity of the relative paucity of pathological findings in patients with rather prominent, and often fluctuating, clinical findings has precipitated a search for other pathophysiological mechanisms by which the function of the central nervous system could be compromised (Bluestein, 1987; Mitchell *et al.*, 1994). One process that has been heavily canvassed as a probable mechanism underlying the ephemeral neuropsychiatric symptoms is an immune-complex-mediated 'vasculitis' associated with complement activation. This process could be very short lasting and produce tissue ischaemia short of infarction. The vascular endothelial damage attendant on ischaemia has been shown to be associated with platelet deposition in small vessels (Jafar *et al.*, 1989). The presence of antiphospholipid antibodies has also been associated with cerebral infarction in SLE (Asherson & Lubbe, 1988; Asherson *et al.*, 1989), and this could be a further mechanism by which tissue ischaemia could develop in the brain. Another more diffuse mechanism

that has been suggested to have a role in the production of the neuropsychiatric symptoms of SLE is antineuronal antibodies, which are hypothesized to gain access to the cerebral parenchyma as a consequence of breakdown of the blood–brain barrier following the immune-mediated vasculitis. Hanson *et al.* (1992) reported the presence of antibodies to a 50 kD neuronal membrane protein in 19 of 20 patients with lupus and CNS involvement but in only 8 of 23 where there was no CNS involvement and 1 of 34 patients with other neurological diseases. It is quite plausible to imagine that access to the brain by an antibody to a widely expressed neuronal protein, particularly if the protein was involved in synaptic transmission, could produce widespread and variable effects on CNS function. Nevertheless, as emphasized by Mitchell *et al.* (1994), the pathogenesis of cerebral lupus is likely to be multifactorial.

Cocaine and other stimulants

Cerebral vasculitis can either be stimulated or mimicked by both cocaine and amphetamines. Cocaine use is associated with an increased frequency of transient ischaemic attacks, cerebral infarcts and haemorrhages which may be subarachnoid or intraparenchymal (Levine *et al.*, 1990). The strokes and intraparenchymal haemorrhages, while usually producing focal neurological symptoms may, if they affect appropriate regions of the brain, also cause cognitive defects. A prominent example would be thalamomesencephalic infarcts (Rowley *et al.*, 1989) that, depending on the precise thalamic structures involved, (Graff-Redford *et al.*, 1985) may have a wide variety of neuropsychological and cognitive problems. Although the vast majority of lesions associated with cocaine abuse are probably manifestations of the acute vasospastic effects of cocaine, there are a few reports where cocaine seems to be associated with a histologically demonstrated vasculitis (Krendal *et al.*, 1990; Tapia & Golden, 1993). A vasculitis with vessel wall necrosis has also been described in association with amphetamine abuse (Citron *et al.*, 1970).

Lymphomatoid granulomatosis

This condition was first described by Liebow, Carrington and Friedman (1972) and is a lymphoreticular proliferative disorder with an angiocentric and angiodestructive polymorphic cellular infiltrate. In a significant minority of cases the condition evolves into, or is associated with, a non-Hodgkin's lymphoma. Although the lung is usually the primary site of disease, the CNS is involved in between a fifth and a quarter of the cases and neurological symptoms may be the mode of presentation (Katzenstein, Carrington & Liebow, 1979). In a very small number of cases, the disease is clinically restricted to the nervous system (Schmidt *et al.*, 1984; Kerr *et al.*, 1987), although there may be pathological evidence of disease in the lungs. Within the brain the lesions may be multiple and show mass effect (Simon *et al.*, 1981). Histologically, there is often necrosis and haemorrhage with parenchymal involvement by a markedly angiocentric and angiodestructive mixed inflammatory infiltrate composed of lymphocytes (often with marked nuclear pleomorphism and irregularity), histiocytes, plasma cells and plasmacytoid lymphocytes together with other bizarre mononuclear cells (Anders *et al.*, 1989; Ironside *et al.*, 1984). The vasculopathic nature of the condition means that its nervous system presentation very much resembles that of a cerebral arteritis with a wide spectrum of neurological abnormalities, including cognitive decline.

Angiotropic (intravascular) large cell lymphoma

This is a rare and generally fatal disease characterized by mononuclear tumour cell growth within the lumens of small vessels that affects predominantly the skin and central nervous system. This condition has had a number of different names including neoplastic angioendotheliomatosis, a portmanteau term that reflects an earlier confusion over the nature of the neoplastic cells (Sheibani *et al.*, 1986). In more modern publications, it is more correctly called angiotropic large cell lymphoma or malignant intravascular lymphoma. How these patients present depends on the location of the disease, but if the principal burden of disease is in the cerebral hemispheres, it can take the form of a subacutely progressive dementia that may mimic a vasculitis (Strouth *et al.*, 1965; Bots 1974; Reinglass *et al.*, 1977; Petito *et al.*, 1978; Fulling & Gersell, 1983; LeWitt, Forno & Brant-Zawadski, 1983). As might be suspected from the nature of the underlying condition, survival tends to be measured in months rather than years.

As a pendant to this list of unusual vascular causes of cognitive decline and dementia, a final and perhaps unique cause of vascular dementia, encountered by one of us, is illustrated in Fig. 5.14. The dementia in this case was the result of a very large number of cavernous angiomas. The multiple and recurrent haemorrhages from the angiomas produced, along with focal symptoms and signs, widespread cerebral damage and a progressive cognitive decline, the cause of which, in the pre-MRI era, was obscure until post-mortem examination.

In this section on aetiology, as is usual, a quite disproportionate amount of space has been devoted to the rarer vascular causes of cognitive decline. It is perhaps worth reemphasizing at the end of this section that the overwhelming majority of cases of cognitive decline due to vascular disease are a result of the combined and interacting effects of hypertension and atherosclerosis.

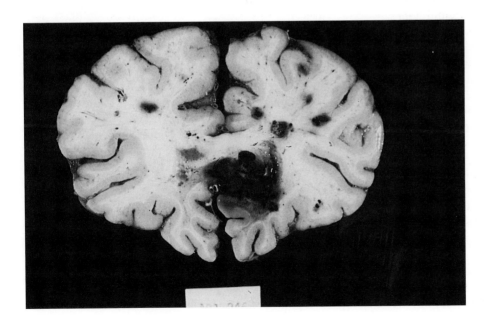

Fig. 5.14. An unusual cause of vascular dementia: This patient, who developed a slowly progressive dementia, with other focal neurological signs, had the syndrome of multiple carvernous angiomas.

NEUROPATHOLOGIC CRITERIA FOR VASCULAR DEMENTIA

Introduction

As noted in the opening paragraphs of this chapter, one of the big three questions in dementia associated with cerebrovascular disease is 'what are the neuropathological criteria for the diagnosis of vascular dementia?' At present, although the matter has been extensively discussed, there are no accepted neuropathological criteria on which to make this diagnosis. The inability of the neuropathological community to produce diagnostic criteria is not solely the result of insouciance since the problems of arriving at a generally agreed set of criteria are not inconsiderable.

Proposed neuropathologic assessment scheme

For the neuropathologist, the challenge is to find a reasonably concise yet meaningful way to describe the distribution and severity of cerebrovascular disease that is useful for correlative clinico-pathological studies of dementia.

The essential components of any workable assessment scheme for cerebrovascular disease are that it should be:

1. Based on clear morphological criteria.
2. Simple to perform.
3. Repeatable.

At a practical level it requires:

1. Description of the vascular morbid anatomy: particularly the presence, distribution and severity of atherosclerosis or other vascular process.
2. Description of the focal lesions (infarcts and lacunes) in terms of the vascular territory(ies), number, and volume of tissue (including the major anatomical structures involved).
3. Description of the diffuse non-occlusive small vessel disease.

Both the description of the vascular morbid anatomy and the focal lesions can be accomplished by gross examination of the brain, while description of the diffuse non-occlusive small vessel disease requires microscopic examination of selected regions of the brain.

CERAD, although principally concerned with the problem of Alzheimer's disease, have produced a protocol that is perfectly adequate to describe the vascular morbid anatomy and focal lesions that are detectable on gross examination. Encouragingly, in the latest revision of the CERAD guide, the Consortium is beginning to approach methods of describing small vessel disease by asking for a record of white matter pallor and Binswanger change on microscopic examination of specific white matter regions. What is proposed here is an extension of these recommendations.

In diffuse, non-occlusive cerebrovascular disease the problem is to define the locations within the brain that are most consistently affected and which therefore need to be sampled, the morphological features to be recorded and a severity rating scale for the features selected.

Selection of blocks for microscopic examination

The most generally affected regions of white and grey matter are:

White matter

Centrum semiovale – at level of striatum.
Parietal lobe – at level of pulvinar.
Occipital lobe – at occipital pole of lateral ventricle.

Grey matter

Basal ganglia
Thalamus

Pons

Basis pontis

In the assessment of dementia associated with cerebrovascular disease, blocks from these regions should always be submitted together with any other relevant regions. A general scheme of block section for the brain in dementia was outlined in Chapter 3.

Morphological features

The major morphological features of diffuse non-occlusive small vessel disease have already been described. They differ somewhat in grey and white matter.

In grey matter, in terms of progressive severity they are:

Arteriolar sclerosis (vascular thickening),
Expansion of the Virchow–Robin spaces
Perivascular gliosis and rarefaction.

While in white matter the changes are:

Arteriolar sclerosis
Expansion of the Virchow–Robin spaces

Diffuse myelin pallor and gliosis (Binswanger change).

Severity rating scale

As has been discussed, a semi-quantitive scale of severity is required for each of the morphological features that we have suggested as possibly significant. Although imperfect, probably the most effective way of defining the various grades of severity in a semi-quantitive scheme such as this is to provide representative illustrations of each grade of severity as has been done in this chapter (Figs. 5.5–7, 5.10).

A possible assessment proforma for recording the aspects of cerebrovascular disease that have been mentioned is provided on pages 166–7. It is the nature of these protocols that they teeter unsteadily along a fine line between over- and under-specification. Upon which side they are considered to err is entirely governed by the level of interest of the user; what is absurd over-simplification to one person is gross information overload to another. We make no advance apologies for our suggestions, but if they seem over-prescriptive, it is because specific pathological information in this area is hard to come by.

Laudable as these proposals may be, they do not address the final component of a diagnostic protocol which must be verification of the diagnostic significance of the pathological changes that are recorded. The pathological changes that we have suggested for recording seem to us to include at least some that are likely to be diagnostically significant and some that are not, but this remains to be demonstrated. Pressed for our own opinion, we think it likely that in brains without concomitant Alzheimer change and where the bulk of the disease is of the diffuse type, changes *restricted to* the arteriolar sclerosis and Virchow–Robin space expansion are not likely to be diagnostically significant, however severe. At the other end of the spectrum, patients with severe white matter pallor and gliosis are very likely to be symptomatic. A major uncertainty is the significance of perivascular gliosis and parenchymal attenuation in the deep grey nuclei, and particularly the thalamus, which can be very prominent in some patients.

REFERENCES

Aharon-Peretz J, Cummings JL, Hill MA (1988) Vascular dementia and dementia of the Alzheimer type: Cognition, ventricular size and leuko-araiosis. *Arch Neurol* 45: 719–21.

Alzheimer A (1902) Die Seelenstörung auf arteriosclerotischer Grundlage. *Z Psychiatr* 59: 695–711.

Anders KH, Harrison L, Change BS, Tomiyasu U, Quddisi AS, Vintners HV (1989) Lymphomatoid granulomatosis and malignant lymphoma of the central nervous system in the acquired immunodeficiency syndrome. *Hum Pathol* 20: 326–34.

Asherson RA, Lubbe WF (1988) Cerebral and valve lesions in SLE: association with antiphospholipid antibodies. *J Rheumatol* 15: 539–43.

Asherson RA, Khamashta MA, Gil A *et al* (1989) Cerebrovascular disease and antiphospholipid antibodies in systemic lupus erythematosus, lupus-like disease and the primary phospholipid syndrome. *Am J Med* 86: 391–9.

Awad IA, Johnson PC, Spetzler RF, Hodak JA (1986) Incidental subcortical lesions identified on magnetic resonance imaging in the elderly. II Postmortem pathological findings. *Stroke* 17: 1090–7.

Babikian V, Ropper AH (1987) Binswanger's disease: a review. *Stroke* 18: 2–12.

Barclay L, Zemcov A, Blass JP *et al* (1985) Survival in Alzheimer's disease and vascular dementia. *Neurology* 35: 834–40.

Bennett DA, Wilson RS, Gilley DW, Fox JH (1990) Clinical diagnosis of Binswanger's disease. *J Neurol Neurosurg Psychiat* 53: 961–5.

Blass JP, Hoyer MD, Nitsch R (1991) A translation of Otto Binswanger's article 'The delination of the generalized progressive paralysis.' *Arch Neurol* 48: 961–72.

Blessed DG, Tomlinson BE, Roth M (1968) The associations between quantitative measures of dementia and of senile change in the cerebral grey matter of elderly subjects. *Br J Psychiat* 114: 797–811.

Bluestein HG (1987) Neuropsychiatric manifestations of systemic lupus erythematosus. *N Engl J Med* 317: 309–11.

Boller F, Lopez OL, Moossy J (1989) Diagnosis of dementia: clinicopathologic correlations. *Neurology* 38: 76–9.

Bots GThAM (1974) Angioendotheliomatosis of the central nervous system. *Acta Neuropath (Berl)* 28: 75–8.

Brun A, Englund E (1986) The white matter disorder in dementia of the Alzheimer type: a pathoanatomical study. *Ann Neurol* 19: 253–62.

Brust JCM (1983) Vascular dementia – still overdiagnosed. *Stroke* 14: 298–300.

Brust JCM (1988) Vascular dementia is overdiagnosed. *Arch Neurol* 45: 799–801.

Burger PC, Burch JG, Kunze U (1976) Subcortical arteriosclerotic encephalopathy (Binswanger's disease): a vascular etiology of dementia. *Stroke* 7: 626–31.

Calabrese LH, Mallek JA (1987) Primary angiitis of the central nervous system. Report of 8 cases, review of the literature and proposal for diagnostic criteria. *Medicine (Baltimore)* 67.

Caplan LR, Schoene WC (1978) Clinical features of subcortical arteriosclerotic encephalopathy (Binswanger's disease). *Neurology* 28: 1206–15.

Chui HC, Victoroff JI, Margolin D et al (1992) Criteria for the diagnosis of ischaemic vascular dementia proposed by the State of California Alzheimer's disease diagnostic and treatment centers, *Neurology* 42: 473–80.

Citron BP, Halpern M, McCarron M et al (1970) Necrotising angiitis associated with drug abuse. *N Engl J Med* 283: 1003–11.

Corsellis JAN (1962) *Mental Illness and the Aging Brain. The Distribution of Pathological Change in a Mental Hospital Population.* Oxford University Press, London.

Cupps TR, Moore PM, Fauci AS (1983) Isolated angiitis of the central nervous system. Prospective diagnostic and theraputic experience. *Am J Med* 74: 97–105.

Davous P, Fallet-Bianco C (1991) Démence sous-corticale familiale avec leucoencephalopathie artériopathique. Observatione clinico-pathologique. *Rev Neurol (Paris)* 147: 376–84.

del Ser T, Bermejo F, Portera A, Arredondo JM, Bouras C, Constantinidis J (1990) Vascular dementia. A clinico-pathological study. *J Neurol Sci* 96: 1–17.

De Reuck J, Crevits L, DeCoster W et al (1980) Pathogenesis of Binswanger chronic progressive subcortical encephalo-pathy. *Neurology* 30: 920–8.

Dubas F, Gray F, Roullet E, Escarolle R (1985) Leucoencé-phalopathies artériopathiques *Rev Neurol (Paris)* 141: 93–108.

Ellis SG, Verity MA (1979) Central nervous system involvement in systemic lupus erythematosus: a review of neuro-pathologic findings in 57 cases, 1955–77. *Semin Arthritis Rheum* 8: 212–21.

Ellison D, Gatter K, Heryet A, Esiri M (1993) Intramural platelet deposition in cerebral vasculopathy of systemic lupus erythematosus. *J Clin Pathol* 46: 37–40.

Erkinjuntti T, Haltia M, Palo J, Sulkava R, Paetau A (1988) Accuracy of the clinical diagnosis of vascular dementia: a prospective clinical and post-mortem neuropathological study. *J Neurol Neurosurg Psychiat* 51: 1037–44.

Esiri M, Wilcock GK (1986) Cerebral amyloid angiopathy in dementia and old age. *J Neurol Neurosurg Psychiat* 49: 1221–6.

Evans DA, Funkenstein HH, Albert MS et al (1989) Prevalence of Alzheimer's disease in a community population of older persons. *JAMA* 262: 2551–6.

Feigin I, Popoff N (1963) Neuropathological changes late in cerebral edema: the relationship of trauma, hypertensive disease and Binswanger's encephalopathy. *J Neuropathol Exp Neurol* 22: 500–11.

Fischer P, Jellinger K, Gatterer G, Danielczyk W (1991) Prospective neuropathological validation of Hatchinski's Ischaemic Score in dementias. *J Neurol Neurosurg Psychiat* 54: 580–3.

Fisher CM (1965) Lacunes: small deep cerebral infarcts. *Neurology* 15: 774–84.

Fisher CM (1968) Dementia in cerebral vascular disease. In Siekert R, Whisnant J (eds) *Cerebral Vascular Disease, Sixth Conference.* Grune and Stratton Inc. NY pp 232–6.

Fisher CM (1969) The arterial lesions underlying lacunes. *Acta Neuropathy (Berl)* 12: 1–15.

Fisher CM (1982) Lacunar strokes and infarcts: a review. *Neurology* 32: 871–6.

Fisher CM (1989) Binswanger's encephalopathy: a review. *J Neurol* 236: 65–79.

Fisher M, Sotak CH, Minematsu K, Li L (1992) New magnetic resonance techniques for evaluating cerebrovascular disease. *Ann Neurol* 32: 115–22.

Fulling KH, Gersell DJ (1983) Neoplastic angioendo-theliomatosis. Histological, immunohistochemical and ultrastructural findings in two cases. *Cancer* 51: 1107–18.

Garcia JH, Brown GG (1992) Vascular dementia: neuro-pathologic alterations and metabolic brain changes. *J Neurol Sci* 109: 121–31.

George AE, DeLeon MJ, Gentes CI, Miller J, London E, Budzilovitch GN, Ferris S, Chase N (1986) Leukoen-cephalopathy in normal and pathologic aging. I CT of brain lucencies. *Am J Neuroradiol* 7: 561–6.

Gorelick PB, Brody J, Cohen D, Freels S, Levy P, Dollear W, Forman H, Harris Y (1993) Risk factors for dementia associated with multiple cerebral infarcts. A case control analysis in predominantly African-American hospital-based patients. *Arch Neurol* 50: 714–20.

Goto K, Ishii N, Fukasawa H (1981) Diffuse white-matter disease in the geriatric population: a clinical, neuro-pathological and CT study. *Radiology* 141: 678–95.

Graff-Redford NR, Damasio H, Yamada T, Eslinger PJ, Damasio AR (1985) Nonhaemorrhagic thalamic infarction. Clinical, neuropsychological and elecrophysiological findings in four anatomical groups defined by computerized tomography. *Brain* 108: 485–516.

Gray F, Robert F, Labreque R et al. (1994) Autosomal dominant arteriopathic leukoencephalopathy and Alz-heimer's disease. *Neuropathol Appl Neurobiol* 1994; 22: 22–30.

Gray F, Dubas F, Roillet E, Escourolle R (1985) Leukoen-cephalopathy in diffuse hemorrhagic cerebral amyloid an-giopathy. *Ann Neurol* 18: 54–9.

Hachinski VC, Lassen NA, Marshall J (1974) Multi-infarct dementia: A cause of mental deterioration in the elderly. *Lancet* ii: 207–10.

Hachinski VC, Iliff LD, Zilhka E et al (1975) Cerebral blood flow in dementia. *Arch Neurol* 32: 632–7.

Hanson VG, Horowitz, M, Rosenbluth D, Speira H, Puszkin S (1992) Systemic Lupus Erythematosus patients central nerv-ous system involvement show antibodies to a 50 kD neur-onal membrane protein. *J Exp Med* 176: 565–73.

Harrison PE Jr (1976) Granulomatous angiitis of the central nervous system. Case report and review. *J Neurol Sci* 29: 335–41.

Howard GF, Ho SU, Kim KS, Wallach J (1984) Bilateral

corotid artery occlusion resulting from giant cell arteritis. *Ann Neurol* 15: 204–7.

Hughes JT, Brownell B (1966) Granulomatous giant-celled angiitis of the central nervous system. *Neurology* 16: 250–6.

Ironside JW, Martin JF, Richmond J, Timperley W (1984) Lymphomatoid granulomatosis with cerebral involvement. *Neuropathol Appl Biol* 10: 397–406.

Jafar JJ, Menoni R, Feinberg H, LeBreton G, Crowell RM (1989) Selective platelet deposition during focal ischaemia in cats. *Stroke* 20: 664–7.

Janota I (1981) Dementia, deep white matter damage and hypertension: 'Binswanger's disease' *Psychiat Neurol* 11: 39–48.

Jellinger K (1977) Giant cell granulomatous angiitis of the central nervous system. *J Neurol* 215: 175–90.

Jellinger K, Danielczyk W, Fischer P, Gabriel P (1990) Clinicopathological analysis of dementia disorders of the elderly. *J Neurol Sci* 95: 239–58.

Joachim CL, Morris, JH, Selkoe DJ (1988) Clinically diagnosed Alzheimer's disease: Autopsy results in 150 cases. *Ann Neurol* 24: 50–6.

Johnson RT, Richardson EP (1968) The neurological manifestations of systemic lupus erythematosus. A clinical pathological study of 24 cases and a review of the literature. *Medicine (Baltimore)* 47: 337–69.

Jung HH, Bassetti C, Tournier-Lasserve E et al (1995) Cerebral autosomal dominant arteriopathy with subcortical infarcts and leukoencephalopathy: a clinicopathological and genetic study of a Swiss family. *J Neurol Neurosurg Psychiat* 59: 138–43.

Kawamura J, Meyer JS, Ichijo M, Kobari M, Terayama Y, Weathers S (1993) Correlations of leuko-araiosis with cerebral atrophy and perfusion in elderly normal subjects and demented patients. *J Neurol Neurosurg Psychiat* 56: 182–7.

Katzenstein A-LA, Carrington CB, Liebow AA (1979) Lymphomatoid granulomatosis: a clinicopathologic study of 152 cases. *Cancer* 43: 360–73.

Kerr RSC, Hughes JT, Blamires T, Teddy PJ (1987) Lymphomatoid granulomatosis apparently confined to one temporal lobe. *J Neurosurg* 67: 612–15.

Kolodney EH, Rebeiz JJ, Caviness VS, Richardson EP (1968) Granulomatous angiitis of the central nervous system. *Arch Neurol* 19: 510–24.

Krendal DA, Ditter SM, Frankel MR, Ross WK (1990) Biopsy proven cerebral vasculitis associated with cocaine abuse. *Neurology* 40: 1092–4.

Lammie GA, Rakshi J, Rossor MN, Harding AE, Scaravilli F (1995) Cerebral autosomal dominant arteriopathy with subcortical infarcts and leukoencephalopathy (CADASIL)– confirmation by cerebral biopsy in 2 cases. *Clin Neuropathol* 14: 201–6.

Lechner-Scott J, Engelter S, Steck A J et al. (1996) A patient with cerebral autosomal dominant arteriopathy with sub-cortical infarcts and leukoencephalopathy (CADASIL) confirmed by sural nerve biopsy. *J Neurol Neurosurg Psychiat* 60: 235–6.

Levine SR, Brust JCM, Futrell N, Ho K-L, Blake D, Millikan CH, Brass LM, Fayad P, Schultz LR, Selwa JF, Welch KMA (1990) Cerebrovascular complications of the use of the 'crack' form of alkoidal cocaine. *N Engl J Med* 323: 699–704.

LeWitt PA, Forno LS, Brant-Zawadski M (1983) Neoplastic angioendotheliomatosis: a case with spontaneous regression and radiographic appearance of cerebral arteritis. *Neurology* 33: 39–44.

Lie JT (1988) Thromboangiitis revisited. *Pathol Annu* 23(II): 257.

Liebow AA, Carrington CRB, Friedman PJ (1972) Lymphomatoid granulomatosis, *Hum Pathol* 3: 457–558.

Lim L, Ron MA, Omerod IE et al (1988) Psychiatric and neurological manifestations in systemic lupus erythematosus. *Quart J Med* 66: 27–38.

Lindenberg R, Spatz H (1940) Über die Thromboendarteriitis obliterans der Hirngefäße (cerebrale form der v. Winiwarter-Buerger'scen Krankheit). *Virchows Arch. (A)* 305: 531–57.

Liston EH, La Rue A (1983) Clinical differentiation of primary degenerative and multi-infarct dementia: a critical review of the evidence. Part II: pathological studies. *Biol Psychiat* 1983: 18: 1467–84.

Liu CK, Miller BL, Cummings JL, Mehringer CM, Goldberg MA, Howng SL, Benson DF (1992) A quantitative MRI study of vascular dementia. *Neurology* 42: 138–43.

Loeb C (1990) Vascular dementia. *Dementia* 1: 175–84.

Loeb C, Gandolfo C (1983) Diagnostic evaluation of degenerative and vascular dementia. *Stroke* 14: 399–401.

Loizou LA, Jefferson JM, Smith WT (1982) Subcortical arteriosclerotic encephalopathy (Binswanger type) and cortical infarcts in a young normotensive patient. *J Neurol Neurosurg Psychiat* 45: 409–17.

Lotz PR, Ballinger WE, Quisling RG (1986) Subcortical arteriosclerotic encephalopathy: CT spectrum and pathologic correlation. *Am J Neuroradiol* 7: 817–22.

Malamud N (1972) Neuropathology of organic brain syndromes associated with aging. In Gaitz CM (ed) *Aging and the Brain*. Plenum Press, New York, pp 63–87.

Marie P (1901) Des foyers lacunaires de désintégration de différents autres états cavitaires du cerveau. *Rev Méd* 21: 281–98.

Mas JL, Dilouya A, de Recondo J (1992) A familial disorder with subcortical ischaemic strokes, dementia, and leukoencephalopathy. *Neurology* 42: 1015–19.

Mielke R, Herholz K, Grond M, Kessler J, Wolf-Dieter H (1992) Severity of vascular dementia is related to volume of metabolically impaired tissue. *Arch Neurol* 49: 909–13.

Mitsias P, Levine SR (1994) Large cerebral vessel occlusive disease in systemic lupus erythematosus. *Neurology* 44: 385–93.

Mitchell I, Hughes RAC, Maisey M, Cameron S (1994) Cerebral lupus. *Lancet* 343: 579–82.

Mölsä PK, Paljärvi L, Rinne UK, Säkö E (1985) Validy of clinical diagnosis of dementia: a prospective clinico-pathological study. *J Neurol Neurosurg Psychiat* 48: 1085–90.

Moore PM (1989) Diagnosis and management of isolated angiitis of the central nervous system. *Neurology* 39: 167–73.

Moore PM, Cupps TR (1983) Neurological complications of vasculitis. *Ann Neurol* 14: 155–67.

Natowicz M, Kelly RI (1987) Mendelian etiologies of stroke. *Ann Neurol* 22: 175–92.

Nishino H, Rubino FA, DeRemee RA, Swanson JW, Parisi JE (1993) Neurological involvement in Wegener's granu-lomatosis: an analysis of 234 consecutive patients at the Mayo Clinic. *Ann Neurol* 33: 4–9.

O'Brien MD (1988) Vascular dementia is underdiagnosed. *Arch Neurol* 45: 797–8.

Okeda R (1973) Morphometrische Vergleichsuntersuchungen an Hirnarterien bei Binswangerscher Encephalopathie und Hochdruckencephalopathie. *Acta Neuropathol (Berl.)* 26: 23–43.

Parnetti L, Mecocci P, Santucci C *et al* (1990) Is multi-infarct dementia representative of vascular dementias? A retrospec-tive study. *Ann Neurol Scand* 81: 484–7.

Petito CK, Gottleib GJ, Dougherty JH, Petito FA (1978) Neoplastic angioendotheliosis: Ultrastructural study and review of the literature. *Ann Neurol* 3: 393–9.

Petroff OAC, Graham GD, Blamire AM, Al-Rayess M, Roth-man DL, Fayad PB, Brass LM, Shulman RG, Pritchard JW (1992) Spectroscopic imaging of stroke in humans: histopath-ology correlates of spectral changes. *Neurology* 42: 1349–54.

Reinglass JL, Muller J, Wissman S, Wellman H (1977) Central nervous system angioendotheliosis: A treatable multiple infarct dementia. *Stroke* 8: 218–21.

Révész T, Hawkins CP, du Boulay EPGH, Barnard RO, McDonald WI (1989) Pathological findings correlated with magnetic resonance imaging in subcortical arteriosclerotic encephalopathy (Binswanger's disease) *J Neurol Neurosurg Psychiat* 52: 1337–44.

Rocca WA, Hofman A, Brayne C, Breteler MMB, Clarke M, Copeland JRM, Dartigues J-F, Engedal K, Hagnell O, Heeren TJ, Jonker C, Lindesay J, Lobo A, Mann AH, Mölsä PK, Morgan K, O'Connor DW, da Silva Droux A, Sulkava R, Kay DWK, Amaducci L (1991) The prevalence of vascular dementia in Europe: facts and fragments from 1980–1990 studies. *Ann Neurol* 30: 817–24.

Román GC, Tatemichi TK, Erkinjuntti T *et al* (1993) Vascular dementia: diagnostic criteria for research studies. Report of the NINDS-AIREN International workshop. *Neurology* 43: 250–60.

Rosen WG, Terry RD, Fuld PA, Katzman R, Peck A (1980) Pathologic verification of ischaemic score in differentiation of dementias. *Ann Neurol* 7: 486–8.

Rosenberg GA, Kornfeld M, Stovring J, Bicknell J (1979) Subcortical arteriosclerotic encephalopathy (Binswanger): computerised tomography. *Neurology* 29: 1102–6.

Rowley HA, Lowenstein DH, Rowbotham MC, Simon RP (1989) Thalamomesencephalic strokes after cocaine abuse. *Neurology* 39: 428–30.

Ruchoux M M, Chabriat H, Bousse M-G *et al.* (1994) Presence of ultrastructural arterial lesions in muscle and skin vessels of patients with CADASIL. *Stroke* 25: 2291–2.

Scheinberg P (1988) Dementia due to vascular disease – a multifactorial disorder. *Stroke* 19: 1291–9.

Schmidt BJ, Meagher-Villemure K, Del Carpio J (1984) Lymphomatoid granulomatosis with isolated involvement of the brain. *Ann Neurol* 15: 478–81.

Schröder J M. Sellhaus B, Jörg J. (1995) Identification of the characteristic vascular changes in a sural nerve biopsy of a case with cerebral autosomal arteriopathy with subcortical infarcts and leukoencephalopathy (CADASIL). *Acta Neuro-pathol* 89: 116–21.

Segarra JM (1970) Cerebral vascular disease and behaviour. I The syndrome of the mesencephalic artery (basilar artery bifurcation) *Arch Neurol* 22: 408–18.

Sheibani K, Battifora H, Winberg CD, Burke JS, Ben-Ezra J, Ellingwer GM, Quigley NJ, Fernandez BB, Morrow D, Rappaport H (1986) Further evidence that 'Malignant angioendotheliomatosis' is an angiotropic large cell lym-phoma. *N Engl J Med* 314: 943–8.

Simon RH, Abeles M, Farber NJ, Grunnet M, Brennan T (1981) Lymphomatoid granulomatosis with multiple intra-cranial lesions. *J Neurosurg* 55: 293–8.

Sonninen V, Savontaus ML (1987) Hereditary multi-infarct dementia. *Eur Neurol* 27: 209–15.

Sourander P, Wallinder J (1977) Hereditary multi-infarct dementia. *Acta Neuropath (Berl)* 39: 247–54.

Sourander P, Sjogren H (1970) The concept of Alzheimer's disease and its clinical implications. In Wolstenholme GEW, O'Connor M (eds) *Alzheimer's Disease and Related Condi-tions*. Churchill Livingston Inc. New York, pp 11–32.

Stevens DL, Hewlett RH, Brownell B (1977) Chronic familial vascular encephalopathy. *Lancet* ii: 1364–5.

Strouth JC, Donshue S, Ross A, Aldred A (1965) Neoplastic angioendotheliosis *Neurology* 15: 644–8.

Sulkava R, Haltia M, Paetau A *et al* (1983) Accuracy of clinical diagnosis in primary degenerative dementia: correlation with neuropathological findings. *J Neurol Neurosurg Psychiat* 46: 9–13.

Tapia JF, Golden JA (1993) Case records of the Massachusetts General Hospital. case 27 – 1993. *N Engl J Med* 329: 117–24.

Tatemichi TK (1990) How acute brain failure becomes chronic: a view of the mechanisms of dementia related to stroke. *Neurology* 40: 1652–9.

Tatemichi TK, Desmond DW, Mayeux R, Paik M, Stern Y, Sano M, Remien RH, Williams JBW, Mohr JP, Hauser WA, Figueroa M (1992) Dementia after stroke: Baseline frequency, risks, and clinical features in a hospitalised cohort. *Neurology* 42: 1185–93.

Tatemichi TK, Desmond DW, Stern Y, Paik M, Sano M, Bagiella E (1994) Cognitive impairment after stroke: frequency, patterns, and relationship to functional abilities. *J Neurol Neurosurg Psychiat* 57: 202–7.

Todorov AB, Go RC, Constantinidis J, Elston RC (1975) Specificity of the clinical diagnosis of dementia. *J Neurol Sci* 26: 81–98.

Tohgi H, Chiba K, Sasaki K, Hiroi S, Ishibashi Y (1991) Cerebral perfusion patterns in vascular dementia of Binswanger type compared with senile dementia of Alzheimer type: a SPECT study. *J Neurol* 238: 365–70.

Tomlinson BE, Henderson G (1976) Some quantitative cerebral findings in normal and demented old people. In Terry RD, Gershon S (eds) *Neurobiology of Aging*. Raven Press Publishers, New York, pp 183–204.

Tomlinson BE, Blessed G, Roth M (1970) Observations on the brains of demented old people. *J Neurol Sci* 11: 205–42.

Tomlinson BE, Blessed G, Roth M (1968) Observations on the brains of nondemented old people. *J Neurol Sci* 7: 331–56.

Tomonaga M, Yamanouchi H, Toghi H, Kameyama M (1982) Clinicopathologic study of progressive subcortical vascular encephalopathy (Binswanger type) in the elderly. *J Am Geriat Soc* 30: 524–9.

Tournier-Lasserve E, Iba-Zizen MT, Romero N, Bouser MG (1991) Autosomal dominant syndrome with stroke-like episodes and leukoencephalopathy. *Stroke* 22: 1297–1302.

Tournier-Lasserve E, Joutel A, Melki J, Weissenbach J, Lathrop GM, Chabriat H, Mas J-L, Dabanis E-A, Baudrimont M, Maciazek J, Bach M-A, Bousser M-G (1993) Cerebral autosomal dominant artiopathy with subcortical infarcts and leukoencephalopathy maps to chromosome 19q12. *Nature Genet* 3: 256–9.

Ulrich J, Probst A, Wuest M (1986) The brain diseases causing senile dementia. *J Neurol* 233: 118–22.

Wilkinson IMS, Russell RWR (1972) Arteries of the head and neck in giant cell arteritis. A pathological study to show the pattern of arterial involvement. *Arch Neurol* 27: 378–91.

Yao H, Sadoshima S, Kuwabara Y, Ichiya Y, Fujishima M (1990) Cerebral blood flow and oxygen metabolism in patients with vascular dementia of the Binswanger type. *Stroke* 21: 1694–9.

Zhan S-S, Beyreuther K, Schmitt HP (1993) Vascular dementia in Spatz-Lindenberg's disease (SLD): cortical synsptophysin immunoreactivity as compared with dementia of Alzheimer type and non-demented controls. *Acta Neuropathol* 86: 259–64.

Proforma

Cerebrovascular disease: 0 = *No*   1 = *Yes*

1. *Vascular morbid anatomy*
   Atherosclerosis – % occlusion

	none	20%	50%	80%	100%
	= 0	= 1	= 3	= 5	= 7

			Left	Right
Location:	ACA	27	☐	☐
	MCA	28	☐	☐
	PCA	29	☐	☐
	Carotid	30	☐	☐
	Vertebral	31	☐	☐
	Carotid bifurcation	32	☐	☐
	Basilar			

   Other surface vascular pathology   23 ☐
   If Yes, Describe

2. *Focal lesions*
   a. Infarcts
      Infarct present   23 ☐

      Number: + > 10 mm diameter   24 ☐

			Left	Right
Arterial territory:	ACA	27	☐	☐
	MCA	28	☐	☐
	PCA	29	☐	☐
	Vertebro-basilar	30	☐	☐
	Watershed	31	☐	☐
	Other	32	☐	☐

			Left		Right	
			%	Age	%	Age
Location:	Frontal	27	☐	☐	☐	☐
	Parietal	28	☐	☐	☐	☐
	Temporal	29	☐	☐	☐	☐
	Hippocampus	30	☐	☐	☐	☐
	Occipital	31	☐	☐	☐	☐
	Thalamus	32	☐	☐	☐	☐
	Other	32	☐	☐	☐	☐

   b. Lacunes:
      Lacune(s) (< 10 mm diameter) present   22 ☐

Location:	Dp.Gr	WhMtr	Bstem	Othr	Mult	33	☐
	= 1	= 2	= 3	= 4	= 5		

Number:	1–4	5–9	10 >	34	☐
	= 1	= 3	= 5		

c. Haemorrhages
    Haemorrhage present   24 ☐

    Number: Single|Multiple   35 ☐
                                = 1   = 3

    Size of largest: < 5 mm |6–10 mm| > 10 mm   36 ☐
                          = 1   = 3   = 5

    Loc. of largest: CTx |WhMtr|Dp.Gr|Bstem| Cbm   37 ☐
                  = 1   = 2   = 3   = 4   = 5

3. *Diffuse small vessel disease*
    a. Grey matter
        Mild = 1, Moderate = 3, Severe = 5

	27/28/29	BG	Thal	Pons
Arteriolar sclerosis	27	☐	☐	☐
Virchow-Robin space expansion	28	☐	☐	☐
Perivascular gliosis and attentuation	29	☐	☐	☐

    b. White matter

		Front	Par	Occ
Arteriolar sclerosis	27	☐	☐	☐
Virchow–Robin space expansion	28	☐	☐	☐
Diffuse myelin loss and WM gliosis	29	☐	☐	☐

    f. Other micro vascular disease   47 ☐
        If yes, describe:

Neuropathologic diagnosis:
    1. Character
        Infarcts only   27 ☐
        Multiple lacunes   28 ☐
        'Diffuse small vessel disease'   29 ☐
        Binswanger's disease   30 ☐
        Haemorrhage only   31 ☐
        Other   32 ☐
    If other please specify

    2. Aetiology
        Hypertension   27 ☐
        Atherosclerosis   28 ☐
        Embolism   29 ☐
        Ischaemic (other)   30 ☐
    If other, please specify

CHAPTER SIX

Parkinson's disease and dementia

M. M. Esiri and R. H. McShane

Problems of clinical ascertainment of dementia
Problems of clinical ascertainment of Parkinson's disease (PD)
Prevalence and incidence of dementia in clinical Parkinson's disease
Clinical correlates of dementia in Parkinson's disease
Neuropsychology of Parkinson's disease
Extrapyramidal signs and dementia
Pathology of classical Parkinson's disease
Prevalence of Lewy body pathology in normal elderly and patients with dementia
Neurochemical findings in Parkinson's disease
Pathological correlates of dementia in Parkinson's disease
Cortical Lewy body dementia
Towards a clinico-pathological definition of cortical Lewy body dementia (CLBD)
Aetiological considerations
Pathological differential diagnosis

James Parkinson, in his original description of the shaking palsy (1817), thought that 'The senses and intellect (are) uninjured'. Fifty years later, Charcot asserted 'in general, psychic faculties are definitely impaired' (Charcot & Vulpian, 1862). The debate about the strength of association between the clinical syndromes of dementia and Parkinson's disease (PD) was often fuelled as much by loyalty to the views of dogmatic and charismatic teachers as by the evidence. The more recent debate about the clinicopathological correlations of dementia in PD has at times seemed no less polarized. Such disagreements reflect the difficulty in organizing studies, particularly those involving post-mortem pathology, which are big enough to allow for several different potentially confounding factors to be controlled.

The complexity of the relationship between PD and dementia is partly due to the diversity of pathology seen in such cases. For example, many patients with PD and dementia have co-exisiting AD-type pathology, and a few have little or no obvious cortical pathology. In this chapter, we outline some of the work on the pathology in the cortex and subcortical nuclei. We focus particularly on recent descriptions of cases of cortical Lewy body disease (CLBD), in which Lewy bodies, which are a cardinal feature of brainstem pathology in PD, are also found in cortical neurons.

Further complexity is added by problems of definition. Difficulties in defining a threshold above which a certain pathology is regarded as important, and in using valid clinical constructs bedevil all research into clinico-pathological correlations. The problem is compounded when investigating the overlap of two conditions since each clinical and pathological entity requires definition. For example, the reported extent of the AD pathology in patients with PD and dementia varies greatly depending on the criteria adopted for the neuropathological definition of AD. Similarly, clinical definitions may be difficult to apply since the presence of PD complicates the assessment of dementia. In attempting to summarize what is known of the complex inter-connections between dementia and PD we therefore begin by outlining some of these problems of clinical assessment before describing the prevalence, clinical features and pathology of dementia in this context.

PROBLEMS OF CLINICAL ASCERTAINMENT OF DEMENTIA

The assessment of dementia in patients who are thought

to have PD is confounded by four factors. First, the DSM3R criteria, which have been used for many studies of clinicopathological correlations, include criteria relating to the patient's ability to perform certain everyday activities as well as cognitive function. Some activities, such as the ability to wash or maintain urinary continence may be affected by problems such as rigidity, bradykinesia and tremor. The motor phenomena of PD may also interfere with performance on tests in the widely used Minimental State Examination, for example, writing or copying drawings, or result in patients becoming relatively understimulated with consequences on their orientation in time. 'On–off phenomena', in which patients on L-DOPA show rapid, marked changes in motor functions and which may be due to fluctuations in functional dopamine levels may complicate this assessment. Secondly, many, and perhaps all, patients with Parkinson's disease develop circumscribed cognitive impairments which do not necessarily progress, are not global and are insufficient, on their own, to justify a label of dementia. Thirdly, patients with PD are prone to becoming depressed. This will influence motivation and may result in the typical 'I don't know' responses of the patient with pseudodementia. Finally, anti-Parkinsonian medication, particularly anti-cholinergics, causes deficits in memory and other cognitive functions in normal subjects and patients with Parkinson's disease (Nishiyama et al., 1993; Cummings, 1991; Sadeh, Brahim & Modan, 1982). All these factors may combine to result in Parkinsonian patients meeting criteria for dementia with relatively less severe cognitive deficits than patients with other causes of dementia.

PROBLEMS OF CLINICAL ASCERTAINMENT OF PARKINSON'S DISEASE (PD)

Two of the more reliably identified defining features of PD, tremor and L-DOPA responsiveness, are less common in the subgroup of PD patients who are at risk of becoming demented. The accurate identification during life of patients with pathological PD is not always possible, particularly among the demented. Even when clinical criteria have been strictly applied by experienced neurologists about 20% of cases do not fulfil neuropathological criteria for PD (Rajput, Rozdilsky, & Rajput, 1991; Hughes et al., 1992). Of these, 25% have AD-type pathology. Conversely, 20% of cases with a clinical diagnosis of AD have additional Lewy body pathology, a cardinal feature of PD, at autopsy (Galasko et al., 1994), and patients with PD-related pathology

form the biggest group of patients misdiagnosed as AD (Gearing et al., 1995). Patients with other conditions such as progressive supranuclear palsy (PSP) which may be confused with PD are less likely to be incorrectly diagnosed if the clinical follow-up has been for more than five years (Rajput et al., 1991) and additional criteria have been proposed to improve diagnostic accuracy of PD (Larsen, Dupont & Tandberg, 1994).

PREVALENCE AND INCIDENCE OF DEMENTIA IN CLINICAL PARKINSON'S DISEASE

In population studies, the prevalence of dementia is 1.4% in those aged 65 to 69, rising exponentially to 20.8% in 85 to 89 year-olds (Jorm, Kortem & Henderson, 1987). The range of estimates for the prevalence of clinical Parkinson's disease is 0.25–0.94% in those aged 60 to 69 rising to 0.7–1.58% (Mutch et al., 1986; Sutcliffe et al., 1985; Gudmundsson, 1967) in those aged 70 to 79. Determing whether the two clinical syndromes occur together more frequently than would expected by chance is a first step in ascertaining whether the two are aetiologically related.

Methods of ascertainment and population selection are of critical importance in prevalence studies. Most, if not all, patients with PD have worse cognitive function than age, sex and education matched controls (Pirozzolo, Hansch & Mortimer, 1982), although, in many cases, this represents mild impairment and patients with extrapyramidal symptoms and AD may be misdiagnosed as PD. The range of prevalence estimates for dementia in patients with PD is 8–81% with the majority of population-based (as opposed to clinic-based) surveys reporting rates of 20–40% (Marttila & Rinne, 1976; Ebmeier et al., 1991; Mayeux et al., 1992). In their review of 1984, Brown and Marsden found an overall excess of dementia in PD of just over twofold and argued that the frequency of dementia was over-estimated because of the lack of specific criteria for the diagnosis of dementia. However, the association of the two conditions is age related and more recent population studies using standardized criteria for dementia have shown a marked excess of dementia in elderly patients with PD. For example, of the 1.14% of the population aged 80 or over who had PD in the study of Mayeux et al. (1992), 68.7% fulfilled neuropsychological and functional criteria for dementia. PD with and without dementia was commoner in men than women and in whites than non-whites.

Prevalence studies are liable to give an under-estimate of the co-occurrence of the two conditions because those PD patients with dementia die more quickly than those with only one of the conditions. Alternatively, higher estimates may be due to low thresholds for dementia 'caseness'. In addition, there may be differences in the rate at which patients with dementia are referred to specialist clinics. A more powerful epidemiological tool for addressing whether the conditions are aetiologically associated is to ask whether the incidence of dementia is greater in those with PD, or vice versa (Marder et al., 1991). There are, as yet, no population-based incidence studies, but the range of incidence of dementia in large cohorts of PD patients of all ages is 48–69/1000 person–years of follow-up (Biggins et al., 1992; Mayeux et al., 1990). This compares with an overall annual incidence of dementia of about 1000/100 000 at age 70 (Jorm, 1990). More recent studies have tended to confirm this figure. The possibility that it is an artefact due to relatively high rates of identification of dementia in PD compared to the general population remains open.

CLINICAL CORRELATES OF DEMENTIA IN PARKINSON'S DISEASE

The age of onset of motor signs in PD has been shown many times to be an important determinant of the rate and type of cognitive decline, irrespective of disease duration (Hietanen & Tervainen, 1988). Up to 83% of those with onset after 70 develop dementia (Reid, 1992). Later onset of PD is also associated with more axial symptoms such as truncal rigidity, dysarthria, bradykinesia, postural instability and gait difficulty (PIGD) as suggested by Zetusky, Jankovic and Pirozzolo (1985) and confirmed in the DATATOP study (Jankovic et al., 1990). Patients with this form of the illness also have a more rapid rate of progression, greater occupational disability and more problems with motivation and depression. In groups matched for disease duration, motor severity and medication (as well as age and sex), demented patients also have a shorter life expectancy (Piccirilli et al., 1994).

Of all the motor signs, bradykinesia and gait disturbance are the most consistently related to dementia, a relationship that holds in the unmedicated as well as in patients on treatment (Marttila & Rinne, 1976; Liberman, 1974). Bradykinesia is also the motor sign most consistently associated with specific cognitive deficits such as visuospatial problems, attention, word fluency and information processing speed (Mortimer et al., 1982, 1988; Reid et al., 1989). Presentation with masked facies,

a form of bradykinesia, has been shown to predict the onset of dementia (Stern et al., 1993). The severity of cognitive decline is related to the severity of motor symptoms in some (Levin et al., 1991a,b) but not all studies. Associations of cognitive function with tremor and rigidity are less reproducible and may be non-specific, reflecting disease severity or co-exisiting bradykinesia.

Several authors have found that patients with late-onset PD are more vulnerable to developing psychosis on L-DOPA and such symptoms are predictors of subsequent dementia (Horiguchi et al., 1991; Friedman & Barcikowska, 1994; Stern et al., 1993). All anti-Parkinsonian medication can precipitate confusion and psychosis, and up to 30% are affected by visual hallucinations. Anticholinergic medication is more likely than dopaminergic drugs to have this effect (Cummings, 1991), particularly in those with incipient or actual dementia (De Smet et al., 1982). The onset of hallucinations with L-DOPA is also predicted by a psychological profile characterized by hypochondriacal ideas, anxiety, self-doubt and general dissatisfaction (Glantz, Bieliauskaus & Paleologos, 1986). Psychotic symptoms were observed in patients before anti-parkinsonian medication had been introduced, but it is not clear whether these patients were also demented or whether they had cortical Lewy body pathology (see below).

Depression is more common in PD than in other chronic disorders and may precede the development of PD. Amongst patients without overt dementia, the severity of depression correlates with measures of cognitive function in the early onset group and with functional ability in the late-onset group (Mayeux et al., 1981; Starkstein et al., 1989). Depression is also a predictor of more rapid cognitive decline and dementia in PD (Starkstein et al., 1992; Stern et al., 1993).

Anti-parkinsonian medication has effects on cognition which may be clinically important as well as being of theoretical interest in helping to illuminate which cognitive functions are mediated by which neurotransmitter systems. As in AD, anticholinergic medication has been shown to result in deficits of recent memory in PD patients (Koller, 1984), but there may also be a specific effect on frontal lobe function in PD (Dubois et al., 1990). Levin has suggested in a substantial series that anticholinergic medication does not have a uniform effect on memory in PD at all stages of the illness but is more important in those with dementia (Levin et al., 1991a,b), who already have a greater cholinergic deficit. Several investigators have used the phenomenon of on–off fluctuations in longstanding PD to make within-subject comparisons of the effects on cognition of dopamine. Increases in depression and anxiety accompany the switch to 'off', are not just a response to increased motor disability, and may be responsible for the apparent decrement in cognitive function during 'off' periods (Brown et al., 1984; Nissenbaum et al., 1987). Withdrawal of exogenous dopamine also impairs frontal lobe functions such as planning and selective attention (Lange et al., 1993). Selegiline, which is metabolized to an amphetamine derivative, improves symptoms of vitality and depression, attention and episodic memory (Lees, 1991).

NEUROPSYCHOLOGY OF PARKINSON'S DISEASE

Most patients with PD perform less well than normal controls on a variety of neuropsychological tests. However, amongst patients with PD, the cognitive scores of groups of patients show no evidence of a bimodal distribution; there is no clear-cut division between demented and non-demented cases (Pirozzolo et al, 1982). The main cognitive deficits in patients with PD are slowness of thought or 'bradyphrenia' (which may be responsible for deficits in effortful recall of information (Appollonio et al., 1994)), and difficulties in shifting attention (which may be responsible for deficits in planning, sequencing and 'executive function' (Cooper, Sagar & Sullivan, 1993; Beatty & Monson, 1990)). In samples of demented and non-demented PD patients matched for overall level of cognitive function with probable AD subjects, PD patients also perform significantly worse on tasks of verbal fluency and visuospatial tasks (Stern et al., 1993).

These differences are apparent in samples matched for age and IQ and are not accounted for by depression or motor impairment (Boyd et al., 1991). They are also present amongst untreated patients (Cooper et al., 1991) and across a broad range of overall cognitive dysfunction (Pate & Margolin, 1994).

Since most patients with PD are not demented but all of them, by definition, have subcortical pathology, study of these patients has helped to show that subcortical pathology may be associated with specific cognitive impairments. Slowness in performing verbal, perceptuo-motor and memory tasks, impaired concentration and drive, mild forgetfulness and a tendency to repetition are among the defining features of the syndrome of 'subcortical dementia', a term first coined by Albert in describing patients with PSP (Albert, Feldman & Willis, 1974).

Comparisons of the neuropsychological deficits seen in PD with those of other conditions in which subcortical nuclei are affected have indeed shown many similarities in the pattern of deficits. However, there are also some differences between the different 'subcortical' dementias (Massman et al., 1990; Pillon, Dubois & Agid, 1991) and the syndrome bears a striking resemblance to the cognitive deficits seen in retarded depression (Rogers et al., 1987) and following frontal lobe lesions (Brown & Marsden, 1988).

EXTRAPYRAMIDAL SIGNS AND DEMENTIA

Extrapyramidal signs (EPSs) which fall short of those required for a diagnosis of PD are common in patients with clinical AD and become more frequent in late dementia (Burns, Jacoby, & Levy, 1991; Stern et al., 1987; Molsa, Marttila, & Rinne, 1984; Bakchine et al., 1989; Chui et al., 1985; Girling & Berrios, 1990). In series restricted to cases of early AD, 40% of cases have mild EPSs, but this rises to 79–92% in unselected groups. More prominent symptoms reaching criteria for parkinsonism are less common, occurring in 15–23% of cases (Merello et al., 1994; Molsa et al, 1984; Stern et al., 1993). These figures represent a significant excess over non-demented age-matched controls (Bell et al., 1992; Franssen et al., 1991; Galasko et al., 1990). Conversely, subjects with gait abnormalities and diminished spontaneous movement are up to six times more likely to have AD (Funkenstein et al., 1993).

There is now a considerable weight of evidence to support Mayeux and Stern's suggestion (1985) that there is a subgroup of patients with AD who have EPSs, are prone to developing psychotic symptoms and have a faster rate of cognitive decline. Two prospective studies (Chui et al., 1994; Stern et al., 1994) have recently demonstrated that the presence of EPSs and psychosis in AD predict a more rapid rate of cognitive and functional decline, and that this association is independent of the severity of dementia when these signs occur. Neuroleptic medication may contribute to the speed of decline.

EPSs not only predict faster decline in those who already have dementia, but undemented healthy elderly people with mild EPSs are also at an increased risk of going on to develop dementia (although not PD). Furthermore, healthy individuals who have isolated EPS but do not have dementia or overt PD show widespread cognitive changes on most of the tests which are affected in patients with PD (Richards, Stern & Mayeux, 1993).

These findings are of interest because they suggest that damage to the extrapyramidal system may result in cognitive decline without causing overt PD. Some of the EPSs may be due to involvement of the basal ganglia by AD or vascular damage. However, EPSs, particularly rigidity, have also been shown to be associated with Lewy body formation and cell loss in the substantia nigra in patients with AD (Förstl *et al.*, 1992; Ditter & Mirra, 1987) suggesting that the sizeable subgroup of AD with EPSs may include many who have dual pathology of both AD and PD.

PATHOLOGY OF CLASSICAL PARKINSON'S DISEASE

The pathological changes in this condition are centred on, though not confined to, the pars compacta of the substantia nigra, where the hallmarks are loss of pigmented neurons, gliosis and the presence of Lewy bodies (LB), laminated, cytoplasmic inclusion bodies, in some of those pigmented neurons that remain (Figs. 3.12, 6.1 and 6.2). LB may also sometimes be found lying free in the neuropil. Other brain stem and diencephalic structures also show the same features. These structures include the hypothalamus, basal nucleus of Meynert, locus ceruleus, dorsal nucleus of the vagus, ventral tegmentum, pedunculo-pontine nucleus, thalamus and

peripheral autonomic system (Fig. 6.3). The widespread dissemination of LB in brain stem nuclei, particularly neuromelanin-containing nuclei, has long been recognized. More recently the amygdala has been found to be invariably affected by LB formation in classical PD. The amygdaloid nuclei particularly affected are the accessory cortical and central nuclei (Braak *et al.*, 1994).

Thorough examination of the cerebral cortex in cases of classical PD has also recently established that a few LB can always be found in the cerebral cortex (Schmidt *et al.*, 1991; Hughes *et al.*, 1993) though this is disputed (Pollanen, Dickson & Bergeron, 1993; Sugiyama *et al.*, 1994). LB may be missed in the substantia nigra unless several sections are examined, particularly in cases where cell loss is severe. Similarly, examination of several brain areas using stains optimal for detecting LB is necessary to exclude the presence of cortical LB (see below); a study that included examination of just a single section of temporal lobe cortex found cortical LB in 30% of PD patients (Gibb & Lees, 1987) and one that examined multiple cortical sections found them in 66% of PD cases (Perry *et al.*, 1990).

Lewy bodies

LB, a defining pathological characteristic of PD, are usually spherical, intracytoplasmic structures 15–30 mm

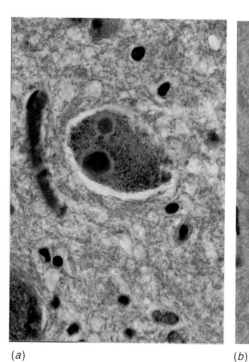

(a)

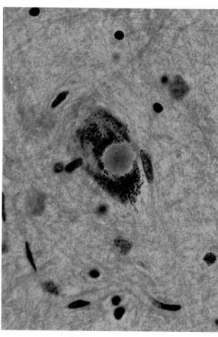

(b)

Fig. 6.1. Appearance of Lewy bodies in pigmented cells of the substantia nigra.

across (Figs. 6.1 and 6.4). However, they may be oval or curved in shape. In the substantia nigra they have a concentric, laminated appearance by light microscopy with an outer paler halo and an inner more intensely stained, eosinophilic core as seen with the haematoxylin and eosin stain (Lewy, 1912). With Lendrum's stain the core is pink and the halo yellow. LB are also argyrophilic, staining well with silver impregnation methods such as Bielschowsky (Tiller-Borcich & Forno, 1988; Love & Nicoll, 1992). Single or multiple LB may be found in substantia nigra neurons in PD. Immunostaining (Galloway *et al.*, 1988; Lennox *et al.*, 1989; Bancher *et al.*, 1989; Arai *et al.*, 1992) has revealed the presence of many antigens in LB. Most regularly demonstrable are phosphorylated neurofilament and ubiquitin (see Table 6.1). Other antigens detectable in some LB include

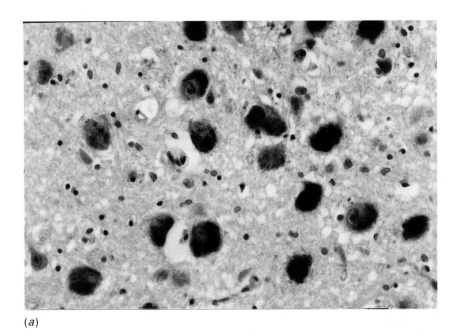

(a)

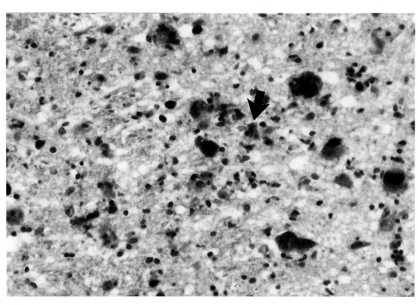

(b)

Fig. 6.2. Microscopic appearance of (a) normal substantia nigra, show typical neuron density and absence of pigment incontinence; (b) substantia nigra from a case of Parkinson's disease showing reduced density of pigmented neurons, an increase in the density of small glial nuclei and some pigment incontinence (arrow).

tubulin, amyloid precursor protein, microtubule-associated proteins, α/β crystallin, a gelsolin-related antigen, complement proteins (Yamada, McGeer & McGeer, 1992) and amyloid P component. A faint reaction for iron may be seen in the halo (Jellinger *et al.*, 1990). No tau protein or β/A4 amyloid protein is present. Ultrastructurally LB are non-membrane bound structures with a dense osmiophilic core composed of granular material and an outer rim containing filamentous fragments 8–20 nm in diameter (Duffy & Tennyson, 1965; Forno, 1986; Galloway, Mulvihill & Perry, 1992; Hill *et al.*, 1991; Pappolla, 1986). In the substantia nigra LB may be accompanied by the presence of less distinctive 'pale bodies' in the central cytoplasm of neurons (Dale *et al.*, 1992; Hayashida *et al.*, 1993).

The mechanism of formation of LB is not understood.

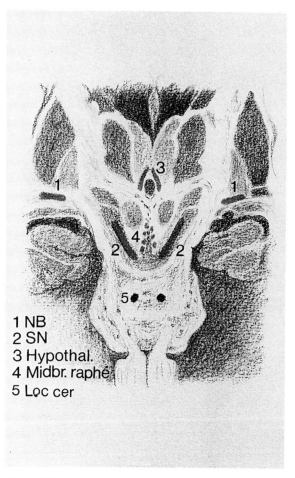

Fig. 6.3. Diagrammatic representation of some of the main sites of pathology in Parkinson's disease.

1 NB
2 SN
3 Hypothal.
4 Midbr. raphé
5 Loc cer

They appear to be associated with a distinctive disruption in neurofilament metabolism and contain ubiquitinated neurofilament protein. They are thought to result from cellular reactions in affected neurons provoked in response to stress. Aggregated neurofilament protein is present in an insoluble form in LB, suggesting that the protein is cross-linked, a configuration that can be provoked in vitro by metal cations (Shea, Beermann & Nixon, 1992). Although inclusion bodies are seen in animal models of Parkinsonism induced by the toxin 1-methyl-4-phenyl-1236-tetra hydropyridine (MPTP), and they share the same sites of predilection as LB, they lack the convincing morphological and immunocytochemical features of LB.

PREVALENCE OF LEWY BODY PATHOLOGY

It is not known if AD predisposes to the formation of LB. Large autopsy series of patients with dementia have found a remarkably consistent rate of about 20% having LBs in the substantia nigra (Joachim *et al.*, 1988; Gibb *et al.*, 1989; Gearing *et al.*, 1995). This figure is only approached in studies at the upper end of the range of estimates of the prevalence of LBs in the non-demented elderly from general autopsy series (Lipkin, 1959; Forno, 1969; Jellinger & Grisold, 1982; Woodard, 1962; Gibb *et al.*, 1989). Amongst the elderly Gibb *et al.* found that 12.8% of those dying in their ninth decade had brainstem LBs. In a small survey confined to the very old, 4 of 27 centenarians with no apparent symptoms had pathological changes of PD, including brain stem LB formation (Mizutani & Shimada, 1992). However, in an autopsy survey of 138 cases aged 51–100, confined to those who lacked psychiatric symptoms or extrapyramidal signs Smith, Irving and Perry (1991) found only three cases (2.2%) with LB, all of whom were over 80. Similarly, there are at least eight case reports of individuals aged less than 60 in whom coexisting AD and LB pathology was found (Delisle *et al.*, 1987; Gibb *et al.*, 1989; Okeda *et al.*, 1982; Kosaka *et al.*, 1973; Popovitch *et al.*, 1987; Kayano *et al.*, 1980). In such cases it is unlikely that the association was one of chance.

Gibb and co-workers have argued that, in the majority of cases, the apparent increased prevalence of LB formation in AD is an artefact (Gibb *et al.*, 1989). They suggest that cases with AD which also have LB will be identified more rapidly because of an additive effect on cognitive function of LB pathology in the nucleus basalis or cortex and cortical AD pathology. It is also

Table 6.1. *Immunoreactions of Lewy bodies and Pick bodies compared*

	Lewy bodies	Pick bodies
Phosphorylated neurofilament	+	+
Tubulin	+	−
Amyloid precursor protein	+	−
Microtubule-associated proteins	+	variable
α/β crystallin	+	−
Gelsolin-related antigen	+	?
Complement proteins	+	?
Amyloid P component	+	−
Ubiquitin	+	+
Tau	−	+
β/A4	−	−
Paired helical filaments	−	+

possible that such cases will die more quickly. Population-based, prospective neuropathological surveys which complement the clinical surveys of dementia prevalence in PD will be necessary to resolve this important question.

Neuronal loss

Neuronal loss accompanied by gliosis in the subcortical nuclei that develop LB is a second essential feature for the diagnosis of PD, though it is less specific than LB being found also in other diseases associated with parkinsonism. These diseases include PSP, striatonigral degeneration, corticobasal degeneration, frontal lobe dementia and post-encephalitic parkinsonism. Neuronal loss in PD is variable but in the substantia nigra is usually about 60–90% (Agid, 1991). It is more severe in the central and caudal part of the nucleus than in the rostral part (Halliday *et al.*, 1990; Hirsch, Graybiel & Agid, 1988). PD symptoms are thought to arise only after nigral cell loss exceeds 50–60%.

NEUROCHEMICAL FINDINGS IN PARKINSON'S DISEASE

The main neurochemical deficiency that develops in PD is of dopamine in the striatum which shows a 70–80% decrease (Hornykiewicz, 1982). Dopamine is released normally by projections of the neuromelanin-containing cells of the pars compacta of the substantia nigra. Loss of dopamine in the striatum in PD tends to be more severe than the loss of dopaminergic cells in the substantia nigra, and is more severe in the putamen than the caudate (Nyberg *et al.*, 1983). In the cortex there is less reduction in dopamine than in the striatum since cortically projecting dopaminergic cells of the ventral tegmental area are less affected than those projecting to the striatum (Javoy-Agid & Agid, 1980). Many other neurotransmitter systems are affected in PD (Agid, Javoy-Agid & Ruberg, 1987). The cell loss in the cholinergic basal nucleus occurs independently of any concomitant AD and, as with the cortical deficit in acetylcholinesterase, correlates with the severity of dementia (Nakano & Hirano, 1984; Perry *et al.*, 1985). Cell loss in the locus ceruleus is reflected in a 40–70% reduction of noradrenaline levels in neocortical and limbic areas such as the nucleus accumbens, amygdala and hippocampus. Although CSF levels of the major noradrenaline metabolite 3-methoxy-4-hydroxyphenylglycol (MHPG) (Stern, Mayeux, & Cote, 1984) and cell loss in the locus ceruleus (Cash *et al.*, 1987) correlate with some deficits in intellectual performance, the reduction of cortical and limbic noradrenaline concentrations is no greater in demented than non-demented cases (Scatton *et al.*, 1983). There is a 50% depletion of serotonin in the striatum and cortex in PD. The concentration in CSF of 5-hydroxy-indoleacetic acid (5HIAA) is reduced in depressed PD patients compared to those with no mood disorder (Mayeux *et al.*, 1984) but there is no direct association with cognitive decline. Alterations are also seen in the concentrations of certain neuropeptides including somatostatin, and corticotrophin releasing factor in the cortex, substance P met-enkephalin and leu-enkephalin in the striatum and cholecystokinin in the substantia nigra.

PATHOLOGICAL CORRELATES OF DEMENTIA IN PARKINSON'S DISEASE

The argument in favour of a dominant role for cortical pathology in the causation of the clinical picture of AD is reviewed in Chapter 1 by Grabowski and Damasio. In that chapter it was emphasized that neither the pathology nor the cognitive deficits of dementia are truly global or uniformly diffuse. Thus, some of the variability in clinical presentation can be accounted for on the basis of variation in the distribution of cortical pathology. For example, cases of AD with an emphasis on pathology in the occipital lobe have prominent visual problems, and the early memory deficits may be explained by the bilateral functional isolation of the hippocampi resulting from early neurofibrillary tangle formation in the entorhinal cortex. The hypothesis underpinning much of the clinicopathological correlative research in PD is that a similar principle applies in PD: the diversity of cognitive dysfunction might reflect the diversity of pathology. In PD, the focus of research has been on four different subcortical sites, the substantia nigra, nucleus basalis of Meynert, locus ceruleus and raphe, as well as on the limbic and neocortex.

It is rare for only one subcortical site to be affected in PD and this complicates the attribution of symptoms to pathology in a particular area. Nevertheless, a tentative synthesis of the available evidence has started to emerge (Chang, Chui & Perlmutter, 1992). This suggests, first, that the mild, circumscribed deficits which are apparent in most patients (bradyphrenia and problems with selective attention) are attributable to loss of dopaminergic cells in the midbrain and their projections to the basal ganglia and thence to the frontal cortex. Secondly, cell loss in the basal nucleus of Meynert, locus ceruleus and median raphe result in further deficits of memory, attention and depression. Thirdly, co-existing Alzheimer's pathology may account for the 'cortical' symptoms of aphasia, apraxia and agnosia and is associated with more severe dementia. The recognition that cortical neurons, particularly those of the 'limbic' cortex, may develop inclusions similar to the LBs of the brain stem occured after much of the clinicopathological work on the association between PD dementia and AD and subcortical pathology was done and has therefore complicated these attributions.

By analogy with the motor symptoms of PD, it is possible that cognitive effects of neurodegeneration only become apparent when a threshold of cell loss in one or more of the subcortical areas or when a threshold level of cortical AD or LB pathology is reached. It is not im-plausible to suggest that, if the tonic regulatory activity of any one of the substantia nigra, locus ceruleus, basal nucleus of Meynert or dorsal raphe is disturbed, some aspect of cognitive function will be affected, and the more nuclei which are affected the more global will be the nature of the deficit. Thus, it is perhaps not surprising that, for both the basal nucleus and the locus ceruleus, the number of publications in favour of it having a role in the dementia is greater than the number against.

In so far as it is possible to tease out these relationships, the single commonest cause of dementia in clinical PD appears to be AD, found pathologically in up to 35% of PD cases (Ditter & Mirra, 1987; Jellinger et al., 1990; Hughes et al., 1993). Some additional cases may be due to vascular disease affecting the striatum and to cortical LB pathology but the importance of the subcortical contribution may be judged by the fact that, in one large series (Hughes et al., 1993), no definite cortical cause of dementia was established in 55% of cases. Cell depletion of the nucleus basalis of less than 40% is uncommon in PD patients with dementia (Ezrin-Waters & Resch, 1986) and a threshold of 60–70% for the emergence of symptoms has been suggested (Jellinger, 1986). The lack of association of cell loss in the nucleus basalis with severity of motor symptoms or coexisting AD supports the idea that nucleus basalis cell loss makes a specific contribution to dementia in PD (Tagliavini & Pilleri, 1983; Gaspar & Gray, 1984; Nakano & Hirano, 1984; Arendt et al., 1983). The question of whether age-related cell loss in the basal nucleus makes a contribution to cognitive decline in PD is unresolved (McGeer et al., 1984). In the locus ceruleus, neuron loss in PD ranges from 26–94% and is greater in cases with dementia (Chan Palay & Asan, 1989; Cash et al., 1987) independently of the presence of AD (Zweig et al., 1993).

CORTICAL LEWY BODY DISEASE

As described above, the pathology of PD extends to a large number of widespread extra-nigral nuclei. However, the main damage is borne by the catecholaminergic nuclei of the brain stem. The more distant nuclei and cerebral cortex are relatively less severely affected. With the increasing recognition of more widespread pathology, facilitated in part by improved methods of detecting LB, has come a realization that the presence of LB in the cortex may be common and may be associated with a distinct clinical syndrome. Several neuropathological series have found that about 20% of cases of dementia have cortical LB which would make it at least as common a cause of dementia as vascular disease (Perry et al., 1990; Hansen et al., 1990; Lennox et al., 1989; Joachim, Morris & Selkoe, 1988; Lennox, 1992). The current debate about whether this syndrome should be regarded as a separate condition is reflected by the number of terms used in the literature to describe it: diffuse or cortical LB dementia, senile dementia of LB type, the LB variant of AD or simply LB dementia. In this chapter it will be referred to as cortical LB dementia (CLBD).

The clinical syndrome of CLBD consists of dementia, extrapyramidal symptoms, episodes of fluctuating cognitive ability for which no cause is found and persistent hallucinations, which are often visual and may be exacerbated by poor eyesight (McKeith et al., 1994; Byrne et al., 1990; Crystal et al., 1990; Hansen et al., 1990; McShane et al., 1995). Other clinical associations which have been described include relatively impaired visuospatial awareness and attention and relatively good recognition memory compared to patients with AD matched for overall severity of dementia. In the early phase of the illness, the dementia may be mild and psychiatric symptoms may result in a diagnosis of functional illness particularly a paranoid or depressive illness. The point at which patients develop symptoms suggestive of temporoparietal involvement such as aphasia, agnosia and apraxia is variable. The degree of parkinsonism also varies greatly but tends to become more severe with time. CLBD can occur in patients with classical clinical PD but in 10% of cases there are no signs of parkinsonism. Cognitive and psychiatric symptoms tend to precede the motor signs, which may respond poorly to L-DOPA. The fluctuating course may give rise to a misdiagnosis of vascular dementia, particularly because insight into the hallucinations and nature of the memory deficit may be retained. Patients with this syndrome may be prone to particularly acute deterioration when given neuroleptic drugs (McKeith et al., 1992) and tend to have more severe cognitive deficits at the time of death. Frontal accentuation of cerebral atrophy, evident on CT scanning (Förstl et al., 1993) and early electroencephalographic abnormalities (Crystal et al., 1990) have also been reported.

Pathology of cortical Lewy body dementia
LB in the cerebral cortex are smaller than those in the substantia nigra and are commonest in small and medium-sized pyramidal cells in the deeper cortical layers (Fig. 6.4). They occur with relatively high density in the parahippocampal and inferior and middle temporal gyri, cingulate gyrus and insula. An even higher density is seen in the amygdaloid nucleus. LB are less frequently seen in parietal and occipital lobe cortex and are not usually present in the hippocampus. Some cortical neurons containing LB have been shown to be immuno-reactive for tyrosine hydroxylase as are the LB-bearing neurons of the substantia nigra and locus ceruleus (Kuljis, Martin-Vasallo & Peress, 1989). Some authors have pointed out that cortical LB develop at sites with a mesolimbic dopamine projection (Eggertson & Sima, 1986; De Keyser, Herregodts & Ebinger, 1990). LB are rarely found in the cortex if they are not present in the substantia nigra. In cases where this does occur, LBs are likely to be found in other subcortical nuclei such as the nucleus basalis or locus ceruleus. Neuron loss and gliosis in the pars compacta in the substantia nigra are also found but may not be as profound as seen in patients with longstanding PD, particularly among those with less severe extrapyramidal symptoms.

LB in cortical neurons have a less distinctive appearance than those in the substantia nigra, usually lacking any lamination (Fig. 6.4). They can thus be mistaken for Pick bodies using routine stains, though these have a different distribution, being, for example, commonly seen in the hippocampus where LB are very rare or absent. Distinction between Pick bodies and cortical LB is readily made using immunocytochemical stains since Pick bodies are tau-positive whereas LB are tau-negative (Table 6.1). The same immunocytochemical reaction distinguishes LB from tau-positive spherical neurofibrillary tangles in cortex. In their immunocytochemical profile cortical LB resemble substantia nigra LB, though there may be minor differences (Schmidt et al., 1991).

Some less constant pathological features have been described in a few reports of CLBD. These include spongy change in layer 2 of the temporal lobe cortex resembling that found in frontal lobe dementia (Chapter 10) (Burkhardt et al., 1988; Hansen et al., 1989); dystrophic axons reminiscent of those seen in neuroaxonal dystrophies (Sugiyama et al., 1993); LB in the cerebellum (Yamamoto & Imai, 1988) and neuron loss in the basal ganglia (Bugiani et al., 1980; Akashi, Maruyama & Sawayama, 1991).

The first description of CLBD was made by Okazaki, Lipkin and Aronson (1961) and many of the early clinico-pathological studies were made in Japan (Kosaka, 1990). The disease was considered to be a rare form of dementia with Parkinsonism, sometimes with onset in middle age. In such early onset cases the cortical LB were not generally associated with other cortical pathology. However, in the much commoner form of the disease in elderly subjects, the cortical LB are far fewer and are often accompanied by argyrophilic plaques of the type found in AD, and in some cases also by relatively sparse neurofibrillary tangles. Many cases of CLBD were pathologically classified in the past as AD, particularly plaque-only AD (Hansen *et al.*, 1993) and most of the plaques in CLBD are of the diffuse type containing no, or only a few, neuritic elements.

The clinical and pathological features of CLBD are still in the process of being defined. Some authors distinguish between the pronounced form in which there are widespread and abundant LB in cortex, mainly in younger patients in whom extrapyramidal motor features of PD are prominent and AD pathology absent or mild, and the more common form seen in older patients in whom cortical LB are scarcer, argyrophilic plaques and sometimes neurofibrillary tangles are also present, and extrapyramidal features milder. This distinction

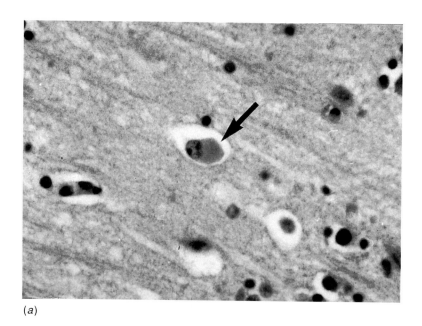

(*a*)

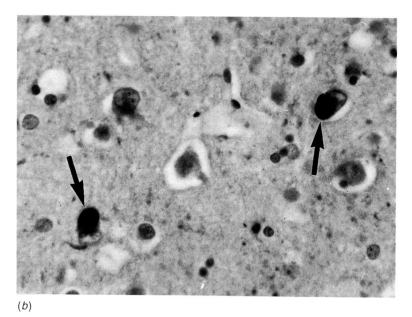

(*b*)

Fig. 6.4. Appearance of cortical Lewy bodies (arrows) stained (*a*) with haematoxylin and eosin and (*b*) immunocytochemically with an antibody to ubiquitin.

seems to us somewhat reminiscent of the division some-times made between AD and senile dementia of Al-zheimer type (SDAT). While such subdivisions empha-size variations in clinical and pathological features and perhaps therapeutic potential, decisions about where to place the divisions between them in order to arrive at definitions of these diseases seem arbitrary and therefore difficult to apply consistently. It therefore seems prefer-able to us that they are considered as one disease. Even then, questions arise about how to distinguish CLBD from AD and from PD.

Relationship between cortical Lewy body disease and Alzheimer's disease

The view of some authors that CLBD, when accom-panied by argyrophilic plaques, should be classified as a variant of AD gains support from the observation that demented subjects in a family with autosomal dominant inheritance of dementia and a missense mutation at codon 717 in the amyloid precursor protein gene have cortical LB as well as typical AD plaques and neurofib-rillary tangles (Lantos et al., 1992, 1994). This strongly suggests that a single gene mutation can generate both types of pathology.

There are several lines of argument against the classifi-cation of CLBD as a form of AD. First, the clinical presentation of CLBD that has been proposed (McKeith et al., 1992) is said to distinguish such cases from cases of AD. Although there are no series restricted to cases with no neuritic or diffuse plaques, there are certainly cases which seem to fulfil the clinical criteria of CLBD but which have no AD pathology. On the other hand, some cases, particularly those with severe dementia, are likely to remain indistinguishable clinically from AD. Further-more, since there is, as yet, no agreed neuropathological definition of CLBD, there is no 'gold standard' against which to judge the strength of the clinicopathological correlations on which the clinical diagnostic criteria are based. Most studies refer to cases of 'PD + dementia' as being distinct from CLBD, even though some of such cases are reported as having cortical LB.

Secondly, these cases have a different pattern of AD pathology. It has already been noted that, in many cases of CLBD, there are sufficient argyrophilic plaques pres-ent to meet some criteria (Khachaturian, 1985) for the diagnosis of AD. Since such plaques are more conspicu-ous than cortical LB in traditionally stained sections of cortex, for many years cases with sparse cortical LB and many argyrophilic plaques were diagnosed as 'plaque-only' AD, and the presence of cortical LB was over-looked (Hansen et al., 1993). Criteria for the pathological diagnosis of AD have been modified recently to require the presence of a minimum number of neuritic rather than diffuse or neuritic plaques (Mirra et al., 1991). This new definition excludes some, but not all, cases that previously have been considered to be 'plaque-only' AD. Even if such cases are no longer regarded as cases of AD, because they lack sufficient neuritic pathology, they do commonly show extensive diffuse deposits of β/A4 amyloid in cerebral cortex (Lippa, Smith & Swearer, 1994). Such deposits are also very common in non-PD, undemented elderly subjects. The extent to which this and neuritic AD-like pathology is over-represented in the brains of subjects with PD and CLBD, compared with undemented controls, is unclear. This question will only be clarified by population-based neuropathological studies of the elderly.

Recent studies have demonstrated an association between possession of the apolipoprotein E (ApoE) ε4 allele and AD (Saunders et al., 1993). An association of similar magnitude between possession of this ApoE ε4 allele and senile dementia of LB type (i.e. cases with a characteristic clinical profile and moderate numbers of cortical LB and β/A4 amyloid deposits but little neuritic pathology) has also been reported (Pickering Brown et al., 1994; Harrington et al., 1994). PD, and pure cortical LB in contrast, are not associated with presence of the ApoE ε4 allele (Harrington et al., 1994). Thus, ApoE ε4 is linked primarily to β/A4 deposition and not to LB formation. However, in as much as cortical LB are commonly associated with β/A4 amyloid deposits, cases with dementia accompanied by cortical LB share with AD an association with the ApoE ε4 allele.

Neurochemical findings in cortical Lewy body disease

One of the best reasons for suggesting that AD and CLBD may usefully be regarded as separate disorders is that they appear to show different neurochemical char-acteristics, which gives an indication of diagnostic valid-ity that is independent of clinical symptoms or neuro-pathology. At present, the most detailed neurochemical research relates to the cholinergic system (Perry et al., 1990; Lennox, 1992; Lennox et al., 1989) and has been performed on elderly subjects with argyrophilic plaques as well as LB. Cases of CLBD show a severe loss of choline acetyl transferase (ChAT) in cerebral cortex, a loss that is more severe than that found in AD (consist-ent with the greater cell loss in the nucleus basalis (Förstl et al., 1991)), but may be less severe than that found in classical PD (Perry et al., 1990; Langlais et al., 1993). In

CLBD the ChAT loss is not correlated with severity of cortical plaque pathology nor prevalence of LB, but is correlated with severity of dementia (Perry et al., 1990). CLBD patients with hallucinations have been found to have lower cortical ChAT levels than patients without hallucinations. The low affinity muscarinic acetylcholine receptor in cortex is reported to be increased in CLBD and PD while it is unchanged or decreased in AD. Somatostatin levels are decreased to a similar extent in CLBD as in AD (Hansen et al., 1990). Cortical markers of serotonin (5HT) show decreased levels with increased turnover of the transmitter as reflected in an increased ratio of the metabolite 5HIAA to 5HT in CLBD. This ratio is particularly increased in CLBD subjects who had suffered hallucinations. In turn, this ratio expressed as a ratio to cortical ChAT levels is even more markedly elevated in CLBD with hallucinations. In contrast, dopamine and its metabolite are hardly altered in the cortex in CLBD (Perry et al., 1993). In the basal ganglia dopamine, derived from pigmented neurons of the substantia nigra, is reduced in CLBD (Langlais et al., 1993) and even more so in PD. Serotonin levels in the caudate in CLBD, as in PD and AD, are reduced. In summary, loss of cholinergic markers in the cortex and increased turnover of 5HT are implicated in the mental impairment and hallucinations of CLBD.

These neurochemical findings give rise to what may turn out to be one of the more important reasons for focusing on CLBD and refining the clinical and pathological requirements for its diagnosis: this condition may be more amenable to cholinomimetic therapy than AD (Perry et al., 1990; Perry et al., 1994; Levy et al., 1994). As stated above, cortical ChAT levels are lower in CLBD than in AD and muscarinic receptors in cerebral cortex are increased in CLBD whereas they are unchanged or decreased in AD. Consistent with this is the finding that the cholinergic nucleus basalis cell loss is more severe in CLBD than AD. By contrast, cortical neuron loss is less severe in CLBD than AD and there is therefore an opportunity for replacement cholinergic therapy to have a better chance of restoring cortical activity. It will therefore be particularly important to differentiate CLBD from AD when examining the possible differential effects of cholinergic therapy in dementia.

CLBD and PD

Another way of fitting CLBD into existing classifications is to regard it as part of a spectrum of LB-associated conditions that also includes PD. Thus, Yoshimura (1988) distinguished three groups of patients

with PD on clinical and pathological grounds: group A (diffuse), relatively rare, in which there was progressive dementia clinically and cortical LB and Alzheimer pathology; group B (intermediate) containing patients with clinical PD, frequent brain stem and diencephalic LB with sparser cortical LB and Alzheimer pathology; and group C, the commonest cases, that had PD clinically without dementia and in which LB were confined to the diencephalon and brain stem. Group A may possibly be subdivisible into the rare cases with numerous cortical LB and the commoner cases with a few cortical LB and usually some features of AD pathology. The finding of Hughes et al. (1993) that all cases with PD had cortical LB, even those with short disease duration, suggests that cortical LB may be formed concurrently with those in the substantia nigra and supports the classification of CLBD as part of the spectrum of PD. Finally, a mutant allele of a cytochrome P450 enzyme which is increased in frequency in PD but not AD is also increased in frequency in patients with AD and cortical LB (Saitoh et al., 1995).

TOWARDS A CLINICO-PATHOLOGICAL DEFINITION OF CORTICAL LEWY BODY DISEASE (CLBD)

At the pathological level there is no widely agreed definition of CLBD as yet. A range of criteria have been used or suggested (Table 6.2). There remains a question mark over whether quantification of cortical LB alone will ever provide a satisfactory definition of CLBD. Ideally, a pathological disease definition requires that the pathology be only and always found in the disease. Prospective studies of demented and control subjects with sufficient information to document whether suggested clinical features of CLBD were present and neuropathological examination are needed to reach a satisfactory definition of CLBD. Studies of PD have shown that cortical LB occur in the absence of dementia but even so it might be possible to define a threshold density of cortical LB above which CLBD is present. Cortical LB density should be closely correlated with the severity of dementia in CLBD if LB density is to form a sound basis for such a quantitative pathological definition of CLBD. One study of fourteen cases of CLBD (Lennox et al., 1989) and a study of 13 cases of PD without AD (Zweig et al., 1993) have shown such a correlation. Others have failed to confirm this finding.

The important point for pathologists to be aware of is that, in every case of progressive dementia the pathology of CLBD as well as that of AD needs to be positively

Table 6.2. *Explicit and implied neuropathological criteria for cortical LB disease*

Reference	Neuropathological criteria
(Crystal *et al.*, 1990)	> 2 LB per × 10 neocortical field using ubiquitin immunostaining
(Perry *et al.*, 1990)	> 2 LB but < 20 LBs/ cm^2 in temporal lobe using H&E or ubiquitin immunostaining
(Lennox *et al.*, 1989)	> 5 LB using H&E or > 12 LB using ubiquitin immunostaining in transversely sectioned anterior cingulate gyrus
(Zweig *et al.*, 1993)	> 0.1 LB/mm^2 in anterior cingulate using ubiquitin immunostaining
(Kosaka, 1990)	> 5 LBs in each × 100 field in predilection sites using H&E
(Hansen *et al.*, 1990)	LB present in three neocortical sites using H&E and in superior temporal cortex using ubiquitin immunostaining
(McShane *et al.*, 1995)	LB present in two limbic cortical sites using H&E and blind to assessment of substantia nigral pathology
(Hughes *et al.*, 1993)	LB easily found in anterior cingulate or parahippocampal gyrus within 5 minutes using H&E

searched for. Since almost all cases of CLBD appear to have LB in the substantia nigra, it is reasonable to scan this structure as a screening procedure. It should be noted that cases with severe nigral cell loss need to have three nigral sections examined for LB. It is particularly cases that have nigral LB that need to have the cortex searched for LB. Conversely, absence of nigral LB makes it unlikely that cortical LB will be found.

AETIOLOGICAL CONSIDERATIONS
The causes of PD and other diseases in which LB develop are unknown. There is little evidence for inherited factors in PD, and so environmental causes are thought to be of potential importance. No environmental toxins have been shown to be clearly implicated in the aetiology of PD. However, there is a proven neurotoxic effect on the substantia nigra of 1-methyl-4-phenyl-1236-tetra hydropyridine (MPTP) in man and animals, and carbon monoxide and manganese poisoning in man can produce a parkinsonian syndrome.

The common occurrence with CLBD of argyrophilic β/A4 amyloid plaques in cortex suggests some aetiological overlap between CLBD, PD and AD. Each is closely linked with ageing. Recent interest has centred on the cytotoxic effect of free radicals and the capacity these may have to damage neurons in these diseases (Agid, 1991;

Jenner, 1994; Friedlich & Butcher, 1994). A further current line of enquiry is the possible role of neurotrophic factors though these are probably more directly relevant to treatment than to aetiology in PD and CLBD. Defective mitochondrial metabolism with decreased activity of respiratory enzyme complex 1 has been found in the substantia nigra in PD (Mizuno *et al.*, 1989; Shapira, 1995). This enzyme is inhibited by MPP +, the active metabolite of the neurotoxin MPTP, so an MPTP-like toxin could be responsible for this finding in man (Jacobs & Le Quesne, 1992). Finally, production of an endogenous toxin, for example, linked to changes in metabolism of sulphur-containing compounds as suggested by work by Steventon *et al.* (1989) has also been suggested to contribute to development of PD.

PATHOLOGICAL DIFFERENTIAL DIAGNOSIS
Dementia with parkinsonism raises several other diagnostic possibilities in addition to CLBD or AD with PD. Vascular dementia in association with PD or with lacunes in the basal ganglia accounts for some cases. Other diseases to consider are PSP (p 241), corticobasal degeneration (p 254), Pick's disease (Chapter 8), frontal lobe dementia (p 245), and rare cases of dementia with multiple system atrophy (p 256). Occasionally cases of

PD and dementia also have clinical and pathological features of motor neuron disease. In PSP there are neurofibrillary tangles (but not LB) in the substantia nigra as well as in other subcortical nuclei not usually affected in PD, notably the subthalamic nucleus and globus pallidus. The cerebellar dentate nuclei and red nuclei are also commonly depleted of neurons in PSP but not in PD. In corticobasal degeneration, Pick's disease and frontal lobe dementia parkinsonian symptoms are not usually prominent clinically. Pathologically these conditions lack LB or neurofibrillary tangles. Frontal lobe dementia shows cortical neuronal loss in frontal and temporal lobes with spongy change in cortical layer 2. In corticobasal degeneration there is cortical neuronal loss in layers 3 and 5 and the presence of pale, swollen neurons like those found in Pick's disease. There is also widespread subcortical neuron loss particularly affecting subthalamic nucleus, striatum, globus pallidus, red nucleus and postero-lateral thalamic nuclei. Pick's disease is distinguished by the presence of severe lobar cortical atrophy and by the microscopic features of Pick cells and/or Pick bodies. Pick bodies can be immunocytochemically characterized as distinct from LB (Table 6.1).

REFERENCES

Agid Y (1991) Parkinson's disease: pathophysiology. *Lancet* 337: 1321–4.

Agid Y, Javoy-Agid F, Ruberg M (1987) Biochemistry of neurotransmitters in Parkinson's disease. In Marsden CD, Fahn S (eds) *Movement Disorders*. 2, Butterworths, London, pp 166–230.

Akashi T, Maruyama N, Sawayama H (1991) An autopsy case of idiopathic parkinsonism with numerous Lewy bodies in the cerebral cortex–diffuse Lewy body disease. *Brain and Nerve* 43: 175–81.

Albert ML, Feldman RG, Willis AL (1974) The 'subcortical dementia' of progressive supranuclear palsy. *J Neurol Neurosurg Psychiat* 37: 121–30.

Appollonio I, Grafman J, Clark K, Nichelli P, Zeffiro T, Hallett M (1994) Implicit and explicit memory in patients with Parkinson's disease with and without dementia. *Arch Neurol* 51: 359–67.

Arai H, Lee VM, Hill WD, Greenberg BD, Trojanowski JQ (1992) Lewy bodies contain beta-amyloid precursor proteins of Alzheimer's disease. *Brain Res* 585: 386–90.

Arendt R, Bigl V, Arendt A, Tennstedt A (1983) Loss of neurons in the nucleus basalis of Meynert in Alzheimer's disease, paralysis agitans, and Korsakoff's disease. *Acta Neuropathol* 61: 101–8.

Bakchine S, Lacomblez L, Palisson E, Laurent M, Derouesne C (1989) Relationship between primitive reflexes, extrapyramidal signs, reflective apraxia and severity of cognitive impairment in dementia of the Alzheimer type. *Acta Neurol Scand* 79: 38–46.

Bancher C, Lassmann H, Budka H, Jellinger K, Grundke-Iqbal I, Iqbal K, Wiche G, Seitelberger F, Wisniewski HM (1989) An antigenic profile of Lewy bodies: immunocytochemical indication for protein phosphorylation and ubiquitination. *J Neuropathol Exp Neurol* 48: 81–93.

Beatty WW, Monson N (1990) Picture and motor sequencing in Parkinson's disease. *J Geriatr Psychiatry Neurol* 3: 192–7.

Bell K, Marder K, Sano M, Richards M, Miller L, Lafleche G, Mayeux R, Stern Y (1992) Comparison of medical conditions and neurological examination in early Alzheimer's disease and normal elderly. *Neurology* 42(suppl 3): 199–200.

Biggins CA, Boyd JL, Harrop FM, Madeley P, Mindham RH, Randall JI, Spokes EG (1992) A controlled, longitudinal study of dementia in Parkinson's disease. *J Neurol Neurosurg Psychiat* 55: 566–71.

Boyd JL, Cruickshank CA, Kenn CW, Madeley P, Mindham RH, Oswald AG, Smith RJ, Spokes EG (1991) Cognitive impairment and dementia in Parkinson's disease: a controlled study. *Psychol Med* 21: 911–21.

Braak H, Braak E, Yilmazer D, De Vos RAI, Jansen ENH, Bohl J, Jellinger K (1994) Amygdala pathology in Parkinson's disease. *Acta Neuropathol* (*Berl*) 88: 493–500.

Brown RG, Marsden CD (1984) How common is dementia in Parkinson's disease? *Lancet* ii: 1262–5.

Brown RG, Marsden CD (1988) 'Subcortical dementia': the neuropsychological evidence. *Neuroscience* 25: 363–87.

Brown RG, Marsden CD, Quinn N, Wyke MA (1984) Alterations in cognitive performance and affect-arousal state during fluctuations in motor function in Parkinson's disease. *J Neurol Neurosurg Psychiat* 47: 454–65.

Bugiani O, Perdelli F, Salvarini S, Leonardi A, Mancardi GL (1980) Loss of striatal neurons in Parkinson's disease: a cytometric study. *Eur Neurol* 19: 339–44.

Burkhardt CR, Filley CM, Kleinschmidt DeMasters BK, de la Monte S, Norenberg MD, Schneck SA (1988) Diffuse Lewy body disease and progressive dementia. *Neurology* 38: 1520–8.

Burns A, Jacoby R, Levy R (1991) Neurological signs in Alzheimer's disease. *Age Ageing* 20: 45–51.

Byrne EJ, Lennox G, Lowe J, Reynolds G (1990) Diffuse Lewy body disease: the clinical features. *Adv Neurol* 53: 283–6.

Cash R, Dennis T, L'Heureux R, Raisman R, Javoy-Agid F, Scatton B (1987) Parkinson's disease and dementia: norepinephrine and dopamine in locus coeruleus. *Neurology* 37: 42–6.

Chan Palay V, Asan E (1989) Alterations in catecholamine neurons of the locus coeruleus in senile dementia of the Alzheimer type and in Parkinson's disease with and without dementia and depression. *J Comp Neurol* 287: 373–92.

Chang Chui H, Perlmutter LS (1992) Pathological correlates of dementia in Parkinson's disease. In Huber SJ, Cummings JL (eds) *Parkinson's disease. Neurobehavioral aspects.* Oxford University Press, New York, pp 164–77.

Charcot JM, Vulpian A (1862) De la paralysie agitante. *Gaz Hebdomadaire Med Chir* 9: 54–9.

Chui HC, Lyness SA, Sobel E, Schneider LS (1994) Extrapyramidal signs and psychiatric symptoms predict faster cognitive decline in Alzheimer's disease. *Arch Neurol* 51: 676–81.

Chui HC, Teng EL, Henderson VW, Moy AC (1985) Clinical subtypes of dementia of the Alzheimer type. *Neurology* 35: 1544–50.

Cooper JA, Sagar HJ, Jordan N, Harvey NS, Sullivan EV (1991) Cognitive impairment in early, untreated Parkinson's disease and its relationship to motor disability. *Brain* 114: 2095–122.

Cooper JA, Sagar HJ, Sullivan EV (1993) Short-term memory and temporal ordering in early Parkinson's disease: effects of disease chronicity and medication. *Neuropsychologia* 31: 933–49.

Crystal HA, Dickson DW, Lizardi JE, Davies P, Wolfson LI (1990) Antemortem diagnosis of diffuse Lewy body disease. *Neurology* 40: 1523–8.

Cummings JL (1991) Behavioral complications of drug treatment of Parkinson's disease. *J Am Geriatr Soc* 39: 708–16.

Dale GE, Probst A, Luthert P, Martin J, Anderton BH, Leigh PN (1992) Relationship between Lewy bodies and pale bodies in Parkinson's disease. *Acta Neuropathol (Berl)* 83: 525–9.

De Keyser J, Herregodts P, Ebinger G (1990) The mesoneocortical dopamine neuron system. *Neurology* 40: 1660–2.

De Smet Y, Ruberg M, Serdaru M, Dubois B, Lhermitte F, Agid, Y (1982) Confusion, dementia and anticholinergics in Parkinson's disease. *J Neurol Neurosurg Psychiat* 45: 1161–4.

Delisle MB, Gorce P, Hirsch E, Hauw JJ, Rascol A, Bouissou H (1987) Motor neuron disease, parkinsonism and dementia. *Acta Neuropathol* 75: 104–8.

Ditter SM, Mirra SS (1987) Neuropathologic and clinical features of Parkinson's disease in Alzheimer's disease patients. *Neurology* 37: 754–60.

Dubois B, Pillon B, Lhermitte F, Agid Y (1990) Cholinergic deficiency and frontal dysfunction in Parkinson's disease. *Ann Neurol* 28: 117–21.

Duffy PE, Tennyson VM (1965) Phase and electron microscopic observations of Lewy bodies and melanin granules in the substantia nigra and locus coeruleus in Parkinson's disease. *J Neuropathol Exp Neurol* 24: 398–414.

Ebmeier KP, Calder SA, Crawford JR, Stewart L, Cochrane RH, Besson JA (1991) Dementia in idiopathic Parkinson's disease: prevalence and relationship with symptoms and signs of parkinsonism. *Psychol Med* 21: 69–76.

Eggertson DE, Sima AAF (1986) Dementia with cerebral Lewy bodies: a mesocortical dopaminergic defect? *Arch Neurol* 43: 524–7.

Ezrin-Waters C, Resch L (1986) The nucleus basalis of Meynert. *Can J Neurol Sci* 13: 8–14.

Forno LS (1969) Concentric hyaline intraneuronal inclusions of Lewy type in the brains of elderly persons (50 incidental cases): relationship to parkinsonism. *J Am Geriat Soc* 17: 557–75.

Forno LS (1986) The Lewy body in Parkinson's disease. *Adv Neurol* 45: 398–414.

Förstl H, Burns A, Levy R, Cairns N, Luthert P, Lantos P (1992) Neurologic signs in Alzheimer's disease. Results of a prospective clinical and neuropathologic study. *Arch Neurol* 49: 1038–42.

Förstl H, Almeida OP, Owen AM, Burns A, Howard R (1991) Psychiatric, neurological and medical aspects of misidentification syndromes: a review of 260 cases. *Psychol Med* 21: 905–10.

Förstl H, Burns A, Luthert P, Cairns N, Levy R (1993) The Lewy-body variant of Alzheimer's disease. Clinical and pathological findings. *Br J Psychiat* 162: 385–92.

Franssen EH, Reisberg B, Kluger A, Sinaiko E, Boja C (1991) Cognition-Independent neurologic symptoms in normal aging and probable Alzheimer's disease. *Arch Neurol* 48: 148–54.

Friedlich AL, Butcher LL (1994) Involvement of free oxygen radicals in beta amyloidosis: an hypothesis. *Neurobiol Aging* 15: 443–55.

Friedman A, Barcikowska M (1994) Dementia in Parkinson's disease. *Dementia* 5: 12–16.

Funkenstein HH, Albert MS, Cook NR, West CG, Scherr PA, Chown MJ, Pilgrim D, Evans DA (1993) Extrapyramidal signs and other neurologic findings in clinically diagnosed Alzheimer's disease. *Arch Neurol* 50: 51–6.

Galasko D, Hansen LA, Katzman R, Wiederholt W, Masliah E, Terry R, Hill LR, Lessin P, Thal LJ (1994) Clinical–neuropathological correlations in Alzheimer's disease and related dementias. *Arch Neurol* 51: 888–95.

Galasko D, Kwo-on-Yuen PF, Klauber MR, Thal LJ (1990) Neurological findings in Alzheimer's disease and normal aging. *Arch Neurol* 47: 625–7.

Galloway PG, Grundke-Iqbal I, Iqbal K, Perry G (1988) Lewy bodies contain epitopes both shared and distinct from Alzheimer neurofibrillary tangles. *J Neuropathol Exp Neurol* 47: 654–63.

Galloway PG, Mulvihill P, Perry G (1992) Filaments of Lewy bodies contain insoluble cytoskeletal elements. *Am J Pathol* 140: 809–22.

Gaspar P, Gray F (1984) Dementia in idiopathic Parkinson's disease. *Acta Neuropathol* 64: 43–52.

Gearing M, Mirra S, Hedreen JC, Sumi SM, Hansen LA, Heyman A (1995) The Consortium to Establish a Registry for Alzheimer's Disease (CERAD). Part X. Neuropathology confirmation of the clinical diagnosis of Alzheimer's disease. *Neurology* 45: 461–6.

Gibb WR, Mountjoy CQ, Mann DM, Lees AJ (1989) A pathological study of the association between Lewy body disease and Alzheimer's disease. *J Neurol Neurosurg Psychiatry* 52: 701–8.

Gibb WRG, Lees AJ (1987) Dementia in Parkinson's disease. *Lancet* 1: 861.

Girling DM, Berrios GE (1990) Extrapyramidal signs, primitive reflexes and frontal lobe function in senile dementia of the Alzheimer type. *Br J Psychiat* 157: 888–93.

Glantz RH, Bieliauskaus L, Paleologos N (1986) Behavioral indicators of hallucinosis in levadopa-treated Parkinson's disease. *Adv Neurol* 45: 417–20.

Gudmundsson KRA (1967) A clinical survey of Parkinsonism in Iceland. *Acta Neurol Scand* 43(suppl.33): 9–61.

Halliday GM, Li YW, Blumbergs PC, Joh TH, Cotton RG, Howe PR, Blessing WW, Geffen LB (1990) Neuropathology of immunohistochemically identified brainstem neurons in Parkinson's disease. *Ann Neurol* 27: 373–85.

Hansen L, Salmon D, Galasko D, Masliah E, Katzman R, DeTeresa R, Thal L, Pay MM, Hofstetter R, Klauber M *et al.* (1990) The Lewy body variant of Alzheimer's disease: a clinical and pathologic entity. *Neurology* 40: 1–8.

Hansen LA, Masliah E, Galasko D, Terry RD (1993) Plaque-only Alzheimer disease is usually the Lewy body variant, and vice versa. *J Neuropathol Exp Neurol* 52: 648–54.

Hansen LA, Masliah E, Terry RD, Mirra SS (1989) A neuropathological subset of Alzheimer's disease with concomitant Lewy body disease and spongiform change. *Acta Neuropathol* 78: 194–201.

Harrington CR, Louwagie J, Rossau R, Vanmechelen E, Perry RH, Perry EK, Xuereb JH, Roth M, Wischik CM (1994) Influence of apolipoprotein E genotype on senile dementia of the Alzheimer and Lewy body types. *Am J Pathol* 145: 1472–84.

Hayashida K, Oyanagi S, Mizutani Y, Yokochi M (1993) An early cytoplasmic change before Lewy body maturation: an ultrastructural study of the substantia nigra from an autopsy case of juvenile parkinsonism. *Acta Neuropathol* 85: 445–8.

Hietanen M, Tervainen H (1988) The effect of age of disease onset on neuropsychological performance in Parkinson's disease. *J Neurol Neurosurg Psychiat* 51: 244–9.

Hill WD, Lee VM, Hurtig HI, Murray JM, Trojanowski JQ (1991) Epitopes located in spatially separate domains of each neurofilament subunit are present in Parkinson's disease Lewy bodies. *J Comp Neurol* 309: 150–60.

Hirsch E, Graybiel AM, Agid YA (1988) Melanized dopaminergic neurones are differentially susceptible to degeneration in Parkinson's disease. *Nature* 334: 345–8.

Horiguchi J, Nishimatsu O, Inami Y, Sukegawa T, Shoda T (1991) A clinical study on intellectual impairment in

parkinsonian patients during long-term treatment. *Jpn J Psychiatry Neurol* 45: 13–18.

Hornykiewicz O (1982) Brain neurotransmitter changes in Parkinson's disease. In Marsden CD, Fahn S (eds) *Butterworths Int Medical Revs Neurology. Movement disorders.* 2, pp 41–58.

Hughes AJ, Daniel SE, Blankson S, Lees AJ (1993) A clinicopathologic study of 100 cases of Parkinson's disease. *Arch Neurol* 50: 140–8.

Hughes AJ, Daniel SE, Kilford L, Lees AJ (1992) Accuracy of clinical diagnosis of idiopathic Parkinson's disease: a clinico-pathological study of 100 cases. *J Neurol Neurosurg Psychiatry* 55: 181–4.

Jacobs JM, Le Quesne PM (1992) Toxic Disorders. In Adams JH, Duchen LW (eds) *Greenfield's Neuropathology.* 5th edn. Arnold, London, pp 881–987.

Jankovic J, McDermott M, Carter J, Gauthier S, Goetz C, Golbe L, Huber S, Koller W, Olanow C, Shoulson I *et al.* (1990) Variable expression of Parkinson's disease: a baseline analysis of the DATATOP cohort. The Parkinson Study Group. *Neurology,* 40: 1529–34.

Javoy-Agid F, Agid Y (1980) Is the mesocortical dopaminergic system involved in Parkinson's disease? *Neurology* 30: 1326–30.

Jellinger K (1986) Overview of morphological changes in Parkinson's disease. *Adv Neurol* 45: 1–18.

Jellinger K, Grisold W (1982) Cerebral atrophy in Parkinson syndrome. *Exp Brain Res* 26–35.

Jellinger K, Paulus W, Grundke Iqbal I, Riederer P, Youdim MB (1990) Brain iron and ferritin in Parkinson's and Alzheimer's diseases. *J Neural Transm Park Dis Dement Sect* 2: 327–40.

Jenner P (1994) Oxidative damage in neurodegenerative disease. *Lancet* 344: 796–8.

Joachim CL, Morris JH, Selkoe DJ (1988) Clinically diagnosed Alzheimer's disease: autopsy results in 150 cases. *Ann Neurol* 24: 50–6.

Jorm AF (1990) *The Epidemiology of Alzheimer's Disease and Related Disorders.* Chapman and Hall, London, p 79.

Jorm AF, Kortem AE, Henderson AS (1987) The prevalence of dementia: A quantitative integration of the literature. *Acta Psychiatr Scand* 76: 465–79.

Kayano T, Funada N, Okeda R (1980) An autopsy case of Parkinson's disease with dementia and a wide distribution of Lewy-like bodies in the cerebral cortex. *Neuropathology* 1: 27–8.

Khachaturian ZS (1985) Diagnosis of Alzheimer's disease. *Arch Neurol* 42: 796–8.

Koller WC (1984) Disturbance of recent memory function in parkinsonian patients on anticholinergic therapy. *Cortex* 307–11.

Kosaka K (1990) Diffuse Lewy body disease in Japan. *J Neurol* 237: 197–204.

Kosaka K, Shibayama H, Kobayashi L, Hoshino T, Iwase S

(1973) An autopsy case of unclassifiable presenile dementia. *Psychiat Neurol Jap* 75: 18–34.

Kuljis RO, Martin-Vasallo P, Peress NS (1989) Lewy bodies in tyrosine hydroxylase-synthesizing neurons of the human cerebral cortex. *Neurosci Lett* 106: 49–54.

Lange KW, Paul GM, Robbins TW, Marsden CD (1993) L-DOPA and frontal cognitive function in Parkinson's disease. *Adv Neurol* 60: 475–8.

Langlais PJ, Thal L, Hansen L, Galasko D, Alford M, Masliah E (1993) Neurotransmitters in basal ganglia and cortex of Alzheimer's disease with and without Lewy bodies. *Neurology* 43: 1927–34.

Lantos PL, Luthert PJ, Hanger D, Anderton BH, Mullan M, Rossor M (1992) Familial Alzheimer's disease with the amyloid precursor protein position 717 mutation and sporadic Alzheimer's disease have the same cytoskeletal pathology. *Neurosci Lett* 137: 221–4.

Lantos PL, Ovenstone IMK, Johnstone J, Clelland CA, Roques P, Rossor MN (1994) Lewy bodies in the brain of two members of a family with the 717 (Valtolle) mutation of the amyloid precursor protein gene. *Neurosci Lett* 172: 77.

Larsen JP, Dupont E, Tandberg E (1994) Clinical diagnosis of Parkinson's disease. Proposal of diagnostic subgroups classified at different levels of confidence. *Acta Neurol Scand* 89: 242–51.

Lees AJ (1991) Selegiline hydrochloride and cognition. *Acta Neurol Scand Suppl* 136: 91–4.

Lennox G, Lowe J, Landon M, Byrne EJ, Mayer RJ, Godwin-Austen RB (1989) Diffuse Lewy body disease: correlative neuropathology using anti-ubiquitin immunocytochemistry. *J Neurol Neurosurg Psychiatry* 52: 1236–47.

Lennox G (1992) Lewy body dementia. *Baillière's Clin Neurol* 1: 653–76.

Levin BE, Llabre MM, Reisman S, Weiner WJ, Sanchez Ramos J, Singer C, Brown MC (1991a) Visuospatial impairment in Parkinson's disease. *Neurology* 41: 365–9.

Levin BE, Llabre MM, Reisman S, Weiner WJ, Brown MC (1991b) A retrospective analysis of the effects of anticholinergic medication on memory performance in Parkinson's disease. *J Neuropsychiatry Clin Neurosci* 3: 412–16.

Levy R, Eagger S, Griffiths M, Perry E, Honavar M, Dean A, Lantos P (1994) Lewy bodies and response to tacrine in Alzheimer's disease. *Lancet* 343: 176

Lewy FH (1912) Paralysis agitans. 1. Pathologische anatomie. In Lewandowsky M (ed), *Handbuch der Neurologie.* Springer, Berlin, pp 920–33.

Liberman AN (1974) Parkinson's disease: a clinical review. *Am J Med Sci* 267: 66–80.

Lipkin LE (1959) Cytoplasmic inclusions in ganglion cells associated with parkinsonian states. *Am J Pathol* 35: 1117–33.

Lippa CF, Smith TW, Swearer JM (1994) Alzheimer's disease and Lewy body disease: a comparative clinicopathological study. *Ann Neurol* 35: 81–8.

Love S, Nicoll JA (1992) Comparison of modified Bielschowsky silver impregnation and anti-ubiquitin immunostaining of cortical and nigral Lewy bodies. *Neuropathol Appl Neurobiol* 18: 585–92.

Marder K, Leung D, Tang M, Bell K, Dooneief G, Cote L, Stern Y, Mayeux R (1991) Are demented patients with Parkinson's disease accurately reflected in prevalence surveys? A survival analysis. *Neurology* 41: 1240–3.

Marttila RJ, Rinne UK (1976) Dementia in Parkinson's disease. *Acta Neurol Scand* 54: 431–41.

Massman PJ, Delis DC, Butters N, Levin BE, Salmon DP (1990) Are all subcortical dementias alike? Verbal learning and memory in Parkinson's and Huntington's disease patients. *J Clin Exp Neuropsychol* 12: 729–44.

Mayeux R, Chen J, Mirabello E, Marder K, Bell K, Dooneief G, Cote L, Stern Y (1990) An estimate of the incidence of dementia in idiopathic Parkinson's disease. *Neurology* 40: 1513–17.

Mayeux R, Denaro J, Hemenegildo N, Marder K, Tang MX, Cote LJ, Stern Y (1992) A population-based investigation of Parkinson's disease with and without dementia. Relationship to age and gender. *Arch Neurol* 49: 492–7.

Mayeux, R, Stern Y, Cote L, Williams JBW (1984) Altered serotonin metabolism in depressed patients with Parkinson's disease. *Neurology* 34: 642–6.

Mayeux R, Stern Y, Rosen J, Leventhal J (1981) Depression, intellectual impairment, and Parkinson's disease. *Neurology* 31: 645–50.

Mayeux R, Stern Y, Spanton S (1985) Heterogeneity in dementia of the Alzheimer type. Evidence of subgroups. *Neurology* 35: 453–61.

McGeer PL, McGeer EG, Suzuki J *et al.* (1984) Aging, Alzheimer's disease, and the cholinergic system of the basal forebrain. *Neurology* 34: 741–5.

McKeith I, Fairbairn A, Perry R, Thompson P, Perry E (1992) Neuroleptic sensitivity in patients with senile dementia of Lewy body type. *Br Med J* 305: 673–8.

McKeith IG, Fairbairn AF, Perry RH, Thompson P (1994) The clinical diagnosis and misdiagnosis of senile dementia of Lewy body type (SDLT). *Br J Psychiat* 165: 324–32.

McKeith IG, Perry RH, Fairbairn AF, Jabeen S, Perry EK (1992) Operational criteria for senile dementia of Lewy body type (SDLT). *Psychol Med* 22: 911–22.

McShane R, Gedling K, Reading M, McDonald B, Esiri MM, Hope T (1995) Prospective study of relations between cortical Lewy bodies, poor eyesight and hallucinations in Alzheimer's disease. *J Neurol Neurosurg Psychiat* 59: 185–8.

Merello M, Sabe L, Teson A, Migliorelli R, Petracchi M, Leiguarda R, Starkstein S (1994) Extrapyramidalism in Alzheimer's disease: prevalence, psychiatric, and neuropsychological correlates. *J Neurol Neurosurg Psychiat* 57: 1503–9.

Mirra SS, Heyman A, McKeel D, Sumi SM, Crain BJ, Brownlee LM, Vogel FS, Hughes JP, Van Belle G, Berg L (1991) The consortium to establish a registry for Alzheimer's disease (CERAD). II. Standardisation of neuropathological assessment of Alzheimer's disease. *Neurology* 41: 479–86.

Mizuno Y, Ohta S, Tanaka M, Takamiya S, Suzuki K, Sato T, Oya H, Ozawa T, Kagawa Y (1989) Deficiencies in complex 1 subunits of the respiratory chain in Parkinson's disease. *Biochem Biophys Res Commun* 163: 1450–5.

Mizutani T, Shimada H (1992) Neuropathological background of twenty-seven centenarian brains. *J Neurol Sci* 108: 168–77.

Molsa PK, Marttila RJ, Rinne UK (1984) Extrapyramidal signs in Alzheimer's disease. *Neurology* 34: 1114–16.

Mortimer JA, Pirozzolo FJ, Hansch EC, Webster DD (1982) Relationship of motor symptoms to intellectual deficits in Parkinson's disease. *Neurology* 32: 133–7.

Mortimer JA, Pirozzolo FJ, Hansch EC, Webster DD (1988) Relationship of motor symptoms to intellectual decline in Parkinson's disease. *Neurology* 51: 757–66.

Mutch WJ, Dingwall Fordyce I, Downie AW, Paterson JG, Roy SK (1986) Parkinson's disease in a Scottish city. *Br Med J* 292: 534–6.

Nakano I, Hirano A (1984) Parkinson's disease: Neuron loss in the nucleus basalis without concomitant Alzheimer's disease. *Ann Neurol* 15: 415–18.

Nishiyama K, Mizuno T, Sakuta M, Kurisaki H (1993) Chronic dementia in Parkinson's disease treated by anticholinergic agents. Neuropsychological and neuroradiological examination. *Adv Neurol* 60: 479–83.

Nissenbaum H, Quinn NP, Brown RG, Toone B, Gotham AM, Marsden CD (1987) Mood swings associated with the 'on-off' phenomenon in Parkinson's disease. *Psychol Med* 17: 899–904.

Nyberg P, Nordberg A, Webster P, Winblad B (1983) Dopaminergic deficiency is more pronounced in putamen than nucleus caudatus in Parkinson's disease. *Neurochem Pathol* 1: 193–202.

Okazaki H, Lipkin LE, Aronson SM (1961) Diffuse intracytoplasmic ganglionin inclusion (Lewy type) associated with progressive dementia and quadraparesis in flexion. *J Neuropathol Exp Neurol* 20: 237–44.

Okeda R, Kayano T, Funata N, Kojima T, Miki M, Iwama H (1982) An autopsy case of Parkinson's disease associated clinically with dementia terminating in akinetic mutism and pathologically with multiple Lewy bodies in the cerebral cortex. *Brain and Nerve* 38: 761–7.

Pappolla MA (1986) Lewy bodies of Parkinson's disease: immune electron microscopic demonstration of neurofilament antigens in constituent filaments. *Arch Pathol Lab Med* 110: 1160–3.

Parkinson J (1817) *An Essay on the Shaking Palsy.* Sherwood, Neely and Jones, London.

Pate DS, Margolin DI (1994) Cognitive slowing in Parkinson's and Alzheimer's patients: distinguishing bradyphrenia from dementia. *Neurology* 44: 669–74.

Perry EK, Curtis M, Dick DJ, Candy JM, Atack JR, Bloxham

CA, Blessed G, Fairbairn A, Tomlinson BE, Perry RH (1985) Cholinergic correlates of cognitive impairment in Parkinson's disease: comparison with Alzheimer's disease. *J Neurol Neurosurg Psychiatry* 48: 413–21.

Perry EK, Marshall E, Perry RH, Irving D, Smith CJ, Blessed G, Fairbairn AF (1990) Cholinergic and dopaminergic activities in senile dementia of Lewy body type. *Alzheimer Dis Assoc Disord* 4: 87–95.

Perry EK, Marshall E, Thompson P, McKeith IG, Collerton D, Fairbairn AF, Ferrier IN, Irving D, Perry RH (1993) Monoaminergic activities in Lewy body dementia: relation to hallucinosis and extrapyramidal features. *J Neural Transm Park Dis Dement Sect* 6: 167–77.

Perry EK, Court JA, Pigott MA, Perry RH (1994) Cholinergic component of dementia and aging. In Huppert FA, Brayne C, O'Connor DW (eds) *Dementia and Normal Aging.* Cambridge University Press, pp 437–69.

Perry RH, Irving D, Blessed G, Fairbairn A, Perry EK (1990) Senile dementia of Lewy body type. A clinically and neuropathologically distinct form of Lewy body dementia in the elderly. *J Neurol Sci* 95: 119–39.

Piccirilli M, D'Alessandro P, Finali G, Piccinin GL (1994) Neuropsychological follow-up of parkinsonian patients with and without cognitive impairment. *Dementia* 5: 17–22.

Pickering Brown SM, Mann DM, Bourke JP, Roberts DA, Balderson D, Burns A, Byrne J, Owen F (1994) Apolipoprotein E4 and Alzheimer's disease pathology in Lewy body disease and in other beta-amyloid-forming diseases. *Lancet* 343: 1155.

Pillon B, Dubois B, Agid Y (1991) Severity and specificity of cognitive impairment in Alzheimer's, Huntington's, and Parkinson's diseases and progressive supranuclear palsy. *Ann N Y Acad Sci* 640: 224–7.

Pirozzolo FJ, Hansch EC, Mortimer JA (1982) Dementia in Parkinson's disease: a neuropsychological analysis. *Brain Cogn* 1: 71–83.

Pollanen MS, Dickson DW, Bergeron C (1993) Pathology and biology of the Lewy body. *J Neuropathol Exp Neurol* 52: 183–91.

Popovitch ER, Wisniewski HM, Kaufman MA, Grundke Iqbal I, Wen GY (1987) Young adult-form of dementia with neurofibrillary changes and Lewy bodies. *Acta Neuropathol Berl* 74: 97–104.

Rajput AH, Rozdilsky B, Rajput A (1991) Accuracy of clinical diagnosis in parkinsonism – a prospective study. *Can J Neurol Sci* 18: 275–8.

Reid WG, Broe GA, Hely MA, Morris JG, Williamson PM, O'Sullivan DJ, Rail D, Genge S, Moss NG (1989) The neuropsychology of *de novo* patients with idiopathic Parkinson's disease: the effects of age of onset. *Int J Neurosci* 48: 205–7.

Reid WG (1992) The evolution of dementia in idiopathic Parkinson's disease: neuropsychological and clinical evidence in support of subtypes. *Int Psychogeriatr*, 4 Suppl 2: 147–60.

Richards M, Stern Y, Mayeux R (1993) Subtle extrapyramidal signs can predict the development of dementia in elderly individuals. *Neurology* 43: 2184–8.

Rogers D, Lees AJ, Smith E, Trimble M, Stern GM (1987) Bradyphrenia in Parkinson's disease and psychomotor retardation in depressive illness. An experimental study. *Brain* 110: 761–76.

Sadeh M, Brahim J, Modan M (1982) Effects of anticholinergic drugs on memory in Parkinson's disease. *Arch Neurol* 39: 666–7.

Saitoh T, Xia MS, Chen X, Masliah E, Galasko D, Shults C, Thal LJ, Hansen LA, Katzman R (1995) The CYP2D6B mutant allele is overrepresented in the Lewy body variant of Alzheimer's disease. *Ann Neurol* 37: 110–12.

Saunders AM, Strittmatter WJ, Schmechel D, St George-Hyslop PH, Pericak-Vance MA, Joo SH, Rosi BL, Gusella JF, Crapper-McLachlan DR, Alberts MJ, Hulette C, Crain B, Goldgaber D, Roses AD (1993) Association of apolipoprotein E allele epsilon-4 with late-onset familial and sporadic Alzheimer's disease. *Neurology* 43: 1467–72.

Scatton B, Javoy Agid F, Rouquier L, Dubois B, Agid Y (1983) Reduction of cortical dopamine, noradrenaline, serotonin and their metabolites in Parkinson's disease. *Brain Res* 275: 321–8.

Schmidt ML, Murray J, Lee VM, Hill WD, Wertkin A, Trojanowski JQ (1991) Epitope map of neurofilament protein domains in cortical and peripheral nervous system Lewy bodies. *Am J Pathol* 139: 53–65.

Shapira AHV (1995) Oxidative stress in Parkinson's disease. *Neuropathol Appl Neurobiol* 21: 3–9.

Shea TB, Beermann ML, Nixon RA (1992) Aluminium alters the electrophoretic properties of neurofilament proteins. Role of phosphorylation state. *J Neurochem* 58: 542–7.

Smith PEM, Irving D, Perry RH (1991) Density, distribution and prevalence of Lewy bodies in the elderly. *Neurosci Res Commun* 8: 127–35.

Starkstein SE, Berthier ML, Bolduc PL, Preziosi TJ, Robinson RG (1989) Depression in patients with early versus late-onset of Parkinson's disease. *Neurology* 39: 1441–5.

Starkstein SE, Mayberg HS, Leiguarda R, Preziosi TJ, Robinson RG (1992) A prospective longitudinal study of depression, cognitive decline, and physical impairments in patients with Parkinson's disease. *J Neurol Neurosurg Psychiat* 55: 377–82.

Stern Y, Folstein M, Albert M, Richards M, Miller L, Bylsma F, Lafleche G, Marder K, Bell K, Sano M et al. (1993) Multicenter study of predictors of disease course in Alzheimer disease (the 'predictors study'). I. Study design, cohort description, and intersite comparisons. *Alzheimer Dis Assoc Disord* 7: 3–21.

Stern Y, Albert M, Brandt J, Jacobs DM, Tang M-X, Marder K, Bell K, Sano M, Devanand DP, Bylsma F, Lafleche G (1994)

Utility of extrapyramidal signs and psychosis as predictors of cognitive and functional decline, nursing home admission, and death in Alzheimer's disease: prospective analyses from the predictors study. *Neurology* 44: 2300–7.

Stern Y, Marder K, Tang MX, Mayeux R (1993) Antecedent clinical features associated with dementia in Parkinson's disease. *Neurology* 43: 1690–2.

Stern Y, Mayeux R, Cote L (1984) Reaction time and vigilance in Parkinson's disease: possible role of norepinephrine metabolism. *Arch Neurol* 41: 1086–9.

Stern Y, Mayeux R, Sano M, Hanser WA, Bush T (1987) Predictors of disease course in patients with probable Alzheimer's disease. *Neurology* 37: 1649–53.

Stern Y, Richards M, Sano M, Mayeux R (1993) Comparison of cognitive changes in patients with Alzheimer's and Parkinson's disease. *Arch Neurol* 50: 1040–5.

Steventon GB, Heathfield MTE, Waring RH, Williams AC (1989) Xenobiotic metabolism in Parkinson's disease. *Neurology* 39: 883–7.

Sugiyama H, Hainfellner JA, Schmid Siegel B, Budka H (1993) Neuroaxonal dystrophy combined with diffuse Lewy body disease in a young adult. *Clin Neuropathol* 12: 147–52.

Sugiyama H, Hainfellner JA, Yoshimura M, Budka H (1994) Neocortical changes in Parkinson's disease, revisited. *Clin Neuropathol* 13: 55–9.

Sutcliffe RL, Prior R, Mawby B, McQuillan WJ (1985) Parkinson's disease in the district of the Northampton Health Authority, United Kingdom. A study of prevalence and disability. *Acta Neurol Scand* 72: 363–79.

Tagliavini F, Pilleri G (1983) Neuronal counts in basal nucleus of Meynert in Alzheimer disease and in simple senile dementia. *Lancet* i: 469–70.

Tiller-Borcich JK, Forno LS (1988) Parkinson's disease and dementia with neuronal inclusions in the cerebral cortex: Lewy bodies or Pick bodies. *J Neuropathol Exp Neurol* 47: 526–35.

Woodard JS (1962) Concentric hyaline inclusion body formation in mental disease analysis of twenty-seven cases. *J Neuropathol Exp Neurol* 21: 442–9.

Yamada T, McGeer PL, McGeer EG (1992) Lewy bodies in Parkinson's disease are recognized by antibodies to complement proteins. *Acta Neuropathol Berl* 84: 100–4.

Yamamoto T, Imai T (1988) A case of diffuse Lewy body and Alzheimer's diseases with periodic synchronous discharges. *J Neuropathol Exp Neurol* 47: 536–48.

Yoshimura M (1988) Pathological basis for dementia in elderly patients with idiopathic Parkinson's disease. *Europ Neurol* 28: Suppl 1: 29–35.

Zetusky WJ, Jankovic J, Pirozzolo F (1985) The heterogeneity of Parkinson's disease: clinical and prognostic implications. *Neurology* 35: 522–6.

Zweig RM, Cardillo JE, Cohen M, Giere S, Hedreen JC (1993) The locus ceruleus and dementia in Parkinson's disease. *Neurology* 43: 986–91.

CHAPTER SEVEN

Amyotrophic lateral sclerosis/parkinsonism-dementia complex of Guam

D. P. Perl

Introduction
Neuropathological features
Aetiology
Summary

INTRODUCTION

Guam is the largest of the Marianas islands, a chain of volcanic islands situated in the western Pacific Ocean. It lies about 1500 miles (2400 km) south of Tokyo and a similar distance east of Manila. Guam is about 30 miles (48 km) long and 4 to 9 miles (6 to 14 km) wide, with total land area of approximately 225 square miles (580 sq. km). Guam is a territory of the US, and has a civilian population of approximately 110 000 people. Of this population, approximately 55 000 are an indigenous native people referred to as Chamorros, while 20–25 000 are immigrants from the Philippine islands and an additional 20 000 inhabitants originate from other ethnic backgrounds (primarily Caucasians who came from the US mainland, Hawaiians and other Pacific islanders and immigrants from other Asian countries). Additionally, there are several large military installations on the island, and as many as 25 000 military personnel and their dependants can be stationed on Guam at any one time.

For the past 40 years, Guam has been recognized as the site of a remarkable concentration of neurodegenerative disease. Dr Harry Zimmerman, a pathologist assigned to the island by the US Navy in the later part of World War II, first called attention to several cases of amyotrophic lateral sclerosis (ALS) among the native Chamorro population and wondered if this could represent a highly prevalent focus of this relatively uncommon disease (Zimmerman, 1945). Folklore accounts and archival death certificates suggest that the disease had been prevalent on the island for at least a century prior to this observation. Nevertheless, Zimmerman's observations stimulated the initiation of a large series of epidemiological, clinical, neuropathological and aetiological studies which have attempted to characterize the nature, extent and underlying cause of endemic neurodegenerative diseases among the island's inhabitants (Garruto et al., 1983; Garruto & Yase, 1986; Lilianfeld, Perl & Olanow, 1994).

Initially, only ALS was recognized to be highly prevalent in the Chamorro inhabitants of Guam (Kurland & Mulder, 1954). The clinical manifestations of ALS among the Chamorros of Guam are virtually indistinguishable from the sporadic form of the disease, as seen elsewhere in the world. Typically, there is an insidious onset of the disease which begins with weakness and clumsiness and then shows progressive weakness and muscular atrophy accompanied by fasciculations and hyperreflexia in its early phases. Later aspects include a flaccid paralysis with increasing dysphagia and dysphonia. Death is commonly related to aspiration and/or hypostatic pneumonia. The mean length of survival is approximately 4 years following the initial diagnosis, but a small percentage of cases are encountered with survival of 10 years or more.

In a study performed in 1953–54, Kurland and Mulder (Kurland & Mulder, 1954) estimated that the prevalence of ALS among Guamanian Chamorros was approximately 420 per 100 000 inhabitants (as compared to 6 per 100 000 on the US mainland). In surveying the island for additional cases of ALS, another neurodegenerative disease was soon identified, namely a form of parkinsonism associated with severe progressive dementia (Hirano *et al.*, 1961*a*, Hirano, Malamud & Kurland, 1961*b*), now referred to as Parkinsonism–dementia complex of Guam (PDC). This disorder is characterized by rigidity, bradykinesia and, to a lesser extent, resting tremor. The dementia typically involves memory impairment, disorientation, and difficulty with simple calculations. In about 30% of cases, the dementia represents the presenting symptom. More recently, cases of a purely dementing syndrome, in the absence of amyotrophy and parkinsonian features, have been identified among the native population (Perl *et al.*, 1994). This newly described pure dementia variant of the Guam disease has been referred to as Marianas dementia and is currently being studied both clinically and neuropathologically.

Two similar foci of neurodegenerative disease have been identified in this region of the world, namely in the Kii peninsula of Japan and in a remote area in southwestern New Guinea. The Kii peninsula is an isolated region on the southeastern coast of Honshu Island. In this region many cases of ALS were reported by Yase and Shiraki (Shiraki & Yase, 1975). Neuropathological studies of cases from the Kii peninsula revealed neuropathological changes that are virtually identical to those encountered among the ALS patients on Guam. PDC is not as well documented in this population and the prevalence of dementia in the region remains undetermined. A second focus was first identified by Gajdusek (Gajdusek, 1963; Gajdusek & Salazar, 1980) among the Auyu and Jakai people living in a remote part of southwestern New Guinea. This focus has been characterized clinically as consisting of both ALS and Parkinsonism with dementia and closely resembles that seen on Guam. However, as yet, no post-mortem examinations have been done on any cases from the New Guinea focus.

NEUROPATHOLOGICAL FEATURES

General features

The neuropathological features of ALS/PDC of Guam were initially described in the seminal papers of Hirano and co-workers (Malamud *et al.*, 1961; Hirano *et al.*, 1961*b*; Hirano, Arumugasamy & Zimmerman, 1967). The brains of affected individuals show prominent generalized cerebral atrophy, typically with brain weights less than 1000 grams and severely dilated lateral ventricles. In cases of PDC, complete loss of grossly visible pigmentation in the substantia nigra is frequently noted. Cases of ALS typically show marked atrophy of the ventral spinal roots.

Neurofibrillary tangles

In 1961, Malamud and co-workers (Malamud, Hirano & Kurland, 1961) first identified large numbers of neurofibrillary tangles in the brains of Guamanian patients with ALS. Subsequent studies of cases of both Guam ALS and PDC have revealed prominent widespread involvement by neurofibrillary tangles in both forms of the disorder (Hirano *et al.*, 1961*b*). Areas with severe involvement include the hippocampus, entorhinal cortex, amygdala, basal forebrain, and neocortex. The Ammon's horn of the hippocampus may show virtually complete involvement by neurofibrillary tangles, frequently accompanied by marked neuronal loss and the formation of large numbers of extracellular 'ghost' tangles (Figs. 7.1 and 7.2). The periaqueductal grey matter, substantia nigra and locus ceruleus may also be sites of extensive involvement. Neurofibrillary tangles represent the morphological hallmark of Guam ALS/PDC and virtually all cases show prominent involvement by this neuropathological alteration. The immunohistochemical and ultrastructural features of the neurofibrillary tangles seen in cases of Guam ALS/PDC are virtually identical to those encountered in cases of Alzheimer's disease elsewhere in the world (Hirano, 1973; Shankar *et al.*, 1989). In cases of PDC, severe neuronal loss is encountered in the substantia nigra and locus ceruleus and globoid forms of neurofibrillary tangles are seen in the few remaining neurons in these areas.

Anderson and colleagues (Anderson *et al.*, 1979) conducted a neuropathological study of brain specimens obtained from relatively young Guamanian Chamorros who during life had been reported to be neurologically intact. They demonstrated that a sizable number of neurologically intact Guamanians showed significant neurofibrillary tangle formation at autopsy. Indeed, in this study, 29% of individuals dying between ages 30 and 39 years and 40% of those dying between 40 and 49 years showed evidence of neurofibrillary tangle formation in the hippocampus and neocortex. It has been assumed that the subjects with early neurofibrillary tangle formation represent individuals with ALS/PDC in a preclinical phase of the disorder. Presumably, the degree of neuropathologic involvement had not yet reached sufficient intensity for symptomatic features to be identified clinically.

Hof and co-workers (Hof *et al.*, 1991) have identified a

pattern of neocortical involvement by neurofibrillary tangles in Guam ALS/PDC that differs from that of Alzheimer's disease. They demonstrated that, in the Guam cases, there was a striking tendency for severe involvement of layers II–III of the neocortex with a relatively lesser extent of tangle formation in layer V.

This pattern differs from that of Alzheimer's disease, where tangle formation tends to predominate in layer V with relatively less involvement in layers II–III.

Eosinophilic rod-like bodies (Hirano bodies)

In his neuropathological evaluation of cases of Guam

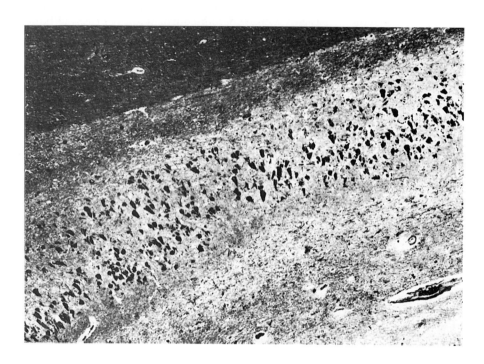

Fig. 7.1. Photomicrograph of the hippocampus (CA1 region) of a case of parkinsonism-dementia complex of Guam showing extensive neurofibrillary tangle formation (modified Bielschowsky stain).

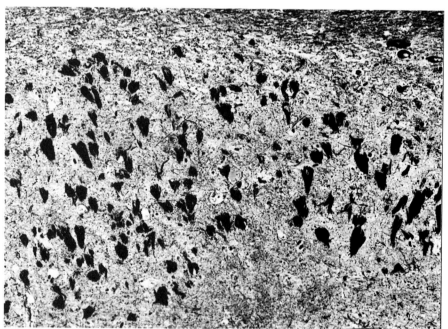

Fig. 7.2. High power photomicrograph of the hippocampus (CA1 region) of a case of parkinsonism-dementia complex of Guam showing extensive neurofibrillary tangle formation (modified Bielschowsky stain).

ALS/PDC, Hirano noted (Hirano, 1965) the presence of large numbers of eosinophilic rod-shaped bodies immediately adjacent to the pyramidal neurons of the hippocampus (Fig. 7.3). These structures, now referred to as Hirano bodies, were initially considered to be specific for the Guam disorder. However, subsequent investigation (Hirano, Dembitzer & Kurland, 1968) revealed similar changes, though in smaller numbers, in the hippocampus of cases of Alzheimer's disease and of Pick's disease. Rare examples of these inclusions may also be found in the brains of elderly non-demented controls elsewhere in the world.

Other neurodegenerative features

Many of the other neuropathological features of the classic neurodegenerative disorders are also encountered in cases of Guam ALS/PDC, whereas other morphological features are specifically absent. For example, granulovacuolar degeneration, a poorly understood alteration consisting of multiple vacuoles each filled with a single basophilic granule, are found in the perikaryal cytoplasm of neurons in the Ammon's horn of the hippocampus (primarily in the boundary zone of the H_1 and H_2 regions) (Simchowicz, 1911) (Fig. 7.4). Although present in small numbers in normal ageing, when prominent granulovacuolar degeneration is encountered in the posterior portion of the hippocampus, this finding correlates highly with a diagnosis of Alzheimer's disease

(Tomlinson & Kitchener, 1972; Ball, 1978). Cases of Guam ALS/PDC show severe granulovacuolar degeneration in this region and although quantitative studies have not been performed, the degree of involvement appears to be much greater than is encountered in Alzheimer's disease (Hirano, 1965).

Cell loss in the nucleus basalis of Meynert is a characteristic feature of Alzheimer's disease (Whitehouse et al., 1982) as well as Parkinson's disease (Whitehouse et al., 1983). Cell loss in the basal forebrain is also encountered in cases of Guam ALS/PDC and two studies (Nakano & Hirano, 1982; Masullo et al., 1989) have documented greater cell loss in this nucleus than is commonly seen in Alzheimer's disease. The remaining neurons in this region typically contain neurofibrillary tangles. The implications of this finding are unclear since, to date, no neurotransmitter studies have been reported on well-characterized cases from Guam. Presumably, such cell loss would lead to a significant neocortical cholinergic deficit.

Studies of the striatum have shown that component neuronal systems remain intact. Immunohistochemical techniques indicate the calbindin-D_{28} (Ito et al., 1992), met-enkephalin, substance P and calcineurin immunoreactive neurons (Goto, Hirano & Matsumoto, 1990; Ito et al., 1993) remain intact in the striatum of cases of PDC. This suggests that, similar to idiopathic Parkinson's disease, the striatum and its efferent

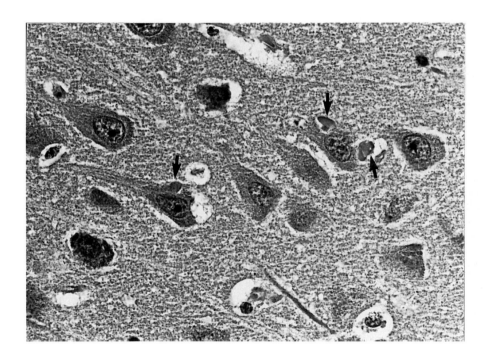

Fig. 7.3. Photomicrograph of the hippocampus, parkinsonism-dementia complex of Guam, showing several Hirano bodies (haematoxylin and eosin stain).

system remains intact despite severe nigral degeneration.

Lewy bodies are not encountered in most cases of PDC. In a large retrospective neuropathological series of Guam cases, less than 10% of cases show evidence of Lewy body formation (Rogers-Johnson *et al.*, 1986). It should be noted that, in these Lewy body positive cases, the number of involved neurons is quite small. In the Guamanian Chamorro, the incidence of true idiopathic Parkinson's disease (that is, with prominent Lewy body formation) is extremely low. Indeed, in the author's exprience, only one case of idiopathic Parkinson's disease has ever been identified in a native Guamanian Chamorro.

Amyloid deposition, senile plaques, congophilic angiopathy

Despite the presence of large numbers of neurofibrillary tangles and other neuropathological features associated with Alzheimer's disease, there is a conspicuous absence of senile plaques and congophilic angiopathy in cases of Guam ALS/PDC. Indeed, the classic neuropathologic descriptions of Guam-derived brain specimens specifically commented on the lack of any evidence of senile plaques (Hirano *et al.*, 1961*b*; Malamud *et al.*, 1961; Hirano *et al.*, 1967). However, occasional cases of Guam ALS/PDC have been identified in which senile plaques are present. Although still relatively uncommon, there is

evidence that the tendency for plaque formation has increased in recent years, compared to what was seen in the immediate post-World War II era. Cases in which plaques are encountered mostly demonstrate diffuse plaques, without evidence of associated neuritic changes. Because the neurofibrillary tangles in such brain specimens predominate in layers II–III, rather than layer V, it is felt that these cases represent examples of ALS/PDC with superimposed diffuse plaques rather than examples of Alzheimer's disease in the at-risk elderly Chamorro population. Amyloid deposition in the leptomeningeal or superficial cerebral cortical vessels is infrequent in Guam-derived brain specimens and when seen, generally is present in only scant amounts.

Evidence of overlap between guam ALS and PDC

ALS and PDC of Guam were originally described as distinct clinical entities. Most of the epidemiological studies of the Guam focus have maintained the concept that these are two separate diseases. Nevertheless, there is substantial evidence of overlap between the two conditions. For example, approximately 45% of cases of Guam ALS show evidence of significant neuronal loss in the substantia nigra (Elizan *et al.*, 1966). Similarly, in 45 cases of PDC, 17 (38%) showed neuropathological evidence of ALS in the spinal cord. Further evaluation of 113 PDC cases revealed that, in 35%, there was evidence of lateral column demyelination and loss of anterior

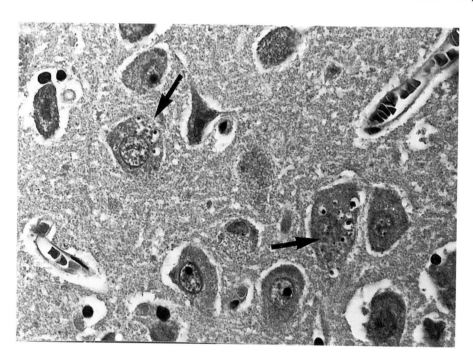

Fig. 7.4. Photomicrograph of the hippocampus, Guam amyotrophic lateral sclerosis, showing prominent granulovacuolar degenerative changes (haematoxylin and eosin stain).

horn cells (Rogers-Johnson *et al.*, 1986). Findings such as these strongly suggest that ALS and PDC of Guam represent the extremes of a spectrum of neurodegeneration and that it is likely, at the very least, that the two forms of the disorder share common pathogenetic mechanisms. Indeed, it may be argued that Guam ALS/PDC actually represents a single entity in which variations in the degree of neuronal system degeneration (e.g. motor system vs. extrapyramidal system) is responsible for observed differences in clinical expression.

AETIOLOGY

Despite extensive investigation, the epidemic of neurodegenerative disease encountered among the native population on Guam has remained an unsolved mystery since it was first characterized in the early 1950s. Over the years it has been recognized that, through a better understanding of specific aetiological mechanisms responsible for the neurodegenerative disorders seen on the island, critical insights could be gained into aetio/pathogenetic factors with relevance to the analogous disorders seen elsewhere in the world, namely ALS, Parkinson's disease and Alzheimer's disease. Over the years, Guam has tended to serve primarily as a model for ALS (Gajdusek, 1982) with analogies less frequently made to Parkinson's disease and Alzheimer's disease. The literature regarding studies of aetiological hypotheses for Guam ALS/PDC are numerous (Garruto & Yase, 1986; Lilienfeld *et al.*, 1994; Garruto & Yanagihara, 1991) and can only be briefly summarized in this chapter.

Genetics

Initially it was assumed that Guam ALS/PDC represented a genetic condition and reflected a mutational event which occurred in a relatively inbred and island-bound population. However, a number of studies have seriously questioned that concept. The Chamorro community living on Saipan (an island 80 miles north of Guam) was extremely small during the nineteenth century and then was repopulated in the early portion of this century by Chamorro immigrants from Guam. Accordingly, the Chamorros of Saipan carry virtually the same genetic markers as those of Guam yet there is little evidence of similar neurodegenerative diseases on this nearby island (Yanagihara *et al.*, 1983). Additionally, epidemiological studies conducted over the past 30 + years have shown a striking change in the clinical characteristics of the epidemic (Garruto, Yanagihara & Gajdusek, 1985; Shankar *et al.*, 1989). In the earliest studies, ALS was a quite common form of the disorder. Over the past 20

years the incidence of ALS has declined markedly and currently new cases are seen relatively infrequently. Cases of PDC remain common on Guam, although the age of onset of the disease has increased by almost 10 years when compared to cases identified and studied in the early 1960s. Clearly, such profound changes in the basic characteristics of a disease outbreak, noted over such a relatively short period of time, would argue strongly against a genetic basis for the problem. Finally, a number of cases of ALS/PDC have been documented among the community of Filipino immigrants who have lived on Guam for more than 20 years (Garruto, Gajdusek & Chen, 1981). These Filipino migrant cases not only manifest all of the clinical features of ALS/PDC but have also shown evidence of the widespread neurofibrillary tangle formation that is typical of the disease in the Guamanian Chamorro. Based on this and other evidence, the importance of environmental factors has been emphasized. Although the possibility that genetic factors may play a role must still be considered, it is most likely that such inherited factors serve to modify susceptibility to the disorder rather than represent the primary etiology of the disease.

Infectious agents

The effects of conventional viral or possibly so-called 'slow latent viral' (i.e. prion-related) infection had been seriously considered as a likely aetiologic candidate for Guam by Gajdusek and colleagues in the 1970s. However, attempts to transmit disease using intracerebral inoculation of a large number of Guam-derived brain tissues into a variety of species, including non-human primates, have yielded entirely negative results (Gibbs & Gajdusek, 1982). Attempts to recover a conventional infectious agent or to identify a consistent serological response have also failed to show evidence of infection in affected patients.

Cycad

The seed of the false sago palm tree (*Cycas circinalis*) serves as a traditional source of food for the Guamanian Chamorro who grind the seeds into flour and use it to prepare dishes such as tortillas and soups. Because the raw seeds contain a severe hepatotoxin, they must be soaked for days in water before they may be safely used. Early in the investigation of the epidemic it was suggested by Whiting (Whiting, 1988) that a putative toxin present in the cycad seed could represent the aetiological factor responsible for the outbreak of neurological disease. This led to an extensive series of toxicological experiments involving both raw cycad from Guam as well as identified chemical constituents of the seeds. The results of these studies (Whiting, 1988; Proceedings of the Third Conference on the Toxicity of Cycads, 1964; Sixth International Cycad Conference, 1972) demonstrated the presence of cycasin, a potent, naturally occurring alkylating agent, and the experimental induction of significant numbers of malignant neoplasms in non-central nervous system organs of experimentally exposed animals. However, despite extensive animal experimentation, involving long- and short-term exposure of a large range of animal species, cycad failed to induce evidence of significant neurologic dysfunction or neuropathologic abnormalities. Based on this negative evidence, support for the cycad hypothesis waned.

However, in 1987, Spencer and colleagues reported the induction of extrapyramidal and motor disfunction in monkeys orally fed large doses of synthetic β-N-methyl-amino-L-alanine (BMAA) (Spencer, 1987). BMAA was employed because it is present in cycad seeds and shares chemical similarities with β-N-oxalylamino-L-alanine (BOAA), which had been implicated in neural lathyrism, a form of acquired non-progressive spastic paraparesis. The findings of Spencer have been questioned on a number of grounds. Loss of substantia nigral neurons or anterior horn cells was not demonstrated in the BMAA-exposed animals nor was evidence presented of a striatal dopaminergic deficit or denervation atrophy. The BMAA doses given to the monkeys were extremely high, particularly since BMAA is present in only small amounts in cycad, is readily removed by brief washing and does not readily cross the blood–brain barrier (Duncan et al., 1990). The role of cycad-containing foods in Guam neurodegeneration remains unsubstantiated and Spencer has subsequently written (Spencer et al., 1990) 'the changes [induced in monkeys fed synthetic BMAA] fall short of a model of the human disease'.

Toxic metals

In 1972, Yase suggested (Yase, 1972) the possibility that Guam neurodegeneration might be related to the abnormal accumulation of potentially neurotoxic trace elements, such as manganese, in the soil of Guam. Using electron probe microanalysis, Perl and Brody (Perl & Brody, 1980) first showed evidence of aluminum accumulation in neurofibrillary tangle-bearing neurons of cases of Alzheimer's disease. Using the microprobe analytic approach they had developed, a dramatic accumulation of aluminium in the tangle-bearing neurons of cases of Guam ALS/PDC was demonstrated (Perl et al.,

1982). These findings have now been confirmed using five different physical methods of analysis (Garruto et al., 1984; Piccardo et al., 1988; Perl et al., 1986). The source of the intraneuronal accumulations of aluminum remains unclear. Gajdusek (Garruto et al., 1983) has hypothesized that a deficiency in calcium and magnesium in soil and water could lead to increased aluminum uptake as an alternative source of cations. However, search for evidence of calcium deficiency has not revealed consistent abnormalities (Steele, Guzman & Driver, 1990; Ashkog et al (1994). As a volcanic bauxite-based island, the soils of Guam are rich in aluminum. It has been suggested that the soil on Guam is different from that of two other bauxite islands, namely Jamaica and Palau, in that Guam soil demonstrates a 42-fold higher level of elutable aluminum (McLachlan et al., 1989). This single study suggests that Guam soils contain more bioavailable aluminium than other volcanic islands. The extent and nature of those differences and, most importantly, their biological significance remains unknown.

More recent studies using laser microprobe mass analysis have demonstrated that the tangle-bearing neurons of Guam contain high concentrations of both aluminum and iron (Good & Perl, 1994), a finding that is paralleled in both the tangles of Alzheimer's disease (Good et al., 1992a) and the neuromelanin granules of neurons of the substantia nigra of idiopathic Parkinson's disease (Good et al., 1992b). We have suggested (Olanow & Perl, 1994) that the combination of iron with aluminium may place a neuron in a state of oxidative stress since aluminium apparently enhances iron's ability to induce lipid peroxidation through the Fenton reaction. It is of interest to note the recent finding of mutations in the Cu/Zn superoxide dismutase (SOD-1) gene in cases of familial ALS (Rosen et al., 1993) and the production of a transgenic mouse model of motor neuron disease through the introduction of such mutations (Gurney et al., 1994). SOD represents one of the important defence mechanisms against oxidative stress. Although cases of Guam ALS/PDC fail to show evidence of mutations in the Cu/Zn SOD gene (Figlewicz et al., 1994), the presence of excess intraneuronal iron and aluminium could overwhelm normal protective mechanisms and induce neurodegeneration. Nevertheless, although the intraneuronal trace element abnormalities in Guam ALS/PDC are striking and potentially are highly toxic to these cells, the mechanism responsible for such accumulations and their potential pathogenetic role in neurodegeneration remains to be elucidated.

SUMMARY

We consider ALS/PDC of Guam to represent the 'Rosetta Stone' of neurodegenerative diseases encountered among the elderly. The Rosetta Stone, a large slab of basalt which was discovered in Egypt in 1799, contains a portion of text which was written in three ancient languages, ancient Greek, the demotic language and Egyptian hieroglyphics. Through an understanding of the ancient Greek inscription the two other ancient languages could finally be decoded leading to the deciphering of numerous other ancient inscriptions. In a similar fashion, it is hoped that, through the deciphering of the clues made available through the study of Guam, its people and its environment, a broader understanding of aetio-pathogenetic factors will be reached for the three major age-related neurodegenerative disorders seen elsewhere in the world, namely Alzheimer's disease, Parkinson's disease and ALS. Despite considerable efforts over many decades by teams of energetic and experienced investigators, the intriguing mystery of Guam ALS/PDC remains to be solved. Nevertheless, it is hoped that through continued studies of affected individuals and patients at risk such insights will finally be achieved.

REFERENCES

Anderson FH, Richardson EP, Okazaki H, Brody JA (1979) Neurofibrillary degeneration of Guam. Frequency in Chamorros and non-Chamorros with no known neurological disease. *Brain* 102: 65–77.

Ashkog JE, Waring SC, Petersen RC *et al* (1994) Guamanian neurodegenerative disease: failure to find abnormal calcium metabolism. *Neurology* 44, S2: 193.

Ball, MJ (1978) Topographic distribution of neurofibrillary tangles and granulovacuolar degeneration in hippocampal cortex of aging and demented patients. A quantitative study. *Acta Neuropathol (Berl)* 42: 73–80.

Duncan MW, Steele JC, Kopin IJ, Markey SP (1990) 2-Amino-3-(methylamino)-propanoic acid (BMAA) in cycad flour: an unlikely cause of amyotrophic lateral sclerosis and parkinsonism–dementia of Guam. *Neurology* 40: 767–72.

Elizan TS, Hirano A, Abrams BM, Need RL, Van Nuis C, Kurland LT (1966) Amyotrophic lateral sclerosis and parkinsonism-dementia complex of Guam. Neurological reevaluation. *Arch Neurol* 14: 356–68.

Figlewicz DA, Garruto RM, Krizus A, Yanagihara R, Rouleau GA (1994) The Cu/Zn superoxide dismutase gene in ALS and parkinsonism–dementia of Guam. *Neuroreport* 5: 557–60.

Gajdusek DC (1963) Motor neuron disease in natives of New Guinea. *N Engl J Med* 268: 474–6.

Gajdusek DC (1982) Foci of motor neuron disease in high incidence in isolated populations of East Asia and the Western Pacific. In Rowland LP (ed) *Human Motor Neuron Disease*. Raven Press, New York, pp 363–93.

Gajdusek DC, Salazar AM (1980) Amyotrophic lateral sclerosis and parkinsonian syndromes in high incidence among the Auyu and Jakai people in West New Guinea. *Neurology* 32: 107–26.

Garruto RM, Fukatsu R, Yanagihara R, Gajdusek DC, Hook G, Fiori C (1984) Imaging of calcium and aluminum in neurofibrillary tangle-bearing neurons in parkinsonism–dementia of Guam. *Proc Natl Acad Sci USA* 81: 1875–9.

Garruto RM, Gajdusek DC, Chen KM (1981) Amyotrophic lateral sclerosis and parkinsonism-dementia among Filipino migrants to Guam. *Ann Neurol* 10: 341–50.

Garruto RM, Yanagihara R (1991) Amyotrophic lateral sclerosis in the Marianas Islands. In deJung JMBV (ed) *Handbook of Clinical Neurology, Vol. 15(59), Diseases of the Motor System*. Elsevier Scientific Publishers, Amsterdam, pp 253–71.

Garruto RM, Yanagihara R, Arion DM, Daum CA, Gajdusek DC (1983) *Bibliography of Amyotrophic Lateral Sclerosis and Parkinsonism–Dementia of Guam*, Bethesda: NIH Publication No. 83–2662.

Garruto RM, Yanagihara R, Gajdusek DC (1985) Disappearance of high-incidence amyotrophic lateral sclerosis and parkinsonism–dementia on Guam. *Neurology* 35: 193–8.

Garruto RM, Yase Y (1986) Neurodegenerative disorders of the western Pacific: the search for mechanisms of pathogenesis. *Trends Neurosci* 9: 368–74.

Gibbs CJ Jr, Gajdusek DC (1982) An update on long-term *in vivo* and *in vitro* studies designed to identify a virus as the cause of amyotrophic lateral sclerosis, parkinsonism dementia and Parkinson's disease. *Adv Neurol* 36: 343–53.

Good PF, Olanow CW, Perl DP (1992a) Neuromelanin-containing neurons of the substantia nigra accumulate iron and aluminum in Parkinson's disease: a LAMMA study. *Brain Res* 593: 343–6.

Good PF, Perl DP (1994) A quantitative comparison of aluminum concentration in neurofibrillary tangles of Alzheimer's disease and parkinsonian dementia complex of Guam by laser microprobe mass analysis. *Neurobiol Aging* 15: S28.

Good PF, Perl DP, Bierer LM, Schmeidler J (1992b) Selective accumulation of aluminum and iron in the neurofibrillary tangles of Alzheimer's disease: a laser microprobe (LAMMA) study. *Ann Neurol* 31: 286–92.

Goto S, Hirano A, Matsumoto S (1990) Immunohistochemical study of the striatal efferents and nigral dopaminergic neurons in parkinsonism–dementia complex on Guam in comparison with those in Parkinson's and Alzheimer's diseases. *Ann Neurol* 27: 520–7.

Gurney ME, Pu H, Chiu AY *et al* (1994) Motor neuron degeneration in mice that express a human Cu,Zn superoxide dismutase mutation. *Science* 264: 1772–5.

Hirano A (1965) Pathology of amyotrophic lateral sclerosis. In Gajdusek DC, Gibbs CJ Jr, Alpers M (eds) *Slow, Latent, and Temperate Virus Infections.* NINDB Monograph No. 2, US Govt. Printing Office, Washington, DC, pp 23–37.

Hirano A (1973) Progress in the pathology of motor neuron diseases. *Prog Neuropathol* 2: 181–215.

Hirano A, Arumugasamy N, Zimmerman HM (1967) Amyotrophic lateral sclerosis. A comparison of Guam and classical cases. *Arch Neurol* 16: 357–63.

Hirano A, Dembitzer HM, Kurland LT (1968) The fine structure of some intraganglionic alterations. Neurofibrillary tangles, granulovacuolar bodies and 'rod-like' structures as seen in Guam amyotrophic lateral sclerosis and parkinsonism–dementia complex. *J Neuropathol Exp Neurol* 27: 167–82.

Hirano A, Kurland LT, Krooth RS, Lessell S (1961a) Parkinsonism–dementia complex, an endemic disease on the island of Guam I. Clinical features. *Brain* 84: 642–61.

Hirano A, Malamud N, Kurland LT (1961b) Parkinsonism–dementia complex, an endemic disease on the island of Guam II. Pathological features. *Brain* 84: 662–79.

Hof PR, Perl DP, Loerzel AJ, Morrison JH (1991) Neurofibrillary tangle distribution in the cerebral cortex of parkinsonism–dementia cases from Guam: differences with Alzheimer's disease. *Brain Res* 564: 306–13.

Ito H, Goto S, Sakamoto S, Hirano A (1992) Calbindin-D28k in the basal ganglia of patients with parkinsonism. *Ann Neurol* 32: 543–50.

Ito H, Goto S, Sakamoto S & Hirano A (1993) Striasomal arrangement of met-enkephalin and substance P expression in parkinsonism–dementia complex on Guam. *Acta Neuropathol* 85: 390–3.

Kurland LT, Mulder DW (1954) Epidemiologic investigations of amyotrophic lateral sclerosis. 1. Preliminary report on geographic distribution with special reference to the Mariana Islands, including clinical and pathologic observations. *Neurology* 4: 355–78, 438–48.

Lilienfeld DE, Perl DP, Olanow CW (1994) Guam Neurodegeneration. In Calne DB (ed) *Neurodegeneration.* Saunders, Philadelphia, pp 895–908.

Malamud N, Hirano A, Kurland LT (1961) Pathoanatomic changes in amyotrophic lateral sclerosis on Guam. *Neurology* 5: 401–14.

Masullo C, Pocchiari M, Mariotti P et al (1989) The nucleus basalis of Meynert in parkinsonism–dementia of Guam: a morphometric study. *Neuropathol Appl Neurobiol* 15: 193–206.

McLachlan DR, McLachlan CD, Krishnan B, Krishnan SS, Dalton AJ, Steele JC (1989) Aluminum and calcium in soil and food from Guam, Palau and Jamaica: implications for amyotrophic lateral sclerosis and parkinsonism–dementia syndromes of Guam. *Env Geochem and Health* 11: 45–53.

Nakano I, Hirano A (1982) Neuron loss in the nucleus basalis of Meynert in parkinsonism-dementia complex of Guam. *Ann Neurol* 13: 87–91.

Olanow CW, Perl DP (1994) Free radicals and neurodegeneration. *Trends Neurosci* 17: 193–4.

Perl DP, Brody AR (1980) Alzheimer's Disease: X-ray spectrographic evidence of aluminum accumulation in neurofibrillary tangle-bearing neurons. *Science* 208: 297–9.

Perl DP, Gajdusek DC, Garruto RM, Yanagihara RT, Gibbs CJ Jr (1982) Intraneuronal aluminum accumulation in amyotrophic lateral sclerosis and parkinsonism–dementia of Guam. *Science* 217: 1053–5.

Perl DP, Hoff PR, Steele JC et al (1994) Marianas dementia: a purely dementing form of ALS/parkinsonism-dementia complex of Guam. *Soc Neurosci Abs* 20: 1649.

Perl DP, Munoz-Garcia D, Good PF, Pendlebury WW (1986) Calculation of intracellular aluminum concentration in neurofibrillary tangle (NFT)-bearing and NFT-free hippocampal neurons of ALS/parkinsonism dementia of Guam using laser microprobe analysis. *J Neuropathol Exp Neurol* 45: 379.

Piccardo P, Yanagihara R, Garruto RM, Gibbs, CJ Jr, Gajdusek DC (1988) Histochemical and X-ray microanalytical localization of aluminum in amyotrophic lateral sclerosis and parkinsonism-dementia of Guam. *Acta Neuropathol* 77: 1–4.

Proceedings of the Third Conference on the Toxicity of Cycads (1964) *Fed Proc* 23.

Rogers-Johnson P, Garruto RM, Yanagihara R, Chen K, Gajdusek DC, Gibbs CJ Jr (1986) Amyotrophic lateral sclerosis and parkinsonism–dementia on Guam: a 30-year evaluation of clinical and neuropathologic trends. *Neurology* 36: 7–13.

Rosen DR, Siddique T, Patterson D et al (1993) Mutations in Cu/Zn superoxide dismutase gene are associated with familial amyotrophic lateral sclerosis. *Nature* 362: 59–62.

Shankar SK, Yanagihara R, Garruto RM, Grundke-Iqbal I, Kosik KS, Gajdusek DC (1989) Immunocytochemical characterization of neurofibrillary tangles in amyotrophic lateral sclerosis and parkinsonism-dementia of Guam. *Ann Neurol* 25: 146–51.

Shiraki H, Yase Y (1975) Amyotrophic lateral sclerosis in Japan. In Vinken PJ and Bruyn GW (eds) *Handbook of Clinical Neurology, Volume 22.* Elsevier, New York, pp 353–419.

Simchowicz T (1911) Histologische studien über die senile dementz in histol. und histopathol. *Arbeiten Åber die Grosshirnrinde* 4: 267.

Sixth International Cycad Conference (1972) *Fed Proc* 31.

Spencer PS (1987) Guam ALS/parkinsonism-dementia: a long-latency neurotoxic disorder caused by 'slow toxin(s)' in food? *Can J Neurol Sci* 14: 347–57.

Spencer PS, Allen RG, Kisby GE, Ludolph AC (1990) Excitotoxic disorders. *Science* 248: 144.

Steele JC, Guzman TQ, Driver MG (1990) Nutritional factors in amyotrophic lateral sclerosis on Guam: observations from Umatac. In Hudson AJ (ed) *Amyotrophic Lateral Sclerosis: Concepts in Pathogenesis and Etiology* Univ. of Toronto Press, pp 193–223.

Tomlinson BE, Kitchener D (1972) Granulovacuolar degeneration of hippocampal pyramidal cells. *J Pathol* 106: 165–85.

Whitehouse PJ, Hedreen JC, White CL, Price DL (1983) Basal forebrain neurons in the dementia of Parkinson's disease. *Ann Neurol* 13: 243–8.

Whitehouse PJ, Price DL, Struble RG, Clark AW, Coyle JT, Delong MR (1982) Alzheimer's disease and senile dementia: loss of neurons in the basal forebrain. *Science* 215: 1237–9.

Whiting M (1988) *Toxicity of Cycads: Implications for Neurodegenerative Diseases and Cancer. Transcripts of Four Cycad Conferences,* Third World Medical Research Foundation, New York.

Yanagihara RT, Garruto RM, Gajdusek DC (1983) Epidemiological surveillance of amyotrophic lateral sclerosis and parkinsonism-dementia in the Commonwealth of the Northern Mariana Islands. *Ann Neurol* 13: 79–86.

Yase Y (1972) The pathogenesis of amyotrophic lateral sclerosis. *Lancet* ii: 292–6.

Zimmerman HM (1945) Monthly report to Medical Officer in Command. *US Naval Medical Research Unit No 2.*

CHAPTER EIGHT

Pick's disease

J. H. Morris

Introduction
Clinical manifestations
Pathological findings
Neurochemistry
Problems in Pick's disease
Related conditions

INTRODUCTION

In papers published in 1892, 1904 and 1906 Alfons Pick, in collaboration with the pathologist Chiari, described the clinical features of the dementia and the characteristic circumscribed frontal and temporal lobe atrophy of the brain of the disease that now bears his name. By a pleasing coincidence, it fell to another great name in dementia, Alois Alzheimer, to produce the first account of the microscropic pathology of the brain in Pick's disease in 1911. Alzheimer described the principal features that we recognize in Pick's disease including the gross depletion of neurons from the affected areas and both Pick's cells and Pick bodies.

There are a number of accounts of the neuropathology of Pick's disease (Constantinidis, Richard & Tissot, 1974; Esiri & Oppenheimer, 1989; Tissot, Constantinidis & Richard, 1975; Tomlinson, 1992) and the description given here will not be found to differ significantly from these. Although usually bracketed with Alzheimer's disease as a type of cortical dementia, Pick's disease is very much rarer, having a prevalence of less than 1% of that of Alzheimer's disease (Lüers & Spatz, 1957; Delay & Brion, 1962; Jervis, 1971). The rarity of Pick's disease has had a considerable and adverse impact on the growth of knowledge and understanding of the disease and continues to hamper efforts to study it. At the most basic level it means that no single individual ever experiences a large number of these cases and much of the information about the disease is derived from the examination of rather small series of cases. From the standpoint of pathological description, there is even a measure of disagreement

(discussed later) about which cases should be included as examples of the condition.

As far as can be determined, given its rarity, Pick's disease has a similar incidence in all countries. Both sporadic and familial cases occur and there appears to be slight excess of female patients, the largest survey indicating a ratio of approximately 5:4 females to males (van Mansvelt, 1954). Other than the genetic component, studies of which suggest transmission as an autosomal dominant with polygenetic influence (Sjögren, Sjögren & Lindgren, 1952), no predisposing or precipitating factors have been demonstrated. The age of onset varies very widely, cases having been recorded in all decades from the third to the tenth, although the sixth and seventh seem to be the most common. In Alzheimer's disease there is a marked increase in frequency with increasing age, but no such increase has been demonstrated in Pick's disease.

CLINICAL MANIFESTATIONS

It can be said with some confidence at the beginning of this section that there are no certain criteria invariably to distinguish between patients with Alzheimer's and Pick's disease. Patients with Pick's disease have been reported to show earlier and more prominent frontal lobe signs and language disturbance than the usual patient with Alzheimer's disease, but the variation in clinical presentation is sufficient to preclude definitive identification in all but the most typical cases. A comparative study by Mendez et al. (1993) suggested that roaming behaviour (which they distinguished from wandering in that it had a more exploratory component), disinhibition and hyperoral behaviour with features of the Kluver–Bucy syndrome (Cummings & Duchen, 1981) were features of Pick's disease that could be used clinically to distinguish Pick's from Alzheimer's disease. However, at present, neuropathological examination is required for certainty (though see below for diagnostic problems). The distinction between Pick's disease and the frontal lobe degenerations (Brun, 1987; Neary et al., 1988; Brun et al., 1994) can be impossible to make on clinical grounds alone, since the fact that similar regions of the brain are affected means that there is a great overlap in the neurological phenomenology in the two groups of conditions.

Conventional CT (Munoz-Garcia & Ludwin, 1984) and MRI scanning can define the regions of cortical and subcortical atrophy, but, as will be discussed below, the pattern of cerebral atrophy is not an invariably reliable way of distinguishing between Pick's disease and Alzheimer's disease (this being the principal differential). A more metabolically based investigation, single photon emission computed tomography (SPECT) scanning, has been reported to show an anterior prominence of blood flow deficits that, in at least some cases, serves to distinguish Pick's disease from the characteristic parietal flow defects seen in Alzheimer's disease (Neary et al., 1987). Similarly, positron emission tomography (PET) (Kamo et al., 1987) scanning is also reported to demon-

strate a frontal hypometabolism markedly different from the temporo-parietal hypometabolism seen in Alzheimer's disease.

PATHOLOGICAL FINDINGS

The external appearance of the brain in classic Pick's disease is one of the most arresting in all neuropathology with, in its most archetypal manifestation, a remarkable degree of cortical atrophy that is severe enough to have attracted the description 'knife blade' atrophy (Fig. 8.1). In addition to being very pronounced, the atrophy is also geographically restricted, being confined to the frontal and temporal lobes and it is this circumscription that has given rise to the alternative designation of lobar atrophy. The unaffected regions in Pick's disease are also conspicuous. Although most of the temporal lobe is atrophic, there is conspicuous sparing of the posterior two thirds of the superior temporal gyrus, the occipital lobe and, in most of the cases, the parietal lobe.

As illustrated in Fig. 8.1 this pattern of selective cortical atrophy produces a readily recognizable appearance but it is important to appreciate that, although eminently recognizable, this gross appearance is not diagnostic. To external examination and gross inspection, occasional cases of Alzheimer's disease have sufficiently pronounced frontal or fronto-temporal atrophy to closely resemble the lobar atrophy of classic Pick's disease (Joachim, Morris & Schoene, 1986). This similarity can extend to apparent preservation of the posterior two-thirds of the superior temporal gyrus. In these cases microscopic examination quickly gives the lie to the diagnosis of Pick's disease, and shows both that the disease is much more widespread than the gross appearance would seem to indicate and that the microscopic features are an indication of Alzheimer's disease with numerous plaques and tangles. However, it is worth remembering that there are a few cases in which the features of both Alzheimer's and Pick's disease can be present in the same brain (Smith & Lantos, 1968).

Analyses of the variation in gross appearance of the brain in Pick's disease (van Mansvelt 1954; Lüers & Spatz, 1957) suggest that the atrophy is symmetrical in about one-third of the cases, and that in the asymmetrical cases the left hemisphere is more affected about three times more frequently than the right. In relation to the balance of atrophy between the frontal and temporal lobes, in just over half the cases both frontal and temporal lobes were affected, the frontal lobes only a quarter of the time and the temporal lobes only in about a fifth of the cases. Although the atrophy is usually

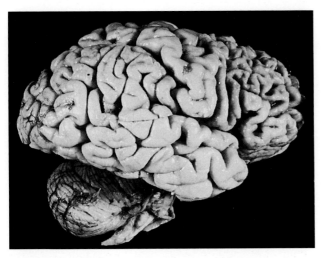

Fig. 8.1. External appearance of a brain with Pick's disease. Compared to the usual appearance of a case of Alzheimer's disease, the atrophy is notably focal cf. Fig. 3.4. In this particular case the atrophy is essentially confined to the frontal lobes, the temporal lobes being spared.

thought of as being restricted to the frontal and temporal lobes, there are a small number of well-described cases that show atrophic changes in the parietal lobe (Cambier *et al.*, 1981; Lang *et al.*, 1994). The supramarginal and angular gyri are the most usually affected. The marked atrophy is accompanied by loss of brain weight, which often falls below 1000 g (Sjögren, Sjögren & Lindgren, 1952).

Brain slices amply confirm the presence of selective atrophy with marked attenuation of the cortical ribbon in the affected regions of cortex and an equally conspicuous sparing of some regions of the cortex (Fig. 8.2). Perhaps the most noticeable sparing occurs in the superior temporal gyrus where the atrophy of the middle temporal gyrus on one side and the insular cortex on the other emphasizes the preservation of the intervening superior temporal gyrus (Fig. 8.3). Outside of the frontal and temporal regions, the anterior cingulate gyrus may also be atrophic. Of the subcortical nuclei, the amygdala is probably the most frequently atrophic in those cases with temporal lobe degeneration. There is no readily evident scheme that would explain the character of this selectivity. As has been remarked by many authors, including Pick himself, many of the atrophic regions are in association cortex and are also among the later developing parts of the cortex. However, the frequent and severe involvement of the hippocampus and parahippocampal gyrus in Pick's disease indicates that this can hardly be a sufficient explanation.

Elsewhere in the brain, the basal ganglia are some-times obviously atrophic (Akelatis, 1944; Kosaka *et al.*, 1991). This can affect the caudate and putamen and be sufficiently severe to produce a concave outline similar to that seen in advanced Huntington's disease. Atrophy of the basal ganglia is also readily identified on CT scans of the brain (Munoz-Garcia & Ludwin, 1984). Cases have also been described where there is atrophy of the

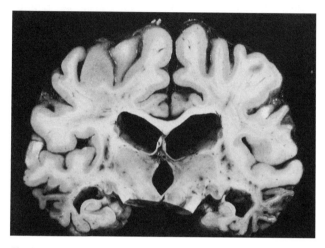

Fig. 8.3. More posterior transverse section of a case of Pick's disease with prominent temporal lobe atrophy. The Superior temporal gyrus is notably spared, but the middle and inferior temporal gyri are very atrophic.

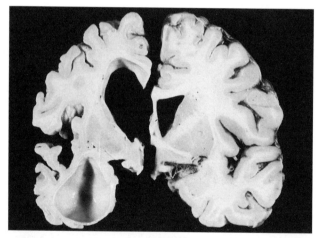

Fig. 8.4. Comparison of the proportions of a slice of normal brain (R) with that of a case of Pick's disease (L) with frontal and temporal atrophy at almost the same anteroposterior level. The extreme dilatation of the temporal pole of the lateral ventricle in this case of Pick's disease is very conspicuous, but the frontal horn of the lateral ventricle is also very dilated.

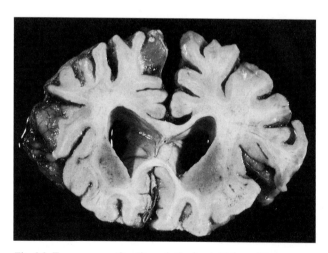

Fig. 8.2. Transverse section through the frontal lobes of the case illustrated in Fig. 8.1. showing marked widening of the sulci and expension of the frontal horns of the lateral ventricles.

caudate and globus pallidus, but not the putamen (Akelatis, 1944). Elsewhere in the brain there may be obvious pallor in the substantia nigra (Hori *et al.*, 1983). In their survey of 32 cases from the University Hospital for Chronic Nervous Diseases in Geneva, Tissot, Constantindis and Richard (1975) noted that atrophy of the basal ganglia and degeneration of the substantia nigra was more frequent in the cases with a predominantly frontal lobe degeneration.

Probably because of the severity of the cortical destruction there is very extensive loss of white matter from the affected lobes. The texture of the white matter is rubbery as a result of the subcortical gliosis. In appearance, the white matter of the affected lobes is reduced in volume and has a granular and often translucent appearance that is a result of the axonal degeneration and reduction in density of parenchymal elements. The gross reduction in volume of the white matter is reflected in a correspondingly dramatic degree of ventricular dilatation of the frontal and/or temporal horns of the lateral ventricles (Fig. 8.4).

Microscopically, the affected areas of cortex show severe neuronal loss and reactive gliosis (Fig. 8.5). In the less severely affected regions of cortex the neuronal loss is most evident in the outer layers and the loss of neurones has been described (Vogt, 1928; Schiffer, 1955) as starting in layer 3 of the cortex and then progressing to layers 2 and 5 with increasing severity of damage. However, there are considerable variations from this pattern and it does not provide a reliable diagnostic

guide, although a recent comparison of cortical changes in Alzheimer's disease and Pick's disease showed that, in Pick's disease, there was extensive neuronal loss from all layers of the cortex which appeared to be most severe in layer III (Arnold, Hyman & Van Hoesen, 1994). In the most severely affected cortex the neuronal loss is so complete as to preclude identification of the normal cortical architecture. Accompanying the neuronal loss is a marked fibrillary astrocytosis that extends through the cortex and into the subcortical white matter. In regions of severe atrophy the degree of attenuation of the neuropil is very marked. The end result is a markedly atrophic cortex in which there may be very few recognizable neurons embedded in a very spongiotic glial meshwork (Fig. 8.6). In the context of such severe damage it comes as no surprise that there is a profound reduction in the number of both presynaptic terminals and dendritic spines. In many respects this appearance is that of 'end-stage cortical degeneration' that is not particularly revealing from either a diagnostic or neurochemical standpoint. The severity of cortical neuronal loss is reflected in a correspondingly severe axonal loss in the white matter where there may be only occasional preserved myelinated axons (Fig. 8.7).

In addition to the cortical atrophy, a proportion of cases also show atrophy of the basal ganglia. A number of studies have examined this phenomenon with estimates of its frequency that have ranged from 40 to 72%. A recent study by Kosaka and colleagues (1991) of an autopsy series of 41 cases from Japan (all of which were

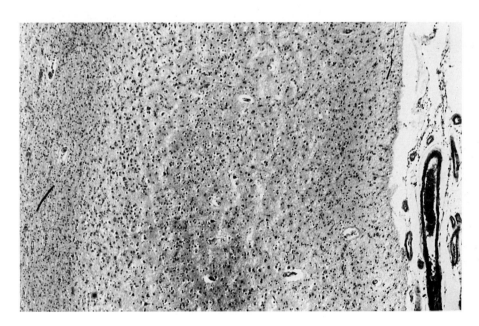

Fig. 8.5. Low power micrograph of an haematoxylin and eosin stained section of the cortical ribbon in a case of Pick's disease (H&E ×50). There is considerable narrowing of the cortical ribbon and attenuation of the density of the neuropil.

sporadic) 8(19.5%) showed severe degeneration, 9(22%) moderate and 15(36.5%) mild degeneration of the striatonigropallidal system. In all, 17 of the 41 cases exhibited definite degeneration of this system. In accordance with the other studies they found that the caudate nucleus was most severely affected. Within the putamen, the dorsomedial part adjacent to the internal capsule was the most severely degenerate and in the globus pallidus, the dorsomedial part adjacent to the internal capsule was again the most vulnerable. The general

histological appearance of the degeneration is also not altogether dissimilar from that seen in Huntington's disease (Kosaka *et al.*, 1991). There is gross loss of neurons from the putamen and caudate and a marked reactive astrocytosis. The neuronal degeneration is reflected in the accompanying degeneration of the pencil fibres that form the output of the putamenal and caudate neurones to the globus pallidus. Some cases of Alzheimer's disease also show marked atrophy of the caudate and putamen but in Alzheimer's disease there is

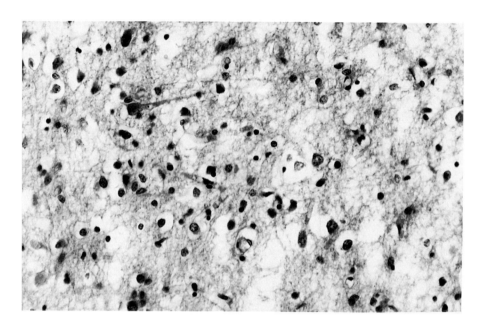

Fig. 8.6. Higher power view of the atrophic cortex. There is very severe neuronal loss and marked reactive astrocytosis. The attenuation of the density of cell processes in the neuropil, which is a reflection of the degree of neuronal loss, is very marked. (H&E ×125)

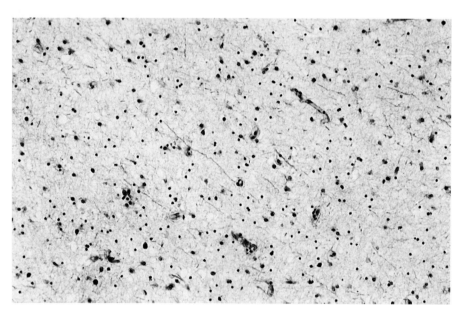

Fig. 8.7. White matter in Pick's disease. The loss of neurons from the cortical ribbon is also reflected in the loss of axons in the white matter. In this micrograph, taken from frontal lobe white matter of the same case as is illustrated in Figs. 8.5 and 8.6, only occasional preserved myelinated axons are present. (LFB/CV ×50)

a loss of neuropil rather than neurones, and the atrophy has a very different microscopic appearance with an apparently increased density of neurones and no marked degeneration of the pencil fibres. It is likely that, in Alzheimer's disease, the atrophy is a reflection of loss of incoming fibres.

The degeneration in the substantia nigra tends to parallel that in the striatum and Pick bodies or Pick's cells may be formed. Lewy bodies and neurofibrillary tangles are not usually present. Within the substantia nigra the medial and the central portions are reputed to be most affected (Kosaka et al., 1991), and the pars reticulata to a greater extent than the pars compacta.

There are conflicting reports about changes in large cholinergic neurones of the basal nucleus of Meynert (nbM) in Pick's disease. Tagliavini and Pilleri (1983) reported five cases of Pick's disease with no significant loss of neurons from the nbM. Uhl et al. (1983), by contrast, showed depletion of nbM neurones to 24 and 31% of control values in two cases, a finding echoed in a single case by Rogers, Brogan and Mirra (1985) and in two cases of 'classic' and one of 'generalized' Picks disease by Munoz-Garcia and Ludwin (1984) where the maximum neuronal density of the nbM was reduced to approximately one-third of that in five age-matched control subjects.

Pick bodies and Pick's cells

The diagnostic histological features of Pick's disease are Pick bodies and Pick cells. Pick bodies are sharply circumscribed generally spherical neuronal intracyto-plasmic inclusions that are slightly basophilic on H&E stains and strongly argyrophilic (Figs. 8.8, 8.9). Pick's cells are found in about half of all cases of lobar atrophy. They are neurons in which the cell body has become swollen and pear shaped with the nucleus usually displaced to one side of the ballooned cytoplasm (Fig. 8.10). With Cresyl violet (Nissl) the expanded cytoplasm remains unstained and residual Nissl substance is displaced to the periphery of the cell. This change is usually seen in large pyramidal neurones, but similar changes can occur in neurones in the basal ganglia and brain stem.

Tissot and colleagues (1975) found that Pick bodies tended to occur preferentially in those cases where there was degeneration in the temporal lobe. Within the temporal lobe, Pick bodies were found most easily in the medial temporal lobe and hippocampus, where they may be present in both the pyramidal cell layer and, most conspicuously, in the neurons of the dentate

fasciculus (Brion et al., 1973; Constantinidis, 1985). This preference for the dentate fasciculus sharply distin-guishes Pick bodies from Alzheimer neurofibrillary tangles which rarely involve the dentate gyrus, although Dickson et al. (1986a) report Pick body-like inclusions in the dentate fascia in Alzheimer's disease. By contrast with Pick bodies, Pick's cells were more frequent in cases where the principal burden of degeneration fell upon the frontal lobes.

Immunocytochemically, Pick bodies are positive for ubiquitin, tau, paired helical filament, neurofilament and Alz 50 antibodies (Perry et al., 1987; Rasool & Selkoe, 1985; Lowe et al., 1988; Love et al., 1988, Munoz-Garcia & Ludwin, 1984; Ulrich et al., 1987) and thus have many of the staining characteristics of neurofibril-lary tangles. However, unlike tangles, extracellular Pick bodies are not seen. It appears that the degeneration of the Pick body-containing neurone results in the dissol-ution of the Pick body. Pick's cells express neurofila-ment (Dickson et al., 1986b) tau and ubiquitin epitopes. Recently, αB crystallin, a protein with a close structural resemblance to small heat shock proteins but with a currently uncertain function, has been shown to be present in Pick cells and in ballooned neurones in several other neurodegenerative diseases, as well as in spheroids adjacent to cerebral infarctions (Lowe et al., 1992; Kato et al., 1992).

With the electron microscope, despite their sharply circumscribed appearance on light microscopy, the Pick body does not have a limiting membrane (Re-wcastle & Ball, 1968; Schochet, Lampert & Lindenberg, 1978). Unsurprisingly in the light of its immunochemi-cal reactions, ultrastructural examination of the Pick body discloses a mixture of filaments, paired helical filaments, and microtubules. Electron microscopic examination of Pick's cells shows many elements simi-lar to those seen in Pick bodies together with granular material and some degenerate organelles Schochet, Lampert & Earle, 1968; Wisniewski, Coblenz & Terry, 1972; Munoz-Garcia & Ludwin, 1984). As with the Pick bodies, they are not present in all cases that show the typical gross appearance of lobar atrophy, and are not usually seen in the most severely degenerated regions of the cortex.

The pathogenetic significance of Pick's cells is un-clear. Their resemblance to chromatolytic neurones has been frequently commented upon, and there has been considerable discussion of the similarities between the ballooned neurones in Pick's disease and rather similar appearing cells seen in corticobasal degeneration (neuronal achromasia) (Gibb, Luthert & Marsden, 1989), and ballooned cells can also be seen in Creutzfeldt–Jakob disease (Nakazato *et al.*, 1990), Alzheimer's disease (Dickson *et al.*, 1986*a,b*) and in a small number of cases of the frontal lobe degeneration with superficial neuronal loss (Brun, 1987). Lippa *et al.* (1991) also described the presence of what were called ach-

romasic neurones in a case of primary progressive aphasia.

NEUROCHEMISTRY

As with other areas of research into Pick's disease, the rarity of the condition has been a significant impediment to systematic study and information is very sparse (Yates

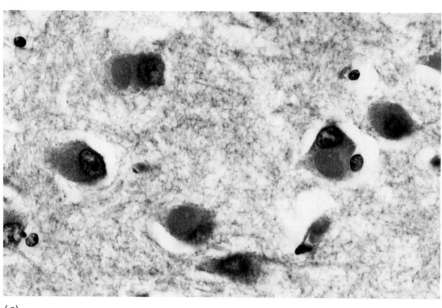

(*a*)

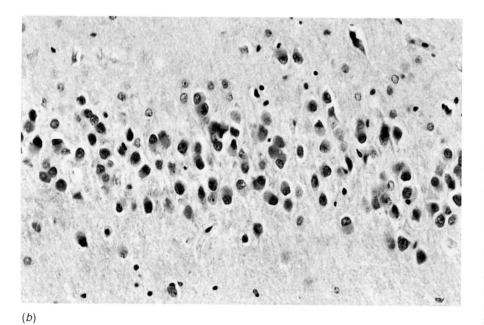

(*b*)

Fig. 8.8. (*a*) Pick bodies visible in an H&E stained section of hippocampal pyramidal neurons. The Pick bodies are mildly basophilic sharply circumscribed cytoplasmic bodies. H&E × 250

(*b*) Pick bodies in the neurons of the dentate fasciculus of the hippocampus in an H&E stained section. At low power, the neurons have much more cytoplasm than is usually the case and have become more spread out. (H&E × 125)

et al., 1980). Cortical choline acetyl transferase has been reported to be normal in Pick's disease, a finding that accords well within the reported preservation of the cholinergic neurones of the basal nucleus of Meynert. Somatostatin and glutamic acid decarboxylase are also reported to be preserved.

PROBLEMS IN PICK'S DISEASE

Definition
In our current state of ignorance, no real discussion about the aetiology or pathophysiology of Pick's disease can occur. However, the lack of substantive information has not proved to be a bar to pathological debate which

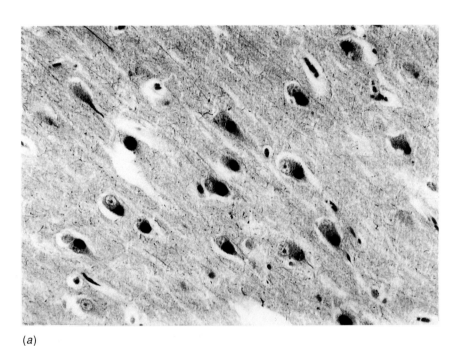

(a)

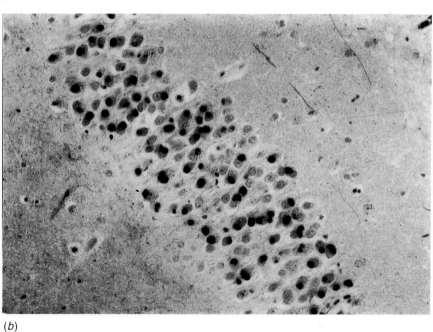

(b)

Fig. 8.9. In silver stained sections of (a) hippocampal pyramidal cells. (Cross × 125) (b) dentate fasciculus neurons the Pick bodies are densely stained and very conspicuous. (Cross × 125)

has focused on the question of what features are necessary for the diagnosis of Pick's disease. The debate about definition, can be summarized as 'Can you make the diagnosis of Pick's disease without the presence of either Pick cells or Pick bodies?'. As has been described, the features of classic Pick's disease can be summarized as gross frontal and temporal atrophy with microscopic findings of severe neuronal loss and gliosis with Pick cells and Pick bodies. Some authors consider that, to be Pick's disease, the case must exhibit one of the two eponymous features of the disease, Pick bodies or Pick cells. This school of thought holds that, since the other gross and microscopic features of Pick's disease can all be found in other conditions, their presence alone is insufficient for a diagnosis of Pick's disease and hence only those cases that exhibit either Pick bodies or Pick cells can be accepted as the genuine article (Heston, White & Mastri, 1987; Muramaya *et al.*, 1990). There is, undoubtedly, a certain rigour about this position that commends itself to many. Also, given our current ignorance about the aetiology of the disease and the pathophysiology of Pick bodies and/or cells, it can be argued that there is no reason to enlarge the concept of Pick's disease to include cases that do not possess the specific features. However, there are cases which have the focal atrophy and severe neuronal loss found in Pick's disease but lack either Pick bodies or Pick cells, and these cases have to be categorized somehow. Such cases are often called non-Pick lobar atrophy but other authors (Hori *et al.*, 1983; Winkleman & Book, 1949),

relying on the distribution of the atrophy and the absence of diagnostic features of other dementing conditions, would include them in the diagnostic category of Pick's disease. Most take up an intermediate position that classifies the cases into those without Pick bodies and cells along with Pick's disease, but gives some alternate designation such as 'atypical' Pick's disease. The most elaborate of such classifications is that of Constantinidis *et al.* (1974) who divided Pick's disease into groups A, B and C. In Group A, both Pick bodies and Pick's cells are present, Group B had only Pick's cells and predominantly frontal atrophy while in Group C, neither Pick bodies or Pick cells was present. Group C was, in fact, further subdivided into Group C1, where the atrophy was restricted to the temporal lobe and Group C2, with more widespread cortical atrophy and involvement of the basal ganglia and thalamus.

A corollary of the requirement for the presence of Pick cells and Pick bodies before the diagnosis can be made is that there must be something pathophysiologically specific about Pick bodies and/or Pick cells. Many neuropathologists can only reluctantly be induced to accept the idea that the Pick body might be no more than a sort of cytoplasmic dustbin. However, as far as can be detected, there is no specific morphological component in the Pick body and the variety of ubiquitin associated degenerate organelles and paired helical filaments seen within it has a disturbing resemblance to what might be expected in cellular garbage. Although these observations seem to suggest that not too much weight should

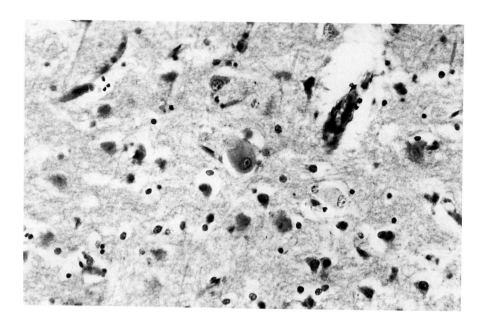

Fig. 8.10. A Pick's cell showing the characteristic ballooned eosinophilic cytoplasm. (H&E × 125)

be placed on the presence or absence of Pick bodies, they are not entirely conclusive, since their occurrence could reflect a systematic defect in the turnover and processing of cytoplasmic organelles. Further, as noted by Hulette and Crain (1992), unlike neurofibrillary tangles, Pick bodies do not remain present in the extracellular space after the death of the cell. Their absence at autopsy in cases of 'lobar atrophy' or 'atypical Pick's disease' may therefore not be definitive evidence that they were not present at some time during the disease.

Perhaps the most persuasive argument for the inclusion of cases with the general macroscopic and microscopic features of Pick's disease, but without Pick cells or Pick bodies, into the general category of Pick's disease is the fact that cases of 'Pick's disease' without the specific inclusions (the non-Pick lobar atrophy of the splitters) have similar clinical features and a similar epidemiological profile as the cases with Pick bodies and/or Pick cells. This would seem to suggest that they all belong to one group of cases. In the present state of ignorance, there is no unequivocally right answer to the question of whether the cases of lobar atrophy without the specific inclusions can, or cannot, be included in the category of Pick's disease. Hulette and Crain (1992) prefer to call such cases lobar atrophy without Pick's bodies or Pick's cells. Our position is that we would include such cases in the category of Pick's disease, although with the rider that neither Pick bodies nor Pick's cells were seen. Whatever designation is used, the most important aspect is that it should clearly indicate what is present on the slides.

RELATED CONDITIONS
Although the diagnosis and neuropathological characteristics of classical and atypical Pick's disease are generally agreed upon, there are still a number of nosologic issues that need to be considered.

The Pick–Alzheimer spectrum and hereditary dysphasic dementia
One clinico-pathological concept that has not really come to fruition is that of the 'Pick–Alzheimer spectrum' which was most forcefully elucidated by Cole and Banker (Cole, Wright & Bank, 1979; Morris et al., 1984) together with their colleagues. In this concept, the pathology of hereditary dysphasic dementia and some other rare dementing diseases that exhibit some of the features of both Alzheimer's and Pick's disease were considered to be intermediate cases that could act as a conceptual bridge between Alzheimer's and Pick's dis-

ease. There are considerable attractions to this idea, not least because of the substantial morphological variation that is seen in the various causes of cortical degenerative dementia. However, it is also possible that many of these apparent similarities are merely a result of the lack of real pathophysiological specificity in so many of the morphological features of the degenerative dementias. Neuronal loss, for example, can occur as the end result of a number of different pathophysiological processes, and gliosis is probably largely a reactive change rather than a primary inciting event. Local atrophy, upon which considerable diagnostic reliance is sometimes placed, is known to be unreliable. Even neurofibrillary tangles and Pick bodies, which seem to be rather specific morphological entities, are likely to be a considerable way along the pathophysiological process and therefore rather less aetiologically specific than might at first sight be thought (Dickson et al., 1986a,b). This is most clearly exemplified by the neurofibrillary tangle, which is known to occur in a variety of diseases, notably Alzheimer's disease, progressive supranuclear palsy, subacute sclerosing panencephalitis (SSPE) and Gerstmann–Sträussler syndrome (GSS) that have clearly different aetiologies.

As regards the relationship between Pick's disease and Alzheimer's disease, the concept of a Pick–Alzheimer spectrum has become rather more difficult to sustain with the widespread recognition of amyloid deposition as an integral part of the pathophysiological process in Alzheimer's disease (Selkoe 1994). Although not clearly established as the cause of all cases of Alzheimer's disease, the association of a specific amyloid protein with the neurofibrillary pathology of Alzheimer's disease clearly distinguishes this disease from both the 'non-specific' neuronal degenerations and Pick's disease, neither of which is associated with amyloid deposition. Although not universally accepted, the amyloid hypothesis of Alzheimer's disease provides a rather specific pathophysiological process to account for the development of the neurofibrillary pathology of Alzheimer's disease. In so doing, it, so to speak, removes one end of the Pick–Alzheimer spectrum.

The conceptual bridge in the Pick–Alzheimer spectrum is seen as hereditary dysphasic dementia. In this condition there is a severe and usually asymmetric fronto-temporal atrophy that manifests microscopically in correspondingly severe neuronal loss and a fibrillary gliosis that extends through the cortex into the underlying white matter. The severe depletion of the neuropil in such cases gives a spongiform appearance to the affected cortex that to some degree resembles the severe cortical damage seen in Pick's disease. However, in the same way that severe kidney disease from a variety of causes can result in a rather similar histological appearance of the so-called 'end-stage kidney', the severity of the cortical damage in these cases is such that it would seem unwise to ascribe too much significance to the details of the microscopic appearances of 'end-stage cerebral cortex'. Most of the cases also exhibit degeneration of the substantia nigra, similar to that which occurs in some cases of Pick's disease. However, the familial character, clinical features and progression of these cases is quite distinct from most cases of Pick's disease and, on these grounds, it seems sensible to distinguish them from Pick's disease until, and unless, a clear aetiological connection between the two conditions is demonstrated.

Slowly progressive aphasia with and without dementia

The exclusion of hereditary dysphasic dementia from the discussion does not resolve all the taxonomic difficulty raised by the focal atrophies. It has been suggested that Pick's disease could have a relationship to the cases of slowly progressive aphasia without dementia such as those described clinically by Mesulam (1982) and Mesulam and Weintraub (1992) and pathologically by Pogacar & Williams (1984) Green et al. (1990) Kempler et al. (1990), Graf-Redford et al. (1990), Benson & Zaias (1991), Holland et al. (1985), Salmon et al. (1989), Mesulam (1982) Calpan and Richardson (1986), Mehler et al. (1987), Snowden et al. (1992). In the cases described by Kirschner (1987), although there is focal cortical atrophy, the degree of cortical damage is much less and the principal burden of neuronal loss falls in layer 2 of the cortex. The superficial spongiosus generated by this neuronal loss has many similarities to that described in the so-called frontal atrophies, and it may be that these cases can be thought of more appropriately as geographically restricted forms of this condition. A possible relationship to cortical–basal ganglionic degeneration (see below) is postulated in the case described by Lippa et al. (1991) where there were numerous achromatic neurons in the affected cortex. Kobayashi et al. (1990) described a single apparently non-familial case of a progressive dysphasic dementia with focal cortical atrophy that affected the pars opercularis and triangularis and, to a lesser extent, the inferior parietal lobe of the left hemisphere. In the degenerate regions of cortex there was neuronal loss affecting all the cortical layer and a fibrillary gliosis that extended through the degenerate cortex and into the immediately subcortical white mat-

ter although the deep white matter was preserved. Occasional ballooned neurones were present in the degenerate cortex, but nothing resembling a Pick body was identified. There was gliosis but no apparent neuronal loss in the hippocampus and amygdala bilaterally. In addition, the left substantia nigra had marked depletion of neurones from the pars compacta. Kobayashi did not consider that this case could fit into the spectrum of Pick's disease principally because of the lack of the characteristic pattern of atrophy, the absence of Pick's cells, and the relative preservation of the deep lobar white matter.

Mendez and Zander (1991), examining cases of dementia presenting with a period of progressive language impairment concluded that the group was pathologically heterogenous. This was confirmed by Scheltens, Rivka and Kamphorst (1994) who reported a case of primary progressive aphasia with 'non-specific' cortical degeneration and reviewed published reports of 15 other cases of primary progressive aphasia where pathological findings are included. Of the 15 cases, 4 had pathology compatible with Alzheimer's disease, 3 with Pick's disease and there were 'non-specific' changes in the remaining 8. This seems to indicate that the clinical syndrome of primary progressive aphasia is not pathologically specific and that the diagnosis will, in most cases, have to depend on post-mortem neuropathological examination.

Corticobasal degeneration

Another disease that has been linked to Pick's disease has had a variety of designations including corticodentatonigral degeneration with neuronal achromasia but is now most commonly called corticobasal degeneration (Rebeiz, Kolodny & Richardson, 1968; Gibb et al., 1989; Riley et al., 1990; Lang, Riley & Bergeron, 1994). The link between Pick's disease and these cases is the presence of ballooned (achromasic) neurones that have a very similar microscopic appearance to Pick's cells. In respect of the distribution of achromasic cells, there are both similarities and differences to Pick's disease. The major difference is in the cortical distribution. In Pick's disease, the Pick's cells are fronto-temporal (most frequently frontal) while, in corticobasal degeneration, the principal burden of disease falls on the rolandic and parietal regions. However, the substantia nigra can be affected in both categories of disease and recent findings indicate that there are also considerable similarities in tau containing glial inclusions found in the two conditions (Chin & Goldman, 1996). Notwithstanding the similarity of appearance of the Pick/achromasic cells, argyrophilic Pick bodies do not seem to occur in the neuronal achromasias. Another major difference between the two conditions is the absence in corticobasal degeneration of the very severe damage to the white matter underlying the degenerate cortex that is so characteristic of Pick's disease. Given the significant similarities in microscopic appearance between Pick's disease and cortico-basal degeneration, it is perhaps worth emphasizing the differences in the gross appearance of the brain in the two conditions. In typical cortico-basal degeneration the atrophy is concentrated in the pre- and post-central gyri, while that in Pick's disease is fronto-temporal.

It also needs to be emphasized that the usual clinical syndrome associated with corticobasal degeneration (neuronal achromasia) is that of a progressive motor and cortical sensory disorder with dementia as a late and inconstant finding. This is quite different from the progressive dementia of Pick's disease. However, Lerner et al. (1992) have described two cases of cortico-basal ganglionic degeneration presenting with dementia and further cases have been encountered masquerading as a fronto-temporal dementia with moderate fronto-temporal atrophy on gross examination of the brain (Jackson, Lennox & Lowe, 1996). The other exceptions are the very rare cases of Pick's disease with parietal predominance (Cambier et al., 1981; Lang et al., 1994). In these cases, the clinical syndrome in Pick's disease can mimic corticobasal degeneration. From this it can be seen that there are cases where the microscopic pathological findings and the clinical picture do not provide a clear differentiation between the two conditions (Feany, Mattiace & Dickson, 1996). It may be that re-evaluation of cases of Pick's disease without Pick bodies, and particularly those cases with degeneration of the substantia nigra, will show that there is a need to widen the spectrum of what is called cortico-basal degeneration and correspondingly narrow that of Pick's disease. However, it does not seem reasonable to group corticobasal degeneration and Pick's disease together on the basis of a perceived similarity of microscopic appearance until, and unless, the pathogenesis of these ballooned cells in the two conditions is shown to have a similar basis. Indeed, using the analogy of the neurofibrillary tangle which is present in a number of different diseases of unequivocally different aetiology, it can be argued that, even if achromasic neurones and Pick's cells can be shown to be identical, this finding alone would not provide a reason to conclude that there is any underlying aetiological or pathophysiological

relationship between the two conditions (see also Chapter 10).

Frontal lobe degeneration of non-Alzheimer's type

The final major group of diseases with a possible link to Pick's disease are the cases described as frontal lobe degeneration of non-Alzheimer type by Brun (1987), Neary et al. (1988) and Neary (1990a). Pathologically, these patients show mild to moderate atrophy of frontal and temporal lobes with loss of cortical neurons, moderate reactive astrocytosis and a characteristic spongy degeneration affecting the upper layers of the affected cortex. As with Pick's disease itself (Brion et al., 1980; Sam et al., 1991; Hamada et al., 1995), some cases are apparently associated with motor neurone disease (Salazar et al., 1983; Horoupian et al., 1984; Neary et al., 1990b; Caselli et al., 1993).

In 1994, the Lund and Manchester groups (Brun et al., 1994) attempted to marry the so-called frontal lobe degeneration and Pick's disease in a consensus statement in which they advocated a definition of an entity they called fronto-temporal dementia. Pathologically this would include a 'frontal lobe degeneration type' and a 'Pick type'. The authors neatly side-step problems with the definition of Pick's disease by suggesting that 'Cases of frontotemporal dementia with a similar level of astrocytosis (to that seen in Pick's disease) but without inclusions or inflated neurons should be best included in this Pick-type category pending a more definitive histological identification' The difficulty with this concept is that it is driven by clinical phenomenology which is not pathologically specific. Since both Pick's disease and frontal lobe degeneration affect the frontal and temporal lobe almost exclusively, it is not surprising that they have many clinical features in common. Pathologically, however, the findings in the cerebral cortex are really quite different in detail and severity. In frontotemporal dementia, the morphological changes are most pronounced in the upper layers of the cortex with a rather characteristic microvacuolation of the neuropil in layers I–III, and the overall impression is that the neuropathological changes are relatively inconspicuous in relation to the severity of the clinical syndrome. By contrast, as has been described, in Pick's disease and 'Pick-type lobar atrophy' the whole thickness of the cortical ribbon is severely degenerate with massive neuronal loss and very marked reactive astrocytosis. The severity of the pathological change is also quite commensurate with the severity and duration of the clinical symptoms. On the basis of personal experience and review of the literature it does not appear that there are many 'transitional' cases where there is significant uncertainty about the neuropathological category in which the case belongs and there is therefore no compelling evidence of a pathological spectrum with typical Pick's disease at one end and archetypal frontal lobe degeneration at the other. Consequently, until a more specific aetiological connection between the conditions can be demonstrated, there does not seem to be any particular benefit to be gained from amalgamating them conceptually except in the sense that it may ease their distinction from other causes of dementia such as Alzheimer's disease where the burden of disease is more widely distributed in the brain (see also Chapter 10).

REFERENCES

Akelatis A (1944) Atrophy of the basal ganglia in Pick's disease: a clinico-pathologic study. *Arch Neurol Psychiat* 51: 27–34.

Alzheimer A (1911) Über einenartige Krankheitsfälle des späteren alters. *Z Gesamte Neurol Psychiate* 4: 356–85.

Arnold SE, Hyman BT, Van Hoesen GW (1994) Neuropathologic changes in the temporal pole in Alzheimer's disease and Pick's disease. *Arch Neurol* 51: 145–50.

Benson DF, Zaias BW (1991) Progressive aphasia: a case with post-mortem correlation. *Neuropsychiat Neuropsychol Behav Neurol* 4: 215–23.

Brion S, Mikol J, Psimaris A (1973) Recent findings in Pick's disease. In Zimmerman HM (ed) Progress in Neuropathology, vol 2. Grune & Stratton, New York, pp 421–45.

Brion S, Psimaras A, Chevalier JF *et al* (1980) L'association maladie de Pick et sclerose laterale amyotrophique. *L'Encephale* 6: 259–86.

Brun A (1987) Frontal lobe degeneration of non-Alzheimer type. I. Neuropathology. *Arch Gerontol Geriatr* 6: 193–208.

Brun A, Englund B, Gustafson L, Passant U, Mann DMA, Neary D, Snowden JS (1994) Clinical and neuropathological criteria for frontotemporal dementia. *J Neurol Neurosurg Psychiat* 57: 416–18.

Calpan LR, Richardson EP Jr (1986) Case records of the Massachusetts General Hospital (case 16 –1986) *N Engl J Mèd* 314: 1101–11.

Cambier J, Masson M, Dairou R, Henin D (1981) Etude anatomoclinque d'une form pariétale de maladie de Pick. *Rev Neurol (Paris)* 147: 693–740.

Caselli RJ, Windebank AJ, Peterson RC, *et al.* (1993) Rapidly progressive aphasic dementia and motor neurone disease. *Ann Neurol* 33: 200–7.

Chin DS-M, Goldman JE. (1996) Glial inclusions in CNS degenerative diseases. *J Neuropathol Exp Neurol* 55: 499–508.

Cole M, Wright D, Banker B (1979) Familial aphasia: the Pick-Alzheimer Spectrum. In Duvoisin RC (ed) *Transactions of the American Neurological Association*, Vol 104. Springer, New York, pp 175–9.

Constantinidis J (1985) Pick dementia: anatomoclinical correlations and pathophysiological considerations. In Modern approaches to the dementias, part I: etiology and pathophysiology. Rose FC, (ed) *Interdisciplinary Topics in Gerontology*. Vol 19, Karger, Basel, pp 72–97.

Constantinidis J, Richard J, Tissot R (1974) Pick's Disease: histological and clinical correlations. *Eur Neurol* 11: 208–17.

Cummings JL, Duchen LW (1981) Kluver–Bucy syndrome in Pick disease: Clinical and pathologic correlations. *Neurology* 31: 1415–22.

Delay J, Brion S (1962) *Les Démences Tardives* Mason, Paris.

Dickson DW, Yen S-H, Suzuki KI, Davies P, Garcia JH, Hirano A (1986a) Ballooned neurons in selected neurodegenerative diseases contain phosphorylated neurofilament epitopes. *Acta Neuropath (Berl)* 71: 216–23.

Dickson DW, Yen S-H, Houruopian DS (1986b) Pick body-like inclusions in the dentate fascia of the hippocampus in Alzheimer's disease. *Acta Neuropathy (Berl)* 71: 38–45.

Esiri MM, Oppenheimer DR (1989) *Diagnostic Neuropathology* Blackwell Scientific Publications. London.

Feany MB. Mattiace LA, Dickson DW. (1996) Neuropathologic overlap of progressive supranuclear palsy, Pick's disease and corticobasal degeneration. *J Neuropathol Exp Neurol* 55: 53–67.

Gibb WRG, Luthert PJ, Marsden CD (1989) Corticobasal degeneration. *Brain* 112: 1171–92.

Graf-Redford NR, Damasio AR, Hyman BT *et al* (1990) Progressive aphasia in a patient with Pick's disease: a neuropsychologic, radiologic and anatomic study. *Neurology* 40: 620–6.

Green J, Morris JC, Sandson J, McKeel DW Jr, Miller JW (1990) Progressive aphasia: a precursor of global dementia? *Neurology* 40: 394–405.

Groen JJ, Endtz LJ (1982) Hereditary Pick's disease: second reexamination of a large family and discussion of other hereditary cases with particular reference to electroencephalography and computerised tomography. *Brain* 105: 443–60.

Hamada K, Fukazawa T, Yanagihara K, Yoshida K, Hamada T, Yoshimura N, Tashiro K (1995) Dementia with ALS features and diffuse Pick bodylike inclusions (atypical Pick's disease). *Clin Neuropathol* 14: 1–6.

Heston LL, White JA, Mastri AR (1987) Pick's disease: clinical genetics and natural history. *Arch Gen Psychiat* 44: 409–11.

Holland AL, McBurney DH, Moossy J, Reinmuth OM (1985) The dissolution of language in Pick's disease with neurofibrillary tangles: a case study. *Brain Lang* 24: 36–58.

Hori A, Volles E, Witzke R, Spaar FW (1983) Pick's disease of early onset with neurologic symptomatology, rapid course and nigrostriatal degeneration. *Clin Neuropathol* 2: 8–15.

Horoupian DS, Thal L, Katzman R, *et al.* (1984) Dementia and motor neuron disease: Morphometric, biochemical and Golgi studies. *Ann Neurol* 16: 305–13.

Hulette CM, Crain B (1992) Lobar atrophy without Pick bodies. *Clin Neuropathol* 11: 151–6.

Jackson M, Lennox G, Lowe J. (1996) Isolated fronto-temporal dementia due to cortico-basal degeneration. *Neuropathol Appl Neurobiol* in press.

Jervis GA (1971) Pick's disease In Minckler J (ed) *Pathology of the Nervous System* vol 2, McGraw-Hill, New York, pp 1395–404.

Joachim CL, Morris JH, Schoene WC (1986) Neuropathological findings in six cases of dementia with severe focal atrophy. *J Neuropathol Exp Neurol* 45: 361 (abst).

Kamo H, McGeer PL, Harrop R, McGeer EG, Calne DB, Martin WRW, Pate BD (1987) Positron emission tomography and histopathology in Pick's disease. *Neurology* 37: 439–45.

Kato S, Hirano A, Umahara T, Kato M, Herz F, Ohama E (1992) Comparative immunohistochemical study on the expression of αβ cystallin, ubiquitin and stress response protein 27 in ballooned neurons in various disorders. *Neuropathol Appl Neurobiol* 18: 335–40.

Kempler D, Metter EJ, Riege WH, Jackson CA, Benson DF, Hanson WR (1990) Slowly progressive aphasia: three cases with language, memory, CT and PET data. *J Neurol Neurosurg Psychiat* 53: 987–93.

Kirschner HS, Tanridag O, Thurman L, Whetsell WO (1987) Progressive aphasia without dementia: two cases with focal spongiform degeneration. *Ann Neurol* 22: 527–32.

Kobayashi K, Kurachi M, Gyoubu T, Fukutani Y, Inao G, Nakamura I, Yamaguchi N (1990) Progressive dysphasic dementia with localised cerebral atrophy: report of an autopsy. *Clin Neuropathol* 5: 254–61.

Kosaka K, Oyabagi S, Matsushita M, Hori A (1976) Presenile dementia with Alzheimer, Pick and Lewy body changes. *Acta Neuropathol (Berl)* 36: 221–33.

Kosaka K, Ikeda K, Kobayashi K, Mehraein P (1991) Striatopallidonigral degeneration in Pick's disease: a clinico-pathological study of 41 cases. *J Neurol* 238: 151–60.

Lang AE, Bergeron C, Pollanen MS, Ashby P (1994) Parietal Pick's disease mimicking Cortico-basal ganglionic degeneration. *Neurology* 44: 1436–40.

Lang AE, Riley DE, Bergeron C (1994) Cortical–basal ganglionic degeneration. In Calne DB (ed) *Neurodegenerative Disease.* WB Saunders, Philadelphia, pp 877–94.

Lerner A, Friedland R, Riley D *et al.* (1992) Dementia with pathological findings of cortico-basal ganglionic degeneration. *Ann Neurol* 32: 271 [abstract].

Lippa CF, Cohen R, Smith TW, Drachman DA (1991) Primary progressive aphasia with focal neuronal achromasia. *Neurology* 41: 882–6.

Love S, Saitoh T, Qijada S, Cole GM, Terry RD (1988) Alz50, ubiquitin and tau immunoreactivity of neurofibrillary tangles, Pick bodies and Lewy bodies. *J Neuropath Exp Neurol* 47: 393–405.

Lowe J, Blanchard A, Morrell K, Lennox G, Reynolds Ll, Billett M, Landon M, Mayer RJ (1988) Ubiquitin is a common factor in intermediate filament inclusion bodies of diverse type in man including those of Parkinson's disease, Pick's disease, and Alzheimer's disease, as well as Rosenthal fibres in cerebellar astrocytomas, cytoplasmic bodies in muscle and Mallory bodies in alcoholic liver disease. *J Pathol* 155: 9–15.

Lowe J, Errington DR, Lennox G, Pike I, Spendlove I, Landon M, Mayer RJ (1992) Ballooned neurons in several neurodegenerative disease and stroke contain αβ crystallin. *Neuropathol Appl Neurobiol* 18: 341–50.

Lüers T, Spatz UH (1957) Picksche Krankheit. In Lubarsch O, Henke F, Rössle R, Scholz W (eds) *Handbuch der speziellen pathologischen Anatomie und Histologie,* vol XIII 1A, Springer, Berlin, pp 614–716.

Mehler MF, Horoupian DS, Davies P, Dickson DW (1987) Reduced somatostatin-like immunoreactivity in cerebral cortex in non-familial dysphasic dementia. *Neurology* 37: 1448–53.

Mendez MF, Zander BA (1991) Dementia presenting with aphasia: clinical characteristics. *J Neurol Neurosurg Psychiat* 54: 542–5.

Mendez MF, Selwood A, Mastri AR, Frey WH (1993) Pick's disease verus Alzheimer's disease: A comparison of clinical characteristics. *Neurology* 43: 289–92.

Mesulam M-M (1982) Slowly progressive aphasia without generalised dementia. *Ann Neurol* 11: 592–8.

Mesulam M-M, Weintraub S (1992) Primary progressive aphasia: sharpening the focus on a clinical syndrome. In Boller F, Forette F, Khatchaturian Z, Poncet M, Christen Y (eds) *Heterogeneity of Alzheimer's Disease.* Springer-Verlag, Berlin, pp 43–66.

Morris JC, Cole M, Banker BQ, Wright D (1984) Hereditary dysphasic dementia and the Pick-Alzheimer spectrum. *Ann Neurol* 16: 455–66.

Munoz-Garcia D, Ludwin SK (1984) Classic and generalised variants of Pick's disease: a clinicopathological, ultrastructural and immunocytochemical comparative study. *Ann Neurol* 16: 467–80.

Muramaya S, Mori H, Ihara Y, Tomonaga M (1990) Immunocytochemical and ultrastructural studies of Pick's disease. *Ann Neurol* 27: 394–405.

Nakazato Y, Horato J, Yshia I, Hoshi S, Hasegawa M, Fukuda T (1990) Swollen cortical neurones in Creutzfelt–Jakob disease contain a phosphorylated neurofilament epitope. *J Neuropathy Exp Neurol* 49: 197–205.

Neary D, Snowden JS, Shields RA *et al* (1987) Single photon emission tomography using ^{99m}Tc-HM0PAO in the investigation of dementia. *J Neurol Neurosurg Psychiat* 50: 1101–9.

Neary D, Snowden JS, Northen B, Goulding P (1988) Dementia of frontal lobe type. *J Neurol Neurosurg Psychiat* 51: 353–61.

Neary D (1990*a*) Non Alzheimer's disease forms of cerebral atrophy. *J Neurol Neurosurg Psychiat* 53: 929–31.

Neary D, Snowden JS, Mann DMA *et al* (1990*b*) Frontal lobe dementia and motor neurone disease. *J Neurol Neurosurg Psychiat* 53: 23–32.

Neumann MA (1949) Pick's disease. *J Neuropathol Exp Neurol* 8: 255–82.

Perry G, Stewart D, Friedman R, Manetto V, Autilio-Gambetti L, Gambetti P (1987) Filaments of Pick's bodies contain altered cytoskeletal elements. *Am J Pathol* 127: 559–68.

Pick A (1892) Ueber die Beziehungen der senilen Hirnatrophie zur Aphasie. *Prager Med Wochenschr* 17: 165–7.

Pick A (1904) Zur Symptomatologie der linksseitigen Schläfenlappenatrophie. *Monatschr Psychatr Neurol* 16: 378–88.

Pick A (1906) Über einen weiteren Symtomenkomplex im Rahmen der Dementia senilis, bedingt durch umschriebene stärkere Hirnatrophie (gemischte Apraxie). *Monatsschr Psychiatr Neurol* 19: 97–108.

Pogacar S, Williams RS (1984) Alzheimer's disease presenting as slowly progressive aphasia. *RI Med J* 67: 181–5.

Rasool CG, Selkoe DJ (1985) Sharing of specific antigens in Pick's disease and Alzheimer's disease. *N Engl J Med* 312: 700–5.

Rebeiz JJ, Kolodny EH, Richardson EP (1968) Corticodentatonigral degeneration with neuronal achromasia. *Arch Neurol* 18: 20–33.

Rewcastle NB, Ball MJ (1968) Electron microscopy of the inclusion bodies in Pick's disease. *Neurology* 18: 1205–13.

Riley DE, Lang AE, Lewis A, Resch L, Ashby P, Hornykiewicz O, Black S (1990) Cortical-basal ganglionic degeneration. *Neurology* 40: 1203–12.

Rogers JD, Brogan D, Mirra SS (1985) The nucleus basalis of Meynert in Neurological disease: a quantitative morphological study. *Ann Neurol* 17: 163–70.

Salazar AM, Masters CL, Gajdusek C, Gibbs CL (1983) Syndromes of amotrophic lateral sclerosis and dementia: relation to transmissible Creutzfeldt-Jakob disease. *Ann Neurol* 14: 17–26.

Salmon E, Sadzot B, Maquet P, Dive D, Franck G (1989) Slowly progressive asphasia syndrome. A positron emission tomographic study. *Acta Neurol Belg* 89: 242–5.

Sam M, Gutmann L, Schochet SS Jr, Doshi H (1991) Pick's disease: a case clinically resembling amotrophic lateral sclerosis. *Neurology* 41: 1831–3.

Scheltens P, Rivka R, Kamphorst W (1994) Pathologic findings in a case of primary progressive aphasia. *Neurology* 44: 279–82.

Schiffer D (1955) Contribution à l'histologie de la maladie de Pick. *Journal für Hirnforschung* 1: 497–515.

Schochet SS Jr, Lampert PW, Earle KM (1968) Neuronal changes introduced by intrathecal vincristine sulphate. *J Neuropath Exp Neurol* 27: 654–8.

Schochet SS Jr, Lampert PW, Lindenberg R (1978) Fine structure of the Pick and Hirano bodies in a case of Pick's disease. *Acta Neuropath (Berl)* 11: 330–7.

Selkoe DJ (1994) Alzheimer's Disease: a central role for amyloid. *J Neuropath Exp Neurol* 53: 438–47.

Sjögren T, Sjögren H, Lindgren A (1952) Morbus Alzheimer and morbus Pick. Genetic, chemical and patho-anatomical study. *Acta Psychiat Neurol Scand* Suppl 82.

Smith DA, Lantos PL (1968) A case of combined Pick's and Alzheimer's disease. *J Neurol Neurosurg Psychiat* 31: 479–86.

Snowden JS, Neary D, Mann DMA, Goulding PJ, Testa HJ (1992) Progressive language disorder due to lobar atrophy. *Ann Neurol* 31: 174–83.

Tagliavini F, Pilleri G (1983) Basal nucleus of Meynert. A neuropathological study in Alzheimer's disease, simple senile dementia, Pick's disease and Huntington's chorea. *J Neurol Sci* 62: 243–60.

Tissot R, Constantinidis J, Richard J (1975) *La Maladie de Pick.* Masson et Cie, Paris.

Tomlinson BE (1992) Aging and the dementias. In Adams JH, Duchen LW (eds) *Greenfield's Neuropathology*, 5th edn, Oxford University Press, pp 1354–9.

Uhl GR, Hilt DC, Hedreen JC, Whitehouse PJ, Price DL (1983) Pick's disease (lobar sclerosis): depletion of neurons in the nucleus basalis of Meynert. *Neurology* 33: 1470–3.

Ulrich J, Haugh M, Anderton BH, Probst A, Lautenschlager C, His B (1987) Alzheimer dementia and Pick's disease: neurofibrillary tangles and Pick bodies are associated with identical phosphorylated neurofilament epitopes. *Acta Neuropath (Berl)* 73: 240–6.

Van Mansvelt J (1954) Pick's disease: a syndrome of lobar atrophy, its clinico-pathological and histological types. Enschelde, Netherlands, Loeff.

Vogt M (1928) Die Picksche Atrophie als Biespiel für die eunomische Form der Schiichtenpathoklise. *Jahrb Psychol Neurol* 36: 124–9.

Winkleman NW, Book MH (1949) Asymptomatic extrapyramidal involvement in Pick's disease. *J Neuropath Exp Neurol* 8: 30–42.

Wisniewski HM, Coblenz JM, Terry RD (1972) Pick's disease. A clinical and ultrastructural study. *Arch Neurol* 26: 97–108.

Yates CM, Simpson J, Moloney AFJ, Gordon A (1980) Neurochemical observations in a case of Pick's disease. *J Neurol Sci* 48: 257–63.

CHAPTER NINE

Huntington's disease

J. P. G. Vonsattel, P. Ge and L. Kelley

Introduction
Neuropathological history
Epidemiology
Anatomy and nomenclature of the basal ganglia
Physiological considerations
Clinical aspects
Neuropathology
CAG repeats – neuropathology – gene expression
Concomitant neuropathological findings
Clinicopathological discrepancies and differential diagnosis

INTRODUCTION

Huntington's disease (HD) is an autosomal dominant neurodegenerative disease with mid-life onset characterized by involuntary movements, and psychiatric and cognitive alterations (Martin & Gusella, 1986). The course of the disease is relatively slow; death occurs 12–15 years from the time of symptomatic onset (Myers et al., 1988). The gene abnormality is located near the tip of the short arm of chromosome 4 (4p16.3) (Gusella et al., 1983; Gusella, 1991); it consists of an expanded and unstable trinucleotide (CAG) repeat that occurs in the 5' region of the coding sequence (The Huntington's Disease Collaborative Research Group et al., 1993). The number of CAG repeats in the normal population varies between 6 and 34; in contrast, the number of CAG repeats in HD varies between 37 and 121. The number of these repeats is unstable through meiotic transmission (Read, 1993). More than 99% of patients with the clinical and pathological hallmarks of HD have an expanded CAG allele; a few individuals with the clinical diagnosis of HD have been reported to have CAG repeat lengths in the normal range (Andrew et al., 1993; The Huntington's Disease Collaborative Research Group et al., 1993; Persichetti et al., 1994).

Atrophy of the striatum (caudate nucleus [CN], putamen, and globus pallidus [GP]) (Carpenter & Sutin, 1983) is the neuropathological hallmark of HD (Dunlap, 1927; Stone & Falstein, 1938). Neostriatal neuronal loss first involves the medial CN adjacent to the lateral ventricle, the dorsal putamen, and the tail of the caudate nucleus (TCN); the nucleus accumbens is spared until late in the course of the disease (Vonsattel et al., 1985). The rate of degeneration of neostriatal neurons varies according to their class. The aspiny neurons are less prone to degeneration than are the spiny ones (Dawbarn, De Quidt & Emson, 1985; Ferrante et al., 1985, 1987b; Graveland, Williams & DiFiglia 1985a). Biochemical data corroborate these observations (Bird & Iversen, 1974; Aronin et al., 1983; Beal et al., 1984, 1988a, 1988b). To some extent, the neurochemical and neuropathological changes seen in HD striatum can be obtained in animal models following overstimulation of striatal glutamate receptors, supporting an excitotoxic theory of the pathophysioloy of HD (Beal et al., 1986; Ellison et al., 1987; DiFiglia, 1990; Roberts et al., 1993). Efforts are currently devoted to identifying the primary cause of the genetically programmed, premature neuronal death that occurs in HD.

NEUROPATHOLOGICAL HISTORY

Anton (1896), and Lannois & Paviot (1897) were the first to identify striatal abnormalities in HD. These findings gained acceptance with the reports of Jelgersma (1908) and Alzheimer (1911). Much less consistent neuropathological changes in HD were described in the claustrum (Bruyn, 1968; Forno & Jose, 1973; Rodda,

1981), hypothalamus (Bruyn, 1973), hypothalamic lateral tuberal nucleus (Kremer et al., 1990, 1991), amygdala (Davison, Goodhart & Shlionsky, 1932; Bruyn et al., 1979), hippocampal formation (Spargo, Everall & Lantos, 1993), subthalamic region (Alzheimer, 1911; Schroeder, 1931; Lange et al., 1976), thalamus (Pfeiffer, 1913; Dom, Malfroid & Baro, 1976), nucleus coeruleus (Zweig et al., 1989, 1992), red nucleus (Lange, 1981), substantia nigra (Schroeder, 1931; Oyanagi et al., 1989), superior olivary nucleus, pons and medulla oblongata (Alzheimer, 1911; Bonduelle, Gruner & Bouygues, 1953; Forno & Jose, 1973; Byers, Gilles & Fung, 1973; Rodda, 1981; Martin & Gusella, 1986; Zweig et al., 1989), cerebellum (Kiesselbach, 1914; Spielmeyer, 1926; Davison, Goodhart & Schlionsky, 1932; Birnbaum, 1941; Hallervorden, 1957; Fau et al., 1971; Byers et al., 1973; Castaigne, Escourolle & Gray, 1976; Rodda, 1981; Jeste, Barban & Parisi, 1984), and spinal cord (Alzheimer, 1911; Kiesselbach, 1914; Spielmeyer, 1926; Hallervorden, 1957).

Although most observers have suggested the opposite, Pfeiffer (1913) and Dunlap (1927) found the putamen to be more involved than the CN in HD. Kiesselbach (1914) and Dunlap (1927) noted atrophy of the white matter. The neuropathological features characteristic of HD may be summarized as the gradual atrophy (loss of neurons with gliosis) of the neostriatum (Bruyn, 1968). The severity of the neuropathological changes in the neostriatum increases along the antero-posterior, latero-medial and ventro-dorsal axes (Vonsattel et al., 1985). The GP is also affected, but to a lesser extent (Kiesselbach, 1914; Terplan, 1924; Bruyn, 1968). In the cerebral cortex subtle changes, especially neuronal loss, occur (Bruyn, 1968; Forno & Jose, 1973; Roizin, Stellar & Liu, 1979; Cudkowicz & Kowall, 1990; Hedreen et al., 1991; Sotrel et al., 1991). Volumetric loss of the cerebral white matter is gradual with the progression of the disease and may be striking (Kiesselbach, 1914; Dunlap, 1927).

EPIDEMIOLOGY

The diagnostic criteria proposed by Hayden (1981) are threefold: 1) a family history of typical Huntington's chorea; 2) progressive motor disability with chorea or rigidity of no other obvious cause and 3) psychiatric disturbance with gradual dementia of no other obvious cause. The disease is ubiquitous (Hayden, 1981). The prevalence of affected persons in North America and Europe is estimated at about 5–10/100 000; it is highest in populations of western European origin and low in African and Asian populations, suggesting that HD may

have originated in north-western Europe (Conneally, 1984; Folstein, 1989a; Harper et al., 1991c). New mutations rarely occur, and have been confirmed by evaluations of the length of CAG repeats in several family members (Myers et al., 1993). Their rate has probably been underestimated (Goldberg et al., 1993). New mutations are described in families with no history of the disorder in which there is a person (with expanded CAG repeats) diagnosed with HD (Myers et al., 1993; Goldberg et al., 1993).

ANATOMY AND NOMENCLATURE OF THE BASAL GANGLIA

The basal ganglia consists of the corpus striatum and the amygdaloid nucleus or archistriatum, which is part of the limbic system (Carpenter & Sutin, 1983). Because of their functions, it would be reasonable to include the subthalamic nucleus and substantia nigra in the basal ganglia.

The corpus striatum consists of the neostriatum (CN and putamen) and paleostriatum (globus pallidus). The GP is divided into external (GPe) and internal (GPi) segments. The neostriatum is commonly referred to as the striatum (Carpenter & Sutin, 1983). The 'lenticular nucleus' is a descriptive definition of both the putamen and the GP. The substantia nigra has two main zones: the pars reticulata (SNr) and the pars compacta (SNc). The pars reticulata contains neurons morphologically similar to those in the GPi; the pars compacta contains neurons that are pigmented in the adult. The nucleus accumbens is the ventral anterior part of the neostriatum, where the CN and putamen fuse. The fibre systems of the corpus striatum that are readily seen on gross examination of coronal sections of the brain are the ansa lenticularis, the lenticular fasciculus, the thalamic fasciculus, and to a lesser extent, the subthalamic fasciculus. The ansa lenticularis and lenticular fasciculus connect the GPi with the thalamus. The ansa lenticularis lies on the ventral surface of the GP. The lenticular fasciculus transverses the internal capsule and courses along the dorsal capsule of the subthalamic nucleus. Both bundles merge and enter the thalamic fasciculus to project into motor thalamic nuclei including the centrum medianum. The subthalamic fasciculus is composed of pallidosubthalamic and subthalamopallidal fibres. The pallidosubthalamic fibres arise from the GPe and then traverse the GPi and the internal capsule to the subthalamic nucleus. The subthalamopallidal fibres are distributed to both the GPe and GPi.

With cresyl violet at least two groups of neurons can be distinguished in the neostriatum (Bielschowsky,

1919). One group consists of small- or medium-sized type and a second of large neurons (40 μm in diameter and larger). The ratio of small–medium to large neostriatal neurons averages 175:1 (range 130:1–258:1) (Schröder *et al.*, 1975). Golgi and ultrastructural studies identify at least five general categories of neurons. The two main categories consist of neurons with spiny dendrites (spiny neurons) and neurons with smooth dendrites (aspiny neurons) (Graveland, Williams & DiFiglia, 1985*b*; Di Figlia & Carey, 1986). Both the spiny (which are the most numerous) and aspiny neurons are represented by large and small–medium-sized neurons (Graveland *et al.*, 1985*b*). Spiny neurons have distant connections and often are referred to as projection neurons; they contain γ-aminobutyric acid, enkephalin, dynorphin, substance P or calbindin (Steiner & Gerfen, 1993; Graybiel & Ragsdale, 1983; Nieuwenhuys, 1985; Selden *et al.*, 1994). Aspiny neurons or interneurons have local connections and contain nicotinamide adenine dinucleotide phosphate diaphorase, somatostatin, neuropeptide Y, cholecystokinin or acetylcholine (Cooper *et al.*, 1981; Sagar *et al.*, 1984; Nieuwenhuys, 1985; Morton, Nicholson & Faull, 1993; Colmers & Bleakman, 1994; Selden *et al.*, 1994).

The primate neostriatum can be divided into two compartments: the striosomes and the matrix (Graybiel & Ragsdale, 1979; Goldman-Rakic, 1982). However, recent data suggest that this compartmentalization might be more complex (Selemon, Gottlieb & Goldman-Rakic, 1994). The intensity of histochemical staining for acetylcholinesterase is weak in the 300- to 600 μm-wide discrete zones referred to as striosomes. The staining is intense in the matrix, which surrounds the striosomes (Goldman-Rakic, 1982; Graybiel & Ragsdale, 1983). Calbindin, a neuronal cytoplasmic calcium-binding protein, is abundant in the matrix and rare in the striosomes (Gerfen *et al.*, 1987*a,b*). Afferents to the striosomes originate in the SNc, prefrontal cortex and limbic system. Efferents from the striosomes terminate in the SNc. Afferents to the matrix originate in the motor and somatosensory cortices, and in the parietal, occipital and frontal cortices. Efferents from the matrix terminate in the SNr, GPi and GPe (Ragsdale & Graybiel, 1981; Gerfen, Herkenham & Thibault, 1987*b*; Gerfen, Baimbridge & Thibault, 1987*a*).

PHYSIOLOGICAL CONSIDERATIONS

The basal ganglia concerned with motor functions can be conceptualized physiologically as two compartments: one for input (CN and putamen) and one for output (GP, subthalamic nucleus and substantia nigra).

The entire cerebral cortex projects onto the striatum (Selemon & Goldman-Rakic, 1985; Whitworth, LeDoux & Gould, 1991; Graybiel *et al.*, 1994). Specific cortical areas send projections to selected portions of the CN and putamen, or input compartment. The output nuclei are the GPi, SNr and ventral pallidum; their target nuclei are located in the thalamus, which has an excitatory action upon the cortex.

Two major pathways (a direct and an indirect) connect the input compartment to the output nuclei. The direct pathway arises from inhibitory neostriatal (CN and putamen) efferents to the GPi. The indirect pathway also arises from the neostriatum but passes first to the GPe, subthalamic nucleus and SNr, and then to the GPi which sends projections to the thalamus. The two efferent systems of the basal ganglia have apparently opposing effects upon the output nuclei and thalamic target nuclei. It seems likely that decreases in GPi–SNr discharges facilitate movement initiated in the cortex, and increases in GPi–SNr discharges inhibit cortically initiated movements (Garrett & Crutcher, 1990).

There is evidence that early in the course of HD there is a selective loss of striatal neurons that give rise to the indirect pathway (Reiner *et al.*, 1988; Albin, Young & Penney, 1989; Albin *et al.*, 1990*a,b*). This neuronal loss reduces the inhibitory action of the GPe upon the subthalamic nucleus, which becomes hypofunctional and causes reduction of the inhibitory action of the GPi upon the thalamus. This subsequent disinhibition of the thalamus leads to choreiform movements.

Chevalier & Deniau (1990) proposed that the basal ganglia output serves as the spatial movement template; this is achieved by a disinhibitory mechanism arousing motor centres. The changes involving the HD striatum probably decrease the tonic output of GPi–SNr to the thalamus with subsequent reduction of its action upon cortical movement-initiating neurons. Albin *et al.* (1990*a,b*) have shown pathological evidence supporting the hypothesis that chorea might result from preferential loss of striatal neurons projecting to the GPe, and that rigid-akinetic HD might be due to the additional loss of striatal neurons projecting to the GPi.

CLINICAL ASPECTS

Most persons with the expanded CAG repeat develop and function normally into early adulthood. Involuntary movements and abnormalities of voluntary motor control may begin any time after infancy but usually start in middle adult life (Folstein, 1989*b*), with a mean age of onset of 40 years (Koroshetz, Myers & Martin, 1992); the mean age of onset of motor symptoms is 37 years (Myers *et al.*, 1988). In 9% of the patients symptoms are present before the age of 20; in 90% of the patients with age of onset under 10 years the gene is paternally transmitted (Bruyn, 1968; Harper *et al.*, 1991*a*). Went *et al.* (1984) reported that juvenile-onset HD is almost always inherited from the father. Myers *et al.* (1983) have reported that more than twice as many of the late-onset patients (age 50 or later) inherited the HD gene from an affected mother than from an affected father.

Young *et al.* (1986) reported that 94% of the patients were adult-onset, and 6% were juvenile-onset in the Venezuelan cohort they examined. Chorea is usually absent in patients with juvenile-onset. The rigid form of the disease is typical of young patients (Jervis, 1963; Bird & Paulson, 1971). The mean duration is about 17 years (Conneally, 1984; Folstein, 1989*b*).

Early signs include the inability to rapidly tap fingers in sequence, dysdiadochokinesia, abnormal voluntary gaze, and the inability to maintain tongue protrusion. Often these signs are present before the onset of chorea. In some instances depression and psychiatric disturbances precede chorea. Chorea is the most common involuntary movement in HD (Folstein, 1989*b*). Early in the course of the disease it is especially obvious in the hands and feet and is displayed as restlessness or fidgeting; the movements are quick and resemble piano playing, or consist of shrugging of the shoulders or rapid raising of the eyebrows, with time it may cause gait instability and becomes disabling. Chorea is more exuberant with stress

or while walking and is absent during sleep. It may gradually disappear late in the course of the disease and be replaced by bradykinesia or rigidity; eventually the patient becomes bedridden (Rosenthal, 1927). Deficits in concentration, attention, comprehension and memory are often present at the time of onset of chorea and gradually worsen. Visual memory tends to be more impaired than verbal memory (Koroshetz *et al.*, 1992). Dementia is included in the diagnostic criteria proposed by Hayden (1981), as stated previously. The prevalence of dementia in HD is difficult to assess. Indeed, there is no consensus regarding the definition of dementia. Patients perform poorly on tests of short-term memory but their amnesia is never as severe as observed in Alzheimer's disease (Koroshetz *et al.*, 1992). Comprehensive reviews of dementia in HD are provided by Folstein (Folstein, 1989*c*) and Harper (Harper *et al.*, 1991*b*). The role of the striatal degeneration in the occurrence of dementia in HD is unknown.

Since chorea is not a clinical hallmark in juvenile cases and since it tends to disappear during the end stage of the disease in patients with mid-life onset, Spielmeyer (1926), Rosenthal (1927) and Schroeder (1931) suggested abandoning the designation of Huntington's chorea and to adopt the term Huntington's disease instead.

NEUROPATHOLOGY

Atrophy of the striatum is the neuropathological hallmark of HD. Five grades (0–4) of neuropathological severity of striatal involvement can be distinguished

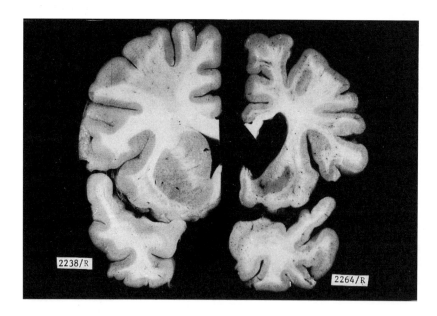

Fig. 9.1. Coronal sections through the head of caudate nucleus (HCN), nucleus accumbens, and putamen (level CAP). The section on the left is that of a 34 year-old man (suicide, brain weight 1680 g); the section on the right is that of a 48 year-old man with HD (brain weight 1100 g, grade 3/4), the atrophy strikingly involves the neostriatum and white matter; cortical thinning is not obvious.

(Vonsattel *et al.* 1985). Grade 0 defines cases of clinically diagnosed HD without discernible abnormality of the striatum as judged by conventional neuropathologic (macroscopical and microscopical) standards. In grade 1, neuropathological changes of the striatum can only be recognized microscopically. In grades 2 and 3, gross striatal atrophy is mild to severe, respectively. In grade 4, the brain is diffusely smaller than normal with the brunt of atrophy involving the striatum, where 95% or more of neurons are lost. There is good correlation between the

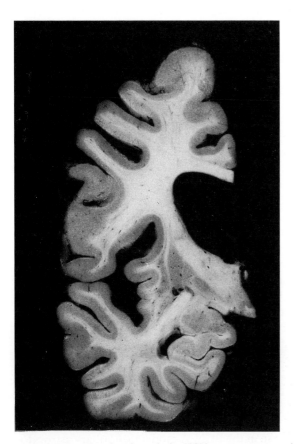

Fig. 9.2. Coronal section through the HCN, putamen, external and internal segments of the globus pallidus (GPe, GPi) and amygdaloid nucleus (level GP) of a 36 year-old man with HD (brain weight 1060 g, grade 4/4). Atrophy of the striatum and white matter is severe. The dorso-medial border of the lenticular nucleus is concave medially. The GPe is relatively more atrophic than the GPi. The pallidal medullary laminae are distinct but thinner than normal. In addition to the striking striatal neuronal loss and gliosis, there was moderate gliosis involving the superior olivary nucleus, subthalamic nucleus, pontine nuclei and red nucleus with mild myelin loss in the central tegmental tract and amiculum of inferior olivary nucleus; these extrastriatal changes are occasionally seen in advanced HD but are not specific.

overall atrophy of the brain and that of the striatum, although there are exceptions. The neuropathological definition of clinically well-established HD can be summarized as a diffuse atrophy of the brain with the brunt of the degenerative changes involving the striatum (Alzheimer, 1911; Vonsattel *et al.*, 1985).

External examination of the brain

Eighty per cent of brains from patients who have died with HD show atrophy on external examination of the brains as evidenced by widened sulci and shrunken gyri, particularly in the frontal lobes. The remaining 20% does not show gross abnormality.

The mean weight of 138 brains was 1067 g (normal about 1350 g) (Vonsattel, 1992). The mean weights of 163 brains that were classified according to grade were as follows: 1240 g for grades 0 and 1, 1140 g for grade 2, 1120 g for grade 3, and 995 g for grade 4 (Vonsattel *et al.*, 1985).

The ventricular system is widened in HD. Measurement of 162 left or right lateral ventricles of HD brains gave a mean volume of 16.3 cm^3 (range: 8–46 cm^3; normal about 7 cm^3). The mean left or right ventricular volume in the series of 138 brains classified according to grade was as follows: 11.7 cm^3 for grade 1, 15.5 cm^3 for grade 2, 16.8 cm^3 for grade 3, 20.2 cm^3 for grade 4 (Vonsattel, 1992). The frontal horns and atria are more widened than the temporal and occipital horns.

Coronal sections

Coronal sections are apparently normal in 5% of the HD brains. Usually, the cerebral cortex is thinner than normal. There is volumetric reduction of the white matter, striatum, and thalamus (Figs. 9.1–9.3). De la Monte, Vonsattel & Richardson (1988) morphometrically evaluated five standardized coronal brain slices in 30 patients with HD. There was a 21–29% loss in the cerebral cortex, a 29–34% loss in the white matter, a 28% loss in the thalamus, a 57% loss in the CN and a 64% loss in the putamen.

Striatum

The most striking changes in HD are exhibited in the striatum, where there is volumetric reduction, neuronal loss and reactive astrogliosis (Figs. 9.1–9.4). The extent and distribution of these changes depend on the degree of illness at the time of death. This pattern is distinctive and probably pathognomonic for HD as judged by our observations of more than 1000 HD brains that we have evaluated systematically during the past ten years. These pathological striatal characteristics are the quintessence of the grading system applied to HD brains, and are invaluable for the differential diagnosis.

As previously stated, five grades of striatal neuropathologic severity can be distinguished, each grade reflecting the extent and distribution of neuronal loss and gliosis. The assignment of a grade is based on striatal

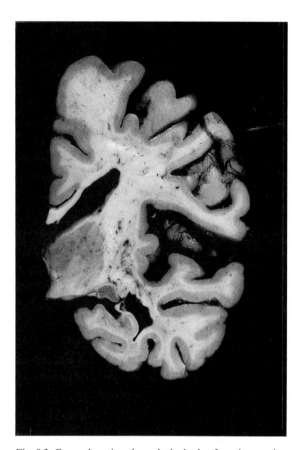

Fig. 9.3. Coronal section through the body of caudate nucleus (BCN), tail of the caudate nucleus (TCN), thalamus with centrum medianum and lateral geniculate body (level LGB) of a 96 year-old man with HD (brain weight 1100 g, grade 3/4). The BCN consists of a thin strip; the TCN is invisible on gross examination. Atrophy of the white matter is moderate; the cortical ribbon is thinner than normal. The hippocampal formation shows mild volumetric reduction. Microscopical changes in the striatum were characteristic of HD. There were occasional Lewy bodies in the nucleus coeruleus, rare neurofibrillary tangles of Alzheimer in the substantia innominata, hippocampal formation and entorhinal cortex. This case illustrates that possession of the HD gene does not prevent an affected person from reaching an advanced age. Furthermore, it illustrates that the extrastriatal atrophy in HD might be in part due to ageing and that it is not always proportional to the striatal atrophy.

findings on both **gross** and **microscopic** examinations of three standardized coronal sections. One coronal section includes the head of the caudate nucleus (HCN), putamen, and nucleus accumbens; this level is referred to as CAP (caudate, accumbens, putamen) (Fig. 9.1). The next coronal section includes the CN, putamen, and both the external and internal segments of the globus pallidus (level GP) (Fig. 9.2). The third coronal section contains the TCN at the level of the lateral geniculate body (LGB); it may provide the only visible change on gross examination early in the course of the disease (Fig. 9.3 and 9.5). In addition, this section contains the body of the caudate nucleus (BCN) and the thalamus (including the centrum medianum) at the midpoint of the sagittal axis between the frontal and occipital poles (Fig. 9.3).

Grade 0

Grade 0 is assigned to brains from patients with unequivocal genetic or clinical evidence for the diagnosis of HD, yet without any gross or microscopic abnormality suggestive of HD on examination of the brain. The grade 0 brains are grossly indistinguishable from normal brains despite a cell count indicating a 30–40% neuronal loss and no significant increase in the number of astrocytes or reactive astrocytosis. These subtle changes might not be appreciated without quantitative study.

No neuropathological change could be identified by conventional examination of 15 brains from patients at risk for HD; three of them turned out to have inherited the HD gene indicating that the striatum of a presymptomatic carrier of the HD mutation appears normal (Persichetti et al., 1994).

Grade 1

Macroscopically, the striatum is apparently normal with the exception of the TCN, which is much smaller than normal; atrophy of the BCN may already be obvious. Neuronal loss and astrogliosis are evident in the TCN and less so in the BCN. A moderate fibrillary astrocytosis is present especially in the medial HCN and in the dorsal half of the putamen; neuronal loss is mild and may be barely perceptible on general survey of the slides. Cell count, however, shows that more than 50% of neurons are lost in the HCN (Vonsattel et al., 1985). The GP is apparently normal on gross and microscopical examination.

Grade 2

Macroscopically, the atrophy of the TCN is severe. The BCN is about half its normal size. At level CAP, atrophy of the HCN and of the putamen might be subtle or is evident; the medial outline of the HCN is only slightly convex but still bulges into the lateral ventricle. At level GP, striatal atrophy ranges from subtle to evident (Fig. 9.6, left).

Neuronal loss and gliosis are severe in the BCN and in the TCN, conspicuous in the medial HCN and in the dorsal half of the putamen; they are less pronounced in the paracapsular portion of the HCN and in the ventral portion of the putamen. The nucleus accumbens and GP are apparently normal.

Grade 3

Macroscopically, the neostriatum is severely reduced in size; however, the atrophy of the nucleus accumbens is less striking. The medial outline of the HCN forms a straight line or is slightly concave medially (Fig. 9.1, right). The BCN is reduced by about 75%; the TCN

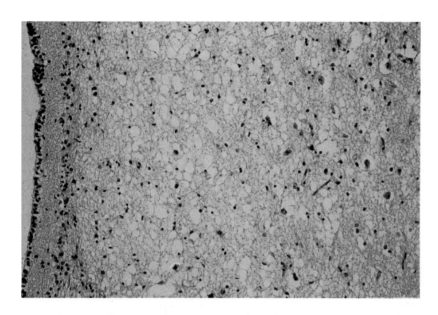

Fig. 9.4. Huntington disease, grade 3/4. Microphotograph of the HCN at midpoint between the dorsal and ventral limits of the neostriatum at level CAP. It shows the ependymal lining, subependymal glial layer and, in continuity, the loosely textured caudate parenchyma, which gradually becomes denser in the opposite direction of the ependymal surface. Neuronal loss is very severe in the loose textured zone, whereas there are scattered neurons in the denser area. LHE, original magnification × 100.

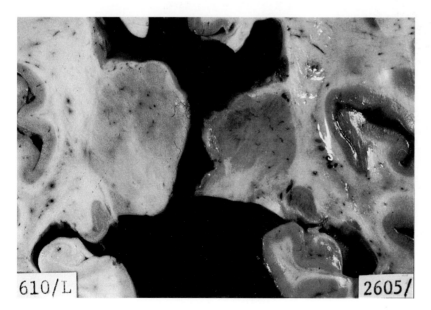

Fig. 9.5. Coronal sections through level LGB. The section on the left is that of a 60 year-old woman with HD (brain weight 1240 g, grade 2/4); the section on the right is that of a 75 year-old man with Alzheimer's disease Lewy body variant (ADLBV) (brain weight 1300 g). The BCN is slightly larger in the HD brain than in the ADLBV brain; however, the TCN is invisible in the HD brain while it is discrete in the ADLBV brain. The HD thalamus is less atrophic than the ADLBV. These examples illustrate the increasing severity of the caudate atrophy along its antero-posterior axis (c.f. Fig. 9.6). The difference in intensity of color between the HD and ADLBV brains is probably due to the different duration of fixation.

consists of a barely visible strip (Fig. 9.3). The dorso-medial outline of the lenticular nucleus is straight or slightly concave medially. The GP is smaller than normal, especially the GPe. The white matter bundles of the lentiform nuclei are thinner than normal or blurred. There is atrophy of the ansa lenticularis, and thinning of the anterior limb of the internal capsule.

The neuronal loss and fibrillary astrocytosis are especially conspicuous in the TCN, BCN, paraventricular portion of the HCN and dorsal half of the putamen

(Fig. 9.4). There is relative preservation of the paracapsular portion of the HCN. The nucleus accumbens is usually normal; however, occasional reactive astrocytes might be present dorsally (Fig. 9.7). Slight fibrillar astrocytosis is present especially in the lateral third of the GPe; the GPi is microscopically within normal limits.

Grade 4
Grade 4 is characterized by extreme atrophy of the

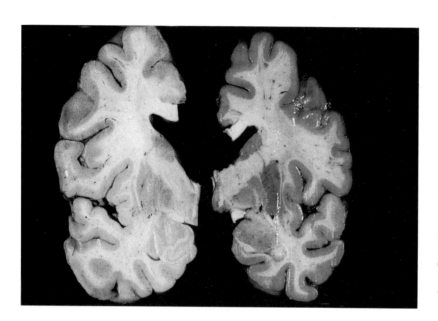

Fig. 9.6. Coronal sections through level GP of the same cases as Fig. 9.5. The striatum of the section on the left (HD, grade 2) is remarkably similar to that of the coronal section on the right (ADLBV). On gross examination, evaluation of the TCN (Fig. 9.5) can be very helpful especially in the early stages of the disease; atrophy of the TCN would support the diagnosis of HD.

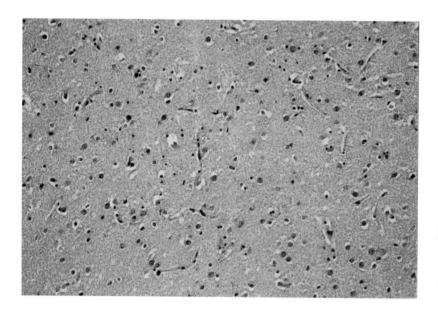

Fig. 9.7. Huntington disease, grade 3/4. Microphotograph of the nucleus accumbens, which is relatively preserved when compared with a more dorsal area of the HCN (Fig. 9.4). Neuronal density and neuropil texture are apparently normal, reactive gliosis is mild. LHE, original magnification × 100.

neostriatum (Fig. 9.2). At level CAP, the HCN is shrunken and yellow-brown. Its medial contour is concave, as is the anterior limb of the internal capsule. The putamen is atrophic with a concave dorso-medial outline. The nucleus accumbens is smaller than normally expected but is relatively prominent in comparison with the adjacent HCN or putamen. At the level of GP, the HCN consists of a thin strip. The putamen is much smaller than normal, often with widened perivascular spaces in its ventral third. The medullary laminae of the

GP are thinner than normal and blurred as are the lenticular white matter bundles (Fig. 9.2 and 9.8 left). There is about a 50% reduction of the GP, the external segment being more involved than the internal segment.

Neuronal loss and gliosis are extremely severe and diffuse throughout the neostriatum; the neuropil is often loosely textured, especially in the paraventricular regions. The bridges between the HCN and the putamen show neuronal loss and gliosis, but less severely than in the main part of the CN or putamen (Fig. 9.9 and 9.10).

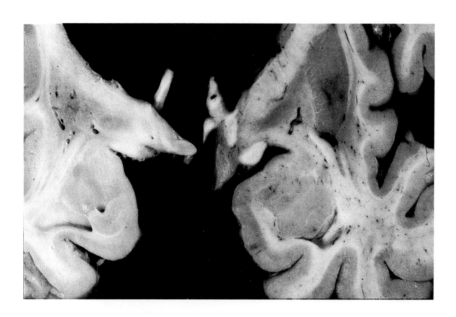

Fig. 9.8. Coronal sections at level GP. The section on the left is that of a 68 year-old man with HD (age of onset 36 years; CAG alleles 43/23, brain weight 1040 g, grade 4), and with Alzheimer's disease (AD). The section on the right is that of a 69 year-old man (brain weight 1340 g) with PSP. Atrophy of the CN and putamen are striking in the HD-AD brain as compared with the PSP one. The distinction between the GPe and the GPi is more discrete, and the GPe atrophy is more striking in the HD-AD than in the PSP brain. Thinning of the entorhinal cortex and atrophy of the amygdaloid nucleus are conspicuous in the HD–AD as compared to the PSP brain.

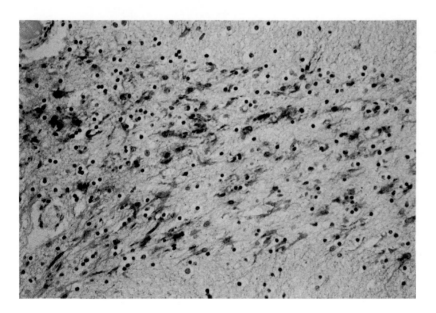

Fig. 9.9. Huntington disease grade 4/4 (same case as Fig. 9.10). Microphotograph of the dorsal, caudo-putaminal grey matter bridge at level CAP showing severe reactive astrocytosis confined to the grey matter bordered dorsally and ventrally by white matter. GFAP, original magnification × 160.

Table 9.1. *Distribution of 245 graded HD brains categorized between 1992 and 1994*

Year (n)	Grade 1	Grade 2	Grade 3	Grade 4
1992 (84)	3 (3.6%)	12 (14.3%)	51 (60.7%)	18 (21.4%)
1993 (73)	4 (5.5%)	13 (17.8%)	39 (53.4%)	17 (23.3%)
1994 (88)	2 (2.3%)	15 (17.0%)	43 (48.9%)	28 (31.8%)
Total (245)	9 (3.7%)	40 (16.3%)	133 (54.3%)	63 (25.7%)

Neuronal depletion and gliosis are less severe in the nucleus accumbens than in the adjacent HCN or putamen. The GP is remarkable for the presence of fibrillary astrocytosis, especially in the GPe; neurons are smaller than usual and are more closely packed together than in age-matched controls.

The distribution of 245 HD brains categorized according to grade between 1992 and 1994 is shown in Table 9.1.

Grade 3 HD brains are those encountered by neuropathologists most frequently; they represent the stage of neuropathological changes that is usually shown in text books, and do not present diagnostic difficulties (Sax & Vonsattel, 1992).

In grade 2, the neostriatal gradients of increased severity of neuronal loss and gliosis along the antero-posterior, ventro-dorsal and latero-medial axes are discrete and probably pathognomonic for HD (Fig. 9.11). The identification of these gradients is crucial in making the diagnosis of HD, especially in the early stages of the disease when there are few if any striatal changes visible on gross examination, with the exception of the TCN. Indeed, the TCN is atrophic early in the course of the disease.

Caution should be exercised in making the diagnosis of grade 1, especially when the tissue is not optimally prepared or when changes due to an acute or remote hypoxic-ischaemic event are present. In these instances, it is advisable to evaluate the length of the CAG repeat for a final diagnostic statement. Careful examination of the TCN is essential in these cases since atrophy is always present early in the course of the disease. However, one should be aware that segments of the TCN might be absent in brains from patients without any neurological or psychiatric disorders (Fig. 9.12). Therefore, prior to concluding that the TCN is atrophic one must scrutinize it in its entirety. In early stages of HD the atrophy of the TCN is always associated with some involvement of the medial half of the BCN, and must be confirmed microscopically. Grade 0 brains are rare. The

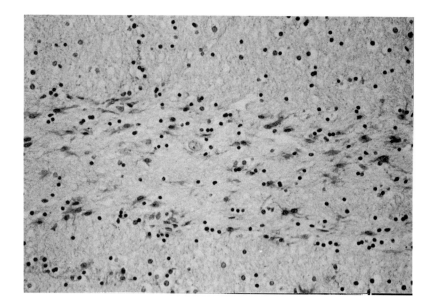

Fig. 9.10. Huntington disease grade 4/4 (same case as Fig. 9.9). Microphotograph of the ventral, caudo-putaminal grey matter bridge at level CAP showing reactive astrocytosis that is less severe than in the dorsal bridge (Fig. 9.9) illustrating the dorsoventral gradient of decreasing neuropathological severity so characteristically present in HD. GFAP, original magnification × 160.

frequency of grade 0 might depend to some extent on the experience of the neuropathologist: the more experienced the neuropathologist, the higher the probability of identifying subtle striatal changes in a very early stage of the disease and, therefore of lowering the frequency of grade 0 brains.

Hedreen & Folstein (1995) have shown that scattered islands of astrocytosis and neuronal loss involve the neostriatum before the ventrally progressive wave of generalized neuronal loss, and that they correspond to striosomes. These islands may be specific for HD; their histological demonstration is important for the pathological differential diagnosis of this disease especially in its early stage.

Unusual neostriatal findings
Less than 5% of the HD brains show unusual neostriatal microscopical changes. They consists of the presence of one to five (rarely more) discrete round or oval islets with ill-defined borders of relatively intact parenchyma present in the anterior neostriatum (Fig. 9.13). The cross sections of the islets measure about 100 mm². They are

readily seen in paraffin-embedded tissue sections stained with Luxol fast blue, counterstained with hematoxylin and eosin (LHE) under low microscopical power (100 ×). The number of neurons in these islets is the same as or slightly lower than in the normal neostriatum, but the number of astrocytes is increased (Vonsattel et al., 1992). These islets are larger than striosomes, but their nature is poorly understood. They are more frequently seen in patients whose symptoms appear earlier and develop faster than in HD patients with the usual neostriatal lesions. Local variation in neuronal loss and gliosis is occasionally noticed in the anterior neostriatum (Terplan, 1924). However, in these instances, the atrophic and relatively spared zones are ill defined. Occasionally there are thin, gliotic bands projecting from the most severely involved areas (dorsal HCN or putamen) into the ventral, relatively preserved parts. These cases might represent intermediary forms between those with the usual neostriatal lesions and those with discrete islets.

Selective or variable rates of degeneration of neostriatal neurons
Spiny or projection neurons bear the brunt of the degenerative process in HD (Graveland et al., 1985a). Aspiny or interneurons tend to be more resistant or to degenerate later in the course of the disease (Ferrante et

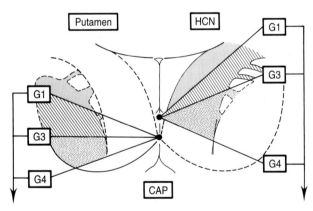

Fig. 9.11. Schematic coronal section at level CAP (caudate, accumbens, putamen) illustrating the topographical progression of the neuropathological changes in the putamen (on the left) and in the HCN (on the right) during the course of the disease (the volumetric changes are not represented). Neuronal loss and gliosis are first seen in the dorsomedial portion of the HCN, dorsal third of the putamen and dorsal caudoputaminal bridges (grade 1 [G1]). Later in the course of the disease, the changes reach the ventral third of the anterior neostriatum with relative preservation of the nucleus accumbens (grade 2 [not shown] and grade 3 [G3]). Most of the ventral third of the anterior neostriatum is involved in the end stage of the disease (grade 4 [G4]), however, to a lesser extent than it is dorsally.

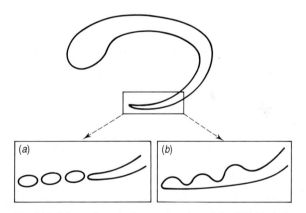

Fig. 9.12. Schematic sagittal representation of the CN. Variations of the TCN are occasionally seen in brains from patients without neurological or psychiatric disorder. The variations include segmental absence of the TCN (A) or focal thinning (B) that mimics HD findings in early stages of the disease. Indeed, in the early stages, the anterior neostriatum and globus pallidus can be unremarkable on gross examination while the TCN may be severely atrophic.

al., 1985, 1987*a,b*; Kowall, Ferrante & Martin, 1987). However, the extreme atrophy of the neostriatum and the loss of 95% of the neostriatal neurons in grade 4 suggest that both the spiny and aspiny neurons are vulnerable.

Of interest is the presence in all grades of HD neostriatum of scattered atrophic neurons referred to as neostriatal dark neurons (NDN), which represent about 5% of the remaining neurons (Fig. 9.14). Neostriatal dark neurons are smaller than normal neurons, and have

scalloped cytoplasmic membranes. The cytoplasm is finely granular and the nucleus is small and lobulated, with finely granular chromatin and an invisible nucleolus. Kiesselbach (1914) and Terplan (1924) mentioned the presence of scattered, atrophic, dark neurons in the HD neostriatum, however, these neurons were not felt to be present consistently. So far, we have not found this type of neuronal change in the neostriatum of normal controls or of patients who have died with non-HD striatal atrophic diseases such as Pick's disease, pro-

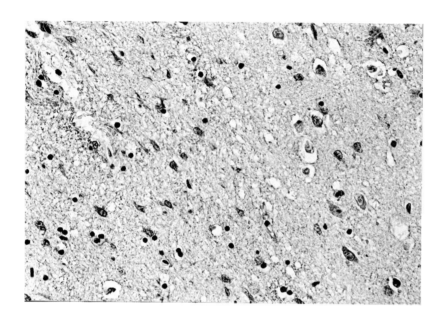

Fig. 9.13. Huntington disease, grade 4/4 (juvenile). Microphotograph showing the (oblique) discrete demarcation between a relatively preserved islet of neostriatal parenchyma (on the right) and the adjacent gliotic area. LHE, original magnification ×250.

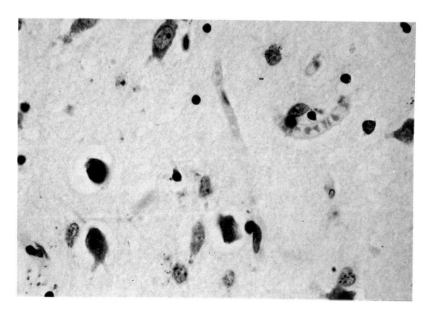

Fig. 9.14. Huntington disease, grade 3/4. Microphotograph from the ventral third of the HCN (level CAP) showing neostriatal dark neurons (NDN) and an apparently normal neuron (upper border). Three NDN are in the lower third, left; two NDN are partially present, one on the right lower border, the other on the left border. These neurons are shrunken and dark, the nucleocytoplasmic demarcation is blurred; the nucleolus is invisible and the cytoplasmic membrane is scalloped. Cresyl violet, original magnification ×400.

gressive supranuclear palsy (PSP), multiple system atrophy, infantile progressive striato-thalamic degeneration, Creutzfeldt–Jakob disease, subacute sclerosing panencephilitis or in acute hypoxic-ischaemic encephalopathy. Therefore, the presence of NDN supports the neuropathological diagnosis of HD. The NDN may be those spiny neurons with degenerative and regenerative changes observed in HD following Golgi impregnation (Graveland *et al.*, 1985*b*); studies to precisely categorize these neurons are in progress.

Reiner *et al.* (1988) evaluated whether there was a differential loss among neostriatal projection neurons in 17 HD brains. They found that enkephalin-containing neurons projecting to the GPe were much more affected than substance P-containing neurons projecting to the GPi. This observation was confirmed by Sapp *et al.* (1995) and Richfield *et al.* (1995). Each of these three studies found a grade-related decline in the striatal enkephalin immunoreactivity or in the number of preproenkephalin-labelled neurons.

Matrix–striosomes

The compartmentalization (matrix–striosomes) is preserved in the HD neostriatum, where the decrease in the surface of the matrix is striking while that of the striosomes is relatively unchanged (Ferrante *et al.*, 1987*b*). However, neuronal loss and gliosis involve both compartments (Ferrante *et al.*, 1989). As mentioned previously, gliosis and neuronal loss were found to first occur in the striosomes, as evidenced by the evaluation of brains of patients who died at an early stage of the disease (Hedreen & Folstein, 1995).

Cerebral cortex and white matter

The cerebral cortex and white matter do not show any specific macroscopical or microscopical changes as judged by conventional neuropathological examination; the exception is a volumetric reduction which is more pronounced in the white matter than in the cortex. It was noted that the loss of white matter was more striking than that of gray matter with the exception of the striatum as early as 1914 (Kiesselbach, 1914; Dunlap, 1927). As stated previously, de la Monte *et al.* (1988) found a 21–29% volumetric cortical loss and a 29–34% loss of white matter in HD. The extent of these losses correlates with the grade of neuropathological severity. However, within the same grade of neuropathological severity, for example, grade 3, the cortical and white matter loss may vary. At times, the atrophy of both cortex and white matter is somewhat proportional to

that of the striatum; there are cases with striatal changes of grade 3 but with only slight volumetric reduction of cortex and white matter.

Dunlap (1927) found the HD cortex (n 30) to be 'slightly thinner than in the controls (n 30), but the difference was very little'. Terplan's illustration in 1924 (reproduced by Hallervorden in his often quoted review published in 1957) compares a normal cerebral cortex with that of a HD patient with severe neuronal loss. The control brain was from a 20 year-old executed convict, the other was from a 38 year-old woman with a 10-year history of chorea and with gangrene of the lungs found at autopsy (these details are to be found in Terplan's publication but not in Hallervorden's review). Zalneraitis *et al.* (1981) found little or no appreciable neuronal loss, normal astrocytes and a relatively normal content of glial fibrillary protein in the cortex of 14 HD brains.

Morphometric studies of the prefrontal cortex in 81 HD brains (grades 2, 3 and 4) and 23 normal age-matched controls showed a loss of large pyramidal neurons in layers III, V and VI in HD; neuronal loss was striking in grade 4; there was no increase in glial cells in the HD cortex (Sotrel *et al.*, 1991). Cudkowicz & Kowall (1990) performed cell counts in the cortex including Brodmann areas 8, 9, and 24 of eleven patients with HD (three grade 2; seven grade 3; and one grade 4) and of six age-matched controls. They found a depletion of long projecting neurons but a normal number of local circuit neurons in HD brains when compared to the controls. Contrary to Sotrel *et al.* (1991), Cudkowicz and Kowall did not find a correlation between the grades and the severity of cortical neuronal loss. Hedreen *et al.* (1991) compared Brodmann area 10 of five HD brains (grade 4) with five age-matched controls. They found cortical thinning, a 57% neuronal loss in layer VI and a 71% loss in layer V in the HD samples.

According to our experience, the extent of cortical atrophy depends on the stage of the disease: it is most pronounced in grades 3 and 4, while the cortex is apparently normal in grades 1 and 2. There is no reactive gliosis across the grades. It can be extremely difficult to identify cortical abnormalities in HD (Richardson, 1990). The volumetric loss of white matter is severe in grades 3 and 4 without any apparent microscopical abnormality.

Thalamus, hypothalamus and substantia nigra

The thalamus is normal on gross and microscopical examination in grades 1 and 2. It is smaller than normal in grade 3 and even more so in grade 4. Astrocytosis and neuronal loss in the centrum medianum are the only microscopical abnormalities regularly observed in grade 4 and, to a lesser extent, grade 3 brains.

Another pathological feature of HD is the neuronal loss that correlates with the grade in both the lateral nucleus of the hypothalamus (Kremer et al., 1990, 1991) and SNr (Richardson, 1990). The SNr is markedly atrophic and the neuronal density is decreased, especially in grades 3 and 4; the SNc is thinner than normal yet its number of neurons remains normal in all grades (Schroeder, 1931; Richardson, 1990). The loss of neuropil results in a relative increased density of pigmented neurons, especially in grades 3 and 4.

Subthalamic nucleus and red nucleus

Personal experience indicates that the subthalamic nucleus and red nucleus show mild to moderate volumetric reduction in grades 3 and 4 without any recognizable microscopical alteration. These nuclei are apparently normal in grades 1 and 2. They were atrophic and gliotic with scattered argyrophilic neurons in a single brain that, in addition to the characteristic features of HD, displayed those of PSP.

Cerebellum

There are no specific cerebellar HD changes recognizable by conventional neuropathological examination. The cerebellum is normal on gross and microscopical examination in grades 1 and 2; there is gross atrophy without microscopical abnormality in grades 3 and 4. Cortical neuronal loss, when present, is often associated with hypoxic-ischaemic events.

We were unable to reliably differentiate 25 HD cases from 25 non-HD cases in a blind evaluation of 50 slides from systematically selected blocks of the dentate nucleus with the cortical ribbon dorsal to it. Dunlap (1927) found the cerebellum to be morphologically normal in 29 of 30 HD cases; one was atrophic.

Juvenile HD patients usually have severe cerebral and cerebeller atrophy with striatal features of grade 4 at the time of autopsy. Byers et al. (1973) reported the neuropathological data of four juvenile HD patients all with severe cerebellar atrophy. The hippocampal formation was available in three of the four patients; of these three hippocampi, two were abnormal. Forty per cent of juvenile HD patients have seizures, which may be accountable for cerebellar or hippocampal neuronal loss (Fau et al., 1971).

The brainstem and spinal cord show volumetric reduction in grades 3 and 4, without any significant microscopical abnormality.

CAG REPEATS – NEUROPATHOLOGY – GENE EXPRESSION

As stated previously, HD appears to be caused by an expansion of an unstable CAG repeat on chromosome 4p16.3 within a coding region of a gene referred to as IT15 (for 'interesting transcript') (Gusella et al., 1993; The Huntington's Disease Collaborative Research Group et al., 1993). Juvenile onset patients typically have repeat lengths of more than 60 units, while most mid-life onset patients have repeat lengths in the 40–50 unit range, and those with very late onset usually have 37–40 units. These numbers of repeats correlate inversely with age of onset or with age at death (Andrew et al., 1993; Snell et al., 1993; Duyao et al., 1993; Persichetti et al., 1994, 1995).

Correlation of CAG repeat lengths and grades using 310 brains from clinically diagnosed HD patients showed that repeat stretches of 37–40 units occurred in all grades and that the largest alleles (> 50 units) occurred only in grades 3 and 4. These observations indicate that there is no larger threshold repeat size associated with grade 4, and that the large alleles influence the rate of striatal atrophy (Persichetti et al., 1994, 1995).

The gene involved in HD may be translated as a variable polyglutamine segment in the cytosolic protein product huntingtin. The HD mutation does not eliminate the expression of huntingtin, as evidenced by its presence in cells from HD homozygotes. The HD huntingtin is larger than the normal huntingtin (Gusella & MacDonald, 1994; Persichetti et al., 1995).

Investigations using in situ hybridization (with RNA probes constructed from cDNA subclones making up the composite sequences of IT15) and immunochemistry (with antisera directed at peptides predicted by the DNA sequence upstream and downstream of the CAG repeats) revealed widespread expression of IT15. Indeed, it is expressed in all brain regions and in other organs of both HD and control samples (Hoogeveen et al., 1993; Duyao et al., 1993; Li et al., 1993; Dure et al., 1994; Strong et al., 1994; Landwehrmeyer et al., 1995; Persichetti et al., 1995). Regional cerebral expression of IT15 is apparently proportional to neuronal density. The highest levels are seen in the cerebellum, hippocampus, cerebral cortex, SNc, and pontine nuclei, with intermediate levels in the neostriatum and with low levels in the GP (Landwehrmeyer et al., 1995). IT15 expression

Table 9.2. *Frequency of concomitant pathologies in 63 of 259 brains with changes of HD that have been evaluated between April 1991 and April 1994. Five brains had two concomitant pathologies; 58 brains had one concomitant pathology*

Alzheimer changes	24
Alzheimer's disease	11
Alzheimer's disease Lewy body variant	1
Amyotrophic lateral sclerosis (motor neuron disease)	1
Cerebritis	1
Grey matter heterotopia	3
Human immunodeficiency virus (HIV) encephalitis	1
Hypertensive encephalopathy (Binswanger disease)	2
Infarcts	21
Metastases	2
Progressive supranuclear palsy	1

Table 9.3. *Clinicopathological discrepancies and clinically unexpected findings: review of 340 brains submitted as HD, possible HD and as at risk for HD evaluated between April 1990 and April 1994*

Amyotrophic lateral sclerosis	1
Alzheimer's disease	1
Multiple system atrophy	3
Progressive, infantile, striato-thalamic degeneration of undetermined type and cause	1
Status cribrosus and lacunaris involving striatum	1

predominates in neurons and is weak in glial cells. The mechanism by which CAG repeats are expanded and translated into a polyglutamine segment in huntingtin leading to neuronal death (especially in the striatum) is unknown.

CONCOMITANT NEUROPATHOLOGICAL FINDINGS

The presence of neuropathological changes of HD does not preclude simultaneous occurrence of cerebral abnormalities other than those characteristic for HD. Between April 1991 and April 1994, we evaluated 259 brains with the pathognomonic changes of HD. Among them 63 brains had one, and five brains had two additional concomitant pathologies other than those of HD. The frequencies of the concomitant pathologies are shown in Table 9.2. The reactive gemistocytic gliosis is apparently indistinguishable from that expected in non-HD brains when, in addition to the HD pathology, another lesion such as infarct or metastasis simultaneously involves the neostriatum.

CLINICOPATHOLOGICAL DISCREPANCIES AND DIFFERENTIAL DIAGNOSIS

The accuracy of clinical diagnosis of HD is high. The morbid course of the disease and its symptoms are quite characteristic; the family history is also a contributory diagnostic factor. At the time of death of the patients, clinical evidence of HD is usually well recognized. The family history might be misleading, however. In the past ten years, we evaluated four brains from patients with

the clinical diagnosis of HD, while the neuropathological findings were characteristic of those of Alzheimer's disease in three of them and of Pick's disease in the other. Table 9.3 includes significant clinicopathological discrepancies among the 340 brains submitted as HD, possible HD and as at risk for HD between April 1990 and April 1994.

Extreme caution must be exercised when determining the presence of the gradients of neuronal loss along the ventro-dorsal, latero-medial, and antero-posterior axes of the striatum in the early stages of the disease to mistakenly avoid ruling out HD (Fig. 9.11). These gradients are probably pathognomonic for HD and should be evaluated in all brains from patients with movement disorders.

Alzheimer's disease

The pathological changes of HD and those of Alzheimer's disease were found in 11 instances among 259 brains of patients with the clinical diagnosis of HD (Table 9.2). On gross examination, the anterior striatum is often atrophic in Alzheimer's disease, however, in contrast to HD, there is preservation of the BCN and TCN, which bulge into the lateral ventricle (Fig. 9.5, right). The amygdala and hippocampal formations are relatively normal in HD, nevertheless, when these structures are atrophic together with atrophy of the BCN and TCN the probability of finding microscopical evidence of HD *and* Alzheimer's disease is high (Fig. 9.8, left). In the neostriatum, the association of HD and Alzheimer's disease is expressed by the presence of occasional argyrophilic tangles involving the large neostriatal neurons; these tangles are not present in pure HD.

Progressive supranuclear palsy

On gross examination, changes of the lenticular nucleus in PSP can mimic those of HD. The discolouration of the GP, particularly of the GPi, is more pronounced in PSP than in HD. Blurring of the pallidal lateral and medial medullary laminae is often striking in PSP contrary to HD, although these laminae are less distinct in grades 3 and 4 than normally expected. In PSP, the atrophy of the GP is more striking than that involving the putamen and CN, whereas in HD it is more pronounced in the CN and putamen (Fig. 9.8, right). The brain of one patient with the clinical diagnosis of HD in our series showed not only atrophy of the striatum with the gradients of neuronal loss and gliosis characteristic for HD, but severe atrophy with gliosis and neuronal loss involving the GPe and GPi, subthalamic nucleus, red nucleus, SNc and SNr, dentate nucleus and inferior olivary nucleus. In addition, there were scattered argyrophilic neurons in the atrophic areas. Only large neostriatal neurons were argyrophilic. This brain simultaneously displayed the changes of HD and those of PSP.

Pick's disease
In a series of 32 neuropathologically evaluated brains with circumscribed atrophy, 69% exhibited atrophy of the CN, 56% displayed pallidal atrophy, and 59% showed nigral lesions (Tissot, Constantinidis & Richard, 1975). The atrophy of the Pick striatum topographically matches that of the cortex; therefore, in Pick's disease, the anterior portions of the striatum are more involved than the posterior, which is in contrast to HD (Spatz, 1952). Furthermore, in Pick's disease, the HCN is often more involved than the putamen, and the nucleus accumbens is severely atrophic, in contrast to HD (Lüers & Spatz, 1957; Vonsattel et al., 1985). Both the SNc and SNr are involved in Pick's disease, whereas there is relative preservation of the SNc in HD (Lüers & Spatz, 1957; Richardson, 1990).

Multiple system atrophy and Corticobasal degeneration or corticodentatonigral degeneration with neuronal achromasia
The neuropathological distinction between multiple system atrophy, corticobasal degeneration and HD can easily be made by topographically evaluating the striatal atrophy. In multiple system atrophy or corticobasal degeneration the putamen is usually more involved than the CN; the middle third of the neostriatum along the antero-posterior axis of the cerebral hemisphere is especially atrophic; neuronal loss and gliosis are more strikingly present in the ventro-lateral portion of the putamen than dorsally. The ventro-lateral portion of the

BCN is often involved while the remainder of the BCN, HCN and TCN are preserved. In addition, the SNc shows neuronal loss and gliosis (Rebeiz, Kolodny & Richardson, 1968; Funkenstein & Miller, 1985; Gibb, Luthert & Marsden, 1989; Riley et al., 1990). According to our experience these changes involving the SNc are very rare in pure HD.

Neuroacanthocytosis
Patients with neuroacanthocytosis (also referred to as familial amyotrophic chorea with acanthocytosis, familial neuroacanthocytosis of Levine–Critchley syndrome) have acanthocytes (erythrocytes with spiky, peripheral projections) with or without lipoprotein, and movement disorders such as dystonia, ataxia, parkinsonism, chorea, orolingual tic-like movements, seizures, dementia, and neurogenic muscular atrophy (Yamamoto et al., 1982; Sakai, Iwashita & Kakugawa, 1985; Peppard et al., 1990; Hardie et al., 1991; Rinne et al., 1994b). McLeod syndrome is an X-linked form of neuroacanthocytosis with movement disorders of insidious onset (in the fourth decade) and a type of muscular dystrophy with changes suggesting a non-dystrophin membrane defect; these patients have weak expression of the antigens for the Kell blood group system (Witt et al., 1992; Ho et al., 1994). Chorea is not always present in neuroacanthocytosis, the occurrence of which can be familial or sporadic (Hardie et al., 1991).

The most consistent neuropathological abnormalities described in neuroacanthocytosis are gross atrophy of the striatum and widening of the frontal horns of the lateral ventricles. The published pictures of coronal sections show severe atrophy of the nucleus accumbens. Neuronal loss and gliosis are severe in the CN and slightly less so in the putamen; neuronal loss is also described in the GP, probably in both external and internal segments (Bird et al., 1978; Iwata et al., 1984; Hardie et al., 1991; Rinne et al., 1994b). Details of the neostriatal distribution of neuronal loss and gliosis are not available in the literature, with the exception of the report by Iwata et al. (1984); these authors found the putamen to be involved ventrally while the dorsal portion was barely affected. Neuronal loss and gliosis were occasionally found in the medial thalamus (Rinne et al., 1994b). The substantia nigra was reported as being normal or was remarkable for neuronal loss; in some cases the SNc was more involved than the SNr or vice versa (Bird et al., 1978; Hardie et al., 1991; Rinne et al., 1994b). According to Rinne et al., (1994a) neuronal loss does occur in the substantia nigra, especially in patients who had parkinsonism; loss of pigmented neurons or of tyrosine hydroxylase immunoreactive neurons was documented throughout the substantia nigra with the ventrolateral portion most severely involved. The cerebral and cerebellar cortices, subthalamic nucleus, brainstem and medulla oblongata are all apparently within normal limits.

Our experience with neuroacanthocytosis is limited to the review of slides of two cases including one reported by Bird *et al.* (1978), and has left us with the impression that the neostriatal gradients of neuronal loss and gliosis so characteristically present in HD are lacking in neuroacanthocytosis. In addition, it seems that the nucleus accumbens is severely atrophic in neuroacanthocytosis while it is relatively spared in HD as compared to the dorsal half of the HCN or dorsal putamen. Another difference is that gliosis in the GPi is frequently described in neuroacanthocytosis but occurs very rarely in HD. Finally, the SNc shows neuronal loss in neuroacanthocytosis in contrast to HD.

The pathological spectrum of the neostriatum in neuroacanthocytosis is still incompletely described; systematic evaluation providing topographic data (rostral versus caudal, dorsal versus ventral, medial versus lateral, GPe versus GPi) will be helpful in making the diagnosis of neuroacanthocytosis or of HD.

Of interest are the neuropathological findings of a patient with spontaneous oral–facial dyskinesia reported by Altrocchi & Forno (1983). Atrophy of the CN was slight. Microscopical examination revealed severe, uneven neuronal loss and fibrillary astrocytosis limited to the dorsal half of the CN and putamen throughout, giving a mosaic appearance. Mild gliosis was also present in the dorsal, lateral portion of the GPe; the other deep gray nuclei, cortex, white matter, brainstem and cerebellum were normal.

We encountered several instances in which, on gross examination of the coronal sections only, the atrophy of the striatum mimicked HD, e.g. Creutzfeldt–Jakob disease (Growdon & Vonsattel, 1993), subacute sclerosing panencephalitis and neuronal lipofuscinosis.

Exceptionally, HD-like neuropathology can occur in the absence of expanded CAG repeats (Persichetti *et al.*, 1994). The identification of such brains by careful neuropathological evaluation, by saving fresh frozen samples for nucleic acid studies, and by genotyping family members could unveil an, as yet, unknown subcategory of striatal degeneration. Clarification of this putative subcategory of brains would be invaluable in the process of understanding the mechanism whereby an expanded CAG allele becomes deleterious to certain classes of neurons in specific areas.

ACKNOWLEDGEMENTS
We thank Dr E. D. Bird, director of the Brain Tissue Resource Center, McLean Hospital, Belmont, MA, USA for his support. We thank Timothy Wheelock and Lisa Kanaley-Andrews for their excellent technical assistance. We gratefully acknowledge L. Cherkas for his photography and advice. We also express our appreciation to the numerous pathologists who referred case material to the Brain Tissue Resource Center. We are especially grateful to the families of the patients for providing brain tissue for research.

This work was supported in part by NIH grants NINCDS 31862 (Brain Tissue Resource Center) and NS 16367 (Huntington's Disease Center Without Walls); and by grants from the Vaughn Foundation and Hereditary Disease Foundation.

REFERENCES
Albin RL, Young AB, Penney JB (1989) The functional anatomy of basal ganglia disorders. *Trends Neurosci* 12: 366–75.

Albin RL, Reiner A, Anderson KD, Penney JB, Young AB (1990*a*) Striatal and nigral neuron subpopulations in rigid Huntington's disease: implications for the functional anatomy of chorea and rigidity-akinesia. *Ann Neurol* 27: 357–65.

Albin RL, Young AB, Penney JB, Handelin B, Balfour R, Anderson KD, Markel DS, Tourtellotte WW, Reiner A (1990*b*) Abnormalities of striatal projection neurons and *N*-methyl-D-aspartate receptors in presymptomatic Huntingtons' disease. *New Engl J Med* 322: 1293–8.

Altrocchi PH, Forno LS (1983) Spontaneous oral-facial dyskinesia: neuropathology of a case. *Neurology* 33: 802–5.

Alzheimer A (1911) Über die anatomische Grundlage der Huntingtonschen Chorea und der choreatischen Bewegungen überhaupt. *Neurol Centralblatt* 30: 891–2.

Andrew SE, Goldberg YP, Kremer B, Telenius H, Theilmann J, Adam S, Starr E, Squitieri F, Lin B, Kalchman MA, Graham RK, Hayden MR (1993) The relationship between trinucleotide (CAG) repeat length and clinical features of Huntington's disease. *Nature Genet* 4: 398–403.

Anton G (1896) Über die Beteiligung der grossen basalen Gehirnganglien bei Bewegungstörungen und insbesondere bei Chorea. *Jahrn Psychiatr Neurol (Lpz)*, 14: 141–81.

Aronin N, Cooper PE, Lorenz LJ, Bird ED, Sagar SM, Leeman SE, Martin JB (1983) Somatostatin is increased in the basal ganglia in Huntington's disese. *Ann Neurol* 13: 519–26.

Beal MF, Bird ED, Langlais PJ, Martin JB (1984) Somatostatin is increased in the nucleus accumbens in Huntington's disease. *Neurology* 34: 663–6.

Beal MF, Kowall NW, Ellison DW, Mazurek MF, Swartz KJ, Martin JB (1986) Replication of the neurochemical characteristics of Huntington's disease by quinolinic acid. *Nature* 321: 168–71.

Beal MF, Ellison DW, Mazurek MF, Swartz KJ, Malloy JR, Bird ED, Martin JB (1988*a*) A detailed examination of substance P in pathologically graded cases of Huntington's disease. *J Neurol Sci* 84: 51–61.

Beal MF, Mazurek MF, Ellison DW, Swartz KJ, McGarvey U, Bird ED, Martin JB (1988*b*) Somatostatin and neuropeptide Y concentrations in pathologically graded cases of Huntington's disease. *Ann Neurol* 23: 562–9.

Bielschowsky M (1919) Einige Bemerkungen zur normalen und pathologischen Histologie des Schweif- und Linsenkerns. *J Psychol Neurol* 25: 1–11.

Bird ED, Iversen LL (1974) Huntington's chorea. Post-mortem measurement of glutamic acid decarboxylase, choline acetyltransferase and dopamine in basal ganglia. *Brain* 97: 457–72.

Bird MT, Paulson GW (1971) The rigid form of Huntington's chorea. *Neurology* 21: 271–6.

Bird TD, Cederbaum S, Valpey RW, Stahl WL (1978) Familial degeneration of the basal ganglia with acanthocytosis: a clinical, neuropathological, and neurochemical study. *Ann Neurol* 3: 253–8.

Birnbaum G (1941) Chronisch-progressive Chorea mit Kleinhirnatrophie. *Arc Psychiat Nervenkrankh* 114: 160–82.

Bonduelle M, Gruner J, Bouygues P (1953) Chorée de Huntington avec paraplégie spasmodique. Deux cas familiaux. Étude anatomique. Remarque sur les relations de la surdité et des lésions de l'olive supérieure. *Rev Neurol* 88: 126–31.

Bruyn GW (1968) Huntington's chorea; historical, clinical and laboratory synopsis. In Vinken PJ, Bruyn GW (eds) *Handbook of Clinical Neurology*. Elsevier Science Publishers, Amsterdam, Vol. 6, pp 298–378.

Bruyn GW (1973) Neuropathological changes in Huntington's chorea. In Barbeau A, Chase TN, Paulson GW (eds) *Huntington's Chorea 1872–1972. Advances in Neurology. Volume 1*, Raven Press, New York, pp 399–403.

Bruyn GW, Bots G, Th AM, Dom R (1979) Huntington's chorea: Current neuropathological status. In Chase TN, Wexler NS, Barbeau A (eds) *Advances in Neurology, vol. 23, Huntington's Disease*, Raven Press, New York, pp 83–93.

Byers RK, Gilles FH, Fung C (1973) Huntington's disease in children. *Neurology* 23: 561–9.

Carpenter MB, Sutin J (1983) *Human Neuroanatomy*. Williams & Wilkins, Baltimore/London. 8th edn, pp 579–86.

Castaigne P, Escourolle R, Gray F (1976) Chorée de Huntington et atrophie cérébelleuse. A propos d'une observation anatomo-clinique. *Rev Neurol* 132: 233–40.

Chevalier G, Deniau JM (1990) Disinhibition as a basic process in the expression of striatal functions. *Trends Neurosci* 13: 277–80.

Colmers WF, Bleakman D (1994) Effects of neuropeptide y on the electrical properties of neurons. *Trends Neurosci* 17: 373–9.

Conneally PM (1984) Huntington disease: genetics and epidemiology. *Am J Hum Genet* 36: 506–26.

Cooper PE, Fernstrom MH, Rorstad OP, Leeman SE, Martin JB (1981) The regional distribution of somatostatin, substance P and neurotensin in human brain. *Brain Res* 218: 219–32.

Cudkowicz M, Kowall NW (1990) Degeneration of pyramidal projection neurons in Huntington's disease cortex. *Ann Neurol* 27: 200–4.

Davison C, Goodhart SP, Shlionsky H (1932) Chronic progressive chorea. The pathogenesis and mechanism; a histopathologic study. *Arch Neurol Psychiat (Chicago)* 27: 906–28.

Dawbarn D, De Quidt ME, Emson PC (1985) Survival of basal ganglia neuropeptide y-somatostatin neurones in Huntington's disease. *Brain Res* 340: 251–60.

de la Monte SM, Vonsattel JP, Richardson EP Jr (1988) Morphometric demonstration of atrophic changes in the cerebral cortex, white matter, and neostriatum in Huntington's disease. *J Neuropath Exp Neurol* 47: 516–25.

DiFiglia M (1990) Excitotoxic injury of the neostriatum: a model for Huntington's disease. *Trends Neurosci* 13: 286–9.

DiFiglia M, Carey J (1986) Large neurons in the primate neostriatum examined with the combined Golgi-electron microscopic method. *J Comp Neurol* 244: 36–52.

Dom R, Malfroid M, Baro F (1976) Neuropathology of Huntington's chorea. *Neurology* 26: 64–8.

Dunlap CB (1927) Pathologic changes in Huntington's chorea. *Arch Neurol Psychiat (Chicago)* 18: 867–943.

Dure LSIV, Landwehrmeyer GB, Golden J, McNeil SM, Ge P, Aizawa H, Huang Q, Ambrose CM, Duyao MP, Bird ED, DiFiglia M, Gusella JF, MacDonald ME, Penney JB, Young AB, Vonsattel JP (1994) IT15 gene expression in fetal human brain. *Brain Res* 659: 3341.

Duyao M, Ambrose C, Myers R, Novelletto A, Persichetti F, Frontali M, Folstein S, Ross C, Franz M, Abbott M, Gray J, Conneally P, Young A, Penney J, Hollingsworth Z, Shoulson I, Lazzarini A, Falek A, Koroshetz W, Sax D, Bird E, Vonsattel J, Bonilla E, Albir J, Bickham Conde J, Cha J-H, Dure L, Gomez F, Ramos M, Sanchez-Ramos J, Snodgrass S, de Young M, Wexler N, Moscowitz C, Penchaszadeh G, MacFarlane H, Anderson M, Jenkins B, Srinidhi J, Barnes G, Gusella J, MacDonald M (1993) Trinucleotide repeat length instability and age of onset in Huntington's disease. *Nature Genet* 4: 387–92.

Ellison DW, Beal MF, Mazurek MF, Malloy JR, Bird ED, Martin JB (1987) Amino acid neurotransmitter abnormalities in Huntington's disease and the quinolinic acid animal model of Huntington's disease. *Brain* 110: 1657–73.

Fau R, Chateau R, Tommasi M, Groslambert R, Garrel S, Perret J (1971) Étude anatomo-clinique d'une forme rigide et myoclonique de maladie de Huntington infantile. *Rev Neurol* 124: 353–66.

Ferrante RJ, Beal MF, Kowall NW, Richardson EP, Martin JB (1987*a*) Sparing of acetylcholinesterase-containing striatal neurons in Huntington's disease. *Brain Res* 411: 162–6.

Ferrante RJ, Kowall NW, Beal MF, Martin JB, Bird ED, Richardson EP (1987*b*) Morphologic and histochemical characteristics of a spared subset of striatal neurons in Huntington's disease. *J Neuropath Exp Neurol* 46: 12–27.

Ferrante RJ, Kowall NW, Beal MF, Richardson EP Jr, Bird ED, Martin JB (1985) Selective sparing of a class of striatal neurons in Huntington's disease. *Science* 230: 561–3.

Ferrante RJ, Kowall NW, Richardson EP Jr (1989) Cellular composition of striatal patch and matrix compartments in Huntington's disease. *Soc Neurosci* 15: 935. (Abst)

Folstein SE (1989*a*) Epidemiology. In Folstein SE (ed) *Huntington's Disease. A Disorder of Families*, The Johns Hopkins University Press, Baltimore and London, pp 88–105.

Folstein SE (1989*b*) The diagnosis of Huntington's disease. In Folstein SE (ed) *Huntington's Disease. A Disorder of Families*, The Johns Hopkins University Press, Baltimore and London, pp 125–148.

Folstein SE (1989*c*) The cognitive disorder. In Folstein, SE (ed) *Huntington's Disease. A Disorder of Families*, The Johns Hopkins University Press, Baltimore and London, pp 32–48.

Forno LS, Jose C (1973) Huntington's chorea: a pathological study. In Barbeau A, Chase TN, Paulson GW (eds) *Advances in Neurology, vol. 1, Huntington's Chorea*, Raven Press, New York, pp 453–70.

Funkenstein HH, Miller DC (1985) Case records of the Massachusetts General Hospital. Case 38–1985. *New Engl J Med* 313: 739–48.

Garrett EA, Crutcher MD (1990) Functional architecture of basal ganglia circuits: neural substrates of parallel processing. *Trends Neurosci* 13: 266–71.

Gerfen CR, Baimbridge KG, Thibault J (1987*a*) The neostriatal mosaic: III. Biochemical and developmental dissociation of patch-matrix mesostriatal systems. *J Neurosci* 7: 3935–44.

Gerfen CR, Herkenham M, Thibault J (1987*b*) The neostriatal mosaic: II. Patch- and matrix-directed mesostriatal dopaminergic and non-dopaminergic systems. *J Neurosci* 7: 3915–34.

Gibb RG, Luthert PJ, Marsden CD (1989) Corticobasal degeneration. *Brain* 112: 1171–92.

Goldberg YP, Kremer B, Andrew SE, Theilmann J, Graham RK, Squitieri F, Telenius H, Adam S, Sajoo A, Starr E, Heiberg A, Wolff G, Hayden MR (1993) Molecular analysis of new mutations for Huntington's disease: intermediate alleles and sex of origin effects. *Nature Genet* 5: 174–9.

Goldman-Rakic PS (1982) Cytoarchitectonic heterogeneity of the primate neostriatum: subdivision into island and matrix cellular compartments. *J Comp Neurol* 205: 398–413.

Graveland GA, Williams RS, DiFiglia M (1985*a*) Evidence for degenerative and regenerative changes in neostriatal spiny neurons in Huntington's disease. *Science* 227: 770–3.

Graveland GA, Williams RS, DiFiglia M (1985*b*) A Golgi study of the human neostriatum: neurons and afferent fibers. *J Comp Neurol* 234: 317–33.

Graybiel AM, Aosaki T, Flaherty AW, Kimura M (1994) The basal ganglia and adaptive motor control. *Science* 265: 1826–31.

Graybiel AM, Ragsdale CW Jr (1979) Fiber connections of the basal ganglia. In Cuénod M, Kreutzberg GW, Bloom FE (eds) *Development and Chemical Specificity of Neurons*, Elsevier, Amsterdam, pp 239–83.

Graybiel AM, Ragsdale CW Jr (1983) Biochemical anatomy of the striatum. In Emson PC (ed) *Chemical Neuroanatomy*, Raven Press, New York, pp 427–504.

Growdon JH, Vonsattel JP (1993) Case Records of the Massachusetts General Hospital. Case 17–1993. A 53-year-old woman who died after several years of a dementing illness with intermittent generalized seizures and abnormal movements of the extremities and head. *New Engl J Med* 328: 1259–66.

Gusella JF (1991) Huntington's disease. In Harris H, Hirschhorn K (eds) *Advances in Human Genetics, Vol 20*, Plenum Press, New York, pp 125–51.

Gusella JF, MacDonald ME (1994) Huntington's disease and repeating trinucleotides. *New Engl J Med* 330: 1450–1.

Gusella JF, MacDonald ME, Ambrose CM, Duyao MP (1993) Molecular genetics of Huntington's disease. *Arch Neurol* 50: 1157–63.

Gusella JF, Wexler NS, Conneally PM, Naylor SL, Anderson MA, Tanzi RE, Watkins PC, Ottina K, Wallace MR, Sakaguchi AY, Young AB, Shoulson I, Bonilla E, Martin JB (1983) A polymorphic DNA marker genetically linked to Huntington's disease. *Nature* 306: 234–8.

Hallervorden J (1957) Huntingtonsche Chorea (Chorea chronica progressiva hereditaria). In Lubarsch O, Henke F, Rössle R, Scholz W (eds) *Handbuch der speziellen pathologischen Anatomie und Histologie (XIII/1 Bandteil A)*, Springer Verlag, Berlin, Göttingen, Heildelberg, pp 793–822.

Hardie RJ, Pullon HWH, Harding AE, Owen JS, Pires M, Daniels GL, Imai Y, Misra VP, King RHM, Jacobs JM, Tippett P, Duchen LW, Thomas PK, Marsden CD (1991) Neuroacanthocytosis. A clinical, haematological and pathological study of 19 cases. *Brain* 114: 13–49.

Harper PS, Morris MR, Quarrell OWJ, Shaw DJ, Tyler A, Youngman S (1991*a*) The clinical neurology of Huntington's disease. In Harper PS (ed) *Huntington's Disease. Major Problems in Neurology, 22*, WB Saunders Company Ltd, London, Philadelphia, Toronto, Sydney, Tokyo, pp 37–80.

Harper PS, Morris MR, Quarrell OWJ, Shaw DJ, Tyler A, Youngman S (1991*b*) Psychiatric aspects of Huntington's disease. In Harper PS (ed) *Huntington's Disease. Major*

Problems in Neurology, 22, WB Saunders Company Ltd, London, Philadelphia, Toronto, Sydney, Tokyo, pp 81–126.

Harper PS, Morris MR, Quarrell OWJ, Shaw DJ, Tyler A, Youngman S (1991c) The epidemiology of Huntington's disease. In Harper PS (ed) *Huntington's Disease. Major Problems in Neurology*, 22, WB Saunders Company Ltd, London, Philadelphia, Toronto, Sydney, Tokyo, pp 251–80.

Hayden MR (1981) Epidemiology. In Hayden MR (ed) *Huntington's Chorea*, Springer Verlag, Berlin, Heidelberg, New York, pp 31–44.

Hedreen JC, Folstein SE (1995) Early loss of neostriatal striosome neurons in Huntington's disease. *J Neuropath Exp Neurol* 54: 105–20.

Hedreen JC, Peyser CE, Folstein SE, Ross CA (1991) Neuronal loss in Layers V and VI of cerebral cortex in Huntington's disease. *Neurosci Lett* 133: 257–61.

Ho M, Chelly J, Carter N, Danek A, Crocker P, Monaco AP (1994) Isolation of the gene for McLeod syndrome that encodes a novel membrane transport protein. *Cell* 77: 869–80.

Hoogeveen AT, Willemsen R, Meyer N, De Rooij E, Roose AC, van Ommen GB, Galjaard H (1993) Characterization and localization of the Huntington disease gene product. *Hum Mol Genet* 2: 2069–73.

Iwata M, Fuse S, Sakuta M, Toyokura Y (1984) Neuropathological study of chorea-acanthocytosis. *Jap J Med* 23: 118–22.

Jelgersma G (1908) Neue anatomische Befunde bei Paralysis agitans und bei chronischer Chorea. *Neurol Centralblatt*, 27: 995–6.

Jervis GA (1963) Huntington's chorea in childhood. *Arch Neurol* 9: 244–57.

Jeste DV, Barban L, Parisi J (1984) Reduced Purkinje cell density in Huntington's disease. *Exp Neurol* 85: 78–86.

Kiesselbach G (1914) Anatomischer Befund eines Falles von Huntingtonscher Chorea. *Monatsschr f Psychiat Neurol (Berl)* 35: 525–43.

Koroshetz WJ, Myers RH, Martin JB (1992) The neurology of Huntington's disease. In Joseph AB, Young RR (eds) *Movement Disorders in Neurology and Neuropsychiatry*, Blackwell Scientific Publications, Boston, pp 167–77.

Kowall NW, Ferrante RJ, Martin JB (1987) Patterns of cell loss in Huntington's disease. *Trends Neurosci* 10: 24–9.

Kremer HPH, Roos RAC, Dingjan G, Marani E, Bots AM (1990) Atrophy of the hypothalamic lateral tuberal nucleus in Huntington's disease. *J Neuropath Exp Neurol* 49: 371–82.

Kremer HPH, Roos RAC, Dingjan GM, Bots GThAM, Bruyn GW, Hofman MA (1991) The hypothalamic lateral tuberal nucleus and the characteristics of neuronal loss in Huntington's disease. *Neurosci Lett* 132: 101–4.

Landwehrmeyer GB, McNeil SM, Dure LSIV, Ge P, Aizawa H, Huang Q, Ambrose CM, Duyao MP, Bird ED, Bonilla E, de Young M, Avila-Gonzales AJ, Wexler NS, DiFiglia M, Gusella JF, MacDonald ME, Penney JB, Young AB, Von-

sattel JP (1995) Huntington's disease gene: regional and cellular expression in brain of normal and affected individuals. *Ann Neurol* 37: 218–30.

Lange H, Thörner G, Hopf A, Schröder KF (1976) Morphometric studies of the neuropathological changes in choreatic diseases. *J Neurol Sci* 28: 401–25.

Lange HW (1981) Quantitative changes of telencephalon, diencephalon, and mesencephalon in Huntington's chorea, postencephalitic, and idiopathic parkinsonism. *Verh Anat Ges* 75: 923–5.

Lannois M, Paviot J (1897) Deux cas de la chorée héréditaire avec autopsies. *Arch Neurol (Paris)* 4: 333–4.

Li S-H, Schilling G, Young WS III, Li X-J, Margolis RL, Stine OC, Wagster MV, Abbott MH, Franz ML, Ranen NG, Folstein SE, Hedreen JC, Ross CA (1993) Huntington's disease gene (IT15) is widely expressed in human and rat tissues. *Neuron* 11: 985–93.

Lüers Th, Spatz H (1957) Picksche Krankheit (Progressive umschriebene Grosshirnatrophie). In Lubarsch O, Henke F, Rössle R, Scholz W (eds) *Handbuch der speziellen pathologischen Anatomie und Histologie (XIII/1 Bandteil A)*, Springer Verlag, Berlin, Göttingen, Heidelberg, pp 614–15.

Martin JB, Gusella JF (1986) Huntington's disease. Pathogenesis and management. Seminars in medicine of the Beth Israel Hospital, Boston. *New Engl J Med* 315: 1267–76.

Morton AJ, Nicholson LFB, Faull RLM (1993) Compartmental loss of NADPH Diaphorase in the neuropil of the human striatum in Huntington's disease. *Neuroscience* 53: 159–68.

Myers RH, Goldman D, Bird ED, Sax DS, Merril CR, Schoenfeld M, Wolf PA (1983) Maternal transmission in Huntington's disease. *Lancet* ii: 208–10.

Myers RH, MacDonald ME, Koroshetz WJ, Duyao MP, Ambrose CA, Taylor SAM, Barnes G, Srinidhi J, Lin CS, Whaley WL, Lazzarini AM, Schwarz M, Wolff G, Bird ED, Vonsattel J-P, Gusella JF (1993) De novo expansion of a (CAG)n repeat in sporadic Huntington's disease. *Nature Genet* 5: 168–73.

Myers RH, Vonsattel JP, Stevens TJ, Cupples LA, Richardson EP, Martin JB, Bird ED (1988) Clinical and neuropathologic assessment of severity in Huntington's disease. *Neurology* 38: 341–7.

Nieuwenhuys R (1985) *Chemoarchitecture of the Brain* Springer Verlag, Berlin, Heidelberg, New York, Tokyo.

Oyanagi K, Takeda S, Takahashi H, Ohama E, Ikuta F (1989) A quantitative investigation of the substantia nigra in Huntington's disease. *Ann Neurol* 26: 13–19.

Peppard RF, Lu CS, Chu N-S, Teal P, Martin WRW, Calne DB (1990) Parkinsonism with neuroacanthocytosis. *Can J Neurol Sci* 17: 298–301.

Persichetti F, Ambrose CM, Ge P, McNeil SM, Srinidhi J, Anderson MA, Jenkins B, Barnes GT, Duyao MP, Kanaley L, Wexler NS, Myers RH, Bird ED, Vonsattel JP, MacDonald ME, Gusella JF (1995) Normal and expanded Huntington's disease gene alleles produce distinguishable proteins due to translation across the CAG repeat. *Mol Med* 'in press'.

Persichetti F, Srinidhi J, Kanaley L, Ge P, Myers RH, D'Arrigo K, Barnes GT, MacDonald ME, Vonsattel J-P, Gusella JF, Bird ED (1994) Huntington's disease CAG trinucleotide repeats in pathologically confirmed post-mortem brains. *Neurobiol Dis* 1: 159–66.

Pfeiffer JAF (1913) A contribution to the pathology of chronic progressive chorea. *Brain* 35: 276–92.

Ragsdale CW Jr, Graybiel AM (1981) The Fronto-striatal projection in the cat and monkey and its relationship to inhomogeneities established by acetylcholinesterase histochemistry. *Brain Res* 208: 259–66.

Read AP (1993) Huntington's disease: testing the test. *Nature Genet* 4: 329–30.

Rebeiz JJ, Kolodny EH, Richardson EP Jr (1968) Corticodentatonigral degeneration with neuronal achromasia. *Arch Neurol* 18: 20–33.

Reiner A, Albin RL, Anderson KD, D'Amato CJ, Penney JB, Young AB (1988) Differential loss of striatal projection neurons in Huntington disease. *Proc Natl Acad Sci USA* 85: 5733–7.

Richardson EP Jr (1990) Third Dorothy S. Russell Memorial Lecture. Huntington's disease: some recent neuropathological studies. *Neuropath Appl Neurobiol* 16: 451–60.

Richfield EK, Maguire-Zeiss KA, Cox C, Gilmore J, Voorn P (1995) Reduced expression of preproenkephalin in striatal neurons from Huntington's disease patients. *Ann Neurol* 37: 335–43.

Riley DE, Lang AE, Lewis A, Resch L, Ashby P, Hornykiewicz O, Black S (1990) Cortical–basal ganglionic degeneration. *Neurology* 40: 1203–12.

Rinne JO, Daniel SE, Scaravilli F, Harding AE, Marsden CD (1994a) Nigral degeneration in neuroacanthocytosis. *Neurology* 44: 1629–32.

Rinne JO, Daniel SE, Scaravilli F, Pires M, Harding AE, Marsden CD (1994b) The neuropathological features of neuroacanthocytosis. *Movement Disorders* 9: 297–304.

Roberts RC, Ahn A, Swartz KJ, Beal MF, DiFiglia M (1993) Intrastriatal injections of quinolinic acid or kainic acid: differential patterns of cell survival and the effects of data analysis on outcome. *Exp Neurol* 124: 274–82.

Rodda RA (1981) Cerebellar atrophy in Huntington's disease. *J Neurol Sci* 50: 147–57.

Roizin L, Stellar S, Liu JC (1979) Neuronal nuclear-cytoplasmic changes in Huntington's chorea: electron microscope investigations. In Chase TN, Wexler NS, Barbeau A (eds) *Huntington's Disease Advances in Neurology. Vol. 23*, Raven Press, New York, pp. 95–122.

Rosenthal C (1927) Zur Symptomatologie und Frühdiagnostik der Huntingtonschen Krankheit, zugleich ein Beitrag zur klinischen Erbforschung (Degenerationserscheinungen und Konstitutionsanomalien in einem Huntingtonstamm). *Z Ges Neurol Psychiat* 111: 254–69.

Sagar SM, Beal MF, Marshall PE, Landis DMD, Martin JB (1984) Implications of neuropeptides in neurological diseases. *Peptides* 5: 255–62.

Sakai T, Iwashita H, Kakugawa M (1985) Neuroacanthocytosis syndrome and choreoacanthocytosis (Levine–Critchley syndrome). *Neurology* 35: 1679.

Sapp E, Ge P, Aizawa H, Bird E, Penney J, Young AB, Vonsattel J-P, DiFiglia M (1995) Evidence for a preferential loss of enkephalin immunoreactivity in the external globus pallidus in low grade Huntington's disease using high resolution image analysis. *Neuroscience* 64: 397–404.

Sax DS, Vonsattel J-P (1992) Case Records of the Massachusetts General Hospital. Case 2–1992. Chorea and progressive dementia in an 88-year-old woman. *New Engl J Med* 326: 117–25.

Schroeder K (1931) Zur Klinik und Pathologie der Huntingtonschen Krankheit. *J Psychol Neurol* 43: 183–201.

Schröder KF, Hopf A, Lange H, Thörner G (1975) Morphometrisch-statistische Strukturanalysen des Striatum, Pallidum und Nucleus subthalamicus beim Menschen. I. Striatum. *J Hirnforsch* 16: 333–50.

Selden N, Geula C, Hersh L, Mesulam M-M (1994) Human striatum: chemoarchitecture of the caudate nucleus, putamen and ventral striatum in health and Alzheimer's disease. *Neuroscience* 60: 621–36.

Selemon LD, Goldman-Rakic PS (1985) Longitudinal topography and interdigitation of corticostriatal projections in the rhesus monkey. *J Neurosci* 5: 776–94.

Selemon LD, Gottlieb JP, Goldman-Rakic PS (1994) Islands and striosomes in the neostriatum in the rhesus monkey: non-equivalent compartments. *Neuroscience* 58: 183–92.

Snell RG, MacMillan JC, Cheadle JP, Fenton I, Lazarou LP, Davies P, MacDonald ME, Gusella JF, Harper PS, Shaw DC (1993) Relationship between trinucleotide repeat expansion and phenotypic variation in Huntington's disease. *Nature Genet* 4: 393–7.

Sotrel A, Paskevich PA, Kiely DK, Bird ED, Williams RS, Myers RH (1991) Morphometric analysis of the prefrontal cortex in Huntington's disease. *Neurology* 41: 1117–23.

Spargo E, Everall IP, Lantos PL (1993) Neuronal loss in the hippocampus in Huntington's disease: a comparison with HIV infection. *J Neurol Neurosurg Psychiat* 56: 487–91.

Spatz H (1952) La maladie de Pick, les atrophies systématisées progressives et la sénescence cérébrale prématurée localisée. In *The Proceedings of the First International Congress of Neuropathology, vol. 2*, Rosenberg and Sellier, Torino, pp 375–406.

Spielmeyer W (1926) Die anatomische Krankheitsforschung am Beispiel einer Huntingtonschen Chorea mit Wilsonschem Symptomenbild. *Z Ges Neurol Psychiat* 101: 701–28.

Steiner H, Gerfen CR (1993) Cocaine-induced c-fos messenger RNA is inversely related to dynorphin expression in striatum. *J Neurosci* 13: 5066–81.

Stone TT, Falstein EI (1938) Pathology of Huntington's chorea. *J Nerv Ment Dis* 88: 773–97.

Strong TV, Tagle DA, Valdes JM, Elmer LW, Boehm K, Swaroop M, Kaatz DW, Collins FS, Albin RL (1994) Widespread expression of the human and rat Huntington's disease gene in brain and nonneural tissue. *Nature Genet* 5: 259–63.

Terplan K (1924) Zur pathologischen Anatomie der chronischen progressiven Chorea. *Virchow's Arch f Pathol Anat (Berl)* 252: 146–76.

The Huntington's Disease Collaborative Research Group, MacDonald ME, Ambrose CM, Duyao MP, Myers RH, Lin C, Srinidhi L, Barnes G, Taylor SA, James M, Groot N, MacFarlane H, Jenkins B, Anderson MA, Wexler NS, Gusella JF (1993) A novel gene containing a trinucleotide repeat that is expanded and unstable on Huntington's disease chromosomes. *Cell* 72: 971–83.

Tissot R, Constantinidis J, Richard J (1975) *La Maladie de Pick*. Masson, Paris, pp 1–122.

Vonsattel J-P, Myers RH, Stevens TJ, Ferrante RJ, Bird ED, Richardson EP Jr (1985) Neuropathological classification of Huntington's disease. *J Neuropath Exp Neurol* 44: 559–77.

Vonsattel J-P, Myers RH, Bird ED, Ge P, Richardson EP Jr (1992) Maladie de Huntington: sept cas avec îlots néostriataux relativement préservés. *Rev Neurol* 148: 107–16.

Vonsattel JP (1992) Neuropathology of Huntington's disease. In Joseph AB, Young RR (eds) *Movement Disorders in Neurology and Neuropsychiatry*, Blackwell Scientific Publication, Boston, pp 186–94.

Went LN, Vegter-van der Vlis M, Bruyn GW (1984) Parental transmission in Huntington's disease. *Lancet* i: 1100–2.

Whitworth RH Jr, LeDoux MS, Gould HJ III (1991) Topographic distribution of connections from the primary motor cortex to the corpus striatum in *Aotus trivirgatus*. *J Comp Neurol* 307: 177–88.

Witt TN, Danek A, Reiter M, Heim MU, Disrschinger J, Olsen EGJ (1992) McLeod syndrome: a distinct form of neuroacanthocytosis. Report of two cases and literature review with emphasis on neuromuscular manifestations. *J Neurol* 239: 302–6.

Yamamoto T, Hirose G, Shimazaki K, Takado S, Kosoegawa H, Saeki M (1982) Movement disorders of familial neuroacanthocytosis syndrome. *Arch Neurol* 39: 298–301.

Young AB, Shoulson I, Penney JB, Starosta-Rubinstein S, Gomez F, Travers H, Ramos-Arroyo MA, Snodgress SR, Bonilla E, Moreno H, Wexler NS (1986) Huntington's disease in Venezuela: neurologic features and functional decline. *Neurology* 36: 244–9.

Zalneraitis EL, Landis DMD, Richardson EP Jr, Selkoe DJ (1981) A comparison of astrocytic structure in cerebral cortex and striatum in Huntington's disease. *Neurology* 31: 151.

Zweig RM, Koven SJ, Hedreen JC, Maestri NE, Kazazian HH Jr, Folstein SE (1989) Linkage to the Huntington's disease locus in a family with unusual clinical and pathological features. *Ann Neurol* 26: 78–84.

Zweig RM, Ross CA, Hedreen JC, Peyser C, Cardillo JE, Folstein SE, Price DL (1992) Locus coeruleus involvement in Huntington's disease. *Arch Neurol* 49: 152–6.

CHAPTER TEN

Other neurodegenerative diseases causing dementia

M. M. Esiri

Progressive supranuclear palsy
Non-specific frontal lobe dementia
Dementia with motor neuron disease
Thalamic degeneration and dementia
Progressive subcortical gliosis (of Neumann)
Corticobasal degeneration
Dementia with argyrophilic grains
Neurofibrillary tangles with calcification
Dentatorubro pallidoluysian degeneration
Multiple system atrophies and dementia

In addition to the neurodegenerative diseases with specific neuropathological features in the cerebral cortex (Alzheimer's disease and Pick's disease) and the clinically distinct Huntington's and Parkinson's diseases, there are a number of other less well-defined neurodegenerative diseases in which dementia may be a prominent clinical feature. They are all relatively uncommon, particularly in those over 75 years of age. However, in patients dying younger than 70 years they probably account for 10–12% of cases of progressive dementia. Except for progressive supranuclear palsy (PSP), corticobasal degeneration and dementia with argyrophilic grains, which show no evidence of being inherited diseases, they all have a fairly high familial incidence. Neuropathological diagnosis in these diseases calls for wide sampling for microscopy not only of the cerebral cortex but, equally important, the multiple subcortical nuclei that are typically affected in each condition (Table 10.1). The anatomical location of most of these nuclei is described briefly in Chapter 2. It is very helpful when studying subcortical nuclei from cases of dementia to have readily to hand comparable sections from a normal brain so that densities of neurons of various sizes and of astrocytes can be compared.

PROGRESSIVE SUPRANUCLEAR PALSY (PSP)

This uncommon disease seems to be of relatively recent origin for it was first described by Steele, Richardson and Olszewski in 1965. The incidence is less than 1 per million/year (Golbe *et al.*, 1988). It affects people mainly in the sixth and seventh decades and survival is from 3–10 years. Clinically, it is characterized by limitation of eye movements, particularly upward gaze, nuchal dystonia, extension and rigidity, truncal instability and pseudobulbar palsy with dysarthria and dysphagia. Parkinsonian symptoms are also sometimes prominent. Dementia often appears to accompany these symptoms and is said to be usually of the subcortical type with slowed responses, inertia, apathy and reduced intellectual activity and attention. Memory defects are also commonly apparent but are normally mild. The disease runs a progressive course, generally over several years, resulting in a rigid, sometimes akinetic, state and death is commonly due to aspiration pneumonia.

Neuropathology

The neuropathological abnormalities are mainly to be found in the basal ganglia, brain stem and cerebellum.

Table 10.1. *Subcortical nuclei showing degeneration in diseases discussed in this chapter*

Site	PSP	NSFLD	D + MND	Thal	PSG	CBD	DRPLA	MSA
Globus pallidus	+	−	−	−	∓	+	+	+
Subthalamic nucleus	+	−	−	−	∓	+	+	±
Caudate nucleus	±	±	+	±	+	∓	−	+
Putamen	±	+	+	±	+	∓	∓	+
Thalamus	−	+	+	+	+	+	∓	−
Periaqueductal grey matter	+	−	−	−	−	∓	∓	−
Substantia nigra	+	+	+	−	−	+	∓	+
Red nucleus	+	−	−	−	−	+	+	−
Dentate nucleus	+	−	−	−	−	∓	+	±
Tegmentum of brainstem	+	−	−	−	−	−	+	∓
Vestibular nuclei	+	−	−	−	−	−	+	+
Superior colliculi	+	−	−	−	−	−	+	−
Basal nucleus	±	−	−	±	−	−	−	−
Locus ceruleus	±	−	−	−	−	±	−	+
Pontine nuclei	±	−	−	−	−	−	−	+
Raphe nuclei	±	−	−	−	−	±	−	−
III nucleus	±	−	−	−	−	−	−	−
Edinger-Westphal nucleus	±	−	−	−	−	−	−	∓
IV nucleus	±	−	−	−	−	−	−	−
X nucleus	±	−	−	−	−	−	−	+
XII nucleus	±	±	+	∓	−	−	−	−
Amygdala	−	−	−	−	−	∓	−	−
Inferior olives	−	−	−	∓	+	−	∓	+
Hypothalamus	−	−	−	−	−	−	−	±
Cerebellar cortex	−	−	−	∓	−	−	∓	+
Anterior horn cells	−	−	+	∓	−	−	−	−

PSP   = progressive supranuclear palsy.
NSFLD   = non-specific frontal lobe dementia.
D + MND = dementia with motor neuron disease.
Thal   = thalamic dementia.
PSG   = progressive subcortical gliosis.
CBD   = corticobasal degeneration.
DRPLA   = dentato rubro pallido luysian atrophy.
MSA   = multiple system atrophy.

Macroscopically the features to look for are enlargement of the fourth ventricle that is a result of the atrophy of the superior cerebellar peduncles (Fig. 10.1(a)) and grey discolouration of the white matter in the hilum of the cerebellar dentate nuclei (Fig. 10.1(b)). The cerebrum generally shows no more than mild atrophy. Microscopically pathological changes consist of neuron loss, the presence of neurofibrillary tangles (NFT) in some of the remaining neurons and astrocytic gliosis. The structures regularly affected by these changes are the subthalamic nucleus (see Figs. 10.2 and 3.11 for the location of this nucleus), globus pallidus, substantia nigra, periaqueductal grey matter, superior colliculi (corpora quadrigemina), red nucleus and tegmentum of the pons (Fig. 10.3). (Steele, Richardson & Olszewski, 1964; Behrman *et al.*, 1969; Constantinidis, Tissot & Ajuriaguerra, 1970; Jellinger, 1971; Ghatak *et al.*, 1980). The dentate nuclei of the cerebellum and the vestibular nuclei in the medulla usually show neuron loss and gliosis but no NFT formation (Fig. 10.4). Tracts showing Wallerian degeneration secondary to neuronal loss are principally the superior cerebellar peduncles and the medial longitudinal fasciculus (Fig. 10.5). Less regularly affected are the putamen, basal nucleus of Meynert, locus ceruleus, pontine nuclei, raphe nuclei and the nuclei of some of the cranial nerves originating in the brain stem, notably the

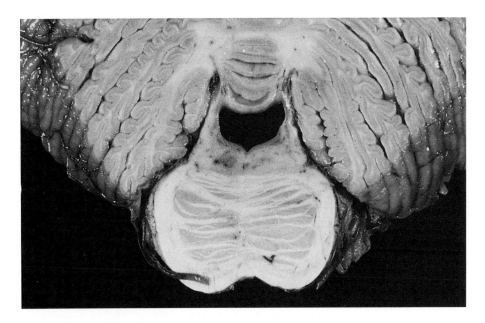

(a)

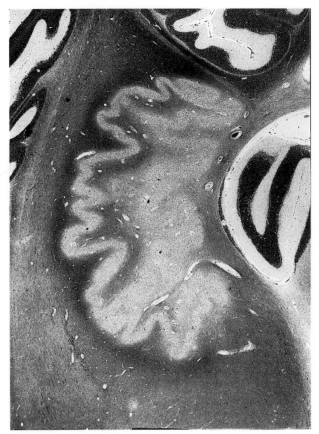

(b)

Fig. 10.1. Progressive supranuclear palsy. (a) Enlarged upper end of the fourth ventricle resulting from atrophy of the superior cerebellar peduncles. (b) Section of the dentate nucleus stained for myelin. Note pallor within the hilum of this nucleus due to loss of fibres in the outflow tract of the dentate nucleus neurons.

Edinger-Westphal nucleus and the nuclei of the III, IV dorsal Xth and XIIth cranial nerves (Behrman et al., 1969; Probst et al., 1988; Shin, Kitamoto & Tateishi, 1991). Exceptionally, even more widespread pathology (neuron loss, gliosis, and/or NFTs) involving the thalamus, amygdala, nucleus accumbens, caudate nucleus and inferior olives may be found. Cerebral atrophy may be profound in these atypical cases (Matsushita et al., 1980; Akashi et al., 1989; Takeuchi et al., 1992).

In addition to developing in subcortical structures, NFT formation is frequently present in the cortex, though the cortical NFT are not so widely distributed as in Alzheimer's disease. In PSP, NFT are found particularly in the entorhinal cortex and hippocampus where the dentate gyrus commonly contains NFT (Fig. 10.6), layers II and III of inferior temporal and frontal cortex and primary motor cortex (Hof, Delacourte & Bouras,

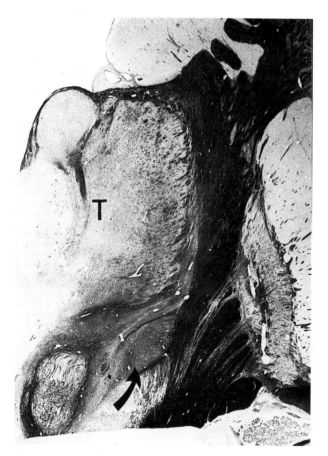

Fig. 10.2. Low power view of myelin-stained section to show the position of the subthalamic nucleus (arrow), medial and adjacent to the internal capsule and beneath the thalamus (T).

1992). Insular cortex and parietal and occipital lobe cortex are less regularly involved. Argyrophilic plaques in cerebral cortex and elsewhere are either absent or sparse. A few cases in which abundant argyrophilic plaques were found, in addition to characteristic clinical and pathological features of PSP, have been interpreted as PSP combined with Alzheimer's disease (David et al., 1968, 1985; Probst, 1977; Takahashi et al., 1988). PSP has also been described in combination with Pick's disease (Arima et al., 1988).

Like the NFT of Alzheimer's disease, NFT in brain stem and basal ganglia in PSP are argyrophilic, congophilic and react with antibodies to tau and ubiquitin. In both PSP and Alzheimer's disease phosphorylated tau polypeptides are the major antigenic components of the NFT, but there are some paired helical filament antigenic determinants detectable in Alzheimer's NFT that are not detected in PSP NFT (Bancher et al., 1987). In addition, the NFT of PSP differ in their ultrastructure from those in Alzheimer's disease, being composed predominantly of bundles of straight tubules or filaments 15 nm in diameter, though there may also be some of the paired helical filaments characteristic of Alzheimer's disease intermixed with these (Powell, London & Lampert 1974; Roy et al., 1974; Tellez-Nagel & Wisniewski, 1973; Tomonaga, 1977; Bugiani et al., 1979; Wisniewski et al., 1979; Yagashita et al., 1979; Ghatak, Nochlin & Hadfield, 1980; Takeuchi et al., 1992).

Biochemical changes in the brain in PSP resemble those in Parkinson's disease with up to 90% reduction in dopamine in the substantia nigra and striatum. There are also reduced choline acetyl transferase and glutamic acid decarboxylase in the striatum (Agid et al., 1987). Levels of cortical dopamine, noradrenalin and 5HT are described as normal.

In our experience, some, but by no means all, cases of PSP are diagnosed clinically. Neuropathologically, the differential diagnosis that most often arises is Alzheimer's disease, particularly if there are modest numbers of argyrophilic plaques as well as NFT present in the cerebral cortex. However, pathological involvement of structures such as the globus pallidus and subthalamic nucleus is not a feature of Alzheimer's disease, and nor is neuron loss in the dentate nuclei of the cerebellum. Even in the cerebral cortex, where NFT are found in both diseases, their distribution differs; most notably the motor cortex contains NFT in PSP but hardly at all in Alzheimer's disease (Hof et al., 1992). Finally, ultrastructural examination of NFT also distinguishes PSP from Alzheimer's disease (see above).

Cases of PSP with severe involvement of the substantia nigra are readily distinguished from Parkinson's disease by the lack of Lewy bodies and the presence of NFT here and at other characteristic subcortical sites. Distinction may be more difficult from post-encephalitic Parkinson's disease, but this does not affect the dentate nuclei of the cerebellum or the cerebral cortex and is clinically different. The substantia nigra may also be severely degenerate in non-specific frontal lobe dementia, cortico-basal degeneration and in some forms of multiple system atrophy, but in these conditions neither NFT nor Lewy bodies are found.

The aetiology of PSP is unknown. The lack of familial cases and its apparently recent appearance casts suspicion on a recently generated environmental toxin, but no candidate has been identified so far, and geographical clustering of cases does not seem to have been noted. The similarities in neurofibrillary pathology to Alzheimer's disease suggest that similar mechanisms disrupting tau metabolism may operate in the two diseases with overlapping but generally distinct populations of neurons at risk.

NON-SPECIFIC FRONTAL LOBE DEMENTIA

With increasing sophistication of psychological testing it has become possible to identify with some confidence patients with dementia of predominantly frontal lobe type (Brun et al., 1994). These patients present with symptoms indicative of a change in their personality and behaviour with disinhibition, neglect of personal appearance, loss of social awareness and impulsive, ill-considered actions. In contrast, memory defects are relatively less marked and alterations in visuo-spatial abilities minimal or absent. Neurological examination is otherwise normal save for the appearance of frontal release signs: grasp and other primitive reflexes. Positron emission tomography (PET) and single photon emission computed tomography (SPECT) scans show reduced uptake of tracer in the frontal lobes. The term dementia of frontal lobe type was suggested by Neary et al. (1988) and Mann et al. (1993) to describe such patients. Similar clinical patients with neuropathology have been described under a variety of terminologies: familial dementia with non-specific findings (Kim et al., 1981); frontal lobe degeneration of non-Alzheimer type (Gustafson, 1987; Brun, 1987; Englund & Brun, 1987); and dementia lacking distinctive histological features (Knopman et al., 1990). Most patients suffering from this condition develop symptoms in their 50s or 60s, and very few cases occur in the over-70 age group. Dysarthria and dysphagia, rigidity and gait disturbance develop during the course of the illness in some patients. Disease duration extends from a few years to a decade or so. A similarly affected close family relative has been noted in approximately half the patients (Gustafson, 1987; Neary et al., 1988; Knopman et al., 1990).

Neuropathology
The neuropathological features of non-specific frontal

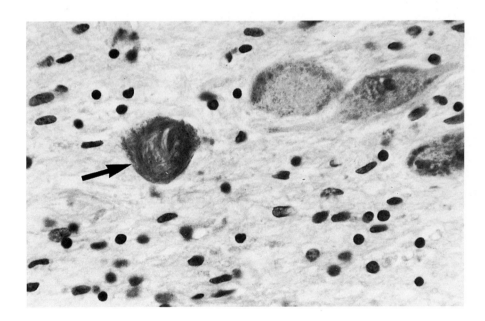

Fig. 10.3. Progressive supranuclear palsy, pigmented neuron in the substantia nigra containing a neurofibrillary tangle (arrow).

lobe dementia are: cerebral atrophy, which is most marked in the frontal lobes but may also affect parietal and anterior temporal lobes, sparing the occipital lobes (Fig. 10.7); mildly to moderately dilated lateral ventricles, particularly of the frontal horns, possibly with some atrophy of the caudate nuclei; histologically, the

most distinctive features of these cases is spongy change with micro-vacuolation in layer II of the cortex particularly in superior and middle frontal gyri and temporal lobes (Fig. 10.8). There is also loss and shrinkage of neurons, mainly pyramidal neurons, of moderate to severe extent, particularly in the frontal lobes; and the

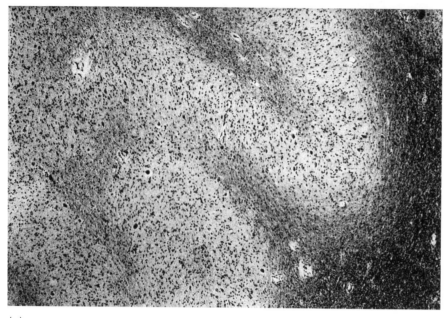

(a)

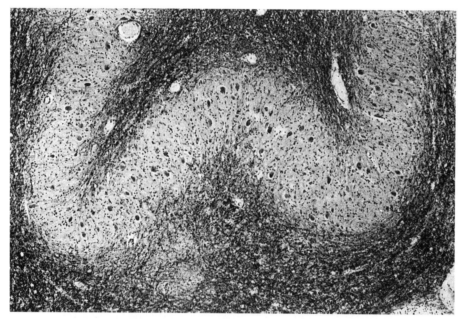

(b)

Fig. 10.4. Low power view of dentate nucleus of the cerebellum in progressive supranuclear palsy (a) and a control case (b). The loss of large neurons and increase in small, glial, nuclei in progressive supranuclear palsy in clearly evident. Haematoxylin and eosin stain.

presence of 'ghost' neurons, shrunken, pale-staining, partially fragmented pyramidal neurons in affected cortex, together with astrocytosis, which is relatively mild in cortex but more severe in immediately subcortical white matter (Fig. 10.9). Argyrophilic plaques and NFT are absent or sparse, and there are no Pick cells, Pick bodies or Lewy bodies; there may be some Wallerian degener-

ation in frontal lobe white matter resulting in secondary demyelination. There is some disagreement in the literature concerning the state of the hippocampus, Knopman *et al.* (1990), stating that it was severely degenerate in 10 of their 14 cases and mildly degenerate in the other 4, with the subiculum and CA1 regions the most severely affected by neuron loss and astrocytosis, while Neary *et*

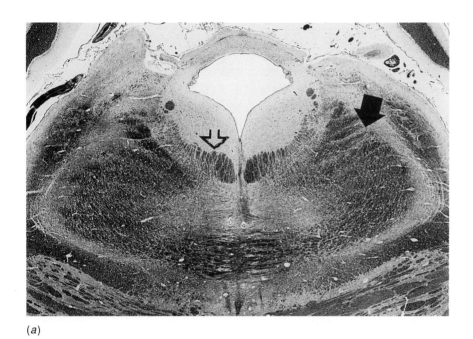

(a)

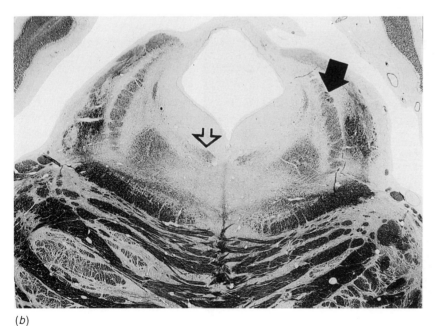

(b)

Fig. 10.5. Tegmentum of the pons in a myelin-stained section from a normal adult (above) and a case of progressive supranuclear palsy (below), both photographed at the same magnification. The entire region is atrophic in progressive supranuclear palsy. Note especially pallor and atrophy of the superior cerebellar peduncles (filled arrows) and medial longitudinal fasciculus (open arrows).

al. (1988) found little or no cell loss in the hippocampus, though some cases showed hippocampal astrocytosis, and Mann *et al.* (1993) found a variable degree of hippocampal pathology. Neuron loss and gliosis may also be present at other sites: the substantia nigra, medial thalamus and striatum; in contrast, the basal nucleus of Meynert and locus ceruleus are well preserved. In keeping with the preservation of the basal nucleus of

Meynert, cortical choline acetyl transferase levels have been normal or only slightly depressed (Knopman *et al.*, 1990).

The clinical and pathological features of non-specific frontal lobe dementia clearly share much in common with Pick's disease, and some cases have macroscopical neuropathological features suggestive of Pick's disease. However, these latter cases are best classified as 'atypi-

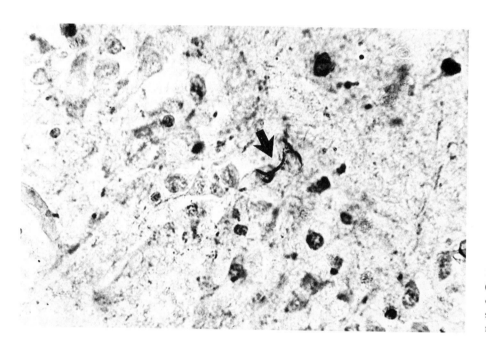

Fig. 10.6. Neurofibrillary tangle (arrow) in the dentate fascia granule cell layer in a case of progressive supranuclear palsy. Cross modification of Palmgren stain.

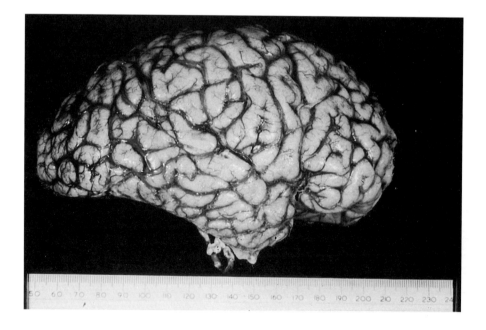

Fig. 10.7. External appearance of the cerebrum in frontal lobe dementia. There is slight atrophy of the frontal lobe and pole of the temporal lobe.

cal' Pick's disease as recommended in Chapter 8 and by Brun *et al.* (1994). Non-specific frontal lobe dementia is probably slightly more common than Pick's disease. The series of 14 cases reported by Knopman *et al.* (1990) represented 10% of cases referred to a brain bank and dying under 70 years, whereas Pick's disease comprised 6.8% of such cases.

In addition to showing clinical and pathological similarities to Pick's disease, non-specific frontal lobe dementia also shares some features in common with dementia with motor neuron disease, discussed below. The absence of ocular palsies clinically, and of neurofibrillary tangles pathologically, clearly distinguishes non-specific frontal lobe dementia from PSP, and lack of Lewy bodies distinguishes it from Parkinson's disease. Absence of NFT and absence or sparsity of argyrophilic plaques and the presence of isolated laminar spongy change in cerebral cortex distinguishes

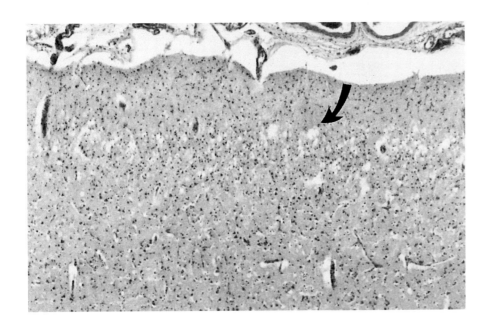

Fig. 10.8. Low power view of frontal lobe cortex from a case of non-specific frontal lobe dementia. Spongiform change is present in layer two (arrow). In addition, there is a shortage of large pyramidal cells in layers 2 and 3. Haematoxylin and eosin stain.

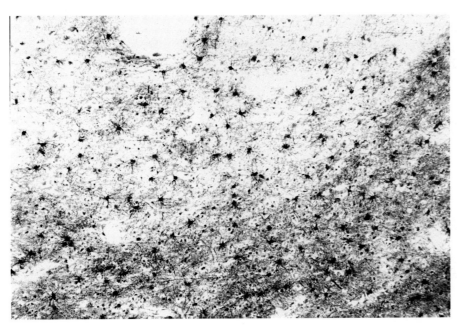

Fig. 10.9. Astrocyte reaction in cortex at the depth of a sulcus and in immediate subcortical white matter (bottom right) in a case of non-specific frontal lobe dementia. Cajal stain.

non-specific frontal lobe dementia from Alzheimer's disease.

DEMENTIA WITH MOTOR NEURON DISEASE

An association between motor neuron disease and dementia has long been recognized in the context of various disease processes. It occurs in the Guam peninsula where the Chamorro tribes of that region are pecularly susceptible to motor neuron disease and a parkinsonian dementia complex in which there is widespread neurofibrillary pathology (Chapter 7). A few cases of Creutzfeldt–Jakob disease show late features of amyotrophy and weakness as well as dementia, myoclonus and ataxia and a single such case has been transmitted (Salazar *et al.*, 1983; Connolly, Allen & Dermott, 1988) (Chapter 12). In addition, dementia is recognized to occur in some few per cent of cases of familial or sporadic motor neuron disease, although it is rare (Finlayson, Guberman & Martin, 1973; Hudson, 1981; Mitsuyama, 1984; Horoupian *et al.*, 1984; Clark *et al.*, 1986*a*,*b*; Morita *et al.*, 1987; Neary *et al.*, 1990). (Such cases are distinct from the occasional co-existence of Alzheimer's disease or another well-defined dementing disease with motor neuron disease.) The clinical and pathological features of dementia with motor neuron disease are reviewed by Kew and Leigh (1992). In these cases, dementia may precede the onset of weakness by as much as several years. Alternatively, weakness may develop first or the two symptoms may arise together. In some patients the dementia progresses very rapidly. Although some cases have been described as having Alzheimer's disease-like dementia, one recent study has emphasized the dementia as being frontal lobe in type and accompanied by reduced SPECT tracer uptake in the frontal lobes (Neary *et al.*, 1990). In another recent report, seven patients were described as having a predominantly aphasic dementia with motor neuron disease (Caselli *et al.*, 1993).

Neuropathology

Neuropathological studies have shown changes in dementia with motor neuron disease very similar to those described above in non-specific frontal lobe dementia. In addition, there are pathological features of motor neuron disease. There is macroscopic cerebral atrophy largely confined to the frontal and anterior temporal lobes (Fig. 10.10), laminar spongy change confined to layer II/III of the frontal and anterior temporal cortex (Fig. 10.11), pyramidal neuron loss in the same regions and also sometimes in the inferior parietal cortex, and more widespread neuronal loss in subcortical nuclei, most frequently the striatum, thalamus and substantia nigra. Gliosis is relatively mild in cortex but more marked in

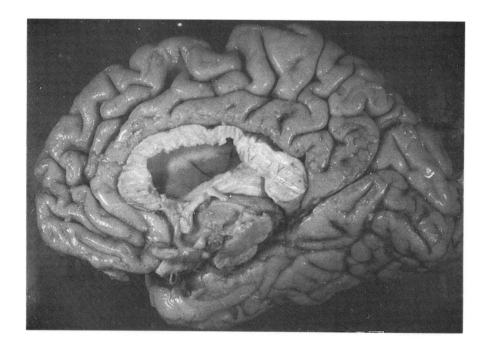

Fig. 10.10. Photograph of the medial aspect of the right cerebral hemisphere from a case of dementia and motor neuron disease. Sulci of the medial frontal lobe, on the left of the picture, show prominent widening. The anterior horn of the ventricle, seen beneath the corpus callosum, is dilated.

subcortical white matter and subcortical grey nuclei. In addition, there are usually the characteristic changes of motor neuron disease with involvement of upper and lower motor neurons, as evidenced by a dying-back type degeneration in pyramidal tracts in the spinal cord, in some cases extending to the medullary pyramids (Fig. 10.12) and loss of anterior horn motor neurons in the spinal cord and of hypoglossal nucleus neurons in the medulla (Fig. 10.13). Some cases have shown only lower motor neuron loss (Morita *et al.*, 1987; Neary *et al.*, 1990). Betz cells in the motor cortex are either lost (Horoupian *et al.*, 1984) or are grossly shrunken (Neary *et al.*, 1990). The nucleus basalis of Meynert, locus ceruleus and dorsal raphe are well preserved. No Lewy bodies, Pick bodies or NFT are present and argyrophilic plaques are scarce or absent. No widespread spongiform changes, as seen in Creutzfeldt–Jakob disease, are present. Pale intracytoplasmic inclusion bodies in anterior horn cells have been described in one case (Neary *et al.*, 1990). These were similar to such bodies found in pure motor neuron disease (Leigh *et al.*, 1988). An interesting recent observation in cases of motor neuron disease with dementia is that ubiquitin-immunoreactive inclusions can be seen in the cell cytoplasm of neurons in frontal, temporal, entorhinal cortex and dentate fascia of the hippocampus (Whiteman *et al.*, 1992). Similar cortical inclusions, as well as filamentous inclusions that are ubiquitin-immunoreactive in the spinal cord and motor cranial nuclei neurons, have been found in motor neuron disease uncomplicated by dementia. The inclusions have a skein-like appearance, consisting of wisps of thread-like material.

The overlap between motor neuron disease with dementia and non-specific frontal lobe dementia is most evident at the psychological and pathological levels. However, there are other indications of links between these conditions. Patients with non-specific frontal lobe dementia may develop progressive dysarthria and dysphagia during the course of their dementing illness, and some cases of this type show hypoglossal nucleus neuron loss (Knopman *et al.*, 1990). Muscle fasciculations have also been noted in some cases of non-specific frontal lobe dementia (Gustafson, 1987). In addition, there is a case recorded of non-specific frontal lobe dementia in which there was a family history of motor neuron disease, though not of dementia (Knopman *et al.*, 1990), and another case of motor neuron disease with dementia who had a family history of frontal lobe dementia without motor neuron disease (Neary *et al.*, 1990). This suggests genetic overlap between the two. The length of disease in dementia with motor neuron disease tends to be shorter by several years than the length of disease in non-specific frontal lobe dementia though there is considerable overlap. Finally, in cases of motor neuron disease without clinical dementia, psychological tests of frontal lobe function have revealed subclinical deficiencies (David & Gillham, 1986). For all these reasons there is circumstantial evidence that there are neurodegenerative processes shared in common and affecting overlapping neuronal populations in non-specific

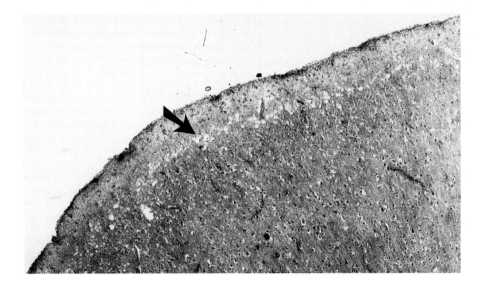

Fig. 10.11. Low power view of frontal lobe cortex from a case of motor neuron disease and dementia. There is spongy change in layer two (arrow). Haematoxylin and eosin stain.

frontal lobe dementia and dementia with motor neuron disease.

THALAMIC DEGENERATION AND DEMENTIA

There are patients described with dementia, among other neuro-psychological abnormalities, who have had pathologies of various types (vascular, neoplastic, inflammatory) largely confined to the thalamus (Martin,

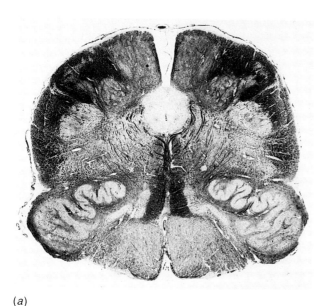

(a)

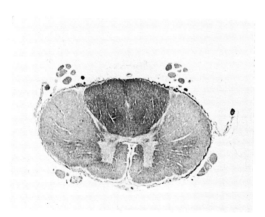

(b)

Fig. 10.12. (a) Pallor of pyramids in a myelin-stained section of the medulla from a case of dementia with motor neuron disease; (b) pallor of myelin staining in the spinal cord, accentuated in the lateral corticospinal tracts, but also evident in all white matter except the posterior columns in a case of dementia and motor neuron disease.

1969). Vascular disease of the thalamus associated with dementia is discussed in Chapter 5. More relevant to this chapter are rare cases of neuron loss and gliosis predominantly, though never exclusively, affecting the thalamus. Such cases are reviewed by Martin (1975) and Deymeer et al. (1989). A high proportion of cases are apparently familial. The most severely affected nucleus in most cases has been the dorsomedial thalamic nucleus (Fig. 2.14). Lesser degrees of cell loss and gliosis have been found in the ventral anterior, centro median, lateral and posterior nuclei. Other subcortical sites outside the thalamus are almost invariably affected to some extent and these have included the striatum, globus pallidus and basal nucleus of Meynert. One case had pathological features of motor neuron disease with dementia as well as severe degeneration of the dorsomedial thalamic nuclei (Deymeer et al., 1989). Some cases have shown laminar spongy change, and neuron loss in the cerebral cortex and cerebral white matter gliosis. No inclusions of any sort are present. As with motor neuron disease and dementia, similarities are to be noted between thalamic dementia and non-specific frontal lobe dementia in which many cases do indeed have thalamic, along with other subcortical, pathology. Cases considered as neurodegenerative thalamic dementia may therefore perhaps be viewed as belonging to the same spectrum of disease as those with non-specific frontal lobe dementia, but with the brunt of the pathology borne by particular thalamic nuclei.

While describing cases of dementia with predominantly thalamic pathology, it should be mentioned that a variant of prion disease (Chapter 12), fatal familial insomnia, has recently been described which is characterized pathologically by selective atrophy of the anterior ventral and dorsomedial thalamic nuclei and inferior olives. Less severe and inconstant involvement of other thalamic nuclei, moderate atrophy of the cerebellar cortex, gliosis of the cerebral cortex and, in one case only, spongy change in cerebral cortex is also described (Lugaresi et al., 1986; Medori et al., 1992; Manetto et al., 1992). In this disease the chief clinical features are intractable insomnia, dysautonomia, myoclonus and ataxia. However, some cases have memory and attention deficits.

Some overlap between a thalamic form of prion disease and thalamic degeneration with spongiform change in the cortex has been suggested by some authors (Kornfield & Seelinger, 1994). Further study of such cases using methods of detecting protease-resistant prion protein will help to clarify the extent of any such overlap.

PROGRESSIVE SUBCORTICAL GLIOSIS (OF NEUMANN)

Neumann and Cohn (1967) described a rare dementing condition with onset usually in the fifth and sixth decades in which variable, but in some cases mild, neuron loss in cerebral cortex, chiefly in frontal and parietal lobes, was accompanied by severe gliosis in subcortical white matter and some subcortical nuclei, principally the basal ganglia, medial and anterior thalamus and brain stem, particularly the inferior olives.

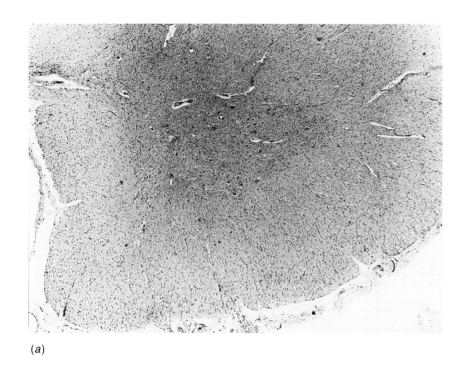

(a)

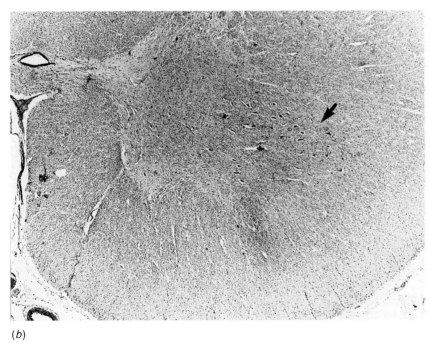

(b)

Fig. 10.13. Anterior horn at the level of the cervical enlargement from a case of dementia with motor neuron disease (a) and a normal control (b). Note large motor neurons, readily seen in (b) (arrow), are largely absent in (a).

Cerebral white matter showed evidence of mild Wallerian degeneration in some cases. Laminar spongy change in cerebral cortex has also been noted in such cases (Verity & Wechsler, 1987) but no ballooned cells, Lewy bodies, neurofibrillary tangles or argyrophilic plaques. The gliosis may extend to the anterior horns of the spinal cord. There are no inclusion bodies found anywhere in the CNS. The main feature of this condition is the apparently excessive gliosis in subcortical nuclei for the evident amount of neuron loss. However, detailed quantitative studies of neuronal populations have not been carried out, and the Wallerian degeneration evident in cerebral white matter in some cases suggests widespread axonal loss. Furthermore, since gliosis occurs as a result of loss of afferent input to a nucleus without the need for neuron loss within it, the grey matter gliosis that occurs in progressive subcortical gliosis may be reflecting a loss of connections of relatively few but widely disseminated axons. Recent studies in some cases have linked progressive subcortical gliosis to abnormal prion protein accumulation in the brain (Petersen et al., 1995; Révész et al., 1995).

CORTICOBASAL DEGENERATION

Corticobasal degeneration is a rare clinico-pathological entity, some 40 cases of which had been described in the literature at the time of review by Rinne et al. (1994). The first cases were described by Rebeiz, Kolodny and Richardson (1968) and Clark et al. (1986a.b). Gibb, Luthert and Marsden (1989) described three further cases. Cortico-dentatonigral degeneration with neuronal achromasia, and cortical degeneration with swollen chromatolytic neurons are alternative terms used to describe the same condition. The clinical features consist of an asymmetrical extrapyramidal and pyramidal slowly progressive disorder with apraxia, rigidity, involuntary movements, dystonia, dysarthria, the alien limb sign and supranuclear palsy. In the later stages of the disease, memory impairment, and dysphasia occur. The cognitive deficit is difficult to assess because of the superimposition of dysarthria and motor incapacity. A few cases have presented with progressive fronto-temporal dementia and did not develop a movement disorder (Jackson M et al., personal communication) (see also p. 214). Onset has been in the sixth to eighth decades, males and females have been equally affected, there is no family history of similar disorder and disease duration has ranged from 7 to 10 years. Brain imaging has shown localized and asymmetric frontoparietal atrophy.

Neuropathology

On gross examination of the brain, the characteristic finding is severe focal cortical atrophy of pre- and post-central gyri with lesser atrophy of other parts of the frontal and parietal lobes and of the temporal and occipital lobes. Secondary degeneration has been described in the corticospinal tracts in the spinal cord in some cases. Cortical atrophy may be asymmetric, being more severe contralateral to the clinically most severely affected limb(s). Microscopically the involved cortex shows loss of neurons, particularly in layers 3 and 5, loss of the normal laminar architecture, severe gliosis and the presence of large pale neurons indistinguishable from Pick cells found in Pick's disease (Chapter 8). These ballooned neurons are found among medium and large pyramidal cells particularly in moderately rather than severely affected cortex. These neurons contain material that is variably argyrophilic but which reacts for phosphorylated neurofilaments and not for tau (Gibb et al., 1989), though this is disputed (Wakabayashi et al., 1994). Ultrastructurally the cells contain aggregates of 10 nm intermediate filaments but no paired helical filaments (Watts et al., 1989). Some affected neurons are vacuolated. The hippocampus is largely free of pathology.

Subcortical structures affected in the disease include the lateral two-thirds of the substantia nigra, the medial third of the subthalamic nucleus, the striatum, globus pallidus, posterolateral thalamic nuclei and red nucleus. Other brain stem nuclei are variably involved, including the locus ceruleus, raphe magnus nucleus and dorsal vagal nucleus. Some swollen neurons, cell loss, and gliosis can be found in the subcortical nuclei that are affected. In the substantia nigra there may be additional intracytoplasmic rounded, basophilic inclusions but no Lewy bodies.

The main differential diagnosis clinically is from progressive supranuclear palsy and Parkinson's disease, though pathologically the greatest similarities are with Pick's disease. However, in Pick's disease the characteristic distribution of maximal atrophy in frontal and temporal poles is different. The hippocampus is usually affected and the substantia nigra is affected in only a relatively small proportion of cases. There is also clear pathological distinction from Parkinson's disease on the basis of an absence of Lewy bodies and presence of ballooned cells and from progressive supranuclear palsy on the basis of absence of brain stem atrophy, absence of neurofibrillary tangles and presence of cortical pathology with ballooned neurons. Cases of corticobasal degeneration that have Wallerian degeneration in pyramidal tracts differ pathologically from cases of dementia with motor neuron disease in the absence of lower motor neuron loss and absence of spongy change in frontal and temporal cortex.

DEMENTIA WITH ARGYROPHILIC GRAINS

Some cases with dementia clinically indistinguishable from Alzheimer's disease are found at autopsy to lack the typical pathology of that disease and, instead, have different and unusual cytoskeletal abnormalities. The most conspicuous of these abnormalities is the presence of small spindle-shaped argyrophilic 'grains', up to 9 μm long and 3 μm across, loosely scattered throughout the neuropil particularly of the CA1 sector of the hippocampus, and entorhinal cortex with lesser quantities in layer III of the temporal, insular and orbitofrontal neocortex (Fig. 10.14). Subcortical structures similarly affected include the amygdala, and hypothalamic lateral tuberal

nucleus. Some cases show additional abnormalities such as abnormal argyrophilic coiled bodies containing dense accumulations of 9 nm straight filaments mainly located in subcortical white matter (Braak & Braak 1987, 1989). Argyrophilic grains, in addition to being the sole pathological change in some cases of dementia may also be seen in association with typical Alzheimer's disease pathology. The grains are reactive with the Alz-50 antibody that recognizes hyperphosphorylated tau (Itagaki et al., 1989), but they do not contain paired helical filaments ultrastructurally.

NEUROFIBRILLARY TANGLES WITH CALCIFICATION

A neurodegenerative condition has been reported principally from Japan presenting as early-onset dementia with mild parkinsonism and, rarely, pyramidal weakness. Autopsies have shown numerous cortical neurofibrillary tangles, frontotemporal lobar atrophy and pro-

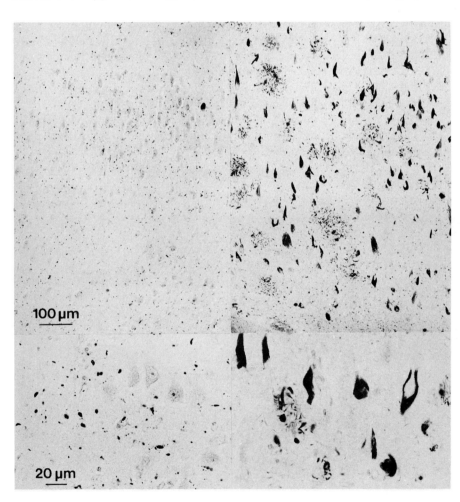

Fig. 10.14. Corresponding portions of sector CA1 of the human hippocampus showing, on the left, a case of dementia with argyrophilic grains scattered throughout the pyramidal layers. There are no plaques and tangles in this case. On the right is shown, for comparison, the appearance in the same region of Alzheimer's disease pathology with numerous plaques and tangles. Gallyas stain on 15 μm sections. (Reproduced by courtesy of Drs H and E Braak and the publishers of *Neuropathology and Applied Neurobiology*.)

nounced calcific deposits (Kosaka, 1994). An absence of senile plaques as well as the calcification distinguishes the condition from Alzheimer's disease and the cortical localization of the tangles, and a clinical picture dominated by dementia distinguishes it from progressive supranuclear palsy.

DENTATORUBRO PALLIDOLUYSIAN DEGENERATION (ATROPHY)

This is a rare sporadic or dominant familial neurodegenerative disease with predominantly motor symptoms of ataxia, epilepsy, chorea, dystonia, dysarthria and opsoclonus. However, some cases, particularly those reported from Japan, also show dementia (Goto *et al.*, 1982; Iizuka, Hirayama & Maehda, 1984; Naito *et al.*, 1977; Takahata *et al.*, 1978). The genetic defect in affected families is an expanded trinucleotide repeat (Warner *et al.*, 1994*a*; Warner, Williams & Harding, 1994*b*). Onset of symptoms occurs over a wide age-span from childhood to late 60s though more than half are affected by the age of 30. Three clinical subtypes of disease have been delineated: toxochoreoathetoid, pseudo-Huntington and myoclonus-epilepsy (Iizuka & Hirayama, 1986), but mixed forms of these phenotypes may be seen within the same family. Dementia occurs in the latter two types. Neurodegenerative changes with neuron loss and gliosis are seen in the globus pallidus, deep cerebellar nuclei, red nucleus, subthalamic nucleus, tegmentum, superior colliculi, reticular formation, and

vestibular nuclei. The pons and medulla are particularly atrophic and gliotic (Fig. 10.15). Substantia nigra and locus ceruleus are generally spared and there are no neurofibrillary tangles, in contrast to PSP. The other main differential diagnoses are Huntington's disease and mitochrondrial encephalopathies, especially MERFF (Warner *et al.*, 1994*a,b*).

MULTIPLE SYSTEM ATROPHIES AND DEMENTIA

The multiple system atrophies are a heterogenous group of progressive neurodegenerative conditions, many with a familial pattern of inheritance, that have in common neuron loss and gliosis at a variety of CNS sites in the absence of any other clearly distinguished features (Oppenheimer & Esiri, 1992). Certain patterns of nuclear involvement commonly occur together and lead to particular clusters of clinical symptoms and signs of which olivo-ponto-cerebellar atrophy and striato-nigral degeneration are the most well known. A few cases are clinically dominated by autonomic failure. Anatomical connections are often known to link the pathologically involved nuclei leading to the suggestion that these are system degenerations, perhaps in this respect akin to motor neuron disease (Saper, Wainer & German, 1987). Severe dementia is not a feature of multiple system atrophy, but subjects may show some impairment on tests of frontal lobe function (Robbins *et al.*, 1992). They may also develop Alzheimer's disease (Trotter, 1973;

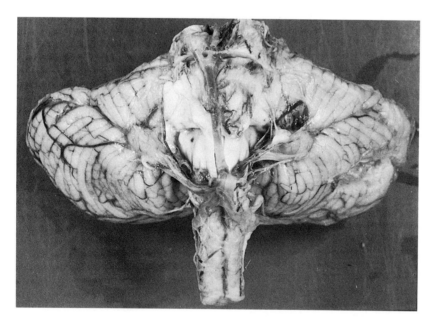

Fig. 10.15. Atrophy of the pons and medulla in a case of dentato rubro pallido luysian atrophy.

Kosaka *et al.*, 1981). The pathological changes in multiple system atrophy consist of neuron loss and gliosis in the subcortical nuclei appropriate to the clinical manifestations, principally the putamen and substantia nigra in striato-nigral degeneration and the pontine nuclei, inferior olives and Purkinje cells of the cerebellum in olivo-ponto-cerebellar atrophy. In affected nuclei and, to a lesser extent in a more widespread distribution, there are argyrophilic fibrillary inclusions in oligodendrocytes. An atypical case with prominent dementia was shown to have the most severe pathology in substantia nigra, pontine tegmentum, and globus pallidus (Wszolek *et al.*, 1992). It will be noted that many of these nuclei are sites that are affected in the other neurodegenerative conditions discussed earlier in this chapter. To this extent non-specific frontal lobe dementia, dementia with motor neuron disease, neurodegenerative thalamic dementia and progressive subcortical gliosis may all perhaps be regarded as further variants of multiple system atrophy. However, it is noteworthy that the restricted cortical laminar spongy change that is rather characteristic of these four conditions does not appear to have been described in cases of more conventional multiple system atrophies with dementia. We believe that understanding of these complex and obscure conditions is better assisted by subdividing them as far as it is reasonable to do so while recognizing that their pathogeneses may eventually turn out to involve common mechanisms. Further details of the pathology of multiple system atrophies can be found in reviews by Oppenheimer and Esiri (1992), Daniel (1992) and Lantos and Papp (1994).

REFERENCES

Agid Y, Ruberg M, Dubois B, Pillon B (1987) Anatomoclinical and biochemical concepts in subcortical dementia. In Stahl SM, Iversen SD, Goodman EC (eds) *Cognitive Neuropharmacology*. Oxford University Press, Oxford, pp 248–71.

Akashi T, Arima K, Maruyama N, Ando S, Inose T (1989) Severe cerebral atrophy in progressive supranuclear palsy: a case report. *Clin Neuropathol* 8: 195–9.

Arima M, Akashi T, Inoset *et al* (1988) An unusual case of Pick's disease, coexistence of PSP tangles with Pick bodies. *29th Japanese Congr Neuropathol* Abst. p 121.

Bancher C, Lasmann H, Budka H, Grundke-Iqbal I, Iqbal K, Wicke G, Seitelberger F, Wisniewski HM (1987) Neurofibrillary tangles in Alzheimer's disease and progressive supranuclear palsy: antigenic similarities and differences. *Acta Neuropathol* 74: 39–46.

Behrman S, Carroll JD, Janota I, Matthews WB (1969) Progressive supranuclear palsy – clinico-pathological study of four cases. *Brain* 92: 663–78.

Braak H, Braak H (1987) Argyrophilic grains: characteristic pathology of cerebral cortex in cases of adult onset dementia without Alzheimer changes. *Neurosci Lett* 76: 124–7.

Braak H, Braak E (1989) Cortical and subcortical argyrophilic grains characterise a disease associated with adult onset dementia. *Neuropathol Appl Neurobiol* 15: 13–26.

Brun A (1987) Frontal lobe degeneration of non-Alzheimer type 1. Neuropathology *Arch Gerontol Geriatr* 6: 193–208.

Brun A, Englund B, Gustafson L, Passant N, Mann DMA, Neary D, Snowden JS (1994) Clinical and neuropathological criteria for frontotemporal dementia. *J Neurol Neurosurg Psychiat* 57: 416–18.

Bugiani O, Moncardi GL, Bursa A, Ederli A (1979) The fine structure of subcortical neurofibrillary tangles in progressive supranuclear palsy. *Acta Neuropathol* 45: 147–52.

Caselli RJ, Windebank AJ, Petersen RC, Komori T, Parasi JE, Okazaki H, Kokmen E, Iverson R, Dinapoli RP, Graff-Redford NR, Svein SD (1993) Rapidly progressive aphasic dementia and motor neuron disease. *Ann Neurol* 33: 200–7.

Clark AW, White CL, Manz HL *et al* (1986*a*) Primary degenerative dementia without Alzheimer pathology. *Can J Neurol Sci* 13: 462–70.

Clark AW, Manz HJ, White CL, Lehmann J, Miller D, Coyle JT (1986*b*) Cortical degeneration with swollen chromatolytic neurons: its relationship to Pick's disease. *J Neuropath Exp Neurol* 45: 268–84.

Connolly JH, Allen IV, Dermott E (1988) Transmissible agent in the amyotrophic form of Creutzfeldt–Jakob disease. *J Neurol Neurosurg Psychiat* 51: 1459–60.

Constantinidis J, Tissot R, De Ajuriaguerra J (1970) Dystonic oculo-cervico-faciale ou paralysie progressive supranucléaire de Steele–Richardson–Olszewski–Pseudo-paralysie du regard, troubles visuo-spatiaux, pseudo-démence, altérations neuronales. *Rev Neurol* 122: 249–62.

Daniel S (1992) The neuropathology and neurochemistry of multiple system atrophy. In Bannister R, Matthias CJ (eds) *Autonomic Failure*, 3rd edn. Oxford University Press, pp 364–85.

David AS, Gillham RA (1986) Neuropsychological study of motor neurone disease. *Psychosomatics* 27: 441–5.

David NJ, Mackey EA, Smith JL (1968) Further observations in progressive supranuclear palsy. *Neurology* 18: 349–56.

Davis PH, Bergeron C, Machachlan DR (1985) Atypical presentation of progresive supranuclear palsy. *Ann Neurol* 17: 337–43.

Deymeer F, Smith TW, De Girolami U, Drachman DA (1989) Thalamic dementia and motor neuron disease. *Neurology* 39: 58–61.

Englund E, Brun A (1987) Frontal lobe degeneration of non-Alzheimer type IV. White matter changes. *Arch Gerontol Geriatr* 6: 235–43.

Finlayson MH, Guberman A, Martin JB (1973) Cerebral lesions in familial amyotrophic lateral sclerosis and dementia. *Acta Neuropathol* 26: 237–46.

Ghatak NR, Nochlin D, Hadfield MG (1980) Neurofibrillary pathology in progressive supranuclear palsy. *Acta Neuropathol* 52: 73–6.

Gibb WRG, Luthert PJ, Marsden CD (1989) Corticobasal degeneration. *Brain* 112: 1171–92.

Golbe L, Davis PH, Schoenberg BS, Duvoisin RC (1988) Prevalence and natural history of progressive supranuclear palsy. *Neurology* 38: 1031–4.

Goto IK, Tobimatsu S, Ohta M *et al* (1982) Dentato rubro-pallidoluysian degeneration: clinical, neuro-ophthalmologic biochemical and pathologic studies on an autosomal dominant form. *Neurology* 32: 1395–9.

Gustafson L (1987) Frontal lobe degeneration of non-Alzheimer type II. Clinical picture and differential diagnosis. *Arch Gerontol Geriatr* 6: 209–33.

Hof PR, Delacourte A, Bouras C (1992) Distribution of cortical neurofibrillary tangles in progressive supranuclear palsy: a quantitative analysis of six cases. *Acta Neuropathol* 84: 45–51.

Horoupian DS, Thal L, Katzman R *et al* (1984) Dementia and motor neuron disease: morphometric biochemical and Golgi studies. *Ann Neurol* 16: 305–13.

Hudson AJ (1981) Amotrophic lateral sclerosis and its association with dementia, parkinsonism and other neurological disorders. *Brain* 104: 217–47.

Iizuka R, Hirayama K, Maehda K (1984) Dentato-rubro-pallido-luysian atrophy: a clinico-pathological study. *J Neurol Neurosurg Psychiat* 47: 1288–9.

Iizuka R, Hirayama K (1986) Dentato-rubro-pallido-luysian atrophy. In Vinken PJ, Bruyn GW, Klawans HL (eds) *Handbook of Clinical Neurology, Vol 5(49). Extrapyramidal disorders.* Elsevier, Amsterdam, pp 437–43.

Itagaki S, McGeer PL, Akiyama H, Beattie BL, Walker DG, Moore GRW, McGeer EG (1989) A case of adult-onset dementia with argyrophilic grains. *Ann Neurol* 26: 685–9.

Jellinger K (1971) Progressive supranuclear palsy (subcortical argyrophilic dystrophy). *Acta Neuropathol* 19: 347–52.

Kew J, Leigh N (1992) Dementia with motor neuron disease. In Rossor MN (ed) *Unusual Dementias. Baillière's Clinical Neurology* Vol 1, No 3 Baillière Tindall, pp 611–26.

Kim RC, Collins GH, Parisi JE *et al* (1981) Familial dementia of adult onset with pathological findings of a 'non-specific' nature. *Brain* 104: 61–78.

Knopman DS, Mastri AR, Frey WH II, Sung J-H, Rustam T (1990) Dementia lacking distinctive histologic features. *Neurology* 40: 251–6.

Kornfield M, Seelinger DF (1994) Pure thalamic dementia with a single focus of spongiform change in cerebral cortex. *Clin Neuropathol* 13: 77–81.

Kosaka K, Iisuka R, Mizutami Y, Kondo T, Nagatsu T (1981) Striato-nigral degeneration combined with Alzheimer's disease. *Acta Neuropath* 54: 253–6.

Kosaka K (1994) Diffuse neurofibrillary tangles with calcifica-tion: a new presenile dementia. *J Neurol Neurosurg Psychiat* 57: 594–6.

Lantos PL, Papp MI (1994) Cellular pathology of multiple system atrophy: a review. *J Neurol Neurosurg Psychiat* 57: 129–33.

Leigh PN, Anderton BH, Dodson A, Gallo J-M, Swash M, Power DM (1988) Ubiquitin deposits in anterior horn cells in motor neuron disease. *Neurosci Lett* 93: 197–203.

Lugaresi E, Medori R, Montagna P *et al* (1986) Fatal familial insomnia and dysautonomia with selective degeneration of thalamic nuclei. *New Engl J Med* 315: 997–1003.

Manetto V, Medori R, Cortelli P *et al* (1992) Fatal familial insomnia: clinical and pathological study of 5 new cases. *Neurology* 42: 312–19.

Mann DMA, South PW, Snowden JS, Neary D (1993) Dementia of frontal lobe type: neuropathology and immunohis-tochemistry. *J Neurol Neurosurg Psychiat* 56: 605–14.

Martin JJ (1969) Thalamic syndromes. In Vinken PJ, Bruyn GW (eds) *Handbook of Clinical Neurology* Vol 2. Amsterdam North Holland, pp 469–96.

Martin JJ (1975) Thalamic degenerations. In Vinken PJ, Bruyn GW (eds) *Handbook of Clinical Neurology* Vol 21. Amsterdam North Holland, pp 587–604.

Matsushita M, Itoh K, Oyanegi S, Uckikoshi T, Ishikawa T, Kase M, Kosaka K (1980) An autopsy case of progressive supranuclear palsy with massive appearance of neurofibril-lary tangles in the limbic system including nuclear accum-bens, septi and nuclear amygdala. *Neuropathology (Kyoto)* 1: 119–32.

Medori R, Tritschler H-J, Le Blanc A *et al* (1992) Fatal familial insomnia, a prion disease with a mutation at Codon 178 of the prion protein gene. *New Eng J Med* 326: 444–9.

Mitsuyama Y (1984) Presenile dementia with motor neuron disease in Japan: clinico-pathological review of 26 cases. *J Neurol Neurosurg Psychiat* 47: 953–9.

Morita K, Kaiya H, Ikeda T, Namba M (1987) Presenile dementia combined with amyotrophy: a review of 34 Japanese cases. *Arch Gerontol Geriatr* 6: 263–77.

Naito H, Tanaka M, Hirose Y, Oyanagi S (1977) Clinico pathological study of two autopsied cases of degenerative type of myoclonus epilepsy with choreo-athetoid movement: proposal of hereditary dentate and pallidal system atrophy. *Psychiat Neurol (Jpn)* 79: 193–201.

Neary D, Snowden JS, Northen B, Goulding P (1988) Dementia of frontal lobe type. *J Neurol Neurosurg Psychiat* 51: 353–61.

Neary D, Snowden JS, Mann DMA, Northen B, Goulding PJ, MacDermott N (1990) Frontal lobe dementia and motor neuron disease. *J Neurol Neurosurg Psychiat* 53: 23–32.

Neumann MA, Cohn R (1967) Progressive subcortical gliosis, a rare form of senile dementia. *Brain* 90: 405–18.

Oppenheimer DR, Esiri MM (1992) Diseases of the basal ganglia, cerebellum and motor neurons. In Adams JH, Duchen LW (eds) *Greenfield's Neuropathology* 5th edn. Arnold, London, pp 988–1045.

Petersen RB, Tabaton M, Chen SG *et al.* (1995) Familial progressive subcortical gliosis: presence of prions and linkage to chromosome 17. *Neurology* 45: 1062–7.

Powell HC, London GW, Lampert PW (1974) Neurofibrillary tangles in progressive supranuclear palsy. *J Neuropathol Exp Neurol* 33: 98–106.

Probst A (1977) Degenerescence neurofibrillaire sous-corticale senile avec présence de tubules contournes et de filaments droits. *Rev Neurol* 133: 417–28.

Probst A, Langui D, Lantenschlager C, Ulrich J, Brion JP, Anderton BP (1988) Progressive supranuclear palsy: extensive neuropil threads in addition to neurofibrillary tangles – very similar antigenicity of subcortical neuronal pathology in progressive supranuclear palsy and Alzheimer's disease. *Acta Neuropathol* 77: 61–8.

Rebeiz JJ, Kolodny EH, Richardson EP (1968) Corticodentatonigral degeneration with neuronal achromasia. *Arch Neurol* 18: 20–33.

Révész T, Daniel SE, Lees AJ, Wil RG (1995) A case of progressive subcortical gliosis associated with deposition of abnormal prion protein (PrP) (letter). *J Neurol Neurosurg Psychiat,* 58: 759–60.

Rinne JO, Lee MS, Thompson PD, Marsden CD (1994) Corticobasal degeneration: a clinical study of 36 cases. *Brain* 117: 1183–96.

Robbins TW, James M, Lange KW, Owen AM, Quinn NP, Marsden CD (1992) Cognitive performance in multiple system atrophy. *Brain* 115: 271–91.

Roy S, Datta CK, Hirano A, Ghatak NR, Zimmerman HM (1974) Electron microscopic study of neurofibrillary tangles in Steele-Richardson-Olszewski syndrome. *Acta Neuropathol* 29: 175–79.

Salazar AM, Masters CL, Gajdusek DC, Gibbs CJ (1983) Syndromes of amyotrophic lateral sclerosis and dementia: relation to transmissible Creutzfeldt–Jakob disease. *Ann Neurol* 14: 17–26.

Saper CB, Wainer BH, German DC (1987) Axonal and transneuronal transport in the transmission system degenerations including Alzheimer's disease. *Neuroscience* 23: 389–98.

Shin RW, Kitamoto T, Tateishi J (1991) Modified tau is present in younger non-demented persons: a study of subcortical nuclei in Alzheimer's disease and progressive supranuclear palsy. *Acta Neuropathol* 81: 517–23.

Steele JC, Richardson EP, Olszewski J (1965) Progressive supranuclear palsy. *Arch Neurol* 10: 333–59.

Takahashi H, Oyanagi K, Takeda S, Hiromac K, Ikuta F (1988) Progressive supranuclear palsy; electron microscopic examination of 2 autopsy cases with diffuse cerebral cortical lesions. *29th Japanese Cong Neuropathol.* Abs p 77.

Takahata N, Ito K, Yoshimura Y *et al* (1978) Familial chorea and myoclonus epilepsy. *Neurology* 28: 913–19.

Takeuchi T, Shibayama H, Iwai H, Xu M, Kitoh J, Kobayashi H, Iwase S, Nakagawa M, Yamada K, Yoshida K, Nambu Y, Ishihara R (1992) Progressive supranuclear palsy with widespread cerebral lesions. *Clin Neuropathol* 11: 304–12.

Tellez-Nagel I, Wisniewski HM (1973) Ultrastructure of neurofibrillary tangles in Steele-Richardson-Olszewski syndrome. *Arch Neurol* 29: 324–7.

Tomonaga M (1977) Ultrastructure of neurofibrillary tangles in progressive supranuclear palsy. *Acta Neuropathol* 37: 177–81.

Trotter JL (1973) Striatonigral degeneration, Alzheimer's disease and inflammatory changes. *Neurology* 23: 1211–16.

Verity MA, Wechsler AF (1987) Progressive subcortical gliosis of Neumann: a clinico pathologic study of two cases with review. *Arch Gerontol Geriatr* 6: 245–61.

Wakabayashi K, Oyanagi K, Makifuchi T, Ikuta F, Homma A, Homma Y, Horikawa Y, Tokiguchi S (1994) Corticobasal degeneration: etiopathological significance of the cytoskeletal alterations. *Acta Neuropathol* 87: 545–53.

Warner TT, Lennox GG, Janota I, Harding AE (1994a) Autosomal-dominant dentato rubro pallidoluysian atrophy in the United Kingdom. *Movement Disorders* 9: 289–96.

Warner TT, Williams L, Harding AE (1994b) DRPLA in Europe. Nature. *Genetics* 6: 225.

Watts RL, Williams RS, Growdon JD, Young RR, Haley EC, Beal MF (1985) Corticobasal ganglionic degeneration. *Neurology* 35 Suppl 1, 178.

Watts RL, Mirra SS, Young RR *et al* (1989) Cortico-basal ganglionic degeneration (CBGD) with neuronal achromasia; clinical pathological study of two cases. *Neurology* 39 suppl: 140.

Wisniewski K, Jervis GA, Moretz RC, Wisniewski HM (1979) Alzheimer neurofibrillary tangles in diseases other than senile and presenile dementia. *Ann Neurol* 5: 288–94.

Wszolek ZK, Pfeiffer RF, Bhart MH, Schelper RL, Cordes M, Snow BJ, Rodnitsky RL, Wolters ECh, Arwert F, Calne DB (1992) Rapidly progressive autosomal dominant parkinsonism and dementia with pallido-ponto-nigral degeneration. *Ann Neurol* 32: 312–20.

Yagashita S, Itoh Y, Amano N, Nakano T, Saitoh A (1979) Ultrastructure of neurofibrillary tangles in progressive supranuclear palsy. *Acta Neuropathol* 48: 27–30.

CHAPTER ELEVEN

Familial cerebral amyloid angiopathies

Gordon T. Plant and M. M. Esiri

Introduction
Historical review
Hereditary cerebral haemorrhage with amyloidosis – Icelandic type (HCHWA-I)
Hereditary cerebral haemorrhage with amyloidosis – Dutch type (HCHWA-D)
Familial CAA with non-neuritic plaque formation
Familial CAA with deafness and ocular haemorrhage (Danish type)
Other familial amyloid angiopathies
Hereditary multi-infarct dementia
Differential diagnosis and neuropathological recommendations

INTRODUCTION

In this chapter we review a number of inherited conditions other than Alzheimer's Disease (Chapter 4) which are associated with cerebral amyloid angiopathy (CAA) (Table 11.1). Dementia may be a major feature in these conditions but, in most, it is the consequences of the vascular damage – haemorrhage or ischaemia – that dominate the clinical picture. A satisfactory classification is as yet incomplete because in not all cases have the amyloid proteins themselves or the genetic defects been identified. Amyloid itself is the result of protein accumulation in a particular quaternary structure, the β-pleated sheet, but the amino acid sequence of the fibrils is not always the same and an increasing number of different peptides are known to produce amyloid in various disorders. In some instances a normally occurring protein may be potentially amyloidogenic but amyloid deposition only occurs if the protein is over-produced or under-metabolized (e.g. light chains in myeloma). In other examples a mutation, for example, a single amino acid residue change in the transthyretin (TTR) molecule, may result in the molecule becoming amyloidogenic. A further important question in the amyloidoses is the extent to which the amyloid deposition is primarily responsible for the clinical features or whether it is epiphenomenal. In Gerstmann–Sträussler–Scheinker disease (GSS) for example, the disease may occur without amyloid deposition: in the case of the cerebral amyloid angiopathies there is a clear direct pathological

consequence of the amyloid deposition, namely vascular damage.

These disorders are rare but of considerable importance because of the relationship to other more common diseases including Alzheimer's disease. For example, hereditary cerebral haemorrhage with amyloidosis-Dutch type (HCHWA-D) is known to result from the deposition of a variant β-protein (β/A4) within the vessel wall, and it is a major challenge to research workers to understand how the same amyloid protein is involved in the causation of two diseases which are very different in clinical manifestations. HCHWA-D, Alzheimer's disease, Down's syndrome, and sporadic CAA are now grouped together as examples of 'β-amyloid diseases'. However, it is important to point out that in studies of Alzheimer's disease cases with a history of stroke are often excluded and it is possible that vascular disease resulting from the amyloid angiopathy may be a more common feature of Alzheimer's disease than is recognized. The British type of hereditary CAA described below shows some resemblance to the Gerstmann–Sträussler–Scheinker disease (Chapter 12) in that non-neuritic, 'kuru' plaques are found, that is to say plaques composed of an amyloid core without dystrophic neurites or reactive cells. There are, however, very few examples of CAA in GSS and these may be co-existent β/A4 deposition (Adam et al., 1982; Plant et al., 1990; Duchen, 1992; Watanabe & Duchen, 1993) and here we seek to understand how two disease processes can give

Table 11.1. *Conditions associated with cerebral amyloid angiopathy (CAA)*

Condition	Clinical features	Amyloid protein	Distribution of amyloid angiopathy
Normal ageing and sporadic CAA. (See Chapter 2)	Cerebral haemorrhage	Aβ and βPP (?ACys)	Cerebral leptomeningeal arteries and arterioles and cortical arterioles, sparing hippocampus
Alzheimer's Disease and Down's Syndrome (see Chapter 4)	Dementia	Aβ and βPP (?ACys)	Cerebral leptomeningeal arteries and arterioles and cortical arterioles, sparing hippocampus, arterioles in leptomeninges over cerebellum
Hereditary cerebral haemorrhage with amyloidosis – Icelandic type (HCHWA-I)	Cerebral haemorrhage Dementia may occur	Variant ACys	Arteries and arterioles of leptomeninges and cerebral cortex, deep grey and white matter of cerebrum, brainstem and cerebellum
Hereditary cerebral haemorrhage with amyloidosis –Dutch type (HCHWA-D)	Cerebral haemorrhage Dementia may occur	Variant Aβ and βPP	Cerebral leptomeningeal and cortical arteries and arterioles, and leptomeningeal vessels over brainstem and cerebellum
Familial CAA with non-neuritic amyloid plaque formation (British type)	Progressive dementia, spasticity and ataxia Strokes occur rarely	Unknown ?tubulin	Small arteries and arterioles of leptomeninges; deep grey and white matter of cerebrum, brainstem, cerebellum and spinal cord
Familial CAA with deafness and ocular haemorrhage (Danish type)	Progressive dementia and ataxia Cataract Ocular haemorrhage Deafness	Unknown	Small arteries and arterioles of leptomeninges; deep grey and white matter of cerebrum, brainstem, cerebellum and spinal cord. Inner retinal arterioles.
CAA in Type 1 Familial amyloid polyneuropathy	Ataxia and spasticity (in addition to polyneuropathy) No dementia	Variant TTR	Leptomeningeal and retinal arterioles
Familial oculo-leptomeningeal amyloidosis	Cerebral haemorrhage Myelopathy No dementia	TTR (by immunochemistry variant not identified in vascular amyloid)	Arterioles in leptomeninges and subependymal vessels in brain and spinal cord. No involvement of parenchymal vessels of brain. Occasional neural and intramuscular vessels affected
Spongiform encephalopathies. (rarely, see Chapter 12)	Progressive dementia No strokes	PrP not yet identified in vascular amyloid in human disease Aβ has been identified by immunohistochemistry in some (?coincidence)	Small arteries and arterioles of cerebral leptomeninges and cortex

The Table summarizes conditions known to be associated with cerebral amyloid angiopathy (CAA). Is also describes the major clinical features, the constituent amyloid protein, where known and the distribution of the amyloid angiopathy in the cerebral vessels.
ACys = Cystatin-C, γ-trace.
Aβ = β-protein, A4 peptide.
βPP = β-protein precursor.
TTR = transthyretin, prealbumin.
PrP = prion protein.

rise to similar plaque morphology but in one vascular amyloid deposition predominates and in the other it is rare.

HISTORICAL REVIEW

Scholz (1938) described in the brains of elderly patients the deposition of amyloid within the media of cortical and meningeal blood vessels. He also coined the term 'drusige entartung' to describe the appearance of the amyloid substance in the parenchyma which appeared to have spread through the walls of the capillaries. (This is often erroneously cited as 'drüsige entartung' which would be translated as 'glandular degeneration' while the term derives from 'druse', a geode, the same word is used to describe hyaline deposits at the optic nerve head.) Fig. 11.6 illustrates the aptness of this description. Scholz' interest was vascular disease but Divry (1927), working on the causes of dementia, had already reported the occurrence of amyloid in the plaques found in Alzheimer's disease and senile dementia. This led him to the discovery of amyloid angiopathy in the same material (Divry, 1941). Other reports of CAA in cases of dementia that followed were considered to be either atypical (Van Bogaert et al., 1940; Luërs, 1947; Corsellis & Brierley, 1954) or typical examples of Alzheimer's disease (Benedek & McGovern, 1949).

Interest in CAA as being of clinical significance increased in the 1970s when it was appreciated that it may be responsible for cerebral haemorrhage in patients without hypertension. One of the earliest reports was a familial example (Gudmundsson et al., 1972) but it became clear that sporadic cases were much more common (for a review see Vinters, 1987) and CAA may account for 5–10% of primary cerebral haemorrhage and a much higher proportion of those which are lobar in elderly patients without hypertension. The significance of CAA in Alzheimer's disease, either with respect to the pathogenesis or the clinical features is an area of current widespread research activity (See Chapter 4). One thing is certain, it provided an important technical breakthrough because it is easier to extract amyloid protein from vessels than from parenchymal plaques and it was in material from amyloid angiopathy that βA4 was first identified in Alzheimer's disease by Glenner and Wong (1984).

As far as the direct consequences of the vascular damage in amyloid angiopathy are concerned, four elements have emerged in sporadic and familial cases. One is lobar cerebral haemorrhage, and this seems to occur particularly in those cases in which fibrinoid

necrosis and microaneurysm formation occur. These are the hallmarks of severe amyloid angiopathy (Vonsattel et al., 1991). Secondly areas of infarction are seen but this rarely dominates the clinical picture. Thirdly, ischaemic white matter changes (leukoencephalopathy or leukoaraiosis) can occur, even when the vessels in the affected white matter do not show evidence of angiopathy, the ischaemia presumably being secondary to involvement of the penetrating cortical vessels (Dubas et al., 1985; Vonsattel et al., 1991). Fourthly, and of major relevance in the present volume is the occurrence of dementia. However, this is multifactorial and may result from the accumulation of strokes, from the subcortical white matter ischaemia or from associated neuronal degeneration in those cases showing parenchymal plaque formation, neurofibrillary change and neuronal loss. Yoshimura et al. (1992) have carried out an autopsy study of a group of 20 patients with cerebral haemorrhage due to CAA (almost all sporadic), 75% of whom were known to have become demented. Of the demented patients, some had changes of Alzheimer's disease while others showed leukoencephalopathy. These factors are reflected in the familial cases described below.

HEREDITARY CEREBRAL HAEMORRHAGE WITH AMYLOIDOSIS – ICELANDIC TYPE (HCHWA-I)

Clinical features

Àrnason in his doctoral dissertation (1935) reported a familial occurrence of cerebral haemorrhage in Iceland, and the pathological finding of CAA was demonstrated by Gudmundsson et al. (1972) who described a pedigree of 116 individuals in which 18 had had cerebral haemorrhage. Seven pedigrees including information on progenitors born up to 200 years ago have more recently been described (Jensson et al., 1987) from small rural communities. All the families may have originated from an area surrounding a large fjord in the West of Iceland but cases are now found throughout Iceland. Dominant transmission with full penetrance has been observed although some carriers may have survived into old age without symptoms. The onset of the disease is relatively early, ranging from 20 to 40 years of age and first strokes proven to be due to CAA are rare in these pedigrees after the age of 50. Death at the first stroke is less common than in the Dutch families described below. Over half may make a good recovery after the first insult. In most, there is a protracted course of multiple strokes and several years may elapse without incident. Progressive cognitive decline has sometimes been observed: such patients are usually bed-ridden or in a wheel chair at the time of the fatal stroke. Àrnason (1935) had noted 3 of 10 patients in whom the progression of their illness was slow and dementia was more prominent than paralysis in those cases. Blöndal et al. (1989) reported on the pathological changes in 19 cases with dementia out of a total of 52 cases studied pathologically. In those 19 cases the duration of the dementia ranged from one to 17 years before death with the mean age of onset being 27.3 years. There was often a history of headache prior to the first vascular accident and the average number of strokes during the course of the disease was 3.2. 25% of the patients developed epilepsy.

Neuropathology

Neuropathological findings were first described by Gudmundson et al. (1972) and later by Blöndal et al. (1989). Very extensive amyloid deposition in small arteries as well as arterioles in grey and white matter of the cerebrum, basal ganglia, brainstem and cerebellum underlies the propensity to multiple severe cerebral haemorrhage. The vascular changes are most pronounced in the leptomeningeal and cortical arterioles, where a double lumen, segmental fibrinoid necrosis and aneurysmal dilatation of arteries are common. Perivascular amyloid deposition is seen in the cortex, in the subpial layer and in the basal ganglia but no argyrophilic plaque or neurofibrillary tangle formation has been found in the brain. Multiple cortical areas of infarction and haemorrhage of different ages are apparent. We are not aware of any published reports describing any white matter pathology, or indicating whether or not there is spinal cord involvement.

Amyloid chemistry and genetics

The protease inhibitor Cystatin-C (ACys) has been demonstrated in the amyloid deposits (Cohen et al., 1983; Ghiso, Jensson & Frangione, 1986). ACys levels in the cerebrospinal fluid are low (Grubb et al., 1984; Shimode et al., 1991) and this has been used as a screening test. Subsequently a point mutation in the ACys gene (Levy et al., 1989) which is located on chromosome 20 (Abrahamsson et al., 1989) has been found: there is a glutamine for leucine substitution at position 68 and this mutation can now be used as a genetic marker for the disease. Recently the same mutation was found in four different families (Abrahamsson et al., 1992). It has been confirmed that the variant of the

protein is found in the amyloid deposits. The presence of the ACys variant has been demonstrated, using immunohistochemical techniques, in skin (Blöndal et al., 1989) although previous reports had not found any evidence of amyloidosis outside the CNS using conventional staining techniques. It has therefore been suggested that 'hereditary ACys amyloidosis' may be a more accurate term but the use of HCHWA-I is likely to continue because the clinical features, the major pathological feature and the relationship to the Dutch cases are emphasized: furthermore, it is not certain that the extracerebral deposits are in the form of amyloid.

There have been some reports suggesting ACys reactivity in sporadic CAA coexisting with βA4-protein reactivity associated with cerebral haemorrhage, (Fujihara et al., 1989; Maruyama et al., 1990) or leukoaraiosis (Vinters et al., 1990). Van Duinen et al. (1987) and Coria et al. (1988) did not find evidence of this in either aged or Dutch cases of CAA and Yamada et al. (1989) failed to find any evidence of ACys deposition in aged Japanese cases of sporadic CAA. Whether or not ACys may be involved in amyloid angiopathy other than in these Icelandic families is at present an open question. ACys production by monocytes has been studied in carriers of the mutation and found to be slower than in unaffected family members (Thorsteinsson et al., 1992). Such studies of the biochemistry of the abnormal gene products have considerable potential in increasing our understanding of the pathogenesis of conditions in which amyloid deposition occurs.

HEREDITARY CEREBRAL HAEMORRHAGE WITH AMYLOIDOSIS – DUTCH TYPE (HCHWA-D)

Clinical features

It has been recognized for some time that there is a familial occurrence of cerebral haemorrhage in the Netherlands and pedigrees from the villages of Katwijk and Scheveningen have been described (Luyendijk & Schoen, 1964). Approximately 500 individuals in Holland are at risk of developing the disease. The presentation is usually between the ages of 45 and 60 years as an acute cerebral haemorrhage often with spread to the subarachnoid space giving rise to typical features: headache, vomiting and focal neurological deficit. Around two-thirds will die as a result of this first episode or soon after, but in others there may be a more prolonged and protracted course in which several minor strokes occur due to cerebral haemorrhage, and such patients may indeed develop dementia. Pathologically it is known that cerebral infarction occurs as well as haemorrhage but it is recurrent haemorrhage that dominates the clinical picture in those patients who survive the first episode. Other associated features may be pre-existing attacks of headache without neurological deficit, of uncertain origin, and some patients develop epilepsy late in the course of the disease. Other neurological features seem simply to reflect the residual damage from the acute episodes, there is no suggestion of a progressive spasticity or ataxia as is seen in the British family described below.

There is also a suggestion that there may be a gradual decline in cognitive functions in some cases and dementia may very occasionally be the presenting feature of the disease (Wattendorff et al., 1982; case 3 of Haan et al., 1989). The existence and characteristics of dementia in this disease are of considerable interest because of the pathological similarities with and differences from Alzheimer's disease, (reviewed below) but it is clearly difficult to decide whether or not dementia has occurred as a result of any process other than the recurrent strokes. Haan et al. (1990b) examined 16 patients between 6 months and 12 years after their first cerebral haemorrhage and found cognitive impairment in 75%. The presence of dementia showed a correlation with the number of focal lesions on CT scan but not with white matter hypodensity. In two cases serial psychological testing revealed progressive deterioration without evidence of further strokes or the acquisition of new lesions on CT scanning. It was not possible to decide on the basis of neuropsychological features whether a dementia of a type occurring in Alzheimer's disease was present in addition to a 'multi-infarct' dementia but the major contribution to the dementia was from the vascular lesions.

Neuro-imaging (Fig. 11.1)

A CT study of 24 patients (Haan, Algra & Roos, 1990a) revealed 99 focal lesions in 59 scans of which 13% were ischaemic and 87% haemorrhagic. Cerebellar and brainstem lesions were not seen. A comparison with lobar haemorrhage in other conditions led to a conclusion that the majority of these lesions were likely to be primary cerebral haemorrhage rather than haemorrhagic transformation of ischaemic strokes, but it was noted that the shape of the haemorrhages was more often irregular rather than the smooth, rounded shape of cerebral haemorrhage due to other causes, and a progression of symptoms after the acute onset was more

likely to occur, furthermore the haemorrhages in the Dutch families are often multiple. A comparison was also made with cases of sporadic CAA presenting with cerebral haemorrhage. In HCHWA-D the haemorrhages tend to spare the frontal lobes whereas this was the most frequent location of the haematomas in sporadic CAA and this correlates with the differences in the distribution of the amyloid angiopathy in the two conditions.

Periventricular white matter lesions were seen in both demented and non-demented patients in the CT study and any contribution to the dementia was uncertain. However, MR imaging in a smaller group of patients showed periventricular white matter changes in all cases (Haan et al., 1990c). The MR studies also demonstrated the different ages of the multiple haemorrhages, most patients having a number of lesions showing different signal characteristics reflecting the age of the lesions.

Neuropathology

Luyendijk and Bots (1980) first demonstrated that the disease was due to extensive amyloid deposition in small leptomeningeal and cortical (both cerebral and cerebellar) arterioles. Complete neuropathological studies have been reported in 63 cases (Wattendorff et al., 1982, 1995; Luyendijk et al., 1988; Van Duinen et al., 1987). Brains were of normal or slightly reduced weight and tended to show thickened leptomeninges externally. Cortical atrophy was not marked. Fixed brain slices showed recent large haemorrhages and remnants of older ones, mainly in the subcortical white matter. In cortex and subcortical white matter recent and old haemorrhagic infarcts were found. These lesions were predominantly located in the temporal, parietal and occipital regions. Extracranial arteries and arteries at the base of the brain showed no marked abnormality.

Histologically, in addition to the presence of multiple vascular lesions, there were small to moderate numbers of cortical amyloid deposits resembling the diffuse plaques seen in Alzheimer's disease. These deposits were missed in the early studies because only more sensitive immunohistochemical staining procedures demonstrated them. Dense plaque cores and neurofibrillary tangles were not seen. Although dystrophic neurites are not prominent some ubiquitin positive structures suggestive of dystrophic neurites are occasionally present in the diffuse amyloid deposits (Tagliavini et al., 1993). Cortical and hippocampal neuronal populations outside the infarcts appeared well preserved. Cerebral and cerebellar white matter showed in varying degrees oedema and demyelination with sparing of the 'U' fibres.

Amyloid chemistry and genetics

Van Duinen *et al.* (1987) examined six brains immunohistochemically using an antibody raised against a region of the βA4 of Alzheimer's disease and Down's syndrome. Both the amyloid angiopathy and the plaque-like lesions showed positive staining. The amyloid protein was also isolated from leptomeningeal vessels and amino acid sequencing has shown it to be βA4 (Van Duinen *et al.*, 1987). Coria *et al.* (1988)

subsequently showed that the positive immunostaining spread out of the blood vessels into the surrounding parenchyma and found the same immunoreactivity in sporadic CAA and CAA due to ageing and coined the term 'the β-amyloid diseases' ('BAD'). βA4 deposits in blood vessel walls were largely confined to leptomeningeal small arteries and cortical arterioles. Among the cortical arterioles affected were the deep penetrating vessels that supply the white matter. The narrowed lumens of these vessels could plausibly account for the incomplete, diffuse infarction in the white matter.

Vascular amyloid deposits, but not the diffuse paren-

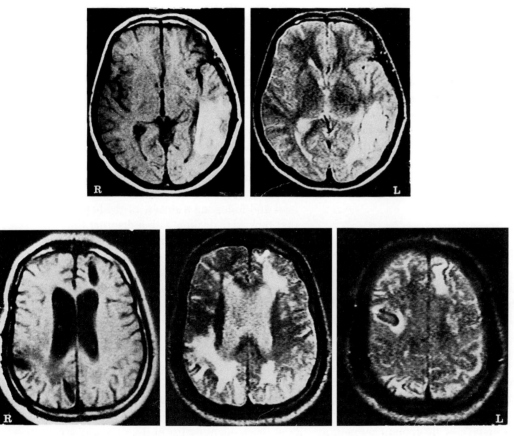

Fig. 11.1. The upper two panels show magnetic resonance (MR) images showing a left temporo-parietal haemorrhage in a case of hereditary cerebral haemorrhage (Dutch type). There is high signal intensity both in the T1- and T2-weighted images (left and right panels, respectively). The haemorrhage had occurred two weeks prior to the scan. The frequency of haemorrhages in this condition is equally distributed over both hemispheres sparing basal ganglia and cerebellum. The lower three panels are MR images of another case of the disease showing multiple haemorrhages of different ages. These show as low intensity regions in the right parietal and left frontal lobes on the T1-weighted image (left panel) and as high intensity on the T2-weighted image (centre). Another old haemorrhage is seen high in the right parietal lobe in the T2-weighted image on the right. This is surrounded by a rim of low signal, indicating the presence of haemosiderin. In addition to the evidence of previous haemorrhage, there is white matter high intensity in the central panel indicating leukoaraiosis. (From Haan *et al.*, 1990c.)

chymal plaques, reacted not only for βA4 but also for its precursor protein (Tagliavini *et al.*, 1990). This suggests that the vascular compartment may be the main source of βA4 that accumulates in the brain in this disease. Parenchymal deposits are in the main a 'halo' around the vessel, a feature less constantly seen in Alzheimer's disease. Linkage to the βA4 precursor gene has been shown in the Dutch families (Van Broeckhoven *et al.*, 1990) and a point mutation has been identified in the gene encoding the Aβ precursor protein (βPP) at codon 618, causing a single amino acid substitution of glutamine instead of glutamic acid in the *extracellular* portion of the βPP (Levy *et al.*, 1990). In a number of families, including one in the United States recently diagnosed as having HCHWA-D (Fernandez-Madrid *et al.*, 1991, the case was a descendant of a Dutch immigrant to the US) it has been shown that the disease segregates with the codon 618 variant. The supposition is that this mutation is responsible for the abnormal processing of the amyloid precursor protein in HCHWA-D. As reviewed by Wisniewski and Frangione (1992), this contrasts with the fact that in familial Alzheimer's disease some of the mutations identified have been at codon 642 in the *intramembrane* region (although some are also in the extracellular portion). The site of the mutation may determine the disease process.

FAMILIAL CAA WITH NON-NEURITIC PLAQUE FORMATION

Clinical features

This term was introduced by Plant *et al.* (1990) to distinguish the condition from familial Alzheimer's disease, from GSS and from the other familial amyloid angiopathies as the combination of CAA and non-neuritic plaque formation is the most distinctive pathological feature of this disorder. To refer to the amyloid angiopathy as 'cerebral' is not strictly accurate because the brainstem, cerebellum and spinal cord are also involved. A further important distinction is that cerebral haemorrhage is unusual and the dementia results to a large extent from neuronal loss in the hippocampus which is associated with parenchymal plaque formation. Any contribution arising as a direct result of the vascular damage is in the form of leukoencephalopathy. As yet the nature of the amyloid protein is not known. An unrelated condition in which familial pseudo-bulbar palsy occurs is now known as the Worster–Drought syndrome (Patton, Baraitser & Brett, 1986) in recogni-

tion of the contribution made by the same neurologist. In the literature the disorder will be found referred to as an example of atypical Alzheimer's disease (e.g. Aikawa *et al.*, 1985); as an example of GSS (Masters, Gajdusek & Gibbs, 1981; Baraitser, 1990); as an atypical form of GSS (Courten-Myers and Mandybur, 1987; Baraitser, 1990) and as a form of primary CAA classified with the Icelandic and Dutch types of HCHWA, (Vinters, 1987); and with the hereditary spastic parapareses (Baraitser, 1990).

A single extensive pedigree with the disease occurring in five generations has been reported (Plant *et al.*, 1990). This family is not without historical interest because the original pathological descriptions (Worster-Drought, Greenfield & McMenemey, 1940; 1944) are the earliest English language descriptions of CAA of any kind but the authors did not recognize it as such and described the vascular changes as 'hyaline degeneration'. It was the discovery by Corsellis and Brierley (1954) of familial cases of dementia with CAA, and the similarity of the pathological changes in the vessels to the earlier descriptions in the French and German literature (Scholz, 1938; Divry, 1941) that led to a review of the pathological material from Worster–Drought's cases and the appropriate stains were then carried out (see McMenemey, 1970). Griffiths *et al.* (1982) described very similar pathological changes in two siblings from Oxford, England and following a review of the literature suggested that they were dealing with a disorder that was 'clearly the same' as that which had affected the brother and two sisters described by Worster-Drought. The correctness of their conclusion has subsequently been affirmed by Plant *et al.* (1990) who demonstrated that both sets of siblings were descended from a common ancestor, a British woman who died in 1883. The link between the two families was established by consulting a family history taken by a House Physician in 1924 when one of the affected family members was admitted to the National Hospital for Nervous Diseases in Queen Square under the care of Dr MacDonald Critchley.

Seventy-five great-great-grand-children of this woman have been identified and 18 of these are at risk of developing the disease. However, at the time of writing none is known to be affected, most are in their fifth decade. Descendants are living in Australia and North America as well as in the United Kingdom. The descendants of two of the common ancestor's children (III 5 and 6 in Fig. 1 of Plant *et al.*, 1990), who both died of the disease in the 1930s (and had between them 15 children) have not been traced and therefore it is highly likely that other affected and at-risk individuals exist among their descendants.

Clinical details of 26 affected individuals in the pedigree are now known and autopsy findings have been published in 5 family members. The clinical features of the disorder may be summarized as being of onset in the fifth decade characterized by progressive dementia and very marked spastic paralysis in all cases and cerebellar ataxia in most. The mean age of onset has been 47 (range 40–57) and the mean age at death 56 (range 50–66).

Psychometric assessment early in the course of the disease has shown marked impairment of memory progressing ultimately to a global dementia. Many of the cases developed personality change as an early manifestation, becoming irritable or in some cases depressed. The spastic paralysis is far more profound than is seen in GSS or in Alzheimer's disease. Pseudo-bulbar palsy and dysarthria are universal and all patients have progressed to a chronic vegetative state; mute, unresponsive, quadraplegic and incontinent. The question of the relative contributions of the vascular pathology and the plaque formation to the clinical course is uncertain but only a small number of the cases have sustained stroke-like episodes, three of those also had hypertension, and there has been no example of a cerebral haemorrhage such as occurs in the Dutch and Icelandic cerebral amyloid angiopathies. One case collapsed in the street and was unconscious for 24 hours. She never left hospital and the story was a slowly progressive one from then on but the initial event was certainly compatible with an acute infarct or cerebral haemorrhage and there was some evidence for minor haemorrhage in the autopsy studies. As well as nystagmus some cases developed other brain stem symptoms such as diplopia. One had a craniotomy because she was thought to have a posterior fossa tumour.

Neuro-imaging

Fig. 11.2 shows coronal images of a magnetic resonance scan of an affected individual at the age of 60, three years following the onset of symptoms. The major features are the moderate ventricular dilatation and relatively preserved cortex with extensive periventricular white matter changes compatible with leukoaraiosis.

Neuropathology

Detailed neuropathology has been reported for five cases of this condition (Worster-Drought et al., 1940, 1944; McMenemey 1952, 1970; Griffiths et al., 1982; Plant et al., 1990). The pathology is confined to the central nervous system in all cases. The brains are of normal or slightly reduced overall weight with leptomeningeal thickening and moderate diffuse atrophy of both the cerebral and cerebellar hemispheres. The cerebral cortex is relatively well preserved in slices of the fixed brain but the white matter is diffusely discoloured and contains small cystic old infarcts (Fig. 11.3). The deep white matter is also atrophied and the lateral ventricles enlarged. Brainstem and spinal cord, when examined, appear normal to the naked eye.

The main histological finding is severe, widespread amyloid deposition in the walls of small leptomeningeal

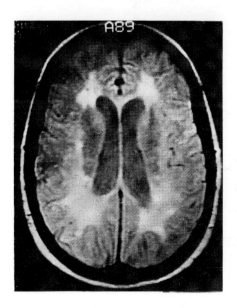 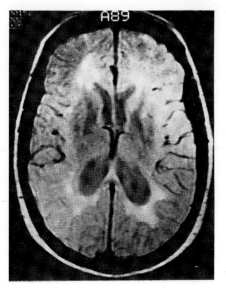

Fig. 11.2. Moderately T2-weighted image of a case of familial cerebral amyloid angiopathy (British type). Extensive leukoaraiosis is shown as periventricular high intensity. White matter changes are more extensive in this disorder than in the Icelandic and Dutch families and evidence of cerebral haemorrhage is rare. The Danish type has very similar MR scan appearances.

arteries and widespread (virtually all) arterioles of grey and white matter. In addition there are numerous parenchymal non-neuritic amyloid plaques, together with ischaemic white matter damage and the presence of neurofibrillary tangles, particularly in the hippocampus. The affected vessels are all of small size, less than 100 microns but are found in most cases in all areas including the spinal cord. Some vessels are narrowed and others completely obstructed (Fig. 11.4). Some show concentric fibrotic thickening, fragmentation of the elastic lamina or splitting to produce a double lumen (Fig. 11.5). Occasional small perivascular haemorrhages or slight inflammation may be seen around the affected vessels and spicules of amyloid radiating from capillaries into the surrounding neuropil (Drusige entartung) are common (Fig. 11.6).

The plaques are of two varieties: large, about 150 micron across, with a central congophilic core with radiating spicules of amyloid emerging from it and a finely fibrillar rim (Fig. 11.7); others are small, with appearances like the cores of the large plaques without a rim (Fig. 11.8). Some of the large plaques are related to a capillary either at its centre or more eccentrically placed within or alongside it, often with an obliterated lumen (Fig. 11.9). Large plaques in one case were most numerous in the fascia dentata and CA3 and CA4 regions of the hippocampus, presubiculum and basolateral nucleus of the amygdala. Perivascular plaques occur chiefly in the cerebral and cerebellar cortex and in white matter, while small plaques are numerous in CA1 and part of CA2 regions of the hippocampus and less common in the granular layer of the cerebellar cortex. An inconsistent feature seen in only some of the cases is neuritic plaque formation in the hippocampus. Neurofibrillary tangles are seen in most of the few remaining pyramidal neurons of the hippocampus. These are also present in the subiculum, entorhinal cortex, amygdala and occasionally elsewhere in the cortex and in the basal nucleus

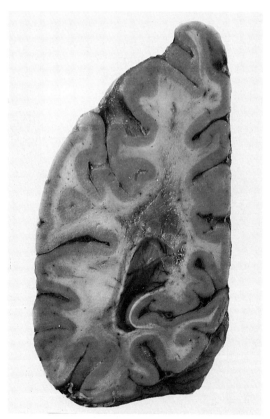

Fig. 11.3. British type CAA: macroscopic view of brain section to show leukoencephalopathy and small white matter infarcts.

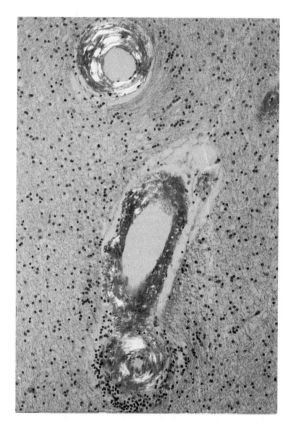

Fig. 11.4. British type CAA: amyloid angiopathy, from white matter. Congo red stain in polarized light × 100.

of Meynert and the raphe nucleus of the brainstem. Ischaemic lesions of microscopic size are also scattered in the cerebral cortex while the deep white matter shows patchy myelin loss and small cystic infarcts. These infarcts show very infrequent evidence of haemorrhage in marked contrast to HCHWA-D and -I. The lentiform and caudate nuclei are relatively well preserved, with few affected vessels, but the thalamus is severely affected as is the cerebellum, particularly near the midline, with many amyloid laden vessels, perivascular amyloid plaques and severe diffuse Purkinje cell loss. Axonal 'torpedoes', milder granule cell loss and severe gliosis are also seen (Fig. 11.10). The dentate nuclei also show neuron loss and deep cerebellar white matter cystic focal ischaemic lesions. In the medulla there is long tract degeneration in the pyramids and inferior cerebellar peduncles, neuron loss and gliosis from the inferior olives and neuron loss and gliosis in the medial accessory olive. The spinal cord shows pallor of myelin staining in all columns of white matter, a few large amyloid plaques in grey and white matter and amyloid containing vessels. However, in one case examined the spinal cord vessels were relatively spared.

The white matter changes are considered to be secondary to the amyloid deposition in arterioles penetrating through the cortex to supply the white matter. The white matter changes may contribute to the dementia. The plaque formation, neurofibrillary tangles and neuron loss in the hippocampus are sufficient to account for amnesia; cerebellar plaques and ischaemic lesions for the ataxia; and cerebral deep white matter and spinal cord long tract involvement, in part, for the spasticity.

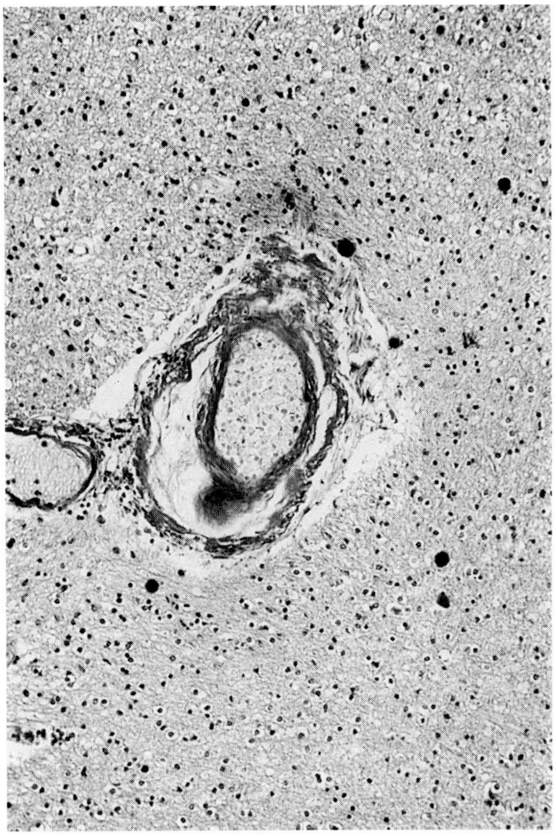

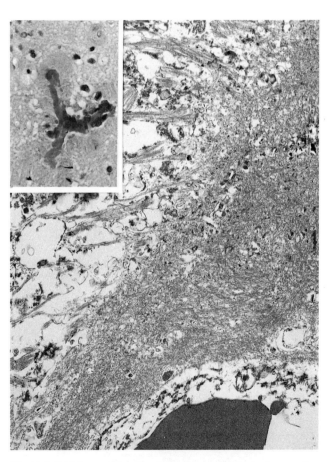

Fig. 11.6. British type CAA: Drusige entatung. Electron micrograph (× 8400) of an arteriole showing a thickened wall composed of amyloid fibrils extending from the capillary wall into the parenchyma. The inset shows a cortical capillary with amyloid (PAS) showing again the extension of the amyloid into the parenchyma.

Fig. 11.5. British type CAA: amyloid angiopathy to show double lumen formation. PAS × 200.

The explanation for the relative rarity of cerebral haemorrhage in this form of familial CAA, despite the severity of the amyloid angiopathy, is not known.

The molecular biology and biochemistry of the disorder is not as well advanced as in the Icelandic and Dutch diseases. Ghiso *et al.* (1995) have shown that the vascular amyloid does not show positive immunostaining for βA4, ACys or transthyretin (TTR). Neither is there currently any evidence for the deposits being prion protein (PrP), despite the resemblance of the plaques to 'kuru' plaques seen in GSS and Creutzfeldt–Jacob disease. The British family appears to be distinct from all other familial diseases associated with cerebral amyloid; distinct from the point of view of clinical manifestation, of pathology and, probably, the constituent amyloid protein. A recent study (Baumann *et al.*, 1996) has demonstrated that C-terminal fragments of tubulin are associated with the amyloid deposits extracted from one case. Whether tubulin is the primary amyloid protein is

not established. The disease which most closely resembles the British family as far as the clinical and pathological features of the cerebral disease are concerned is described in the following section. Very recently a second British family has been described in which two siblings have been affected by a clinically and pathologically indistinguishable disease (Doshi *et al.*, 1996).

FAMILIAL CAA WITH DEAFNESS AND OCULAR HAEMORRHAGE (DANISH TYPE)

Clinical features

Strömgren (1981) described 9 cases in 3 generations of a dominantly inherited disorder originating in the region of Århus in Jutland, Denmark. The clinical picture is unique, there is early (around age 20) cataract formation followed by deafness (around 30) and a progressive ataxia and dementia beginning in the fifth and sixth decades. Progression to death occurs less than ten years

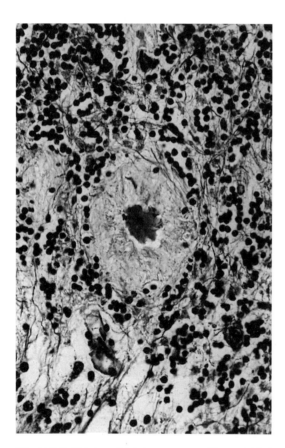

Fig. 11.7. British type CAA: large non-neuritic amyloid plaque, cerebellum. There is a central core PAS × 300.

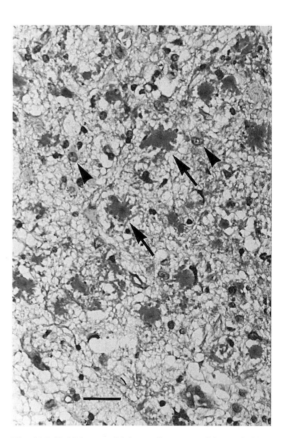

Fig. 11.8. British type CAA: small non-neuritic amyloid plaques, hippocampus. There is no central core. PAS × 400.

following the onset of neurological symptoms. Stroke-like episodes are rare and once the neurological disease becomes established the clinical manifestations are very similar to the British family described above. Some patients have recurrent intra-ocular haemorrhage before the neurological disease becomes apparent.

Neuro-imaging
Neuro-imaging studies show extensive white matter ischaemic change similar to the British family.

Neuropathology
The published report (Strömgren, 1981) noted accumulation of lipid in the vessel walls and parenchyma, but recent studies (H. Braendgaard, personal communication) have established that there is CAA. Material from 3 autopsied family members is available. There is widespread amyloid angiopathy in the cerebrum, cerebellum, spinal cord and retina. Deposits of amyloid are found in the vessels and stroma of the choroid plexus. Drusige entartung is seen in the cerebrum and spinal cord but not in the cerebellum. Neuritic plaques and sparse NFTs are seen in the hippocampus where there is some cell loss. Scarlet red staining revealed the presence of large amounts of fat products in the vessel walls and parenchyma. As in the British family the major consequence of the amyloid angiopathy is demyelination and white matter ischaemia with little or no evidence of haemorrhage.

The retinal involvement presumably accounts for the intraocular haemorrhage in some cases and this feature,

together with the deafness and cataract clearly distinguish the disease from all of the families described above. The eye is involved in a number of hereditary amyloidoses. Corneal lattice dystrophy occurs in the Finnish type of familial amyloid polyneuropathy (FAP type five) first described by Merejota (1969) in which the amyloid protein is gelsolin (Haltia *et al.*, 1990). Vitreous opacities occur in various TTR amyloidoses (see Herbert, 1989 for a review) and ocular microangiopathy has been described in TTR amyloidosis (Ando *et al.*, 1990). Haan *et al.* (1990*d*) have carried out fluorescein angiography in HCHWA-D and have shown some abnormalities. The realization of the importance of the Danish family is very recent and as yet the nature of the amyloid protein is unknown.

OTHER FAMILIAL AMYLOID ANGIOPATHIES
CAA in familial Alzheimer's disease is discussed elsewhere (Chapter 4). There are a few other rare examples of familial disorders in which CAA is found, some of these may be examples of familial Alzheimer's disease and were often described as such in the original reports (Van Bogaert *et al.*, 1940; Lüers, 1947, cases 1 and 2 (siblings); Corsellis and Brierley, 1954, Case 1; Gerhard, Bergener & Homayun, 1972; Aikawa *et al.*, 1985). In addition to the dementia all of these cases had spasticity and sometimes ataxia with death occurring in the range 40 – 60 years. A distinct family has been described from Britain with pathological features very similar to the British family described above but the presentation was

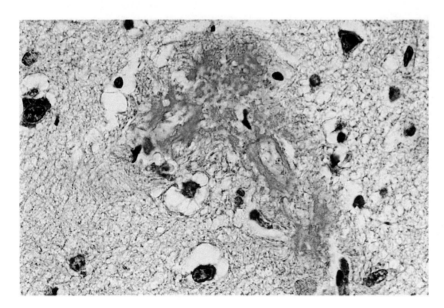

Fig. 11.9. British type CAA: large plaques related to a capillary (PAS × 300).

as a hereditary ataxia without dementia (Love & Duchen, 1982). It would be of considerable interest if some of the pathological material in these cases could be studied by immunohistochemistry for evidence of β/A4, which would confirm the relationship to Alzheimer's disease in those cases showing a positive result.

There is a familial oculoleptomeningeal amyloidosis, due to the deposition of a variant TTR, in which the involvement of meningeal vessels has led to cerebral haemorrhage and myelopathy but not specifically dementia (Uitti et al., 1988). Recently, a Japanese family (the 'K' family) has been reported with TTR related type 1 FAP in which there was, in addition to a sensorimotor and autonomic peripheral neuropathy, cerebellar ataxia and pyramidal tract signs without dementia or stroke (Ikeda et al., 1989) the leptomeningeal and pia-arachnoid vessels are principally involved and the brain parenchyma is spared, most vessels were observed to be free of amyloid shortly after entering the cerebral cortex

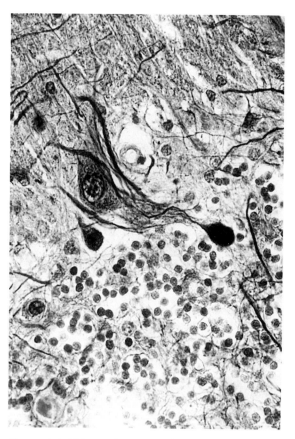

Fig. 11.10. British type CAA: cerebellum – axonal torpedoes and severe gliosis. Bielschowsky. × 300.

(Ushiyama, Ikeda & Yanagisawa, 1991). Characteristically, the amyloid is deposited in the pia-arachnoid membranes and choroid plexus also. CAA of this type may in fact be common in type 1 FAP even without evidence of CNS involvement (Ushiyama et al., 1991) and the variant TTR has been identified in the amyloid fibrils in the 'K' family (Kametani et al., 1992).

GSS or inherited spongiform encephalopathy appears to be rarely associated with CAA (one case in six members of the 'W' family; Adam et al., 1982) and care must be taken in attributing CAA in GSS and Creutzfeldt-Jakob disease to PrP deposition without immunohistochemical confirmation, as β/A4 CAA may coexist with sporadic and familial spongiform encephalopathy (Roberts et al., 1988; Tateishi et al., 1992; Watanabe & Duchen, 1993). As yet there is no example of CAA in a human prion disease in which PrP has been shown to be the constituent protein of the vascular amyloid. Parenchymal plaques of amyloid in GSS are similar to those seen in the British family described above except that many are multi-centric (see Chapter 12).

HEREDITARY MULTI-INFARCT DEMENTIA

The conditions discussed here are not associated with CAA but clearly there is some overlap in the clinical features with familial CAA because vascular disease is responsible in these families for a progressive dementia. Sourander and Walinder (1977), Stevens, Hewlett & Brownell (1977), Yokoi and Nakayama (1985) and Sonninen and Sarontaus (1987) have all described families in which strokes occur progressing to dementia. Cerebral haemorrhage is not a feature. Inheritance is as an autosomal dominant. These conditions are described further in Chapter 5.

DIFFERENTIAL DIAGNOSIS AND NEUROPATHOLOGICAL RECOMMENDATIONS

These conditions should be considered particularly in cases in which there is a positive family history of dementia and in which dementia is accompanied by ataxia and spasticity. Differential diagnosis includes other familial causes of dementia, the most common of which is Alzheimer's disease (Chapter 4) but including Pick's disease (Chapter 8), a wide range of metabolic disease (Chapter 14) and GSS (Chapter 12). Only the latter condition is likely to closely mimic clinically those familial amyloid angiopathies not associated with cerebral haemorrhage. Cases with stroke-like episodes need to be distinguished from other causes of ischaemic dementia and occasionally normal pressure hydrocephalus or paraneoplastic syndromes may overlap clinically. When the naked eye appearances of the brain in a case of familial amyloid angiopathy are considered, the most likely differential diagnosis includes other forms of vascular dementia. If possible, the spinal cord as well as the brain should be examined, since this is unlikely to be abnormal (with the exception of Wallerian degeneration) in other forms of vascular dementia. Histological sampling needs to be widespread, including multiple areas of cerebral cortex, hippocampus, cerebral white matter, basal ganglia, thalamus and multiple levels of the brainstem, cerebellum and spinal cord. It is essential to carry out stains for amyloid if the true nature of these conditions is not to be overlooked; as stated above, in the original descriptions of both the British and Danish families the amyloid deposits were only recognized as such when the pathology was reviewed some years later. It is, in fact, recommended that an amyloid stain be carried out on all cases of vascular dementia (Chapter 5). Once the amyloid has been detected, its biochemical nature should be investigated with immunostain for β/A4, ACys and PrP. In addition, the morphological form of any parenchymal amyloid deposits considerably assists in distinguishing one form of familial CAA form another but this is not an absolute guide.

In conclusion, these rare familial conditions cause dementia partly on the basis of neurodegeneration and partly as a result of recurrent focal ischaemia, recurrent haemorrhage or leucoaraiosis or a combination of these changes. An interesting feature of many of these conditions is the paucity of neuritic pathology in comparison with Alzheimer's disease. Haemorrhage seems to predominate in those families in which the CAA is less extensive, affecting mainly the leptomeningeal and cortical vessels (HCHWA-I and -D), When large and small vessels throughout the brain are involved the vascular consequence is leucoaraioisis rather than haemorrhage (British and Danish families). This distinction cannot be attributed to the sparing of larger vessels in the British and Danish families as vessels of all sizes are extensively involved. Although rare in themselves the identification and study of familial CAA is proving of great importance in increasing our understanding of common neurodegenerations including Alzheimer's disease.

ACKNOWLEDGEMENTS

It is a pleasure to acknowledge the invaluable help of Tom Wisniewski, Blas Frangione and Thomas Révész in the preparation of this article. We are especially grateful to Hans Braendgaard for permission to review unpublished material.

REFERENCES

Abrahamsson M, Islam MQ, Szpirer J, Szpirer C, Levan G (1989) The human Cystatin-C gene (CST3), mutated in hereditary Cystatin-C amyloid angiopathy, is located on chromosome 20. *Hum Gen* 82: 223–6.

Abrahamsson M, Jonsdottir S, Olafsson I, Jensson O, Grubb A (1992) Hereditary Cystatin-C amyloid angiopathy: identification of the disease-causing mutation and specific diagnosis by polymerase chain reaction based analysis. *Hum Genet* 89: 377–80.

Adam J, Crow TJ, Duchen LW, Scaravilli F, Spokes E (1982) Familial cerebral amyloidosis and spongiform encephalopathy. *J Neurol Neurosurg Psychiat* 45: 37–45.

Aikawa H, Suzuki K, Iwasaki Y, Iizuka R. (1985) Atypical Alzheimer's disease with spastic paresis and ataxia. *Ann Neurol* 17: 297–300.

Ando E, Ando Y, Maruoka S, Sakai Y, Watanabe S, Yamashita E, Okamura K, Araki S (1990) Ocular microangiopathy in familial amyloidotic polyneuropathy, type I. *Graefe's Arch* 230: 1–5.

Àrnason A (1935) Apoplexie und ihre Vererbung. Acta Psychiatr Neurol Suppl VII.

Baraitser M (1990) *The Genetics of Neurological Disease.* Oxford Medical Publications, Oxford pp 93, 129, and 284.

Baumann MH. Wisniewski T, Levy E, Plant GT, Ghiso J (1996) C-terminal fragments of α- and β-tubulin form amyloid fibrils *in vitro* and associate with amyloid deposits of familial CAA, British type, *Biochem Biophys Res Commun* 219: 238–42.

Benedek S, McGovern VJ (1949) A case of Alzheimer's disease with amyloidosis of the cerebral cortex. *Med J Aust* 2: 429–30.

Blöndal H, Gudmundsson G, Benedikz E, Johannesson G (1989) Dementia in hereditary Cystatin-C amyloidosis. *Progr Clin Biol Res* 317: 157–64.

Cohen DH, Feiner H, Jensson O, Frangione B (1983) Amyloid fibril in hereditary cerebral haemorrhage with amyloidosis (HCHWA) is related to the gastroentero-pancreatic neuroendocrine protein, γ-trace. *J Exp Med* 158: 623–8.

Coria F, Castaño E, Prelli F, Larrondo-Lillo M, Van Duinen S, Shelanski ML, Frangione B (1988) Isolation and characterisation of amyloid P component from Alzheimer's disease and other types of cerebral amyloidosis. *Lab Invest* 58: 454–8.

Corsellis JAN, Brierley JB (1954) An unusual type of pre-senile dementia: (atypical Alzheimer's disease with amyloid vascular change). *Brain* 77: 571–87.

Courten-Myers G, Mandybur TI (1987) Atypical Gerstmann-Sträussler syndrome or familial spino cerebellar ataxia and Alzheimer's disease? *Neurology* (Cleveland) 37: 269–75.

Divry P (1927) Étude histo-chimique des plaques sénile. *J Belge Neurol Psychatr* 27: 643–57.

Divry P (1941) De l'amylöidose vasculaire cérébral et méningée (méningiopathie amylöide) dans la démence sénile. *J Belge Neurol Psychiat* 42: 141–58.

Doshi RB, Révész T, Harwood G, Plant G (1996) Familial cerebral amyloid angiopathy (British type) with non-neuritic plaque formation is not restricted to a single family *Neuropathol Appl Neurobiol* 22: 163.

Dubas F, Gray F, Roullet E, Escourolle R (1985) Leucoencephalopathy in diffuse haemorrhagic cerebral amyloid angiopathy. *Ann Neurol* 18: 54–9.

Duchen LW (1992) Current status review: cerebral amyloid. *Int J Exp Path* 73: 535–50.

Fernandez-Madrid I, Levy E, Marder K, Frangione B (1991) Codon 618 variant of Alzheimer amyloid gene associated with inherited cerebral haemorrhage. *Ann Neurol* 30: 730–3.

Fujihara S, Shimode K, Nakamura M, Kobayashi S, Tsunematsu T (1989) Cerebral amyloid angiopathy with the deposition of cystatin C (α-trace) and β protein. In Iqbal K, Wisniewski HM, Winblad B (eds) *Alzheimer's Disease and Related Disorders. Progress in Clinical and Biological Research Vol. 317.* Alan R Liss, New York, pp. 939–44.

Gerhard L, Bergener M, Homayun S (1972) Angiopathie bei Alzheimerscher Krankheit. *Z Neurol* 201: 43–61.

Ghiso J, Jensson O, Frangione B (1986) Amyloid fibrils in hereditary cerebral haemorrhage with amyloidosis of Icelandic type is a variant of γ trace basic protein (cystatin-C) *Proc Natl Acad Sci* 83: 2974–8.

Ghiso J, Plant GT, Révész T, Wisniewski T, Frangione B (1995) Familial cerebral amyloid angiopathy (British type) with nonneuritic amyloid plaque formation may be due to a novel protein. *J Neurol Sci* 129: 74–5.

Glenner GG, Wong CW (1984) Alzheimer's disease: initial report of the purification and characterisation of a novel cerebrovascular amyloid protein. *Biochem Biophys Res Commun* 120: 885–90.

Griffiths RA, Mortimer TF, Oppenheimer DR, Spalding JMK (1982) Congophilic angiopathy of the brain: a clinical and pathological report on two siblings. *J Neurol Neurosurg Psychiat* 45: 396–408.

Grubb A, Jensson O, Gudmundson G, Àrnason A, Hofberg H, Malm J (1984) Evidence that abnormal metabolism of γ-trace is the basic defect in hereditary cerebral haemorrhage with amyloidosis. *New Engl J Med* 311: 1547–9.

Gudmundsson G, Hallgrimsson J, Jonasson TA, Bjarnason O (1972) Hereditary cerebral haemorrhage with amyloidosis. *Brain* 95: 387–404.

Haan J, Roos RA (1992) Comparison between the Icelandic and Dutch forms of hereditary cerebral amyloid angiopathy. *Clin Neurol Neurosurg* 94 Suppl: S82–3.

Haan J, Algra PR, Roos RAC (1990a) Hereditary cerebral haemorrhage with amyloidosis – Dutch type: clinical and CT analysis of 24 cases. *Arch Neurol* 47: 649–53.

Haan J, Lanser JBK, Zijdervald I, van der Does IGF, Roos RAC (1990b) Dementia in hereditary cerebral haemorrhage with amyloidosis – Dutch type. *Arch Neurol* 47: 965–7.

Haan J, Roos RAC, Algra PR, Lanser JBK, Bots GTAM, Vegter-van der Vlis (1990c) Hereditary cerebral haemorrhage with amyloidosis – Dutch type: Magnetic resonance imaging findings of seven patients. *Brain* 113: 1251–67.

Haan J, Bollemeijer JG, de Keizer RJW, Roos RAC (1990d) Fluorescein angiography of the retina in hereditary cerebral amyloid angiopathy – Dutch type: a preliminary study. In *Hereditary cerebral haemorrhage with amyloidosis – Dutch type. Clinical, Radiological and Genetical Aspects.* Thesis. Rijksuniversitet te Leiden, pp. 81–6.

Haan J, Roos RAC, Briët PE, Herpers MJHM, Luyendijk W, Bots GTAM (1989) Hereditary cerebral haemorrhage with amyloidosis-Dutch type: clinical characteristics. *Clin Neurol Neurosurg* 91: 285–90.

Haltia M, Prelli F, Ghiso J, Kiuru S, Somer H, Palo J, Frangione B (1990) Amyloid protein in familial amyloidosis (Finnish type) is homologous to gelsolin, an actin-binding protein. *Biochem Biophys Res Commun* 167: 927–32.

Herbert J (1989) Familial amyloidotic polyneuropathies. In Rowland LP, Wood DS, Schou EA, Di Mauro S (eds) *Molecular Genetics in Diseases of the Brain, Nerve and Muscle*, Oxford University Press, pp 299–325.

Ikeda S-I, Allsop D, Glenner GG (1989) The morphology and distribution of plaque and related deposits in the brain of Alzheimer's disease and control cases: an immunohistochemical study using amyloid β-protein antibody. *Lab Invest* 60: 113–22.

Jensson O, Gudmundsson G, Àrnason A, Blöndal H, Petursdottir I, Thorsteinsson L, Grubb A, Löfberg H, Cohen D, Frangione B (1987) Hereditary cystatin-C (γ-trace) amyloid angiopathy of the CNS causing cerebral haemorrhage. *Acta Neurol Scand* 76: 102–14.

Kametani F, Ikeda S, Yanagisawa N, Ishi T, Hanyu N (1992) Characterisation of a transthyretin-related amyloid fibril protein from cerebral amyloid angiopathy in type 1 familial amyloid polyneuropathy. *J Neurol Sci* 108: 178–83.

Levy E, Carmen MD, Fernandez-Madrid IJ, Power MD, Lieberburg I, Van Duinen SG, Bots GTAM, Luyendijk W, Frangione B (1990) Mutation of the Alzheimer's disease amyloid gene in hereditary cerebral haemorrhage, Dutch type. *Science* 248: 1124–6.

Levy E, Lopez-Otin C, Ghiso J. Geltner D, Frangione B (1989) Stroke in Icelandic patients with hereditary amyloid angiopathy is related to a mutation in the Cystatin-C gene, an inhibitor of cysteine proteases. *J Exp Med* 169: 1771–8.

Love S, Duchen LW (1982) Familial cerebellar ataxia with cerebrovascular amyloid. *J Neurol, Neurosurg Psychiat* 45: 271–3.

Luërs T (1947) Über die familiäre juvenile Form der Alzheimerischen Krankheit mit neurologischen Herder-scheinungen. *Arch Psychiat Nervenkrank* 179: 132–45.

Luyendijk W, Bots GTAM (1980) Familial incidence of ICH. In Pia HW, Langmaid C, Zierski J (eds). *Spontaneous Intracerebral Haematomas. Advances in Diagnosis and Therapy.* Springer-Verlag, Berlin/Heidelberg/New York pp 50–5.

Luyendijk W, Bots GTAM, Vegter-an der Vlis M, Went LN, Frangione B (1988) Hereditary cerebral haemorrhage caused by cortical amyloid angiopathy. *J Neurol Sci* 85: 267–80.

Luyendijk W, Schoen JHR (1964) Intracerebral haematomas. A clinical study of 40 surgical cases. *Psychiat Neurol Neurochir* 67: 445–68.

McMenemey WH (1952) Discussion. In *Proceedings of the First International Congress of Neuropathology.* Rome, Volume 2. Turin: Rosenberg and Sellier, pp 432–6.

McMenemey WH (1970) Discussion. In Wolstenholme GEW, O'Connor M (eds) *Alzheimer's Disease and Related Conditions: A Ciba Foundation Symposium.* J and A Churchill, London, pp 132–3.

Maruyama K, Ikeda S, Ishihara T, Allsop D, Yanagisawa N (1990) Immunohistochemical characterisation of cerebrovascular amyloid in 46 autopsied cases using antibodies to beta protein and Cystatin-C. *Stroke* 21: 397–403.

Masters CL, Gajdusek DC, Gibbs CJ (1981) The familial occurrence of Creutzfeldt–Jacob disease and Alzheimer's disease. *Brain* 104: 535–58.

Merejota J (1969) Familial systemic paramyloidosis with lattice dystrophy of the cornea, progressive cranial neuropathy, skin changes and various internal symptoms. *Ann Clin Res* 1: 314–24.

Patton MA, Baraitser M, Brett EM (1986) A family with congenital suprabulbar paresis (Worster-Drought syndrome). *Clin Genet* 29: 147–50.

Plant GT, Révész T, Barnard RO, Harding AE, Gautier–Smith PC (1990) Familial amyloid angiopathy with nonneuritic amyloid plaque formation. *Brain* 113: 721–47.

Roberts GW, Lofthouse R, Allsop D, Landon M, Kidd M, Prusiner SB (1988) CNS amyloid proteins in neurodegenerative diseases. *Neurology, Cleveland* 38: 1534–40.

Scholtz W (1938) Studien zur Pathologie der Hirngefässe; die drusige entartung der hirnarterien und capillaren (eine Form seniler Gefässerkrankung). *Zeit Ges Neurol Psychiat* 162: 694–715.

Shimode K, Fujihara S, Nakamura M, Kobayashi S, Tsunematsu T (1991) Diagnosis of cerebral amyloid angiopathy by enzyme linked immunoabsorbant assay of cystatin-C in cerebrospinal fluid. *Stroke* 22: 860–6.

Sonninen V, Savontaus ML (1987) Hereditary multi-infarct dementia: *Europ Neurol* 27: 209–15.

Sourander P, Wallinder J (1977) Hereditary multi-infarct dementia. *Acta Neuropathol* 39: 247–54.

Stevens DL, Hewlett RH, Brownell B (1977) Chronic familial vascular encephalopathy. *Lancet* ii: 1364–5.

Strömgren E. (1981) Heredopathia opthalmo-oto-encephalica.

In Vinken PJ, Bruyn GW (eds) *Handbook of Clinical Neurology* Vol 42, North Holland Publishing Co. Amsterdam. pp 150–2.

Tagliavini F, Ghiso J, Timmers WF, Giaccone G, Bugiani O, Frangione B (1990) Coexistence of Alzheimer's amyloid precursor protein and amyloid protein in cerebral vessel walls. *Lab Invest* 62: 761–7.

Tagliavini F, Giaccone G, Orso Bugiani O, Frangione B. (1993) Ubiquinated neurites are associated with preamyloid and cerebral amyloid β deposits in patients with HCHWA-D. *Acta Neuropath* 85: 267–71.

Tateishi J, Kitamoto T, Doh-ura K, Boellard JW, Pfeiffer J (1992) Creutzfeldt-Jacob disease with amyloid angiopathy: diagnosis by immunological analysis and transmission experiments. *Acta Neuropath (Berlin)* 83: 559–63.

Thorsteinsson L, Georgsson G, Asgiersson B, Bjarnadottir M, Olafsson I, Jensson O, Gudmundsson G (1992) On the role of monocytes/macrophages in the pathogenesis of central nervous system lesions in hereditary Cystatin-C amyloid angiopathy. *J Neurol Sci* 108: 121–8.

Uitti RJ, Donat JR, Rozdilsky B, Schneider RJ, Koeppen AH (1988) Familial oculoleptomeningeal amyloidosis: report of a new family with unusual features. *Arch Neurol Chicago* 45: 1118–22.

Ushiyama M, Ikeda S, Yanagisawa N (1991) Transthyretin-type cerebral amyloid angiopathy in type 1 familial amyloid polyneuropathy. *Acta Neuropath* 81: 524–8.

Van Bogaert L, Maere M, Smedt E de (1940) Sur les formes familiales précoces de la maladie d'Alzheimer. *Monatssch Psychiat Neurol* 102: 249–301.

Van Broeckhoven C, Haan J, Bakker E, Hardy JA, Van Hul W, Wehnert A, Vegter-Van der Vlis M, Roos RAC (1990) Amyloid β-protein precursor gene and hereditary cerebral haemorrhage with amyloidosis (Dutch) *Science* 248: 1120–2.

Van Duinen SG, Castaño EM, Prelli F, Bots GTAM, Luyendijk W, Frangione B (1987) Hereditary cerebral haemorrhage with amyloidosis in patients of Dutch origin is related to Alzheimer disease. *Proc Natl Acad Sci USA* 84: 5991–4.

Vinters HV (1987) Cerebral amyloid angiopathy: a critical review. *Stroke* 18: 311–24.

Vinters HV, Secor DL, Partridge WM, Gray F (1990) Immunohistochemical study of cerebral amyloid angiopathy. III. Widespread Alzheimer A4 peptide in cerebral microvessel walls colocalises with γ-trace in patients with leucoencephalopathy. *Ann Neurol* 28: 34–42.

Vonsattel JPG, Myers RH, Hedley-White ET, Ropper AH, Bird ED, Richardson EP (1991) Cerebral amyloid angiopathy without and with cerebral haemorrhages: a comparative histological study. *Ann Neurol* 30: 637–49.

Watanabe R, Duchen LW (1993) Cerebral amyloid in human prion diseases. *Neuropath Appl Neurobiol* 19: 253–60.

Wattendorff AR, Bots GTAM, Went LN, Endtz LJ (1982)

Familial cerebral amyloid angiopathy presenting as recurrent cerebral haemorrhage. *J Neurol Sci* 55: 121–35.

Wattendorff AR, Frangione B, Luyendijk W, Bots GTAM (1995) Hereditary cerebral haemorrhage with amyloidosis, Dutch type (HCH-D): clinicopathological studies. *J Neurol Neurosurg Psychiat* 58: 699–705.

Wisniewski T, Frangione B (1992) Molecular biology of Alzheimer's amyloid – Dutch variant. *Mol Neurobiol* 6: 75–86.

Worster-Drought C, Greenfield JG, McMenemey WH (1940) A form of familial presenile dementia with spastic paralysis: (including the pathological examination of a case) *Brain* 63: 237–54.

Worster-Drought C, Greenfield JG, McMenemey WH (1944)

A form of familial presenile dementia with spastic paralysis *Brain* 67: 38–43.

Yamada M, Tsukagoshi H, Wada Y, Otomo E, Hayakawa M, Thorsteinsson L, Jensson O (1989) Absence of the Cystatin-C amyloid in the cerebral amyloid angiopathy, senile plaque and extra-CNS amyloid deposits of aged Japanese. *Acta Neurol Scand* 79: 504–9.

Yokoi S, Nakayama H (1985) Chronic progressive leucoencephalopathy with systemic arteriosclerosis in young adults. *Clin Neuropathol* 4: 165–73.

Yoshimura M, Yamanouchi H, Kuzuhara S, Mori S, Sigiura S, Mizutari T, Shimada H, Tomonaga M, Togokura Y (1992) Dementia in central amyloid angiopathy: a clinico-pathological study. *Lab Invest* 60: 113–22.

CHAPTER TWELVE

Human prion diseases

K. Hsiao

Introduction
Clinical syndromes: infectious, inherited and sporadic prion diseases
Diagnosing human prion diseases

INTRODUCTION

Human prion diseases, despite their rarity, are among the most fascinating and best understood of neurodegenerative disease. The three human prion diseases, kuru, Creutzfeldt–Jakob disease (CJD), and Gerstmann–Sträussler–Scheinker disease (GSS) are also called transmissible encephalopathies, spongiform encephalopathies or slow virus diseases consequent to the discovery that transmission to chimpanzees occurred when brain homogenates from patients with kuru were inoculated (Gajdusek, Gibbs & Alpers, 1966).

Several remarkable discoveries in the past three decades have led to the molecular and genetic characterization of an unusual aetiological agent, a proteinaceous infectious pathogen called a *prion* by Prusiner to distinguish it from viruses and viroids (Prusiner, 1982). An abnormal isoform of the prion protein (PrP), PrP^{Sc}, is the only known component of the prion (Prusiner et al., 1981, 1984; Prusiner, 1991). PrP is encoded by a gene on the short arm of chromosome 20 in humans (Oesch et al., 1985; Basler et al., 1986; Kretzschmar et al., 1986; a Sparkes et al., 1986; Puckett et al., 1991). PrP^{Sc} differs from the normal uninfectious isoform PrP^{C} by its propensity to aggregate and its relative resistance to proteolysis.

Most human prion diseases are associated with the accumulation of PrP^{Sc} in the brain. The presence of PrP^{Sc} implicates prions in the pathogenesis of these diseases. However, in rare patients (and mice) which appear to lack PrP^{Sc} but express mutant PrP, neurodegeneration may, at least in part, be caused by abnormal metabolism of mutant PrP. As the molecular and genetic characteristics of PrP in neurodegenerative diseases have been studied in greater detail, the definition of

human prion disease has evolved to include any neurodegenerative condition in which a pathogenic form of PrP is detected.

CLINICAL SYNDROMES: INFECTIOUS, INHERITED, AND SPORADIC PRION DISEASES

The three human prion diseases, kuru, CJD, and GSS, have infectious, inherited, and sporadic forms (Table 12.1). Infectious forms of prion diseases result from the horizontal transmission of the infectious agent, as occurs in iatrogenic CJD and kuru. Inherited forms, notably GSS and familial CJD, comprise 10–15% of all cases of prion disease. A mutation in the protein-coding portion of the PrP gene has been found in all reported kindreds with inherited prion disease, with the possible exception of a familial progressive subcortical gliosis in which protease-resistant PrP was detected in the brain, but no mutations were found in the PrP open-reading-frame (Petersen et al., 1995). The disease is linked to chromosome 17 in this family. Sporadic forms of prion disease comprise most cases of CJD and possibly some cases of GSS. How prions arise in patients with sporadic diseases is unknown.

Infectious prion diseases

Iatrogenic CJD

Iatrogenic CJD was first reported in 1974 in a 55 year-old woman who developed symptoms 18 months after corneal transplantation (Duffy et al., 1974). Since then, iatrogenic CJD has been described in over three dozen patients infected through a variety of means including neurosurgical instrumentation, stereotactic

Table 12.1. *Human prion diseases*

Disease	Form
Kuru	
Iatrogenic Creutzfeldt–Jakob disease	Infectious
Gerstmann–Sträussler–Scheinker disease	
Familial Creutzfeldt–Jakob disease	Genetic
Fatal familial insomnia	
Creutzfeldt–Jakob disease	Sporadic

electroencephalography, dura mater implantation, pituitary growth hormone injections and pituitary gonadotrophin injections (Brown, Preece & Will, 1992*b*). Patients with CJD transferred through instrumentation and tissue transplantation developed a dementing illness, while patients with CJD transferred through pituitary extracts developed an ataxic syndrome.

Patients' susceptibility to infection may be partially determined by their PrP codon 129 genotype (Collinge, Palmer & Dryden, 1991*a*), analogous in principle to the incubation-time alleles in mice (Carlson *et al.*, 1986, 1988; Westaway *et al.*, 1987). PrP is polymorphic at codon 129, encoding either methionine (met) or valine (val). Population frequencies for this polymorphism in Caucasians are 12% val/val, 37% met/met, and 51% met/val (Collinge *et al.*, 1991*a*). In 16 patients (15 Caucasian, 1 Afro-American) from the UK, USA, and France with iatrogenic CJD from contaminated growth hormone extracts, 8 (50%) were val/val, 5 (31%) were met/met, and 3 (19%) were met/val (Collinge *et al.*, 1991*a*; Brown *et al.*, 1992*b*. A disproportionate number of patients with iatrogenic CJD were homozygous for valine at PrP codon 129. Heterozygosity at codon 129 appears to provide partial protection, as only two of 25 iatrogenic CJD patients in France were heterozygous at codon 129, in contrast to about 50% of the healthy control group (Deslys *et al.*, 1994). Thousands of children who received pituitary growth hormone extracts are still at risk for the development of CJD. Fortunately, the use of genetically engineered growth hormone will eliminate this form of iatrogenic CJD.

New variant CJD

Ten cases of CJD in the United Kingdom afflicting individuals under the age of 40 were recently reported (Will *et al.*, 1996). These ten cases differed clinically and pathologically from classical CJD in several respects: (1) the age of onset occurred in young individuals ranging from 16 to 39 years of age – classical CJD typically begins in individuals 45 to 75 years of age; (2) a longer duration of illness was observed ranging between 7 and > 22 months – classical CJD typically runs a 3 to 6 months course; (3) the early clinical symptoms included limb pain, behavioural and psychiatric disturbances, and ataxia with dementia and myoclonus occurring much later in the course – classical CJD typically presents with dementia and myoclonus; (4) all cases contained kuru plaques staining with antibodies to PrP – only 10% of brains from classical CJD cases contain PrP plaques; and 5) electroencephalographic periodic complexes were absent in the new variant – periodic complexes are present in the majority of classical CJD cases. Since the appearance of the publication on these ten new variant CJD cases, four additional cases have been identified in the UK and two cases in France.

A presumptive link was made between the ten atypical or new variant cases of CJD recently reported in the UK and the outbreak of bovine spongiform encephalopathy (BSE) in that country affecting over 160 000 cattle since the epidemic began in 1986 and peaked in 1992 (Anderson *et al.*, 1996). The initial belief (Department of Health, 1989), when the BSE epidemic was first identified, was that the risk of transmission of the disease to humans was extremely remote. This belief was based on the supposition that BSE represented sheep scrapie transmitted to cows through the inadvertent feeding of scrapie-contaminated sheep offal to cows (following contemporary modifications in the rendering industry), and relied heavily on the failure of all epidemiological studies to link scrapie in sheep to CJD in humans. However, two lines of evidence now call this reasoning into question and enhance the likelihood that new variant CJD is linked to the BSE epidemic. The first of these lines of evidence concerns transmission experiments and, in particular, comparisons between the disease produced in animals by transmission of scrapie with that produced by transmission of BSE. Briefly, scrapie transmitted to mice produces a variable distribution of pathology and variable lengths of incubation period depending both on the source of the scrapie inoculum and the genotype of the mouse (Bruce *et al.*, 1991). In contrast, BSE produces a uniform pattern of pathology and one that does not conform to any of the several variant patterns recognised to result from one of the scrapie 'strains' (Bruce *et al.*, 1994). Furthermore, BSE, even after inoculation into sheep and then transferred to mouse, produces the BSE, and not a scrapie pattern of pathology. The suspicion is therefore growing that BSE may have arisen from an undetected bovine source and not from sheep scrapie. As such, its capacity to cross species barriers may differ from scrapie and it is noteworthy that alongside new variant CJD in humans have arisen in the United Kingdom minor epidemics of spongiform encephalopathy in zoo animals and cats, epidemics that have also been presumptively linked to BSE and the feeding to these animals of BSE-contaminated feed. The second line of evidence concerns the detection of a BSE-distinctive glycosylation pattern of PrP which can be detected by Western blotting performed on brain tissue. This glycosylation pattern differs from that of scrapie and sporadic human CJD, but is identical to that of new variant CJD (Collinge *et al.*, 1996). A further piece of evidence linking new variant CJD with BSE is that BSE transmitted to macaque monkeys, pathologically closely resembles the rather distinctive

new variant CJD in humans (see section below on Diagnosing Prion Diseases) (Lasmézas *et al.*, 1996). Therefore, the circumstantial evidence is growing that new variant human CJD is linked to the epidemic of BSE and may result from oral transmission of the BSE agent during the late 1980s, after onset of the BSE epidemic and before prohibition of the use of certain bovine products (including brain) for use in human food.

Kuru

Kuru is a progressive ataxia accompanied by dementia which affected the Fore linguistic tribe of Papua, New Guinea. It was probably spread by ritualistic cannibalism, since new cases can be traced to the period prior to the cessation of the practice, and no new cases have appeared in individuals who were born after the ritual was eliminated (Gajdusek, 1977). Spongiform degener-

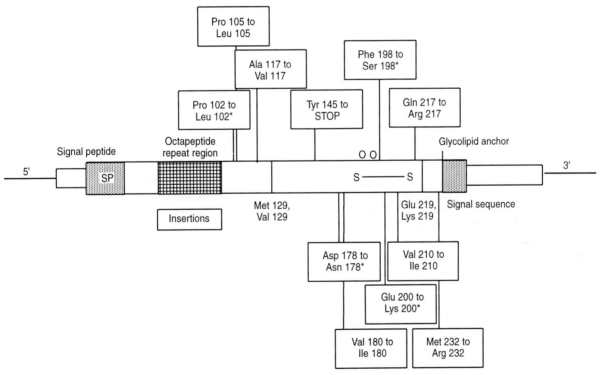

Fig. 12.1. Prion protein mutations in human prion diseases. The PrP open reading frame (ORF) is indicated by an open box, the mRNA untranslated region by a narrower box and the intron by a solid black line. Six point mutations associated with GSS are indicated by boxes drawn above the Figure. Five point mutations associated with CJD are indicated by boxes drawn below the Figure. Normal polymorphisms are located at codons 129 and 219. A 32 aa signal peptide is represented by SP. Five Gly-Pro-rich octapeptide repeats are located between codons 51 and 91. Cysteine 179 and cysteine 214 are linked by disulphide bonds. Asparagine-linked glycosylation sites are located at residues 181 and 197. Residues 231–253 encode a hydrophobic signal sequence which is removed when a glycolipid anchor is attached to serine 230.

ation, astrogliosis and neuronal loss are present as expected. Compact (kuru) plaques are seen in most but not all cases of kuru (Roberts *et al.*, 1986).

Kuru resembles the ataxic form of sporadic CJD, in which compact (kuru) plaques are also present. One may speculate that kuru arose sporadically in a single individual who developed the ataxic form of CJD. The illness might then have become epidemic through endocannibalism. An insufficient number of Fore individuals have been studied to answer whether genetic predisposition to prion infection could have facilitated horizontal transmission of kuru. Two of three patients with kuru were homozygous for valine at PrP codon 129 (Goldfarb *et al.*, 1989). No other mutations were found in these patients. The population frequency of the PrP codon 129 polymorphism in the Fore people would be interesting to know because a high frequency of valine at codon 129 would support the hypothesis that individuals homozygous for valine at PrP codon 129 are genetically predisposed to prion diseases.

Inherited prion diseases

Familial CJD (fCJD) comprises 10–15% of all CJD cases. Most GSS cases are familial. Epidemiologic studies of fCJD and GSS suggested that both diseases are vertically transmitted in an autosomal dominant pattern (Masters *et al.*, 1979; Masters, Gajdusek & Gibbs, 1981*a*,*b*). Yet the diseases can sometimes be horizontally transmitted to rodents and non-human primates through intracerebral inoculation of patients' brain homogenates (Masters *et al.*, 1981*a*,*b*).

The paradox of how a disease could be both inherited and infectious began to make sense when genetic linkage of a missense mutation in the PrP gene to GSS was established (Hsiao *et al.*, 1989). Linkage of a missense mutation resulting in substitution of leucine for proline at PrP codon 102 to GSS in two unrelated pedigrees was strong evidence that GSS is a Mendelian disorder. Two

lines of transgenic mice which expressed the GSS PrP mutation spontaneously developed murine GSS (Hsiao *et al.*, 1990), a neurological illness clinically and histologically indistinguishable from experimental murine scrapie. This provided direct evidence that the mutant prion protein caused disease in transgenic mice and, by inference, humans. The spongiform degeneration and fatal neurologic illness can be transmitted and passaged to hamsters and mice from transgenic mice with murine GSS, indicating that prions can be created *de novo* in transgenic mice expressing mutant prion proteins (Hsiao *et al.*, 1994).

Since 1989, molecular genetic analyses of kindreds around the world have revealed 18 pathogenic PrP mutations: 11 point mutations and 7 insertional mutations (Fig. 12.1). Six PrP missense mutations have been identified in patients with GSS: (1) Pro102 → Leu102 (Hsiao *et al.*, 1989; Doh-ura *et al.*, 1989; Speer *et al.*, 1991; Kretzschmar *et al.*, 1991); (2) Phe198 → Ser198 (Hsiao *et al.*, 1992); (3) Gin217 → Arg217 (Hsiao *et al.*, 1992); (4) Ala117 → Val117 (Doh-ura *et al.*, 1989; Hsiao *et al.*, 1991*b*), (5) Tyr105 → stop codon (Kitamoto *et al.*, 1993*a*,*b*,*c*); and (6) Pro105 → Leu105 (Kitamoto *et al.*, 1993*a*,*b*,*c*; Kitamoto *et al.*, 1993*a*,*b*,*c*), five PrP missense mutations in patients with CJD: (1) Asp178 → Asn178 (Goldfarb *et al.*, 1991*a*; Medori *et al.*, 1992*a*); (2) Glu200 → Lys200 (Goldgaber *et al.*, 1989; Goldfarb *et al.*, 1990; Hsiao *et al.*, 1991*a*), (3) Val180 → Ile180 (Kitamoto *et al.*, 1993); (4) Val210 → Ile210 (Pocchiari *et al.*, 1993; Ripoll *et al.*, 1993), and (5) Met232 → Arg232 (Kitamoto *et al.*, 1993), and a set of seven insertional mutations in the octapeptide coding repeats of PrP (Owen *et al.*, 1989; Goldfar *et al.*, 1991*b*).

There are also three PrP polymorphisms: (1) a deletion of one octapeptide repeat present in about 4% of normal Caucasians (Vnencak-Jones & Phillips, 1992); (2) valine or methionine at codon 129 (Collinge *et al.*, 1991*a*); and (3) glutamate or lysine at codon 219

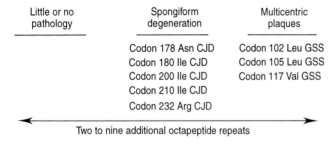

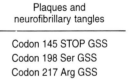

Little or no pathology	Spongiform degeneration	Multicentric plaques	Plaques and neurofibrillary tangles
	Codon 178 Asn CJD	Codon 102 Leu GSS	Codon 145 STOP GSS
	Codon 180 Ile CJD	Codon 105 Leu GSS	Codon 198 Ser GSS
	Codon 200 Ile CJD	Codon 117 Val GSS	Codon 217 Arg GSS
	Codon 210 Ile CJD		
	Codon 232 Arg CJD		

Two to nine additional octapeptide repeats

Fig. 12.2. Spectrum of human inherited prion diseases.

(Furukawa *et al.*, 1995). These polymorphisms have been found in patients with prion diseases. In some instances their significance is uncertain (Laplanche *et al.*, 1990; Vnencak-Jones & Phillips, 1992; Diedrich *et al.*, 1992). In patients with Asp178 → Asn178, the codon 129 polymorphism modulates the phenotypic expression of the disease; patients with methionine at codon 129 exhibit fatal familial insomnia, while patients with valine at codon 129 exhibit CJD (Goldfarb *et al.*, 1992a,b).

A spectrum of clinical and pathological phenotypes are represented by different kindreds with inherited prion diseases (Fig. 12.2). GSS and familial CJD are histologically distinct in this spectrum. Multicentric plaques are pathognomonic for GSS. Plaques are absent in most patients with fCJD; when they are present, in 10–20% of patients, they are compact (kuru) plaques. The duration of disease is usually longer in GSS (1 to 10 years) than in fCJD (2 months to 3 years).

The segregation of GSS and fCJD PrP point mutations is evidence that some interfamilial phenotypic variation can be explained by allelic heterogeneity. But intrafamilial phenotypic variability, when it occurs, and interfamilial variability within the same genotype must be explained by the influence of other genetic or environmental factors which are currently unknown. Because phenotypic variability occurs within families with unique PrP genotypes, the following classification of inherited prion diseases is by genotype rather than by phenotype.

GERSTMANN–STRÄUSSLER–SCHEINKER DISEASE

Codon 102 leucine variant of GSS (102L-GSS): Patients in six kindreds with the PrP codon 102 leucine variant usually develop a neurodegenerative disorder characterized by the onset of ataxia and dementia in the third to seventh decades of life. Significant genetic linkage to the PrP gene was first demonstrated in 102L-GSS; a combined lod score of 4.52 has now been obtained in three families (Hsiao *et al.*, 1989; Speer *et al.*, 1991). Some intrafamilial clinical variation occurs, however, and rare patients develop dementia alone or ataxia alone. Pathological examination of patients in all kindreds have revealed multicentric plaques characteristic of GSS. Spongiform degeneration, gliosis, neuronal loss, and long tract degeneration are variably present. One of the patients with 102L-GSS was a descendant of the original kindred described by the Viennese physicians Gerstmann, Sträussler, and Scheinker (Kretschmar *et*

al., 1991). 102L-GSS has also been called the ataxic form of GSS.

Codon 117 valine variant of GSS (117V-GSS): Patients in an American and an Alsatian kindred with the PrP codon 117 valine variant develop dementia in the third to sixth decades of life (Doh-ura *et al.*, 1989; Hsiao *et al.*, 1991b). The clinical and pathological signs were restricted to the forebrain in the American kindred, hence the appellation, telencephalic variant of GSS (Nochlin *et al.*, 1989). The distribution of pathology has not been described in the Alsatian family, but it may be more widespread since a few patients were reported to have limb ataxia (Warter *et al.*, 1982). Although few or no neocortical neurofibrillary tangles (NFTs) accompanied multicentric plaques in the American kindred, the clinical and pathological picture in this kindred resembled Alzheimer's disease sufficiently for it to be initially misdiagnosed (Heston, Lowther & Leventhal, 1966). The diagnosis was revised when the amyloid plaques were found to react with PrP antiserum but not β-amyloid antiserum (Nochlin *et al.*, 1989).

Codon 198 serine varient of GSS (198S-GSS): Patients in a large American kindred in Indiana with the PrP codon 198 serine variant develop ataxia, dementia, and Parkinsonism in the fifth to seventh decades of life (Farlow *et al.*, 1989). Genetic analysis of linkage between the codon 198 serine mutation and GSS in this pedigree yielded a lod score of 6.37 (Hsiao *et al.*, 1992; Dlouhy *et al.*, 1992). These GSS patients are atypical in possessing neocortical NFTs (Ghetti *et al.*, 1989). Neuritic amyloid plaques reacted with PrP antiserum but not β-amyloid antiserum, with the exception of those found in the eldest patient, 73 years of age at death, which reacted with both antisera (Ghetti *et al.*, 1989; Giaccone *et al.*, 1991). In this patient, β-amyloid peptide deposits were located around PrP plaques.

Codon 217 arginine variant of GSS (217R-GSS): Two patients in a Swedish family with the PrP 217 arginine variant developed dementia and ataxia in the seventh decade of life (Hsiao *et al.*, 1992). As in patients with the codon 198 serine variant, neocortical NFTs were present. In these patients, who were 67 and 71 years old at death, amyloid plaques reacted with both PrP and β-amyloid antiserum (Ikeda *et al.*, 1991).

Codon 105 leucine variant GSS (105L-GSS): Patients with the PrP 105 leucine variant developed spastic paraparesis and progressive dementia without cerebellar signs, myoclonus, or periodic complexes (Kitamoto et al., 1993a).

Codon 145 stop variant of GSS (145STOP-GSS): One patient was described with a progressive dementing illness and neuropathological findings of amyloid plaques with neurofibrillary tangles (Kitamoto et al., 1993b). Interestingly, the amyloid plaques were comprised solely of the truncated form of PrP.

FAMILIAL CREUTZFELDT–JAKOB DISEASE

Codon 178 asparagine variant of CJD (178N-CJD): Patients in several families with the PrP codon 178 asparagine variant develop dementia in the fifth to seventh decades of life (Goldfarb et al., 1991a; Medori et al., 1992a; Brown et al., 1992a). Insomnia was a prominent complaint in one family, where patients were given the descriptive diagnosis of fatal familial insomnia (Medori et al., 1992a). Patients in another family with dementia and thalamic degeneration were given the diagnosis of familial thalamic dementia (Petersen et al., 1992). Yet other patients developed clinically recognizable CJD (Brown et al., 1992a; Goldfarb et al., 1992a). The clinical phenotype is determined by the codon 129 haplotype of the mutant allele (Goldfarb et al., 1992b).

In a comparative study of 45 patients with 178N-CJD and 211 patients with sporadic CJD, the former developed a more protracted disease (mean = 23 months) than the latter (mean = 6 months) (Brown et al., 1992a). Transmission to primates occurred with brain homogenates from 6 to 10 patients with 178N-CJD, a somewhat lower rate than the 80 to 85% transmission rate for sporadic CJD. Plaques have not been found in any patient with 178N-CJD. Although some salient clinical features differed between families, other features were common to all the families. Periodic complexes on electroencephalograms were conspicuously absent in 44 of 45 patients in one series (Brown et al., 1992a) and 4 of 5 patients in another series (Manetto et al., 1992), despite this feature being present in 56% of patients with sporadic CJD. PrP^{Sc} was difficult to detect or absent in some patients with fatal familial insomnia (Medori et al., 1992b; Little et al., 1986; Manetto et al., 1992). PrP genotyping can be invaluable in making the diagnosis of 178N-CJD because of the atypical clinical and histological presentations, electroencephalographic findings, and molecular features of PrP in these patients.

Codon 200 lysine variant of CJD (200K-CJD): Patients in families with the PrP codon 200 lysine variant develop a rapidly progressive dementia in the fourth to seventh decades of life that corresponds well to the established criteria for CJD (Goldgaber et al., 1989; Goldfarb et al., 1990; Hsiao et al., 1991a). Earlier speculation that a large cluster of Libyan Jews with CJD was due to a culinary practice of eating lightly cooked sheep brains and eyes has been proved incorrect by the discovery of the codon 200 lysine variant in every Libyan Jew with CJD examined. One patient, homozygous for the codon 200 lysine variant, developed CJD at the age of 42 (Hsiao et al., 1991a). The age of onset and clinical course of this patient's illness was no different from patients heterozygous for the codon 200 lysine variant, indicating that fCJD, like Huntington's chorea, is a true dominant disorder. Another cluster of CJD cases in the Orava region of Czechoslovakia was traced to the same mutation (Goldfarb et al., 1990).

Octapeptide coding repeats in inherited prion diseases

A set of five insertional mutations in the octarepeat region between codons 51 and 91 are found in patients with progressive neurodegenerative diseases which may resemble CJD, GSS, or an atypical dementia (Owen et al., 1989; Collinge et al., 1990; Goldfarb et al., 1991b). In patients with human prion diseases the octarepeat region, which normally encodes 5 octapeptide repeat sequences, may be extended to encode an additional 5 to 9 octapeptide repeats. A 4-octapeptide repeat insertion was found in an individual with a non-neurologic illness (Goldfarb et al., 1991b).

Histologic examination of patients with 5 to 9 additional octapeptide insertions has revealed the virtual gamut of prion disease pathology, ranging from multicentric plaques, to spongiform change without plaques, to an absence of pathology altogther (Collinge et al., 1990, 1992; Goldfarb et al., 1991b; Brown et al., 1992c). PrP^{Sc} was barely detectable or undetectable in both patients with 7 additional octapeptide repeats from one family (Brown et al., 1992c). PrP genotyping can be very important when making the diagnosis of inherited prion disease in families with octapeptide insertions because of the atypical clinical, pathological, and molecular features.

Sporadic prion diseases

Over 85% of CJD cases are sporadic; no prior exposure to prions can be ascertained and no family history of CJD or GSS elicited. The aetiology of sporadic CJD is

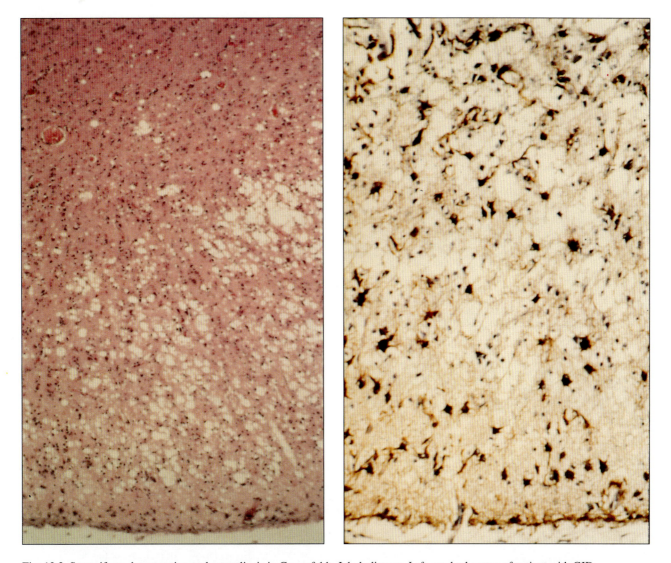

Fig. 12.3. Spongiform degeneration and astrogliosis in Creutzfeldt–Jakob disease. *Left*, cerebral cortex of patient with CJD stained with haematoxylin and eosin shows spongiform changes. *Right*, cerebral cortex of patient with CJD stained for glial fibrillary acidic protein shows astrogliosis.

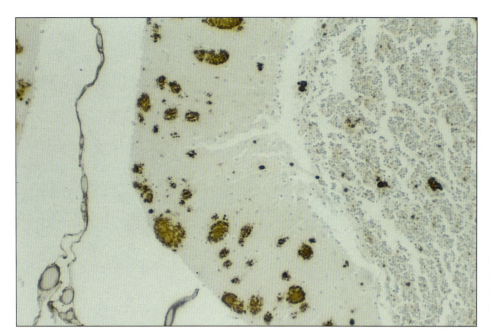

Fig. 12.4.(*a*). Case of Gerstmann–Sträussler syndrome. Immunoreactive Prp plaques in the molecular and granule cell layers of the cerebellar cortex.

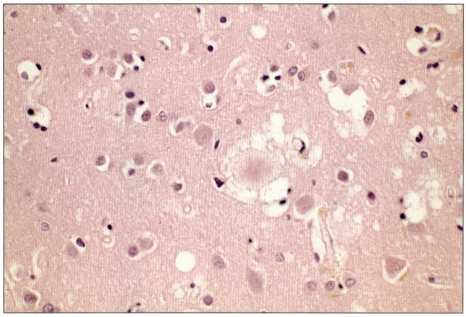

Fig. 12.4.(*b*). Cerebral cortex from a case of the new variant of CJD. At centre is a compact plaque surrounded by spongiform vacuoles. Haematoxylin and eosin stain. (Photograph kindly supplied by Dr J. McLaughlin.)

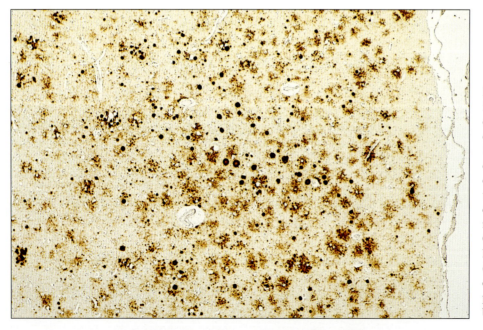

Fig. 12.4.(*c*). Prp immunostained section of cerebral cortex from the same case as that illustrated in Fig. 12.4.(*b*). Note abundant Prp deposits, some in the form of compact, circular plaques while the remainder of the cortex is filled with scattered, more irregular, deposits. Counterstained with haematoxylin. (Immunostaining courtesy of Professor J. Ironside, photograph kindly supplied by Dr J. McLaughlin.)

unknown. One in a million individuals develops CJD regardless of race, sex, occupation, or nationality (Will & Mathews, 1984; Brown et al., 1987). Investigations of geographic clusters of CJD have uncovered mutations in PrP rather than endemic exposure to a common source of prions with the exception of the predominantly UK-located new variant CJD cases discussed above. The evidence that transgenic mice which express a mutant PrP develop murine GSS supports a genetic rather than infectious origin of the other clusters.

Patients with sporadic CJD typically develop symptoms of mental deterioration in the sixth to eighth decades of life and survive 6 months (Brown et al., 1986). Involuntary movements consisting of myoclonus or other movement disorders develop in 90% of patients. 85% of patients develop either 1–2 cycle/s periodic complexes or burst suppression activity on electroencephalograms.

No specific mutations have been identified in the PrP gene of patients with sporadic CJD. However, patients with sporadic CJD are overwhelmingly homozygous at codon 129 (Palmer et al., 1991). This finding supports a model of prion production which favours PrP interactions between homologous proteins, as appears to occur in transgenic mice expressing hamster PrP inoculated with either hamster prions or mouse prions (Scott et al., 1989; Prusiner et al., 1990).

Approximately 15% of patients with sporadic CJD develop ataxia as an early sign, accompanied by dementia (Brown et al., 1984). Most, but not all, patients with ataxia have compact (kuru) plaques in the cerebellum (Pearlman et al., 1988). Patients with ataxia and compact plaques exhibit a protracted clinical course which may last up to 3 years. The molecular basis for the differences between CJD of shorter and longer duration have not yet been fully elucidated. However, some preliminary analyses have suggested that patients with protracted, atypical clinical courses are more likely to be heterozygous at codon 129 (Doh-ura et al., 1991; Collinge et al., 1991b).

There is no completely satisfactory model of how sporadic prion disease is initiated. One model, the exposure to prions in the environment is disfavoured by epidemiologic studies. Another model, the occurrence of a somatic mutation, with the subsequent spontaneous development of prions within a cell or cells expressing a pathogenic mutation, complements epidemiological studies, which suggest a random process. This model is supported by the development of spontaneous neurological disorders in transgenic mice overexpressing wild-type prion proteins (Westaway et al., 1994).

One problem with the somatic mutation model is the observed discrepancy between the incidence of sporadic CJD and sporadic GSS. The model would predict equal incidences of sporadic CJD and sporadic GSS since there are equal numbers of CJD and GSS PrP mutations. Yet virtually all sporadic prion disease is CJD. Another problem with this model is the observation that the mere expression of pathogenic PrP mutations may not be sufficient to achieve the levels of PrP^{Sc} and prions which are observed in all patients with sporadic CJD. PrP^{Sc} is poorly detectable in some patients with the codon 178 asparagine variant associated with CJD (Manetto et al., 1992; Little et al., 1986; Medori et al., 1992b) and in some patients with additional octapeptide repeats (Brown et al., 1992c). An amended model which takes both observations into consideration would restrict somatic mutations resulting in sporadic disease to certain PrP codons. However, it is difficult to rationalize why such a restriction should occur. Unfortunately, the somatic mutation model is difficult to prove because the cell or cells in which the putative mutation arose may have degenerated and become inaccessible for genetic analyses by the time the patient has died.

DIAGNOSING HUMAN PRION DISEASES

Human prion disease should be considered in any patient who develops a progressive subacute or chronic decline in cognitive or motor function. Typically adults between 40 and 70 years of age, patients often exhibit clinical features helpful in providing a premorbid diagnosis of prion disease, particularly sporadic CJD (Brown et al., 1986). There is as yet no specific diagnostic test for prion disease in the cerebral spinal fluid. A definitive diagnosis of human prion disease, which is invariably fatal, can usually be made from the examination of brain tissue. Over the past three years knowledge of the molecular genetics of prion diseases has made it possible to diagnose inherited prion diseases in living patients using peripheral tissues.

Neuropathology

Neuropathological studies have played, and continue to play, an important part in assisting understanding and diagnosis of prion diseases since the first human cases were described in the 1920s (Jakob, 1921). Initially, they were considered to be neurodegenerative diseases. It was the recognition in 1958 by Hadlow (Hadlow, 1959, 1992), a veterinary pathologist, of the similarity in pathology of kuru to sheep scrapie, shown to be transmissible in the 1930s (Cuille & Chelle, 1939), that led to successful attempts to transmit both kuru (Gajdusek, Gibbs & Alpers, 1966) and CJD (Gibbs *et al.*, 1968) to primates. Historically, emphasis on varying clinical phenomenology and distribution of pathological change led to the description of variants such as the cerebellar and Heidenhein types of CJD (Masters & Richardson 1995). However, subsequent studies suggest that the boundaries between these subtypes are ill-defined and of less biological significance than was originally thought (UK National CJD Surveillance Centre report, 1995; Will, 1996).

Neuropathological examination of the brain in cases of human prion diseases continues to provide the basis for confirmation of the diagnosis in most cases, the exceptions being those rare cases of inherited prion diseases that lack any neuropathological changes and in which molecular genetics is essential for diagnosis. For this purpose a sample of frozen brain or spleen should be reserved at autopsy if blood has not been subjected to molecular genetic analysis in life. At the present time, neuropathological examination is essential in investigating and classifying cases that may be new variant CJD in the UK and Europe, since clinical criteria for diagnosing these cases have not yet been clearly formulated, and most cases do not meet clinical criteria for diagnosing probable sporadic CJD. Neuropathology with immunostaining for PrP is also essential for carrying out surveillance for CJD in the wake of the United Kingdom BSE epidemic. Recent reviews of the neuropathology of prion diseases include those of Bell & Ironside (1993), Ironside (1996) and Budka *et al.*, (1995). (See p. 36 and Appendix 3 for safety precautions to take when dealing with cases of possible prion disease.)

Because of the short clinical course of most cases of CJD, the macroscopic appearance of the brain is usually unremarkable. There may be slight, generalized cerebral atrophy or atrophy of the cerebellar cortex but these are not reliable or specific findings. Occasionally, particularly in cases with a prolonged clinical course, atrophy may be more conspicuous. It is important when taking blocks of tissue from brain slices from a case of possible CJD to sample widely since the amount and distribution of the diagnostic microscopic pathology is remarkably variable from case to case (Bell & Ironside, 1993; Lantos 1992; Budka *et al.*, 1995). Our practice is to sample all the main lobes of the cerebrum, basal ganglia, thalamus, brain stem and cerebellum.

The cardinal microscopic features of prion diseases are the presence of spongiform change accompanied by neuronal loss, astrocytosis, microglial cell activation and, in some cases, plaques that immunostain for PrP (Kitamoto *et al.*, 1986; Roberts *et al.*, 1988) (Figs. 12.3 and 12.4). With the exception of immunostaining for PrP, these features are not entirely specific since neuronal loss and astrocytosis occur in many forms of neurodegenerative disease and spongiform change occurs, albeit in very restricted locations, in frontal lobe degeneration and some cases of diffuse Lewy body disease. Spongiform change in cerebral cortex needs to be distinguished from artefactual vacuoles produced by shrinkage of tissue during dehydration for processing, particularly of oedematous brain. This usually produces spaces that surround neurons or small blood vessels, and therefore do not appear empty. Furthermore, artefactual spongy change is more uniformly distributed than spongiform change of CJD. The presence of astrocytosis is also particularly helpful in distinguishing genuine spongiform change for its artefactual mimics. Another pitfall is the spongiform change that is sometimes seen in severely atrophic cortex in which a vacuolar loosening of the parenchyma is produced as a result of neuronal depletion (Fig. 4a.14). This, like the spongiform change of frontal lobe dementia and diffuse Lewy body disease, is confined to the outer layers of the cerebral cortex whereas that seen in prion diseases extends through all the layers of the cortex, although in a patchy manner. Amyloid, PrP-containing plaques have an appearance somewhat reminiscent of the cores of Alzheimer plaques but have finely fibrillar radiating processes that extend into the neighbouring neuropil and are not surrounded by any dystrophic neurites.

As indicated in the foregoing sections on infectious, inherited and sporadic prion diseases, these types of disease differ in the distribution and emphasis on each type of pathology. Another factor that appears to play a part in determining the type of pathology found is the host prion protein genotype with respect to codon 129 of the PrP gene (de Silva *et al.*, 1994; Macdonald *et al.*, 1996).

In sporadic CJD, much the commonest of the prion diseases to be encountered in diagnostic practice, spongiform change is usually widespread but patchy in cerebral cortex, basal ganglia, thalamus and cerebellum. It consists of multiple, empty vacuoles 5–50μm across located mainly in grey matter parenchyma (Fig. 12.3). A few cases with prominent spongiform change or necrosis in cerebral white matter have also been reported (Bastian, 1991; Kawata *et al.*, 1992). Ultrastructurally, the more usual grey matter vacuoles consist of distentions in neural processes (Masters & Gajdusek, 1982; Bastian, 1991; Liberski *et al.*, 1990). Amyloid plaques occur in about 10% of cases of sporadic CJD (Bastian, 1991; Bell & Ironside 1993; Ironside, 1996) and are associated with possession of one or more valine alleles at codon 129 of the PrP gene. They are found almost exclusively in the cerebellum where they form rounded, fibrillary structures with a dense core and pale rim in the granule cell layer or molecular layer of the cortex. They are visible with routine stains but are much more readily seen with PrP immunostaining. After immunostaining, PrP can be seen to be also deposited in a more diffuse fashion in grey matter in a perivacuolar or synaptic distribution. These deposits cannot be appreciated with routine stains. The quantity of PrP immunostaining is not clearly related to the extent of spongiform change (Budka *et al.*, 1995; Hayward *et al.*, 1994). The neuronal loss is variable in extent and astrocytosis may be very noticeable even in the absence of marked neuron loss.

In iatrogenic CJD, studied mainly in those given peripheral injections of cadaveric growth hormone, the clinical form of the disease is often dominated by ataxia with dementia occurring late. The pathology frequently includes the presence of PrP- immunoreactive plaques in cerebellar cortex and white matter and cerebellar pathology dominates over cerebral cortical pathology with the extent of pathology in the basal ganglia and thalamus being intermediate in severity. Iatrogenic cases with prion inoculation into the CNS via insertion of contaminated electrodes, dura mater grafts, etc. show pathology that resembles that of sporadic CJD (Ironside, 1996).

The new variant of CJD has a pathological distinctiveness that is striking and assisted in the recognition of this as a new form of prion disease (Will *et al.*, 1996). There is a marked abundance of PrP immunostaining, part of it in the form of numerous plaques which resemble those seen in the cerebellum in a minority of cases of sporadic CJD and in kuru and which have been described above. These plaques are plentiful in the cerebellum and also in the cerebral cortex. All cerebral lobes can be affected but particularly commonly the occipital lobe (Ironside, 1996). In the cerebral cortex some take the form of 'florid' plaques in which the central core of faintly radiating fibrillary material is surrounded by a halo of spongiform vacuoles (Fig. 12.4b). These plaques are intensely stained by PrP antibodies and there are additional, abundant diffuse or synaptic deposits which are distributed in the cerebral

and cerebellar cortex, particularly the molecular layer of the latter, and to a variable extent in the basal ganglia and thalamus. The more diffuse deposits of PrP bear some resemblance to diffuse deposits of β/A4 in Alzheimer's disease. Basal ganglia and thalamus commonly show severe pathology with spongiform change, neuron loss and astrocytosis. The new variant cases are unusual in the close similarity they all show in their pathology. It is noteworthy that all sufferers so far investigated have been methionine homozygous at codon 129 of the PrP gene (Will *et al.*, 1996).

By contrast, inherited forms of prion disease present the greatest variability in their pathological findings (Fig. 12.2). Even within the same family the phenotypic variation may be marked. As indicated above, GSS is characterized predominantly by cerebellar pathology in which neuron loss and astrocytosis are accompanied by the presence of multifocal clusters of plaques, each individually rather smaller than typical kuru or new variant CJD plaques (Fig 12.4b). Spongiform change tends to be inconspicuous or absent but spinocerebellar tract degeneration may be prominent. As noted above (Fig. 12.2), some cases with GSS develop neurofibrillary tangles in neocortex and in a few individuals β/A4 as well as PrP deposits have accompanied the neurofibrillary tangles. Studies of ApoE genotype in prion diseases have not in general shown the increased prevalence of the e4 genotype found in Alzheimer's disease (Amouyel *et al.*, 1994; Nakagawa *et al.*, 1995; Pickering-Brown *et al.*, 1995).

The diseases with which prion diseases are most often clinically confused are, in our experience, paraneoplastic syndrome, multiple system atrophy (confused with inherited forms of prion disease), rapidly progressive Alzheimer's disease and the calcifying leukoencephalopathy described on page 412. These all have neuropathological findings that are quite distinct from prion diseases. The conditions that need to be distinguished from prion diseases at the pathological level are those mentioned above that give rise to spongy change and Alzheimer's disease which can be readily distinguished from prion diseases with immunostaining for β/A4 and PrP.

Molecular and genetic analyses of PrP

Because it is now possible to perform molecular and genetic examination of PrP in patients with unusual dementing illnesses, diagnoses of inherited prion disease have been established where there was either little or no neuropathology (Collinge *et al.*, 1990), atypical neur-

Table 12.2. *Diagnosis of human prion disease*

1. Neuropathological assessment with immunohistology of amyloid plaques, if present
2. Detection of PrP^{Sc} by dot blot, Western blot, or histoblot
3. PrP genotype by PCR, followed by screening for known mutations, or sequencing for novel mutations

odegenerative disease (Medori *et al.*, 1992a), or misdiagnosed neurodegenerative disease (Azzarelli *et al.*, 1984; Heston *et al.*, 1966), including Alzheimer's disease.

The presence of protease-resistant PrP in the infectious and sporadic forms and most of the inherited forms of prion disease implicates prions in their pathogenesis. However, in some patients with prion diseases PrP^{Sc} is barely detectable or undetectable (Medori *et al.*, 1992b; Manetto *et al.*, 1992; Little *et al.*, 1986; Brown *et al.*, 1992a), a situation mimicked in transgenic mice which express a mutant PrP gene and spontaneously develop

neurologic illness indistinguishable from experimental murine scrapie (Hsiao *et al.*, 1990). In patients (and mice) which appear to lack protease-resistant PrP but express mutant PrP, neurodegeneration may, at least in part, be caused by abnormal metabolism of mutant PrP. Because of these dichotomous pathogenic forms of PrP, making a definitive diagnosis of human prion disease may require both molecular and genetic analyses of PrP.

Molecular studies of PrP assess the presence of PrP^{Sc}. Two sensitive methods are the guanidium dot-blot method and Western immunoblot analysis of brain homogenates treated to limited proteolysis with proteinase-K (Serban *et al.*, 1990) (Appendix 12.1). The more rapid dot blot method exploits exhancement of PrP^{Sc} immunoreactivity following denaturation in the chaotropic salt, guanidium chloride. A third method, the PrP^{Sc} histoblot, combines limited proteolysis and guandidium enhancement for PrP^{Sc} detection with histologic localization on nitrocelluose paper on to which frozen sections of brain tissue have been applied (Taraboulos *et al.*, 1992) (Appendix 12.2).

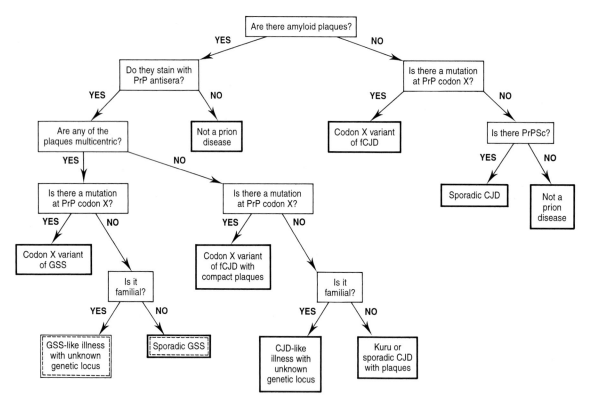

Fig. 12.5. Algorithm for the diagnosis of human prion diseases. All diagnoses are bold framed. Hypothetical diagnoses are represented by dashes within a solid frame, indicating as yet no clearly documented cases of the given diagnosis.

Genetic analyses of PrP are easily performed using the polymerase chain reaction (PCR) (Appendix 12.3). Although the first missense PrP mutation was discovered when the two PrP alleles of a patient with GSS were cloned from a genomic library and sequenced, all subsequent novel missense and insertional mutations have been identified in PrP open reading frames (ORFs) amplified by PCR and sequenced. The 759 base pairs encoding the 253 amino acids of PrP reside in one exon of the PrP gene, providing an ideal situation for the use of PCR. Amplified PrP ORFs may be screened for known mutations using one of several methods, including allele-specific oligonucleotide hybridization. If known mutations are absent, then novel mutations may be found when the PrP ORF is sequenced.

In summary, the diagnosis of prion disease may be made in patients on the basis of: (1) appropriate neuropathology and immunohistology; (2) PrP genotype; and/or (3) the presence of PrP^{Sc} (Table 12.2), and should not be excluded in patients with atypical neurodegenerative diseases until these examinations have been performed. An algorithm for diagnosing human prion diseases is proposed (Fig. 12.5).

REFERENCES

Amouyel P, Vidal O, Launay JM, Laplanche JL (1994) The apolipoprotein E alleles as major susceptibility factors for Creutzfeldt–Jakob disease. *Lancet* 344: 1315–18.

Anderson RM, Donnelly CA, Fergus NM *et al* (1996) Transmission dynamics and epidemiology of BSE in British cattle. *Nature* 382: 779–88.

Azzarelli B, Muller J, Ghetti B, Dyken M, Conneally PM (1984) Cerebellar plaques in familial Alzheimer's disease (Gerstmann–Sträussler–Scheinker variant?). *Acta Neuropathol (Berl)* 65: 235–46.

Basler K, Oesch B, Scott M *et al.* (1986) Scrapie and cellular PrP isoforms are encoded by the same chromosomal gene. *Cell* 46: 417–28.

Bastian FO (ed) (1991) *Creutzfeldt–Jakob disease and other transmissible human spongiform encephalopathies* Mosby Year Book, St. Louis.

Bell JE, Ironside JW (1993) Neuropathology of spongiform encephalopathies in humans. *Brit Med Bull* 49:738–77.

Brown P, Rodgers-Johnson P, Cathala F, Gibbs CJ, Gajdusek DC (1984) Creutzfeldt–Jakob disease of long duration: clinicopathological characteristics, transmissibility, and differential diagnosis. *Ann Neurol* 16: 295–304.

Brown P, Cathala F, Castagne P, Gajdusek DC (1986) Creutzfeldt–Jakob disease: clinical analysis of a consecutive series of 230 neuropathologically verified cases. *Ann Neurol* 20: 597–602.

Brown P, Cathala F, Raubertas RF, Gajdusek DC, Castaigne P (1987) The epidemiology of Creutzfeldt–Jakob disease: conclusion of a 15-year investigation in France and review of the world literature. *Neurology* 37: 895–904.

Brown P, Goldfarb LG, Kovanen J, Haltia M, Cathala F, Sulima M, Gibbs Jr. CJ, Gajdusek DC (1992a) Phenotypic characteristics of familial Creutzfeldt–Jakob disease associated with the codon 178ASN PRNP mutation. *Ann Neurol* 31: 282–5.

Brown P, Preece MA, Will RG (1992b) 'Friendly fire' in medicine: hormones, homografts, and Creutzfeldt–Jacob disease. *Lancet* 340: 24–7.

Brown P, Goldfarb LG, McCombie WR, Nieto A, Squillacote D, Sheremata W, Little BW, Codec MS, Gibbs CJ Jr, Gajdusek DC (1992c) Atypical Creutzfeldt–Jacob disease in an American family with an insert mutation in the PRNP amyloid precursor gene. *Neurology* 42: 422–7.

Bruce ME, McConnell I, Fraser H, Dickinson AG (1991) The disease characteristics of different strains of scrapie in sinc congenic mice lines; implications for the nature of the host agent and host control of pathogenesis. *J Gen Virol* 72: 595–603.

Bruce ME, Chree A, McConnell I, Foster J, Pearson G, Fraser H (1994) Transmission of bovine spongiform encephalopathy and scrapie in mice: strain variation and species barrier. *Phil Trans R Soc London [B Biol Sci]* 343: 405–11.

Budka H, Aguzzi A, Brown P *et al* (1995) Neuropathological diagnostic criteria for Creutzfeldt–Jakob disease (CJD) and other human spongiform encephalopathies (prion diseases). *Brain Pathol* 5: 459–66.

Carlson GA, Kingsbury DT, Goodman PA *et al* (1986) Linkage of prion protein and scrapie incubation time genes. *Cell* 46: 503–11.

Carlson GA, Goodman PA, Lovett M, Taylor BA, Marshall ST, Peterson-Torchia M, Westaway D, Prusiner SB (1988) Genetics and polymorphism of the mouse prion gene complex: control of scrapie incubation time. *Mol Cell Biol* 8: 5528–40.

Collinge J, Owen F, Lofthouse R, Shah T, Harding AE, Poulter M, Boughey AM *et al* (1989) Diagnosis of Gerstmann–Sträussler syndrome in familial dementia with prion protein gene analysis. *Lancet* ii: 15–17.

Collinge J, Owen F, Poulter M, Leach M, Crow TJ *et al* (1990) Prion dementia without characteristic pathology. *Lancet* 336: 7–9.

Collinge J, Palmer MS, Dryden AJ (1991a) Genetic predisposition to iatrogenic Creutzfeldt–Jakob disease. *Lancet* 337: 1441–2.

Collinge J, Palmer M (1991b) Scientific correspondence. *Nature* 353: 802.

Collinge J, Brown J, Hardy J, Mullan M, Rossor MN *et al* (1992) Inherited prion disease with 144 base pair gene insertion: II; Clinical and pathological features. *Brain.*

Collinge J, Sidle KCL, Meads J, Ironside J, Hill AF (1996)

Molecular analysis of prion strain variation and the aetiology of 'new variant' CJD. *Nature* 383: 685–90.

Cuillé J, Chelle PL (1939) Experimental transmission of trembling to the goat. *C R Séances Acad Sci* 208: 1058–60

Department of Health and Ministry of Agriculture, Food and Fisheries (1989) *Report of the Working Party on Spongiform Encephalopathy.*

de Silva R, Ironside JW, McCardle L, Esmonde TFG, Bell JE, Will RG (1994) Neuropathological phenotype and 'prion protein' genotype correlation in sporadic Creutzfeldt–Jakob disease. *Neurosci Lett* 179: 50–52.

Deslys JP, Marce D, Dormont D (1994) Similar genetic susceptibility in iatrogenic and sporadic Creutzfeldt-Jakob disease. *J Gen Virol* 75: 23–7.

Diedrich JF, Knopman DS, List JF, Olson K II WHF, Emory CR, Sung JH, Haase AT (1992) Deletion in the prion gene in a demented patient. *Hum Mol Genet* 1: 443–4.

Dlouhy SR, Hsiao K, Farlow MR, Foroud T, Conneally PM, Johnson P, Prusiner SB, Hodes ME, Ghetti B (1992) Linkage of the Indiana kindred of Gerstmann–Sträussler–Scheinker disease to the prion protein gene. *Nat Genet* 1: 64–7.

Doh-ura K, Tateishi J, Sasaki H, Kitamoto T, Sakaki Y (1989) Pro Æleu change at position 102 of prion protein is the most common but not the sole mutation related to Gerstmann–Sträussler syndrome. *Biochem Biophys Res Commun* 163: 974–9.

Doh-ura K, Kitamoto T, Sakaki Y, Tateishi J (1991) Scientific correspondence. *Nature* 353–801.

Duffy P, Wolf J, Collins G et al (1974) Possible person-to-person transmission of Creutzfeldt–Jakob disease. *NEJM* 290: 692.

Farlow M, Yee RD, Conneally PM, Azzarelli B, Ghetti B (1989) Gerstmann–Sträussler–Scheinker disease. I. Extending the clinical spectrum. *Neurology* 39: 1446–52.

Furukawa H, Kitamoto T, Tanaka, Y, Tateishi J (1995) New varient prion protein in a Japanese family with Gerstmann–Sträussler syndrome. *Brain Res Mol Brain Res* 30: 385–8.

Gajdusek DC, Gibbs CJ Jr, Alpers M (1966) Experimental transmission of a kuru-like syndrome to chimpanzees. *Nature* 209: 794–6.

Gajdusek DC (1977) Unconventional viruses and the origin and disappearance of kuru. *Science* 197: 943–60.

Ghetti B, Tagliavini F, Masters CL, Beyreuther K, Giaccone G, Verga L, Farlow MR, Conneally PM, Dlouhy SR, Azzarelli B, Bugiani O (1989) Gerstmann–Sträussler–Scheinker disease. II. Neurofibrillary tangles and plaques with PrP-amyloid coexist in an affected family. *Neurology* 38: 1453–61.

Giaccone G, Tagliavini F, Bugiani O, Frangione B, Farlow MR, Ghetti B (1991) PrP- and beta-amyuloid coexist in plaques of an aged patient of the Indiana kindred of Gerstmann–Sträussler–Scheinker disease. *Neurol Suppl* 41: 155.

Goldfarb LG, Brown P, Goldgaber D, Asher DM, Strass N, Graupera G, Piccardo P, Brown WT, Rubinstein R, Boellaard JW, Gajdusek DC (1989) Patients with Creutzfeldt–Jakob disease and kuru lack the mutation in the PRIP gene found in Gerstmann–Sträussler syndrome, but they show a different double-allele mutation in the same gene. *Am J Hum Gen* [suppl] 45: A189.

Goldfarb LG, Brown P, Goldgaber D, Garruto RM, Yanaghiara R, Asher DM, Gajdusek DC (1990) Identical mutation in unrelated patients with Creutzfeldt–Jakob disease. *Lancet* 336: 174–5.

Goldfarb LG, Haltia M, Brown P, Nieto A, Kovanen J, McCombie WR, Trapp S, Gajdusek DC (1991a) New mutation in scrapie amyloid precusor gene (at codon 178) in Finnish Creutzfeldt–Jakob kindred. *Lancet* 337: 425.

Goldfarb LG, Brown P, McCombie WR, Goldgaber D, Swergold GD, Wills PR, Cerenakova L, Baron H, Gibbs CJ Jr, Gajdusek DC (1991b) Transmissible familial Creutzfeldt–Jakob disease associated with five, seven, and eight extra octapeptide coding repeats in the PRNP gene. *PNAS* 88: 10926–30.

Goldfarb LG, Brown P, Haltia M, Cathala F, McCombie WR, Kovanen J, Cerenakova L, Goldin L, Nieto A, Godec M, Asher DM, Gajdusek DC (1992a) Creutzfeldt–Jakob disease cosegregates with the codon 178 asparagine PRNP mutation in families of European origin. *Ann Neurol* 31: 274–81.

Goldfarb LG, Petersen RB, Tabaton M, Brown P, LeBlanc AC, Montagna P, Cortelli P, Julien J, Vital C, Pendelbury WW et al (1992b) Fatal familial insomnia and familial Creutzfeldt-Jakob disease: disease phenotype determined by a DNA polymorphism. *Science* **258**: 806–8.

Goldfarb LG, Brown P, Gajdusek DC The molecular genetics of human transmissible spongiform encephalopathy, in Prusiner SB, Collinge J, Powell J, Anderton B (eds) *Prion Diseases in Humans and Animals* (Ellis Horwood, London, in press).

Goldgaber D, Goldfarb LG, Brown P, Asher DM, Brown WT et al (1989) Mutations in familial Creutzfeldt–Jakob disease and Gerstmann–Sträussler–Scheinker's syndrome. *Exp Neurol* 106: 204–6.

Hadlow WJ (1959) Scrapie and kuru *Lancet* 2: 289–90.

Hadlow WJ (1992) The scrapie–kuru connection: recollections of how it came about. In Prusiner S, Collinge J, Powell J, Anderton B (eds) *Prion diseases of humans and animals* Horwood, New York pp 40–46.

Hayward PAR, Bell JE, Ironside JW (1994) Prion protein immunocytochemistry: the development of reliable protocols for the investigation of Creutzfeldt–Jakob disease. *Neuropathol Appl Neurobiol* 20: 375–83.

Heston LL, Lowther DLL, Leventhal CM (1966) Alzheimer's disease. *Arch Neurol* 15: 225–33.

Hsiao KK, Baker HF, Crow TJ, Poulter M, Owen F et al (1989) Linkage of a prion protein missense variant to Gerstmann–Sträussler syndrome. *Nature* 338: 342–5.

Hsiao KK, Scott M, Foster D, Groth DF, DeArmond SJ et al (1990) Spontaneous neurodegeneration in transgenic mice with mutant prion protein. *Science* 250: 1587–90.

Hsiao K, Meiner Z, Kahana E, Cass C, Kahana I, Avrahami D, Scarlato G, Abramsky O, Prusiner SB, Gabizon R (1991a) Mutation of the prion protein in Libyan Jews with Creutz-feldt–Jakob disease. *New Eng J Med* 324: 1091–7.

Hsiao KK, Cass C, Schellenberg GD, Bird T, Devine-Gage E, Wisniewski H, Prusiner SB (1991b) A prion protein variant in a family with the telencephalic form of Gerstmann–Sträussler–Scheinker syndrome. *Neurology* 41: 681–4.

Hsiao K, Dlhouhy SR, Farlow MR, Cass C, Da Costa M, Conneally PM, Hodes ME, Ghetti B, Prusiner S (1992) Mutant prion proteins in GSS disease with NFT. *Nat Genet* 1: 68–71.

Hsiao KK, Growth D, Scott M, Yang S-L, Serban H, Raff D, Foster D, Torchia M, DeArmond SJ, Prusiner SB (1994) Serial transmission in rodents of neurodegeneration from transgenic mice expressing mutant prion protein. *Proc Natl Acad Sci* 91: 9126–30.

Hsiao KK, Groth D, Scott M, Yang SL, Serban A, Raff D, Foster D, Torchia M, DeArmond SJ, Prusiner SB Prusinerr SB, Collinge J, Powell J, Anderton B (eds) Genetic and Transgenic Studies of Prion Proteins in GSS Disease, Ellis Horwood, London, in press.

Ikeda S, Yanagisawa N, Allsop D, Glenner GG (1991) A variant of Gerstmann Sträussler–Scheinker disease with beta-protein epitopes and cystrophic neurites in the peripheral regions of PrP-immunoreactive amyloid plaques. In Natvig J, Forre O, Husby G, Husebekk G, Skogen A, Sletten G, Westermark P (eds) *Amyloid and Amyloidosis* 737–40.

Ironside JW (1996) Creutzfeldt–Jakob disease. *Brain Pathol* 6: 379–88.

Jakob A (1921) Uber eingenartige Erkrankung des Zentralner-vensystems mit bemerkenswertem anatomischen. *Befunde Z Ges Neurol Psych* 64: 42–228.

Kascak RJ, Rubensein R, Merz PA, Tonna-DeMasi M et al (1987) Mouse polyclonal and monoclonal antibody to scrapie-associated fibril proteins. *J Virol* 61: 3688–93.

Kawata A, Masakazu S, Oda M, Hayashi H, Tanabe H (1992) Creutzfeldt–Jakob disease with congophilic kuru plaques: CT and pathological findings of the cerebral white matter. *J Neurol Neurosurg Psychiat* 55: 849–51.

Kitamoto T, Tateishi J, Tashima T, Takeshita I, Barry R, DeArmond SJ, Prusiner SB (1986) Amyloid plaques in Creutzfeldt–Jakob disease stain with prion protein antibo-dies. *Ann Neurol* 20: 204–8.

Kitamoto T, Amano N, Terao Y, Nakazato Y, Isshiki T, Mizutani T, Tateishi J (1993a) A new inherited prion disease (PrP-P105L mutation) showing spastic paraparesis. *Ann Neurol* 34: 808–13.

Kitamoto T, Iizuka R, Tateishi J (1993b) An amber mutation of prion protein in Gerstmann-Sträussler syndrome with mu-tant PrP plaques. *Biochem Biophys Res Commun* 192: 525–31.

Kitamoto T, Ohta M, Doh UK, Hitoshi S, Terao Y, Tateishi J (1993c) Novel missense variants of prion protein in Creutz-feldt–Jakob disease or Gerstmann–Straussler syndrome. *Biochem Biophys Res Commun* 191: 709–14.

Kretzschmar HA, Stowring LE, Westaway D, Stubblebine WH, Prusiner SB, DeArmond SJ (1986) Molecular cloning of a human prion protein cDNA. *DNA* 5: 315–24.

Kretzschmar HA, Honold G, Seitelberger F, Feucht M, Wessely P, Mehraein P, Budka H (1991) Prion protein mutation in family first reported by Gerstmann, Sträussler, and Scheinker. *Lancet* 337: 1160.

Lantos PL (1992) From slow virus to prion: a review of transmissible spongiform encephalopathies. *Histopathology* 20: 1–11.

Laplanche JL, Chatelain J, Launay JM, Gazengel C, Vidaud M (1990) Deletion in prion protein gene in a Moroccan family. *Nuc Acids Res* 18: 6745.

Lasmézas CI, Deslys J-P, Demalmay R, et al (1996) BSE transmission to macaques. *Nature* 381: 743–44.

Liberski PP, Yanagihara R, Asher DM, Gibbs CJ, Gajdusek DC (1990) Reevaluation of the ultrastructural pathology of experimental Creutzfeldt–Jakob disease. *Brain* 113: 121–37.

Little BW, Brown PW, Rodgers-Johnson P et al., (1986) Familial myoclonic dementia masquerading as Creutz-feldt–Jakob disease. *Ann Neurol* 20: 231–9.

MacDonald ST, Sutherland K, Ironside JW (1996) Prion protein genotype and pathological phenotype studies in sporadic Creutzfeldt–Jakob disease. *Neuropathol Appl Neurobiol* 22: 285–92.

Manetto V, Medori R, Cortelli P, Montagna P, Tinuper P, Baruzzi A, Rancurel G, Hauw JJ, Vanderhaeghen JJ, Mail-leux P, Bugiani O, Tagliavini F, Bouras C, Rizzuto N, Lugaresi E, Gambetti P (1992) Fatal familial insomina: clinical and pathologic study of five new cases. *Neurology* 42: 312–19.

Masters CL, Gajdusek DC (1982) The spectrum of Creutzfeldt–Jakob disease and the virus-induced spongiform encepha-lopathies. In Smith WT, Cavanagh JB (eds) *Rec Advs in Neuropathol* Vol 2, Churchill Livingstone, Edinburgh pp 139–64.

Masters CL, Harris JO, Gajdusek DC, Gibbs Jr CJ, Bernoulli C, Asher D (1979) Creutzfeldt–Jakob disease: patterns of worldwide occurrence and the significance of familial and sporadic clustering. *Ann Neurol* 5: 177–88.

Masters CL, Gajdusek DC, Gibbs Jr CJ (1981a) The familial occurrence of Creutzfeldt–Jakob disease and Alzheimer's disease. *Brain* 104: 535–58.

Masters CL, Gajdusek DC, Gibbs CJ Jr (1981b) Creutz-feldt–Jakob disease virus isolations from the Gerstmann–Sträussler syndrome with an analysis of the various forms of amyloid plaque deposition in the virus-induced spongiform encephalopathies. *Brain* 104: 559–88.

Medori R, Tritschler H-J, LeBlanc A, Villare F, Manetto V *et al* (1992*a*) Fatal familial insomnia, a prion disease with a mutation at codon 178 of the prion protein gene. *NEJM* 326: 444–9.

Medori R, Montagna P, Tritschler HJ, LeBlanc A, Cortelli P, Tinuper P, Lugaresi E, Gambetti P (1992*b*) Fatal familial insomnia: a second kindred with mutation of prion protein gene at codon 178. *Neurology* 42: 669–70.

Nakagawa Y, Kitamoto T, Kurukawa H, Ogomori K, Tateishi J (1995) Apolipoprotein E in Creutzfeldt–Jakob disease. *Lancet* 345: 68–69.

Nochlin D, Sumi SM, Bird TD *et al* (1989) Familial dementia with PrP-positive amyloid plaques: a variant of Gerstmann–Sträussler syndrome. *Neurology* 910–18.

Oesch B, Westaway D, Walchli M, McKinley MP, Kent SBH, Aebersold R, Barry R, Tempst P, Teplow DB, Hood LE, Prusiner SB, Weissmann C (1985) A cellular gene encodes scrapie PrP 27–30 protein. *Cell* 40: 735–46.

Owen F, Poulter M, Lofthouse R, Collinge J, Crow TJ *et al* (1989) Insertion in prion protein gene in familial Creutzfeldt–Jakob disease. *Lancet* 1: 51–2.

Palmer MS, Dryden AJ, Hughes JT, Collinge J (1991) Homozygous prion protein genotype predisposes to sporadic Creutzfeldt–Jakob disease. *Nature* 352: 340–2.

Pearlman RL, Towfighi J, Pezeshkpour GH, Tenser RB, Turel AP (1988) Clinical significance of types of cerebellar amyloid plaques in human spongiform encephalopathies. *Neurology* 38: 1249–54.

Petersen RB, Tabaton M, Medori R, Tritschler HJ, Berg L, Schrank B, Torack RM, Julien J, Vital C, Pendlebury W, Montagna P, Lugaresi E, Gambetti P (1992) Familial thalamic dementia and fatal familial insomnia are prion diseases with the same mutation. *Neurobiol Aging* 13 [Suppl 1]: S93.

Petersen RB, Tabaton M, Chen SG, Monari L, Richardson SL, Lynch T, Manetto V, Lanska DJ, Markesbery WR, Currier RD, Autilio-Gambetti L, Wilhelmsen KC, Gambetti P (1995) Familial progressive subcortical gliosis: presence of prions and linkage to chromosome 17. *Neurology* 45: 1062–7.

Pickering-Brown SM, Mann DMA, Owen F *et al* (1995) Allelic variations in apolipoprotein E and prion protein genotype related to plaque formation and age of onset in sporadic Creutzfeldt–Jakob disease. *Neurosci Lett* 187: 127–9.

Pocchiari M, Salvatore M, Cutruzzola F, Genuardi M, Allocatelli CT, Masullo C, Macchi G, Alema G, Galgani S, Yi YG *et al* (1993) A new point mutation of the prion protein gene in Creutzfeldt–Jakob disease. *Ann Neurol* 34: 802–7.

Prusiner SB, McKinley MP, Groth DF *et al* (1981) Scrapie agent contains a hydrophobic protein. *PNAS* 78: 6675–9.

Prusiner SB (1982) Novel proteinaceous infectious particles cause scrapie. *Science* 215: 136–44.

Prusiner SB, Groth DF, Botlon DC, Kent SB, Hood LE (1984) Purification and structural studies of a major scrapie prion protein. *Cell* 38: 127–34.

Prusiner SB, Scott M, Foster D, Pan KM, Groth D *et al* (1990) Transgenetic studies implicate interactions between homologous PrP isoforms in scrapie prion replication. *Cell* 63: 673–86.

Prusiner SB (1991) Molecular biology of prion diseases. *Science* 252: 1515–22.

Puckett C, Concannon P, Casey C, Hood L (1991) Genomic structure of the human prion protein gene. *Am J Hum Gen* 49: 320–9.

Richardson EPJr, Masters CL (1995) The nosology of Creutzfeldt–Jakob disease and conditions related to the accumulation of PrP in the nervous system. *Brain Pathol* 5: 33–41.

Ripoll L, Laplanche JL, Salzmann M, Jouvet A, Planques B, Dussaucy M, Chatelain J, Beaudry P, Launay JM (1993) A new point mutation in the prion protein gene at codon 210 in Creutzfeldt–Jakob disease. *Neurology* 43: 1934–8.

Roberts GW, Lofthouse R, Brown R *et al* (1986) Prion-protein immunoreactivity in human transmissible dementias. *NEJM* 315: 1231–3.

Roberts GW, Lofthouse R, Allsop D, Landon M, Kidd M, Prusiner SB, Crow TJ (1988) CNA amyloid proteins in neurodegenerative diseases. *Neurology* 38: 1534–40.

Saiki R, Gelfand D, Stoffel S, Scharf S, Higuchi R, Horn G, Mullis K, Erlich H (1988) Primer-directed enzymatic amplification of DNA with a thermostable DNA polymerase. *Science* 239: 487–94.

Scott M, Foster D, Mirenda C *et al* (1989) Transgenic mice expressing hamster prion protein produce species-specific scrapie infectivity and amyloid plaques. *Cell* 59: 847–57.

Serban D, Taraboulos A, DeArmond SJ, Prusiner SB (1990) Rapid detection of Creutzfeldt–Jakob disease and scrapie prion proteins. *Neurology* 40: 110–17.

Sparkes RS, Simon M, Cohn VH *et al* (1986) Assignment of the human and mouse prion protein genes to homologous chromosomes. *PNAS* 83: 7358–62.

Speer MC, Goldgaber D, Goldfarb LG, Roses AD, Pericak-Vance MA (1991) Support of linkage of GSS syndrome to the prion protein gene on chromosome 20p12-pter. *Genomics* 9: 366–8.

Taraboulos A, Jendroska K, Serban D, Yang S-L, DeArmond SJ, Prusiner SB (1992) Regional mapping of prion proteins in brain *PNAS* 89.

UK National CJD Surveillance Centre Report, 1995.

Vnencak-Jones Cindy L, Phillips III John A (1992) Identification of heterogeneous PrP gene deletions in controls by detection of allele-specific heteroduplexes (DASH). *Am J Hum Gen* 50: 871–2.

Warter JM, Steinmetz G, Heldt N, Rumbach L, Marescaux Ch, Eber AM, Collard M, Rohmer F, Loquet, Guedenet JC, Gehin P, Weber M (1982) Demence presenile familiale syndrome de Gerstmann–Sträussler–Scheinker. *Rev Neurol (Paris)* 138: 107–21.

Westaway D, Goodman PA, Mirenda CA *et al* (1987) Distinct

prion proteins in short and long scrapie incubation period mice. *Cell* 51: 651–62.

Westaway D, DeArmond SJ, Cayetano-Canlas J, Groth D, Foster D, Yang S-L, Torchia M, Carlson GA, Prusiner SB (1994) Degeneration of skeletal muscle, peripheral nerves, and the central nervous system in transgenic mice overexpressing wild-type prion proteins. *Cell* 76: 117–29.

Will RG, Mathews WB (1984) A retrospective study of Creutzfeldt–Jakob disease in England and Wales 1970–1979. I. Clinical features. *J Neurol Neurosurg Psych* 47: 134–40.

Will RG, Ironside JW, Zeidler M *et al* (1996) A new variant of Creutzfeldt–Jakob disease in the UK. *Lancet* 347: 921–5.

Will RG (1996) Surveillance of prion diseases in humans. In Baker HF, Ridley RM (eds) *Prion diseases* Humana, New Jersey pp 119–37.

APPENDIX 12.1

Immunoblot (Dot and Western) methods of PrP^{Sc} detection

(from Serban *et al.*, 1990)

Preparation of brain extracts. 0.5–1 g unfixed brain (specimens from different brain regions should be assayed) are homogenized in 9 parts lysis buffer (100 mmol of sodium choride per litre, 10 mmol EDTA per litre, 0.5% NP40 [Nonidet P-40, a non-ionic detergent], 0.5% sodium deoxycholate, and 10 mmol TRIS–HCl per litre, pH 7.4). Homogenate is centrifuged at 500 × g for five minutes to remove insoluble debris. (Supernatant may be stored at − 70 °C.)

Two hundred μl supernatant centrifuged at 100 000 × g for one hour. Pellet suspended in 40 μl lysis buffer. Prepare two aliquots, one for dot blot, one for Western blot.

Dot blot. Add an equal volume of electrophoresis-sample buffer to resuspended pellet (0.125 mol of Tris per litre and 4% sodium dodecyl sulphate; pH 6.8). Spot 4 μl of this mixture on a dry nitrocellulose membrane (0.45 μ; Bio-Rad, Richmond, CA). Thoroughly air dry the dots. Wash membranes extensively in TBSB (0.1% Brij 35, 150 mM sodium choride per litre and 10 mM Tris–HCl per litre, pH 7.8). Incubate membranes incubated with 200 μg/ml proteinase K (Beckman, Palo Alto, CA) in TBSB at 38 °C for 2 h on shaker. Stop the reaction by washing the membranes in TBST (0.05% Tween 20, 150 mM sodium choride per litre and 10 mM Tris–HCl per litre, pH 7.8) followed by incubation with 3 mM phenylmethyulsulphonylfluoride (PMSF) per litre in TBST, 20 minutes. Incubate further 10 minutes at room temperature with 3 M per litre GdnSCN (Fluka, Buchs, Switzerland). Wash membranes thoroughly in TBST. Block membranes with 5% non-fat milk in TBST, and incubate overnight with primary polyclonal antiserum R073 (Serban *et al.*, 1990) diluted between 1:1000 and 1:5000, or monoclonal antibodies 3F4 (Kascak *et al.*, 1987) or 5C10 (ref) diluted (1:1000 ascitic fluid: 1:1 supernatant), followed by alkaline phosphatase-conjugated antibodies diluted 1:7500 (Promega, Madison, WI) and developed with 5-bromo-4-chloro-3-indoyl-phosphate and nitro-blue tetrazolium as substrates (Promega).

Western blot: Add an equal volume of electophoresis sample buffer to resuspended pellet and incubate for one hour at 37 °C with or without the addition of proteinase K (5 to 100 μg/ml). Stop the reaction by adding PMSF (final concentration 1 mmol/l). Resolve 5 μl in a 12% acrylamide gel and transfer to immobilon P (polyvinylidine difluroide membrane; Millipore, Bedford, Mass.). Block membrane in 5% non-fat milk and incubate with antiserum R073 or monoclonal antibodies 5C10 or 3F4 diluted as described above. Incubate with alkaline phosphate-conjugated antibodies diluted 1:7500 and develop with 5-bromo-4-chloro-3- indoyl-phosphate and nitroblue tetrazolium as described above.

Histoblot method of PrP^{Sc} detection

(From Taraboulos *et al.*, 1992)

Wet a nitrocellulose membrane in lysis buffer (lysis buffer as described in Appendix 12.1). Lay it upon a double layer of thick blotting paper saturated with lysis buffer. 8 micron-thick cryostat sections of unfixed brain tissue on glass slides are thawed quickly and immediately pressed onto the membrane for 25 seconds, then inspected for complete transfer of the section. The transfer is facilitated by a slow rotary motion that prevents trapping of air bubbles. The membrane is left on the stack of blotting paper for several minutes.

For detection of PrP^{Sc} the membranes are thoroughly air dried, rehydrated for 1 hour in TBST (TBST as described in Appendix 12.1) and then subjected to limited proteolysis in digestion buffer (proteinase K at 100 μg/l for 18 hours at 37°C in 0.1% Brij 35, 100 mM sodium chloride per litre, 10 mM Tris–HCl per litre, pH 7.8). To stop the reaction, the blots are rinsed three times in TBST and incubated for 30 minutes in TBST with 3 mM phenylmethylsulphonyl fluoride per litre. Finally, the blots are incubated in 3 M GdnSCN per litre in 10 mM Tris–HCl per litre, pH 7.8, for ten minutes and rinsed three times before immunostaining. Immunostaining is done as for dot blots and Western blots described in Appendix 12.1.

Detecting novel mutations in PrP

The PrP ORF of genomic DNA can be amplified by the polymerase chain reaction between primers K (5′ AAGAA TTCTC TGACA TTCTC CTCTT CA-3′) and H (5′-AAGGA TCCCT CAAGC TGGAA AAG-3′), which have been designed with EcoRI and BamHI linkers, respectively, for ease of cloning. The PCR products are fractionated on a (3%:1%) Nusieve: Seakem agarose gel and the 864 base-pair product excised and further purified with GeneClean (Bio101). Sequencing reactions are performed on gel-purified inserts of cloned PCR products by the dideoxy method. 'Shuffle clones' (Saiki *et al.*, 1988) have been encountered in about one-third of our studies involving sequences of individual cloned PCR products, with the result that mutations may be missed and phases misinterpreted. We thus favour sequencing the total PCR product rather than cloned individual PCR products when searching for novel point mutations.

Typically, 2 mg of genomic DNA is amplified in a DNA Thermal Cycler (Perkin Elmer Cetus) in a reaction volume of 100 ml with 500 ng each of primers K and H, 10 ml of a 2 mM nucleotide solution (dATP, dCTP, dGTP, dTTP), 10 ml PCR reaction buffer (Cetus), 2 ml of 50 mM EDTA, and 2.5 units Taq polymerase. The cycles are as follows: 96°C for 1 minute, 55°C for 30 seconds, and 72°C for 2 minutes 30 seconds for 5 cycles; then 94°C for 1 minute, 55°C for 30 seconds, and 72°C for 2 minutes 30 seconds for 30 cycles. Double-stranded template DNA is denatured at 98°C for 8 minutes in the presence of primer prior to chain extension and sequenced with the Sequenase deazaG sequencing reagent kit (US Biochemical). Five primers which may be used to sequence the PrP ORF are: KH02 5′ CAGGG CAGCC CTGGA GGCAA 3′ (sense); KHO3 5′ AAGGA GGTGG CACCC ACAGT 3′ (sense); KH06 5′ TCCCT CAAGC TGGAA AAAGA 3′ (antisense); KH07 5′ CTCTG ACATT CTCCT CTTCA 3′ (sense); KH15 5′GAGGA AAGAG ATCAG GAGGA T 3′ (antisense). 100 ng of DNA is used per reaction, with 70 ng of primers KH03 and KH06, 100 ng of primers KH02, KH07, KH15.

CHAPTER THIRTEEN

Alcoholism and dementia

C. Harper and D. Corbett

Introduction
Primary alcoholic dementia
The Wernicke–Korsakoff syndrome
Hepatic encephalopathy
Pellagra

INTRODUCTION

There is little doubt that excessive consumption of alcohol over a considerable period of time leads to an impairment of cognitive function. Specific alcohol-related disorders such as the Wernicke–Korsakoff syndrome, hepatic encephalopathy, and pellagra cause clinical dementia syndromes but when these have been excluded there is still a considerable number of alcoholics who can be classified as demented. This group of cases has been labelled 'Dementia associated with alcoholism 291.20'in DSM-III-R (American Psychiatric Association, 1987) although there is still controversy as to whether such a condition exists. In 1985 Victor and Adams debated the issue and reviewed the clinical, neuropsychological, neuropathological and neuroradiological evidence concerning alcohol specific neurotoxicity and concluded that there was no need to invoke a separate entity due to the toxic effect of alcohol on the brain as they could practically always account for the clinical state of their patients by one or a combination of the Wernicke–Korsakoff syndrome, acute and chronic hepatic encephalopathy, communicating hydrocephalus, Alzheimer's disease, Marchiafava-Bignami disease, ischaemic infarction or anoxic encephalopathy. Moreover they emphasized that no one had established a discrete pathological basis for the syndrome of alcoholic dementia. To their credit they suggested that morphometric and other quantitative techniques might disclose the lesions and this will be discussed below. Nevertheless it must be remembered that not all alcoholics have impairment of cerebral function. Butters and his colleagues (Butters *et al.*, 1987) have shown that 30–50% of alcoholics will perform a range of neuropsychological tests within the normal range for controls. However, as Tuck and Jackson (1991) report, careful study of people who drink excessively (median daily intake of 180 grams per day) and are not overtly demented frequently reveals a cognitive impairment which takes the form of frontal lobe dysfunction and may be relatively subtle. These signs may precede those of other alcohol related neurological disorders such as cerebellar degeneration, peripheral neuropathy and Wernicke–Korsakoff syndrome by more than ten years. Thus there seems to be a wide spectrum of the effects of alcohol on the brain with considerable individual variability in susceptibility which to some extent may be determined genetically (Parsons, 1987).

PRIMARY ALCOHOLIC DEMENTIA

The existence of specific neurotoxic effects of alcohol on the central nervous system (primary alcoholic dementia) can be approached from a number of points of view. Clinical and neuropsychological data point towards such an entity. Moreover, as neuroimaging techniques become more sophisticated, abnormalities at the structural and functional level are being identified in uncomplicated alcoholics who are cognitively impaired (Pfefferbaum, Lim & Rosenbloom, 1992). Nevertheless, the ultimate proof of the existence of this entity rests with the identification of the pathological substrate of alcohol specific neurotoxicity.

There is now a significant literature on animal models of alcohol neurotoxicity. Arendt (Arendt *et al.*, 1988) has shown that rats that are well nourished and given alcohol develop memory deficits. Pathologically, both hippocampal neurons (Walker *et al.*, 1981) and cerebellar Purkinje cells (Cragg & Phillips, 1983) (Pentney, 1982) appear to be damaged by prolonged exposure to alcohol. McMullen and her colleagues (McMullen *et al.*, 1984) made an important observation in this regard when they showed that five months of exposure to alcohol in rats caused a significant reduction in the branching of the dendritic arbour of hippocampal neurons but that the arbour returned towards normality after two months of abstinence.

Human neuropathological studies are far more difficult. Ideally, cases should have been tested clinically and neuropsychologically before death and cognitive deficits documented. Other causes of dementia such as Alzheimer's disease, strokes, Wernicke–Korsakoff syndrome, etc. must be excluded in order to address the question of alcohol specific neurotoxicity. There are only limited data on such uncomplicated alcoholic cases.

Brain weight studies show that a group of uncomplicated alcoholics (drinking more than 80 grams of alcohol per day for more than 15 years) had a significantly reduced brain weight compared to controls (Harper & Kril, 1992). This brain shrinkage has been reported even in social drinkers when studied by CT scan (Cala, 1983). The loss of brain tissue can be more accurately defined by expressing the brain volume as a proportion of intracranial volume. This ratio has been termed the pericerebral space (PICS) (Harper, 1983) and in uncomplicated alcoholics the PICS is 11.3% compared to 8.3% in controls (Harper & Kril, 1985).

Somewhat surprisingly the loss of tissue seems to be largely accounted for by a reduction in the white matter volume of the cerebral hemispheres rather than a loss of cortical tissue (Harper & Kril, 1992). These changes are more severe in those alcoholics with either Wernicke–Korsakoff syndrome or cirrhosis (Harper & Kril, 1985). The explanation for this white matter change has yet to be elucidated but some, at least, appears to be reversible in that after prolonged abstinence the brain shrinkage reverts towards normality (Carlen *et al.*, 1984). Nevertheless there is likely to be a permanent component which could relate to axonal degeneration subsequent to neuronal loss in cortical or subcortical regions.

Although the majority of the tissue loss from the cerebral hemispheres in alcoholics is accounted for by a reduction in the volume of the cerebral white matter, there is also generally a slight reduction in the volume of the cerebral cortex. This has been demonstrated both pathologically (De la Monte, 1988) and using MRI with quantitative morphometry (Jernigan *et al.*, 1991). Not all the alcoholic groups have reduced cortical grey matter.

Although in many alcoholic cases there is an apparent atrophy of the cerebral cortex with widening of cortical sulci and narrowing of gyri, this could be explained on the basis of loss of white matter as discussed above.

At the microscopic level several authors have subjectively described a patchy loss of cortical neurones in alcoholics (Courville, 1955; Victor, Adams & Collins, 1971). The first quantitative study documenting neuronal loss in alcoholics was published in 1987 (Harper *et al.*, 1987). Cortical neurones were counted using a Quantimet 900 image analyser. There was a 22% reduction in the density of neurons in the superior frontal cortex (Brodmann's area 8), but no significant change in the primary motor (area 4), frontal cingulate (area 32) or inferior temporal (areas 20 & 36) cortices (Kril & Harper, 1989).

This finding of severe damage to the frontal cortex in alcoholics is consistent with clinical (Walsh, 1985) and neuroradiological studies (Jernigan *et al.*, 1991) which suggest that the frontal lobe may be more susceptible to alcoholic-related brain damage than other cortical regions. Moreover there may be particular groups of neurons which are more likely to be damaged. An analysis of the pattern of neuronal loss from the superior frontal cortex in alcoholics revealed that large pyramidal neurons, with a somal area greater than $90\mu m^2$ were selectively lost (Harper & Kril, 1989). This population of large neurons has been recognized as being more vulnerable in both Alzheimer's disease (Terry *et al.*, 1981) and the normal ageing process (Terry and Hansen, 1987). There is no evidence to suggest that particular layers of the cerebral cortex are more vulnerable than others (Harper & Kril, 1989). Subpopulations of cortical neurons can now be identified on the basis of their neurochemical content using immunohistochemistry (Beal & Martin, 1986). These techniques have yet to be applied to alcohol-related brain damage. There is some neurochemical and neuropharmacological data to suggest that these techniques might provide useful information (Hakim & Pappius, 1983; Freund and Ballinger, 1988*a,b*).

Ultrastructural studies have not been possible using human material. Harper and Corbett (Harper & Corbett, 1990) have examined and measured the dendritic arbor of cortical neurons in 15 alcoholic subjects using Golgi impregnation techniques. They showed there was a significant reduction in the basal dendritic arbor of layer III pyramidal neurons in both the superior frontal and motor cortices (Harper & Corbett, 1990). This study suggests that, even though there is not a significant reduction in numbers of cortical neurons in the motor cortex, there are cellular structural abnormalities which could have important functional implications.

Analysis of cortical neuronal counts in the different alcoholic groups revealed that there is no significant difference between those alcoholics with Wernicke–Korsakoff syndrome or cirrhosis of the liver and the uncomplicated alcoholics (Harper & Kril, 1989). This finding suggests that alcohol abuse is responsible for the neuronal loss in the superior frontal cortex and that the additional complication of Wernicke–Korsakoff syndrome, although significantly contributing to the brain shrinkage in alcoholics does not accentuate neuronal loss. However, Jensen and Pakkenberg (1993) used stereological techniques to estimate the total number of neurones in the neocortex in eleven alcoholic and control patients. They found no difference in the two groups although it should be noted that selective neuronal loss from particular gyri could be missed using this technique. There are clinical and radiological data which support the finding of selective frontal lobe damage in alcoholics (Jernigan et al., 1991; Oscar-Berman & Hutner, 1993).

One other cortical abnormality which has been described in alcoholics is Morels laminar sclerosis (Victor, Adams & Collins, 1989). This is an uncommon condition and has not been seen by the authors in spite of our specific interest in alcohol-related brain damage. The disease is characterized by necrosis and degeneration of layers III and IV of the cerebral cortex. It is frequently associated with Marchiafava–Bignami disease (Victor et al., 1989). However, it has been reported in isolation (Naeije et al., 1978).

The specific mechanisms linking the long-term abuse of alcohol (ethanol) with the pathological changes described above are still largely unknown. It has, however, been recognized that alcohol or one of the metabolites has a direct neurotoxic effect on the nervous system. Most of the speculation is based on experimental animal models and in vitro tissue culture studies. These models are studied using neurochemical, neuropharmacological and neurophysiological techniques.

Alcohol is thought to be rapidly assimilated into plasma membranes of cells causing a general disturbance of the hydrophobic regions of membrane lipids and proteins (Goldstein, 1983). These facts have been well reviewed by Charness and his colleagues (Charness et al., 1989) in their paper entitled 'Ethanol and the nervous system'.

There are many other factors which can play a role in the long-term effects of alcohol on the nervous system. Some of these will be discussed in the later parts of this chapter but one should not forget that alcoholics are prone to recurrent head injuries, fitting is common, and there is also a close link between alcohol and the sleep-apnoea syndrome (Carlen and Wilkinson, 1987).

THE WERNICKE–KORSAKOFF SYNDROME

The Wernicke–Korsakoff syndrome is a far more common disease than generally realized with an incidence at autopsy ranging from 0.75 to 2.8% (Harper, 1983; Lindboe & Loberg, 1988). There is still considerable debate as to the relationship between Wernicke's encephalopathy and Korsakoff's psychosis. It has been said that Wernicke's encephalopathy and Korsakoff's psychosis are the acute and chronic components of the same pathological process. However, there are many cases of chronic Wernicke's encephalopathy (diagnosed pathologically) who do not have the characteristic clinical syndrome of chronic mental impairment in which memory deficits overshadow other aspects of cognitive failure. The acute syndrome is more straightforward. Patients may develop acute confusion, impairment of consciousness, ophthalmoplegia, nystagmus and ataxia and examination of the brain shows characteristic pathological changes in specific regions. It should be noted that the full clinical triad as outlined above is the exception rather than the rule and many of the patients will present with only one or two of the clinical signs (Harper, Giles & Finlay-Jones, 1986).

Butterworth (1989), in a recent review of the effects of thiamine deficiency on brain metabolism noted that thiamine transport across the blood brain barrier occurs at a rate similar to that calculated for thiamine turnover in the brain. He suggested that thiamine transport may be just sufficient to meet cerebral requirements. Thiamine levels have been found to be reduced in the brain in human and animal studies of alcohol toxicity and thiamine deficiency (Summers et al., 1991), (Abe & Itokawa, 1977). Thiamine deficiency is often noted in alcoholic populations (Darnton-Hill & Truswell, 1990). This may be caused by dietary deficiency, decreased absorption (Thomson, 1978; Hoyumpa, 1980) and increased excretion (Rindi et al., 1987). In thiamine deficiency there is decreased production of thiamine pyrophosphate (TPP). Three important enzyme systems, the pyruvate dehydrogenase complex (PDHC), α-ketoglutarate dehydrogenase (αKGDH) and transketolase (TK) are dependent on TPP. All these enzymes are involved in glucose metabolism and it has been shown that acute Wernicke's encephalopathy can be precipitated when glucose loads are given to patients with thiamine deficiency (Harper, 1980). The activity of all three enzyme systems has been shown to be decreased in thiamine deficient rats, but only levels of αKGDH have been related to cerebral cortical glucose oxidative capacity and reversal of neurological symptoms following thiamine administration, hence αKGDH is the likely biochemical lesion in acute reversible Wernicke's encephalopathy.

Reductions in αKGDH activities are accompanied by decreases in the synthesis of glucose derived neurotransmitters such as aspartate and GABA. The roles of PDHC and TK in the biochemistry of thiamine deficiency are not clear.

Thus, possible mechanisms of brain damage in thiamine deficiency include compromised cerebral energy metabolism (Butterworth, 1989) and focal accumulation of lactate and decreased pH (Hakim & Pappius, 1983). Two other mechanisms which may play a role and which will receive a lot more attention in the next few years include excitotoxins and free radicals. Several authors have recently drawn comparisons between the changes seen in experimental Wernicke's encephalopathy and excitotoxic neuronal damage (Langlais & Mair, 1990; Lancaster, 1992). The principle of this mechanism is that excitatory amino acids such as glutamate are toxic to neurons if present in excessive amounts. The excessive amounts of the excitatory amino acids activate specific groups of receptors on postsynaptic structures (cell soma and dendrites) which leads to an influx of calcium ions (in the case of NMDA receptors). The high levels of intracellular calcium in turn activate a number of calcium dependent enzymes which can cause neuronal degeneration or death (Meldrum & Garthwaite, 1991). The link between thiamine deficiency and the excessive accumulation of excitatory amino acids is unclear but several factors may play a role. First, an important function of astrocytes is the re-uptake of excitatory amino acids. Since these cells appear to be a principal target in the pathology of thiamine deficiency, their damage may permit the accumulation of higher than normal concentrations of excitatory amino acids in the extracellular fluid. Secondly, in the late stages of thiamine deficiency in both animal models and in humans, epileptic fits are quite common. Repeated fitting (status epilepticus) can result in the excessive accumulation of excitatory amino acids and this is a proposed mechanism underlying hippocampal

neuronal death. The most important data which suggests that excitotoxic action plays a role in brain damage associated with thiamine deficiency is that the pathological changes in experimental models can be attenuated by the use of antagonists to the excitotoxins (Langlais & Zhang, 1993). Langlais and his colleagues (Langlais et al., 1994) further suggested that histamine release may contribute to glutamate-N-methyl-D-aspartate (NMDA)-mediated excitotoxic neuronal death in thiamine deficiency. Excitotoxic damage can also be caused by exogenous agents such as domoic acid, an analogue of the excitotoxin kainate. It is sometimes present in mussels that have been fed on seaweed and an outbreak of domoic acid poisoning occurred in Canada in 1987 (Teitelbaum et al., 1990). Currently, this excitotoxic mechanism does not explain the specific susceptibility of the glial and vascular endothelial cells in thiamine deficiency. Cavanagh and his colleagues have found that nicotinamide analogues and nitroheterocyclic compounds can cause neuropathological changes similar to acute Wernicke's encephalopathy in rats (Cavanagh, 1988; Romero et al., 1991). The glio-vascular lesions in the brainstem caused by 1-3 dinitrobenzene are accompanied by regional increases in blood flow similar to those described by Hakim (Hakim, 1986) in his animal models of acute thiamine deficiency. Romero and his colleagues (Romero et al., 1991) postulate that these changes may be caused by free radical generation from the interaction of the 1-3 dinitrobenzene with xanthine oxidase which is found in high concentration in endothelial cells.

Monographs and many papers have been written on the pathology of the Wernicke–Korsakoff syndrome but with new technologies such as quantitative morphometry and immunohistochemistry we are now in a position to study the brains of these patients in much more detail.

The evolution of the disease can be documented both clinically and pathologically. In pathological studies of Wernicke–Korsakoff syndrome approximately 17% of the cases are acute, 66% of the cases are chronic and there is a significant proportion of cases (17%) which show acute on chronic changes (Harper, 1983). These patients have obviously suffered repeated episodes of thiamine deficiency, some of which may have been subclinical (Lishman, 1981). In a Scandinavian study of 45 cases 53% were acute and 47% were chronic (Torvik, 1987).

In most previous studies of the neuropathology of the Wernicke–Korsakoff syndrome the question of the distribution of lesions in the different stages of the disease has not been raised . It has always been assumed that the distribution is the same for acute and chronic cases and that the lesions are largely restricted to the periventricular regions. However, it is extremely difficult to be certain about the presence or absence of more subtle lesions such as gliosis in many of the chronic cases. Moreover, little effort has been made to study either cortex or subcortical regions such as basal nucleus of Meyenert, and locus coeruleus and raphe nuclei which project widely throughout the brain. Damage to these latter regions are thought to give rise to significant memory and cognitive deficits (Wilcock *et al.*, 1988).

The topography of the lesions in acute WE are as previously described in great detail by Victor and his colleagues (Victor *et al.*, 1971). The mamillary bodies are almost invariably affected and the regions around the third and fourth ventricles and aqueduct are frequently involved (Harper, 1979; Victor *et al.*, 1989). In a study by

Torvik (Torvik, 1987) only three of the 24 acute and subacute cases studied had lesions restricted to the mamillary bodies. The diagnosis is not always evident on macroscopic examination of the brain. In studies by two different groups the diagnosis was suspected on gross examination in only 75% of the cases (Harper, 1983; Torvik, 1987). The most easily recognised acute lesions are haemorrhages, often petechial or in some cases only seen on microscopic examination. In the study by Rosenblum & Feigin (Rosenblum and Feigin, 1965) 47% of 41 cases had such haemorrhages. In acute cases red cells are often present in the perivascular spaces, almost as if the vessel walls are leaky. The tissues appear oedematous and spongy. Silver impregnation methods (e.g. Modified Bielschowsky) show disruption of axons and axonal irregularities. After several days the endothelial cells become plump with active looking nuclei and they proliferate so that the lumina of the

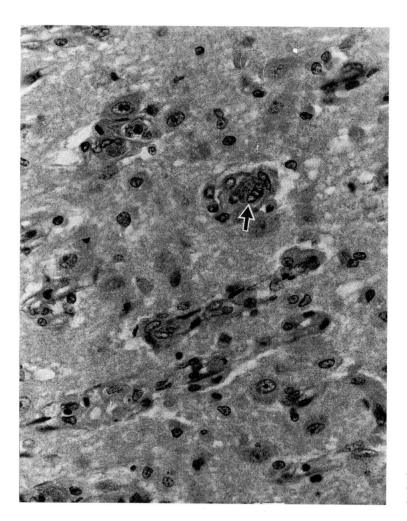

Fig. 13.1. Acute Wernicke's encephalopathy with endothelial proliferation and luminal narrowing (arrow) in the mamillary body. Haematoxin and eosin × 125.

vessels become narrowed (Fig. 13.1). There is evidence of a breakdown in the blood brain barrier in experimental animal models (Phillips & Cragg, 1984) and this may lead to an exudation of protein into the vessel wall which would contribute to the narrowing or obstruction of the lumina of the vessels. At the same time capillary budding commences and by about 7–10 days the affected region has a highly vascular appearance. Rosenblum and Feigin (1965) examined the question of haemorrhage in Wernicke's encephalopathy and concluded that patients who develop severe and extensive haemorrhages are likely to have an additional cause such as a bleeding diathesis due to cirrhosis or uraemia. Such lesions are, in most cases, incompatible with survival and may be the cause of sudden death (Harper, 1979, 1980).

It has been said that there is a relative sparing of the neurons in acute Wernicke's encephalopathy. In the less severe cases this may be correct, but there is sometimes frank necrosis of tissues and destruction of neurons. The most common site for the necrotizing lesion is the medial thalamus as demonstrated by Victor and his colleagues (Victor et al., 1989) in 6 of 45 cases (Fig. 13.2). There is sparing of the immediate subependymal tissues. Several authors have drawn our attention to the fact that a second pattern of pathology is seen in the thalamic nuclei and olives (Victor & Adams, 1985). In these regions the neurons appear to be the principal target and show changes which resemble acute ischaemic cell change with eosinophilia of the cytoplasm and ultimately neuronal disintegration. The endothelial and capillary changes are much less florid than in the mamillary body. It may be that the mechanism underlying this neuronal change is excitotoxic as discussed above. Similar changes in the olivary neurones have been described by Cavanagh (Cavanagh, 1988). Virtually all the neurones in the inferior olive are destroyed following an injection

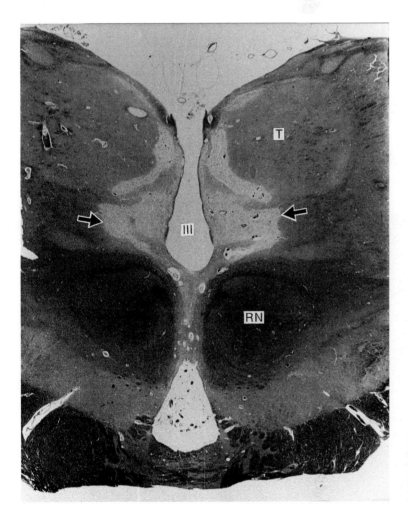

Fig. 13.2. Acute Wernicke's encephalopathy with necrotizing lesions in the medial thalamus (arrows). There is relative sparing of the subependymal tissues. III: third Ventricle, T: thalamus, RN: red nucleus. Nissl × 2.

of 3-acetyl pyridine. This is an analogue of nicotinamide which is readily incorporated into NAD and NADP. Another similar analogue, 6-aminonicatinamide causes a pattern of damage similar to that found in acute Wernicke's encephalopathy. As in these experimental models it is conceivable that variations in the metabolic status of patients with thiamine deficiency may give rise to different patterns of pathology.

In the periventricular lesions one rarely sees any form of inflammatory cell infiltrate. The astrocytes are slow to react and are not easily recognized until the vascular changes begin to subside. They are much more evident in the chronic stages of the disease. Myelin stains show some generalized pallor but there is no definite de-myelination.

In chronic Wernicke–Korsakoff syndrome the characteristic macroscopic lesion is shrinkage and brown discoloration of the mamillary bodies. Microscopically,

the mamillary bodies show spongy degeneration and a relative excess of small blood vessels which can be highlighted by the use of reticulin stains (Fig. 13.3). There is some loss of neurons and gliosis. Occasionally there are haemosiderin laden macrophages, evidence of previous haemorrhages. Neuronal loss, gliosis and pallor of myelin staining are the principal findings in thalamic nuclei and periventricular regions. The thalamic lesions tend to be more severe in dorso-medial, centro-medial and anterior nuclei (Victor et al., 1989).

The incidence of involvement of brain stem nuclei and tracts are quoted in many papers but it must be emphasized that almost all these studies have been subjective evaluations, often using only one section as representative of quite large structures (Victor et al., 1989; Torvik, 1987). Quantitative morphometric studies using serial or step sections and three-dimensional reconstructions provide much more reliable informa-

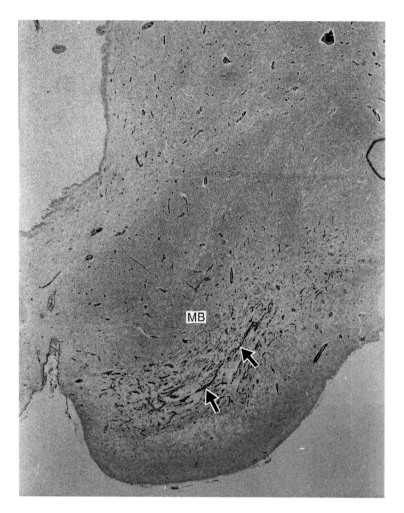

Fig. 13.3. Chronic Wernicke's encephalopathy. There is an increase in the number of blood vessels (arrows) associated with shrinkage and spongiosis of the mamillary body (MB). Reticulin × 10.

tion. Studies of raphe nuclei have shown a significant reduction (56%) in numbers of serotonergic neurons in alcoholics with both Wernicke's encephalopathy and Korsakoff's psychosis (Halliday *et al.*, 1995). It has been suggested that damage to raphe nuclei, which project widely to cerebral cortex, limbic system and hippocampus (Tork & Hornung, 1990), could account for the memory disorders which some of these patients suffer (McEntee & Mair, 1990).

Lesions in the noradrenergic locus coeruleus are said to cause impairment of attention and information processing. There may also be links with learning and memory as indicated by experimental models (Squire *et al.*, 1993). Several groups of workers have emphasised the importance of this nucleus and its noradrenergic pathways in alcoholics with the Wernicke–Korsakoff syndrome (Mair *et al.*, 1979; McEntee & Mair, 1990). Victor *et al.* (1971) noted abnormalities in the locus coeruleus in 19 of the 28 cases studied (67.9%). Various other groups have studied the locus coeruleus in a quantitative fashion but there are contradictory data and further studies will be necessary to determine whether or not neurones in the locus coeruleus are affected in the Wernicke–Korsakoff syndrome (Arango *et al.*, 1994; Halliday *et al.*, 1992; Mayes *et al.*, 1988; McEntee & Mair, 1990).

Pathological studies to date do not adequately explain the difference between the clinical entities of Wernicke's encephalopathy and Korsakoff's psychosis. Lesions in the thalamus correlate best with the amnesia seen in Korsakoff's psychosis (Victor *et al.*, 1971, Warrington & Weiskrantz; Mair, 1979; Mayes *et al.*, 1988). However there is some debate as to the most relevant thalamic nuclei. Damage to the dorsomedial nucleus was first correlated with amnesia by Victor *et al.* (1971). Animal models of Wernicke–Korsakoff syndrome support these findings in that there is degeneration of the dorsomedial thalamic nucleus which correlates with a loss of spontaneous synchronous bursts of activity in the cortex (Armstrong-James *et al.*, 1988). However, detailed studies of four alcoholics with Korsakoff's psychosis have shown that there was damage to the medial thalamus but that the dorsomedial nucleus was largely spared (Mair *et al.*, 1979; Mayes *et al.*, 1988). Despite the differing opinions about the site of thalamic damage, all studies implicate the thalamus as the primary pathological region causing amnesia in Korsakoff's psychosis. More detailed studies of cortical and subcortical structures using immunohistochemistry and quantitative morphometry on well-documented clinical cases may help to characterize the anatomical substrate for the amnestic syndrome.

The mechanisms underlying the pathological changes are unclear and can probably only be addressed using animal models. Alcohol toxicity and thiamine deficiency may well act synergistically.

HEPATIC ENCEPHALOPATHY

The clinical features of hepatic encephalopathy are confusion progressing to drowsiness with inappropriate behaviour, inarticulate speech and ultimately coma. A flapping tremor (asterexis) is often elicitable if looked for carefully (Sherlock, 1981). Deep tendon reflexes are usually increased, as is muscle tone. As the coma deepens the patients may become flaccid. This clinical syndrome is largely reversible with improvement of liver function and reduction of blood ammonia levels. As may therefore be anticipated, pathological changes are relatively minor and, based on experimental studies, appear to be largely reversible. Macroscopically the brain usually appears normal although in fulminant hepatic failure acute brain swelling is a common cause of death (Tholen, 1971). With improved management of hepatic failure this is seen less commonly these days but is a feature of failed liver transplant cases and some cases of acute viral hepatitis. Brain swelling in fulminant hepatic failure appears to be cytotoxic in type and ultrastructural studies show swelling of endothelial cells and perivascular astrocytes. In the astrocytes mitochondria were swollen and there is dilation of endoplasmic reticulum (Kato *et al.*, 1992).

Portal systemic encephalopathy (PSE) is the most common form of hepatic encephalopathy. It accompanies the development of portal-systemic collaterals arising as a result of portal hypertension secondary to liver cirrhosis. The recent use of transjugular intrahepatic portal systemic shunts (TIPS) for the prevention of oesophageal variceal bleeding may precipitate PSE in 30% of patients, particularly the more elderly (Conn, 1993).

The most common pathological finding is at the microscopic level and seems to selectively affect astrocytes. This change was first described by von Hosslin and Alzheimer (von Hosslin & Alzheimer, 1912) and the cells are now called Alzheimer type II astrocytes. These cells have an enlarged pale nucleus, marginated chromatin and often a prominent nucleolus. In patients with long standing hepatic encephalopathy, the astrocyte nuclei also contain glycogen inclusion bodies. The astrocyte nuclei are often lobulated or bean shaped

(Fig. 13.4). Norenberg (Norenberg, 1994), in a review of astrocyte responses to CNS injury, claimed that lobulation is more prominent in certain brain regions including pallidum, substantia nigra and dentate nucleus. With conventional stains, there is no visible cytoplasm, although an excess of lipofuscin can sometimes be identified. There is a marked diminution of the amount of glial fibrillary acidic protein staining using immunohistochemical techniques (Sobel *et al.*, 1981). Characteristically, the astrocyte nuclei occur in pairs suggesting cellular division (Norenberg *et al.*, 1990). These Alzheimer II astrocytes are seen most easily in specific areas of the central nervous system (pontine nuclei of the basis pontis, Ammon's horn, lower layers of the cortex and in the basal ganglia and dentate nucleus). They are occasionally seen in the subcortical white matter. There appears to be a correlation between the severity of the astrocytic change and the severity of the hepatic failure although this has not been well documented scientifically. There is little evidence to suggest significant neuronal loss in this condition. Kril and Harper (1989) found that cirrhosis of the liver does not appear to accentuate the loss of cortical neurons from the superior frontal lobe in alcoholics. Other histopathological studies reveal no evidence of neuronal damage and the measurement of neuronal marker enzymes (Lavoie *et al.*, 1987) or specific binding sites for postsynaptic neuronal ligands (Butterworth *et al.*, 1988) provides no evidence of neuronal loss.

Brumback and Lapham (Brumback & Lapham, 1989), in a study of rats injected with methionine sulphoximine (which causes an elevation in brain ammonia levels), noted the development of Alzheimer type II astrocytes as soon as 18 hours after injection. There was also labelling of these astrocytes by tritiated thymidine given to the rats at the same time as the methionine sulphoximine. This suggests that astrocytes undergo DNA replication and division early in the course of hepatic encephalopathy as part of the Alzheimer type II change. Earlier studies found no increase in the total number of glial cells (Diemer, 1978) and whether or not there is a true astrocytosis still remains unclear.

Interestingly, the changes in the astrocytes are more pronounced following immersion fixation and it has been suggested that this is due to post-mortem fluid shifts, the dimension of the shift being determined by ammonia-induced translocation of ions (Pilbeam *et al.*, 1983).

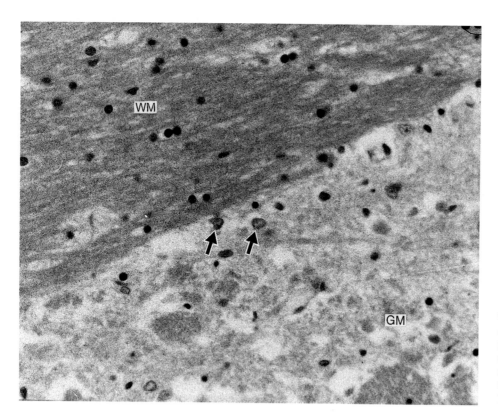

Fig. 13.4. Hepatic encephalopathy showing Alzheimer type II astrocytes in pons (arrows). Note the changes are more pronounced in grey matter (GM) (pontine nucleus) than in white matter (WM). Haematoxin and eosin × 125.

These microscopic changes are seen in other disease states which result in an hyperammonaemia (e.g. inherited metabolic disorders of the urea cycle) and in uraemia, hypercapnia and in the early stages of anoxia (Norenberg, 1994). The basic effect of ammonia on the neuronal membrane is inhibition of chloride extrusion and neuronal depolarization. This disturbs the interaction between individual neurones and the processing of information in neuronal circuits (Rabbe, 1990). There are also changes in brain amino acids. Therrien and Butterworth (Therrien & Butterworth, 1991), in a study of portacaval shunted rats injected with ammonium acetate, observed increases in the cerebrospinal fluid concentrations of glutamine, glutamate, alanine, phenylalanine, and tyrosine. GABA levels were unchanged. Of the amino acids studied alanine best reflected the progression of neurological dysfunction.

Magnetic resonance imaging (MRI) in cirrhotic patients with portal systemic encephalopathy (PSE) reveal bilateral signal hyperintensity of T_1-weighted images in the globus pallidus (Kulisevsky et al., 1992). Direct measurement of tissue removed from the globus pallidus (at autopsy) from patients with chronic liver disease who died in hepatic coma reveal 2 to 7-fold increases of pallidal manganese. This suggests that pallidal magnetic resonance signal hyperintensity is the result of manganese deposition (Butterworth et al., 1995) In positron emmission tomography (PET) studies of patients with PSE, brain ammonia utilisation is increased 2–3 fold and the blood brain barrier appears to be more permeable to ammonia (Lockwood et al., 1991). There is a selective loss of dopaminergic D2 receptors in the globus pallidus of these patients (Mousseau et al., 1993) and it has been suggested that these findings reflect dopaminergic neuronal dysfunction which could contribute to the extrapyramidal signs in these patients.

PELLAGRA

Pellagra is a disease caused primarily by a deficiency of niacin (nicotinic acid). Deficiencies of the amino acid tryptophan, a niacin precursor, may also produce the syndrome. Pellagra is much less common today when compared with the epidemic prevalence during the early part of the twentieth century. Currently pellagra is seen most commonly in the alcoholic population and in patients being treated with isoniazid for tuberculosis (Ishii & Nishihara, 1981; Ishii & Nishihara, 1985). In the standard medical texts the clinical features of pellagra are listed as dermatitis, dementia and diarrhoea (Wilson, 1991). However clinical papers from as early as the 1940s

emphasized that neuropsychiatric features were often the only manifestation of the disorder (Jolliffe et al., 1940; Jolliffe, 1941; Gottlieb, 1944). The diagnoses in most of these cases, were based upon the observed clinical improvement following nicotinic acid therapy (most patients were also given thiamine) and pathological confirmation was the exception. In a more recent study by Serdaru et al. (1988) the cases of pellagra were identified pathologically and then the hospital clinical notes were reviewed. The findings echoed warnings that in the more acute cases of nicotinic acid deficiency the skin and gastrointestinal manifestations of the disease are often absent and may only develop after a prolonged deficiency state allowing structural changes to develop (Jolliffe, 1941; Gottlieb, 1944). The characteristic clinical picture in the 22 cases described by Serdaru et al. (1988) were confusion and/or clouding of consciousness (100%), oppositional hypertonia (100%) and myoclonic jerking (55%). Fluctuations in levels of mentation and consciousness are also a feature. The hypertonia was seen days to weeks before the development of coma. The myoclonus tends to affect face and shoulders. Four of the cases also had Wernicke–Korsakoff syndrome, 8 had Marchiafava–Bignami disease and one had both. This finding emphasizes the close interrelationship between the vitamin B group deficiency states. It may well be that treatment using one of the deficient vitamins (e.g. thiamine only) may precipitate say pellagra by increasing the metabolic demand and requirement for nicotinic acid. Lishman (Lishman, 1981) suggested that such antagonism between thiamine and nicotinic acid may exist.

Pathologically the characteristic feature of pellagra is chromatolytic change in neurons. In particular regions of the central nervous system there is ballooning and enlargement of affected neurons and an apparent clearing of the cytoplasm due to loss of nissl substance (rough endoplasmic reticulum). The nuclei become eccentrically placed and appear smaller than normal. No changes have been noted in the glia, myelin, blood vessels or meninges. The topography of these changes varies to some extent depending upon whether the pellagra is sporadic, endemic or induced by isoniazid. In the latter two cases the cortical neurons, especially the Betz cells are always heavily affected. Hauw and his colleagues (Hauw et al., 1988) deal with this in great detail. They showed that in the sporadic alcoholic cases the central chromatolysis is seen predominantly in the brainstem, especially the pontine nuclei, the nuclei of cranial nerves (third, sixth, seventh and eighth) the reticular nuclei and arcuate nuclei. In the spinal cord posterior horn cells were frequently affected. Cerebellar dentate nuclei were also targeted. Other brain stem and spinal cord changes were described in detail by Hauw et al (Hauw *et al.* (1988).

Although seemingly straightforward, one of us (CH) has had the opportunity of reviewing several of Hauw *et al*'s (1988) cases and it is evident that the chromatolytic change in neurons typical of pellagra could be easily overlooked by even experienced neuropathologists. In our own neuropathological studies of many hundreds of alcoholic cases in Australia we have not identified a single case of pellagra. The explanation for this is unclear but may relate to governmental laws on supplementation of foods with nicotinic acid. In France there is no provision for vitamin supplementation of flour, whereas in Australia it is recommended that nicotinic acid and other vitamins be added to flour and bread (Axford & Williams, 1981).

Potential false positive diagnoses could be made as a result of several factors. It should be noted that in some regions (e.g. third and fourth cranial nerve nuclei) normal neurons often have eccentrically placed nuclei. Excessive lipofuscin in neurons (e.g. olivary nuclei) can also mimic chromatolysis and ischaemic cell change can cause confusion.

REFERENCES

Abe T, Itokawa Y (1977) Effect of ethanol administration on thiamin metabolism and transketolase activity in rats. *Int J Nutr Res* 47: 307–314.

American Psychiatric Association (1987) *Diagnostic and Statistical Manual of Mental Disorders.*

Arango V, Underwood MD, Mann JJ (1994) Fewer pigmented neurons in the locus coeruleus of uncomplicated alcoholics. *Brain Res* 650: 1–8.

Arendt T, Allen Y, Sinden J, Schugens MM, Marchbanks RM, Lantos PL, *et al.* (1988) Cholinergic-rich transplants reverse alcohol-induced memory deficits. *Nature* 332: 448–50.

Armstrong-James M, Ross DT, Chen F, Ebner FF (1988) The effect of thiamine deficiency on the structure and physiology of the rat forebrain. *Metab Brain Dis* 3: 91–124.

Axford DWE, Williams DA (1981) Flour enrichment around the world. *Br Flour Milling Baking Res Ass* 4: 156–63.

Beal MF, Martin JB (1986) Neuropeptides in neurological disease. *Ann Neurol* 20: 547–65.

Brumback RA, Lapham LW (1989) DNA synthesis in Alzheimer type II astrocytosis. The question of astrocytic proliferation and mitosis in experimentally induced hepatic encephalopathy. *Arch Neurol* 46: 845–8.

Butters N, Granholm E, Salmon D, Grant I, Wolfe J (1987) Episodic and semantic memory: a comparison of amnesic and demented patients. *J Clin Exp Neuropsychol* 9: 479–97.

Butterworth R (1989) Effects of thiamin deficiency on brain metabolism: implications for the pathogenesis of the Wernicke–Korsakoff syndrome. *Alcohol Alcohol* 24: 271–9.

Butterworth RF, Lavoie J, Giguere JF, Pomier Layragues G (1988) Affinities and densities of GABA-A receptors and of central benzodiazepine receptors are unchanged in autopsied brain tissue from cirrhotic patients with hepatic encephalopathy. *Hepatology* 8: 1084–8.

Butterworth RF, Spahr L, Fontaine S, Layrargues GP (1995) Manganese toxicity, dopaminergic dysfunction and hepatic encephalopathy. *Metab Brain Dis* 10: 259–67.

Cala LA (1983) Results of computerized tomography, psychometric testing and dietary studies in social drinkers, with emphasis on reversibility after abstinence. *Med J Aust* 2: 264–9.

Carlen PL, Wilkinson DA (1987) Reversibility of alcohol-related brain damage: Clinical and experimental observations. *Acta Med Scand* 222 [suppl 717]: 19–26.

Carlen PL, Wilkinson DA, Wortzman G, Holgate R (1984) Partially reversible cerebral atrophy and functional improvement in recently abstinent alcoholics. *Can J Neurol Sci* 11: 441–4.

Cavanagh JB (1988) Lesion localisation: implications for the study of functional effects and mechanisms of action. *Toxicology* 49: 131–6.

Charness ME, Simon RP, Greenberg DA (1989) Ethanol and the nervous system. *New Engl J Med* 321: 442–54.

Conn HO (1993) Transjugular intrahepatic portal–systemic shunts: the state of the art. *Hepatology* 1: 148–58.

Courville CB (1955) *Los Angeles*: San Lucas Press.

Cragg B, Phillips S (1983) Toxic effects of alcohol on brain cells and alternative mechanisms of brain damage in alcoholism. *Aust Drug/Alc Rev* 2: 64–70.

Darnton-Hill I, Truswell AS (1990) Thiamin status of a sample of homeless clinic attenders in Sydney. *Med J Aust* 152: 5–9.

De la Monte SM (1988) Disproportionate atrophy of cerebral white matter in chronic alcoholics. *Arch Neurol* 45: 990–2.

Diemer NH (1978) Glial and neuronal changes in experimental hepatic encephalopathy. *Acta Neurol Scand* 58 Suppl 71: 1–144.

Freund G, Ballinger WE (1988a) Decrease of benzodiazepine receptors in frontal cortex of alcoholics. *Alcohol* 5: 275–82.

Freund G, Ballinger WE (1988b) Loss of cholinergic muscarinic receptors in the frontal cortex of alcohol abusers. *Alc Clin Exp Res* 12: 630–8.

Gottlieb B (1944) Acute nicotinic acid deficiency (anioacinosis). *Br Med J* 1: 392–3.

Hakim AM (1986) Effect of thiamine deficiency and its reversal on cerebral blood flow in the rat. Observations on the phenomena of hyperfusion, 'no reflow', and delayed hypoperfusion. *J Cereb Blood Flow Metab* 6: 79–85.

Hakim AM, Pappius HM (1983) Sequence of metabolic, clinical, and histological events in experimental thiamine deficiency. *Ann Neurol* 13: 365–75.

Halliday G, Baker K, Harper C (1995) The role of serotonin in alcohol-related brain damage. *Metab Brain Dis* 10: 25–30.

Halliday G, Ellis J, Harper C (1992) The locus coeruleus and memory: a study of chronic alcoholics with and without the memory impairment of Korsakoff's psychosis. *Brain Res* 598: 33–7.

Harper C (1979) Wernicke's encephalopathy: a more common disease than realised. *J Neurol, Neurosurg Psychiat* 42: 226–31.

Harper C, Corbett D (1990) A quantitative Golgi study of cortical neurons from alcoholic patients. *J Neurol Neurosurg Psychiat* 53: 865–1.

Harper C, Kril J (1985) Brain atrophy in chronic alcoholic patients: a quantitative pathological study. *J Neurol, Neurosurg Psychiat* 48: 211–17.

Harper C, Kril J (1989) Patterns of neuronal loss in the cerebral cortex in chronic alcoholic patients. *J Neurol Sci* 92: 81–9.

Harper C, Kril J, Daly J (1987) Are we drinking our neurones away? *Br Med J* 294: 534–6.

Harper CG (1980) Sudden, unexpected death and Wernicke's encephalopathy. A complication of prolonged intravenous feeding. *Aust N Z J Med* 10: 230–5.

Harper CG (1983) The incidence of Wernicke's encephalopathy in Australia – a neuropathological study of 131 cases. *J Neurol, Neurosurg Psychiat* 46: 593–8.

Harper CG, Giles M, Finlay-Jones R (1986) Clinical signs in the Wernicke–Korsakoff complex – a retrospective analysis of 131 cases diagnosed at necropsy. *J Neurol Neurosurg Psychiat* 49: 341–5.

Harper CG, Kril JJ (1992) *Neuropathological Changes in Alcoholics*. Washington, DC: US Department of Health and Human Services.

Hauw J-J, De Baecque C, Hausser-Hauw C, Serdaru M (1988) Chromatolysis in alcoholic encephalopathies. *Brain* 111: 843–57.

Hoyumpa AM (1980) Mechanisms of thiamin deficiency in chronic alcoholism. *Am J Clin Nutr* 33: 2750–61.

Ishii N, Nishihara Y (1981) Pellagra among chronic alcoholics: clinical and pathological study of 20 necropsy cases. *J Neurol, Neurosurg Psychiat* 44: 209–15.

Ishii N, Nishihara Y (1985) Pellagra encephalopathy among tuberculous patients: its relation to isoniazid therapy. *J Neurol, Neurosurg, Psychiat* 48: 628–34.

Jensen GB, Pakkenberg B (1993) Do alcoholics drink their neurons away? *Lancet* 342: 1201–4.

Jernigan TL, Butters N, DiTriaglia G, Schafer K, Smith T, Irwin M *et al* (1991) Reduced cerebral grey matter observed in alcoholics using magnetic resonance imaging. *Alcoholism: Clin Exp Res* 15: 418–27.

Jolliffe N (1941) Treatment of neuropsychiatric disorders with vitamins. *JAMA* 117: 1496–502.

Jolliffe N, Bowman K, Rosenblum L, Fein H (1940) Nicotinic acid deficiency encephalopathy. *JAMA* 114: 307–9.

Kato M, Hughes RD, Keays RT, Williams R (1992) Electron microscopic study of brain capillaries in cerebral edema from fulminant hepatic failure. *Hepatology* 15: 1060–6.

Kril JJ, Harper CG (1989) Neuronal counts from four cortical regions of alcoholic brains. *Acta Neuropath (Berl)* 79: 200–4.

Kulisevsky J, Pujol J, Balauzo J, Junque C, Dues J, Capdevilla AEA (1992) Pallidal hyperintensity on magnetic resonance imaging in cirrhotic patients: clinical correlations. *Hepatology* 16: 1382–8.

Lancaster FE (1992) Alcohol, nitric oxide and neurotoxicity: is there a connection? – a review. *Alc Clin Exp Res* 16: 539–41.

Langlais PJ, Mair RG (1990) Protective effects of the glutamate antagonist MK-801 on pyrithiamine-induced lesions and amino acid changes in rat brain. *J Neurosci* 10: 1664–74.

Langlais PJ, Zhang SX (1993) Extracellular glutamate is increased in thalamus during thiamine deficiency-induced lesions and is blocked by MK-801. *J Neurochem* 61: 2175–82.

Langlais PJ, Zhang SX, Weilersbacher G, Hough LB, Barke KE (1994) Rapid communication: histamine-mediated neuronal death in a rat model of Wernicke's encephalopathy. *J Neurosci Res* 38: 565–74.

Lavoie J, Giguere JF, Pomier Layaragues G, Butterworth RF (1987) Activities of neuronal and astrocytic marker enzymes in autopsied brain tissue from patients with hepatic encephalopathy. *Metab Brain Dis* 2: 283–90.

Lindboe D, Loberg E (1988) The frequency of WKS in alcoholics: a comparison between the 5-year periods 1975–1979 and 1983–1987. *J Neurol Sci* 88: 107–13.

Lishman WA (1981) Cerebral disorders in alcoholism. Syndromes of impairment. *Brain* 104: 1–20.

Lockwood AH, Yap EWH, Wong WH (1991) Cerebral ammonia metabolism in patients with severe liver disease and minimal hepatic encephalopathy. *J Cereb Blood Flow Metab* 11: 337–41.

Mair WGP, Warrington GK, Weiskrantz L (1979) Memory disorder in Korsakoff's psychosis. *Brain* 102: 749–83.

Mayes AR, Meudell PR, Mann D, Pickering A (1988) Locations of the lesions in Korsakoff's syndrome: neuropathological data on two patients. *Cortex* 24: 367–88.

McEntee WJ, Mair RG (1990) The Korsakoff syndrome: a neurochemical perspective. *Trends in Neurosci* 13: 340–4.

McMullen PA, Saint-Cyr JA, Carlen PL (1984) Morphological alterations in rat CA1 hippocampal pyramidal cell dendrites resulting chronic ethanol consumption and withdrawal. *J Comp Neurol* 225: 111–18.

Meldrum B, Garthwaite J (1991) Excitatory amino acid neurotoxicity and neurodegenerative disease. *Trends Pharmacol Sci* 11, Suppl: 54–62.

Mousseau DD, Perney P, Pomier Layargues G, Butterworth RF (1993) Selective loss of pallidal dopamine D_2 receptor density in hepatic encephalopathy. *Neurosci Lett* 162: 192–6.

Naeije R, Jacobovitz LF, Flament-Durand J (1978) Morel's laminar sclerosis. *Eur Neurol* 17: 155–9.

Norenberg MD (1994) Astrocyte response to CNS injury. *J Neuropathol Exp Neurol* 53: 213–20.

Norenberg MD, Neary JT, Norenberg LOB, McCarthy M (1990) Ammonia induced decrease in glial fibrillary acidic protein in cultured astrocytes. *J Neuropath Exp Neurol* 49: 399–405.

Oscar-Berman M, Hutner N (1993) Frontal lobe changes after chronic alcohol ingestion. In: Hunt WA, Nixon SJ. *Alcohol Induced Brain Damage*. Rockville: NIH Publications: 121–56.

Parsons OA (1987) Intellectual impairment in alcoholics: Persistent issues. *Acta Med Scand* 171: 33–46.

Pentney RJ (1982) Quantitative analysis of ethanol effects on Purkinje cell dendritic tree. *Brain Res* 249: 397–401.

Pfefferbaum A, Lim KO, Rosenbloom M (1992) Structural imaging of the brain in chronic alcoholism. In: Zakhari SW E. *Imaging in Alcohol Research*. Washington, DC: US Government Printing Office 99–120.

Phillips SC, Cragg BC (1984) Alcohol withdrawal causes a loss of cerebellar Purkinje cells in mice. *J Stud Alcohol* 45: 475–80.

Pilbeam CM, Anderson RM, Bhthal PS (1983) The brain in experimental portal–systemic encephalopathy. 1. Morphological changes in three animal models. *J Pathol* 140: 331–45.

Rabbe W (1990) *Effects of NH_4 on the Function of the CNS*. New York: Plenum Press.

Rindi G, Comincioli V, Reggiani C, Patrini C (1987) Nervous system thiamine metabolism in vivo. III. Influence of ethanol intake on the dynamics of thiamine and its phosphoesters in different brain regions and sciatic nerve of the rat. *Brain Res* 413: 23–35.

Romero I, Brown AW, Cavanagh JB, Nolan CC, Ray DE, Seville MP (1991) Vascular factor in the neurotoxic damage caused by 1,3-dinitrobenzene in the rat. *Neuropathol Appl Neurobiol* 17: 495–508.

Rosenblum WI, Feigin I (1965) The hemorrhagic component of Wernicke's Encephalopathy. *Arch Neurol* 13: 627–32.

Serdaru M, Hausser-Hauw C, Laplane D, Buge A, Castaigne P, Goulon M, *et al* (1988) The clinical spectrum of alcoholic pellagra encephalopathy. *Brain* 111: 829–42.

Sherlock S, (1981) Hepatic encephalopathy. *Acute (Fulminant) Hepatic failure*. Oxford: Blackwell Scientific Publications.

Sobel RA, DeArmond SJ, Forno LS, Eng LF (1981) Glial fibrillary acidic protein in hepatic encephalopathy: an immunohistochemical study. *J Neuropathol Exp Neurol* 40: 625–32.

Squire LR, Knowlton B, Musen G (1993) The structure and organization of memory. *Ann Rev Psychol* 44: 435–95.

Summers J, Pullan P, Kril J, Harper C (1991) Increased central immunoreactive β-endophin content in patients with Wenicke–Korsakoff syndrome and in alcoholics. *J Clin Pathol* 44: 126–9.

Teitelbaum JS, Zatorre R, Carpenter S, Gendron D, Evans A, Gjedde A *et al* (1990) Neurologic sequelae of domoic acid intoxication due to the ingestion of contaminated mussels. *New Engl J Med* 322: 1781–7.

Terry RD, Hansen LA (1987) Neocortical cell counts in normal human adult aging. *Ann Neurol* 21: 530–9.

Terry RD, Peck A, DeTeresa R, Schechter R, Horoupian DS (1981) Some morphological aspects of the brain in senile dementia of the Alzheimer type. *Ann Neurol* 10: 184–92.

Therrien G, Butterworth RF (1991) Cerebrospinal fluid amino acids in relation to neurological status in experimental portal–systemic encephalopathy. *Metab Brain Dis* 6: 65–73.

Tholen H (1971) Hironeden. Eine todesursache beim endogenen Leberkoma. *Klin Wochenschr* 50: 196–301.

Thomson AD (1978) Alcohol and nutrition. *Clin in Endocrinol Metab* 7: 405–28.

Tork I, Hornung J-P (1990) Raphe nuclei and the serotonergic system. In: Paxinos G. *The Human Nervous System*. San Diego: Academic Press 1001–22.

Torvik A (1987) Topographic distribution and severity of brain lesions in Wernicke's encephalopathy. *Clin Neuropathol* 6: 25–9.

Tuck RR, Jackson M (1991) Social, neurological and cognitive disorders in alcoholics. *Med J Aust* 155: 225–9.

Victor M, Adams RD (1985) *The Alcoholic Dementias*. Amsterdam: Elsevier Science Publishers.

Victor M, Adams RD, Collins GH (1971) *The Wernicke–Korsakoff Syndrome*. Oxford: Blackwell Scientific.

Victor M, Adams RD, Collins GH (1989) The Wernicke–Korsakoff Syndrome. Philadelphia: Davis.

von Hosslin D, Alzheimer A (1912) Ein Beitrag zur Klinik und pathologischen Anatomie der westphal-Strumpellschen Pseudosklerose. *Z Ges Neurol Psychiat* 8: 183–209.

Walker DW, Hunter BE, Abraham WC (1981) Neuroanatomical and functional deficits subsequent to chronic ethanol administration in animals. *Alcoholism: Clin Exp Res* 5: 267–82.

Walsh KW, Walsh KW (1985) *Understanding Brain Damage*. Edinburgh, Churchill Livingstone.

Wilcock G, Esiri M, Bowen D, Hughes A (1988) The differential involvement of subcortical nuclei in senile dementia of Alzheimer's type. *J Neurol Neurosurg Psychiat* 51: 842–9.

Wilson JD, Wilson JD (1991) *Vitamin Deficiency and Excess*. New York: McGraw-Hill Inc.

CHAPTER FOURTEEN

Dementia due to other metabolic diseases and toxins

M. M. Esiri

Conditions associated with hypoxia
Haematological conditions
Chronic renal failure
Hepatic disease
Pancreatic disorders
Vitamin B_{12} and folate deficiencies
Porphyria
Alexander's disease
Adult polyglucosan body disease (Lafora disease)
Kuf's disease (adult onset neuronal ceroid lipofuscinosis)
Cerebrotendinous xanthomatosis
Polycystic lipomembranous osteodysplasia with sclerosing leukoencephalopathy
Hypocalcaemia with calcification of the basal ganglia
Neuronal intranuclear inclusion disease
Adrenoleukodystrophy
GM_1 and GM_2 gangliosidosis
Gaucher's disease type 1
Niemann–Pick disease
Mucopolysaccharidosis type IIIB (San-filippo's disease)
Mitochondrial disorders
Leigh's encephalopathy
Metachromatic leukodystrophy
Fabry's disease
Krabbe's disease (globoid cell leukodystrophy)
Effects of drugs
Effects of environmental toxins

Metabolic derangements of the adult brain are better known for causing acute or subacute confusion or encephalopathy than dementia. Reversible confusion in a patient with bronchopneumonia is a commonplace occurrence in geriatric wards. However, when disturbed brain metabolism develops insidiously and persists for months or years, dementia may be the main clinical manifestation. Symptoms of impaired subcortical function are likely to be prominent: slowed responses, impaired arousal and attention, memory impairment, and mood changes. There may also be disturbance of motor function: tremor, myoclonus, chorea or alterations in limb tone, and epilepsy.

The acquired disorders giving rise to those disturbances are varied and, particularly in the elderly, common (Table 14.1). In addition, there is an increasing number of inherited diseases most commonly associated with mental retardation or dementia in infancy and childhood, that are now recognized occasionally to cause dementia as a presenting feature in adult life (Table 14.1) (Coker, 1991). Some conditions, for example, thyroid, parathyroid and adrenal disturbances, hyper- and hy-

Table 14.1. *Metabolic conditions associated with dementia in adults (modified after Cummings & Benson, 1992; Coker, 1991)*

Conditions associated with hypoxia
Anoxic/hypoxic anoxia*
  Pulmonary insufficiency
Stagnant anoxia*
  Cardiac disease
  Hyperviscosity states
Severe anaemic
  Post-anoxic dementia*
Chronic renal failure
Uraemic encephalopathy
Dialysis dementia
Hepatic diseases
Porto-systemic encephalopathy*
Inherited hepatolenticular degeneration*
Pancreatic diseases
Insulinoma and severe recurrent hypoglycaemia*
Vitamin deficiencies *
Thiamine/B1 (see Chapter 13)
B$_{12}$
Folate
Nicotinic acid (see Chapter 13)
Endocrine disease
Thyroid disturbance
Parathyroid disturbance
Adrenal disturbance
Pan hypopituitarism
Porphyria
Alexander's disease *
Lafora disease *
Kuf's disease *
Cerebrotendinous xanthomatosis *
Polycystic lipomembranous osteodysplasia with sclerosing
  leukoencephalopathy *
Neuronal intranuclear inclusion disease *
Adrenoleukodystrophy *
Gangliosidosis type III (GM$_1$)*
Gangliosidosis type II (GM$_2$)*
Gaucher's disease *
Niemann–Pick disease *
Mucopolysaccharidosis type II-B (San filippo's disease)*
Mitochondrial disorders *
Mitochondrial myopathy with ragged red fibres (MERRF)
Mitochondrial myopathy, encephalopathy, lactic acidosis
  and stroke-like episodes (MELAS)
Kearns–Sayre syndrome (KSS)
Metachromatic leukodystrophy *
Fabry's disease *
Krabbe's disease (Globoid cell leukodystrophy)*

Table 14.1. (*cont.*)

Acid maltase deficiency	
Effects of drugs	
anticholinergics	barbiturates
levodopa	neuroleptics
anticonvulsants	opiates*
methotrexate * and	amphotericin B*
other cancer chemotherapies	cyclosporin*
Effects of toxins	
Alcohol* (see Chapter 13)	
Aluminium*	
Arsenic	
Bismuth*	
Cadmium	
Carbon monoxide* (see Hypoxia, this chapter)	
Chromium	
Ethylene oxide*	
Lead*	
Mercury*	
Methyl bromide*	
Toluene*	
Trimethyl tin*	

*Structural neuropathology described.

pocalcaemia and the effects of a variety of drugs, produce no well-defined neuropathological changes. However, others do, as outlined below.

There are problems for the pathologist anxious not to miss cases of metabolic disease when examining brains from adult cases of dementia, some of which may not have had an adequate neurological work up. Although metabolic diseases are common, those giving rise to dementia with structural pathology are rare, probably comprising less than 2% of adult cases of progressive dementia coming to autopsy and thus, the wide range of inherited diseases is likely to be more familiar to paediatric neuropathologists and pathologists than to those dealing with adult neuropathology. Therefore, the advice of a paediatric pathologist colleague more experienced in diagnosing these diseases can be invaluable. In making a diagnosis of many of the inherited metabolic diseases, it is often necessary to examine snap frozen cryostat sections to search for stored materials that are leached out during fixation or paraffin embedding, so that, if an inherited disease is recognized as a possibility (e.g. there is a family history), it is important to freeze samples at autopsy. Samples taken from the fresh brain at autopsy for this purpose should include white matter as well as cerebral cortex. When taking blocks of fixed tissue for microscopy, areas of brain that appear macroscopically abnormal should be chosen and, in addition, a wide selection of grey and white matter from cerebrum, brainstem and cerebellum should be sampled. For full treatment of the neuropathology of these conditions a general textbook of neuropathology such as *Greenfield's Neuropathology* (Adams & Duchen, 1992) or Davis and Robertson's (1996) *Textbook of Neuropathology* should be consulted.

CONDITIONS ASSOCIATED WITH HYPOXIA

Usually dementia in common conditions associated with hypoxia, such as respiratory or cardiac disease, is reversible when the worst effects of the disease can be relieved. Under these conditions, no obvious structural sequelae in the nervous system result. However, after profound oxygen deprivation of the brain, as may occur following cardio-respiratory arrest or carbon monoxide poisoning, there may be structural pathology and incomplete return of function. Three levels of severity of sequelae can result: *brain death*, in which bodily functions can only be maintained artifically, *persistent vegetative state*, in which autonomic and brain stem function, but no higher cortical activity, is restored, and a *dementia syndrome*, in which a variable degree of loss of higher mental functions is the only sequela. In the latter syndrome there is *loss of neurons* in vulnerable parts of the cerebral cortex and hippocampus and possibly also in basal ganglia and thalamus (Adams & Graham, 1992). Purkinje cells of the cerebellum are also at high risk. In the cerebral cortex, the pyramidal neurons are vulnerable to damage, either in a diffuse, laminar or patchy distribution, or with accentuation at the depths of the cortical sulci and at the boundary zones of the main cortical arterial supply territories. Cortical layers 2, 3 and 5 containing pyramidal neurons are those most at risk (Fig. 14.1). In the hippocampus, the CA1 pyramidal neurons are particularly liable to be damaged or lost (Fig. 14.2). Depending on the severity and chronicity of the damage the macroscopic appearance of the brain may vary from normal to severely atrophic. Carbon monoxide poisoning tends to produce foci of necrosis in the globus pallidus which, when well established, are visible to the naked eye and later form cysts (Fig. 14.3). Neuron loss at these sites is accompanied by local microglial cell activation, capillary proliferation and reactive astrocytosis (Fig. 14.4). Acute neuronal damage is evidenced by eosinophilia and shrinkage of neuronal cytoplasm and basophilia of nuclei. Long after the

hypoxic episode, the remnants of some dead neurons may be seen in mummified form, impregnated with iron and calcium salts and appearing deeply basophilic in haematoxylin and eosin preparations (Fig. 14.5).

Rarely, *white matter damage* may also be seen following severe anoxia, particularly after carbon monoxide poisoning (Lapresle & Fardeau, 1966). White matter damage takes one or more of three forms and may occur in the absence of grey matter lesions. These are (1) perivascular foci occurring throughout the white matter of the corpus callosum, internal and external capsules and optic tracts; (2) diffuse damage to the centrum ovale; (3) plaque-like foci of demyelination in posterior and deep parts of the cerebral white matter, with myelin

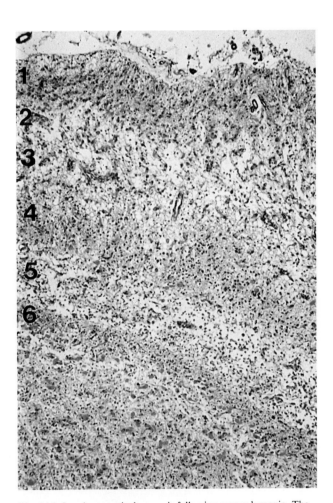

Fig. 14.1. Laminar cortical necrosis following severe hypoxia. The pial surface is at the top. The layers of the cortex are numbered on the left. Layers 2, 3 and 5 show the greatest damage. Haematoxylin and eosin stain.

sheaths around blood vessels being relatively spared. The third pattern tends to be seen in patients who undergo secondary deterioration with neuropsychiatric symptoms after initial recovery. The other two patterns are seen more in patients who remain comatose throughout the course of the illness.

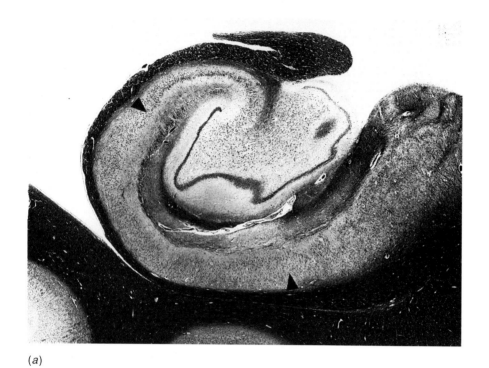

(a)

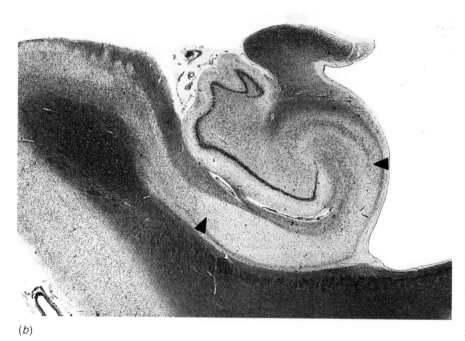

(b)

Fig. 14.2. The effect of severe hypoxia on the hippocampus. Low power view of luxol fast blue/cresyl violet stained sections of (a) normal and (b) hypoxic hippocampus. Note loss of large neurons in the CA1 sector (marked by arrow heads) in (b).

HAEMATOLOGICAL CONDITIONS

Any condition that interferes with the efficient delivery of oxygen and nutrients to the brain and impairs removal of its waste products is likely to adversely affect intellectual function. There are a number of haematological conditions which act in this way by increasing the viscosity of the blood and therefore reducing cerebral blood flow, or by reducing the oxygen carrying capacity of the blood.

Hyperviscosity syndromes which predispose to impaired cerebral blood flow include macroglobulinaemia, myeloma and polycythemia rubra vera. In cases of dementia suffering from such diseases there may be no specific neuropathological changes, or there may be evidence of hypoxia as described above, or of ischaemic damage due to thrombosis and infarction (Chapter 5).

Severe, chronic *anaemia* may give rise to the features of hypoxic damage described above. *Sickle cell anaemia* is, in addition, liable to produce multiple small cerebral infarcts due to sludging of deformed erythrocytes in small blood vessels. Severe anaemia from any cause may be associated with venous thrombosis and consequent haemorrhagic cerebral venous infarction.

CHRONIC RENAL FAILURE

There are many possible causes of altered mental state and dementia in patients with chronic renal failure (Cummings & Benson, 1992) (Table 14.2). As indicated in Table 14.2 the neuropathology of many of these conditions can be found in other parts of this book. In *uraemic encephalopathy* there are no specific changes to be found in the brain. White matter shows a non-specific diffuse astrocytosis. Cerebrovascular disease is common in renal failure so incidental cerebral infarcts may be found. Peripheral nerves may show evidence of a peripheral neuropathy with chronic axonal degeneration.

HEPATIC DISEASE

Acquired portal–systemic encephalopathy most commonly develops in those with cirrhosis of the liver. The pathogenesis of the encephalopathy is not well understood, but there are several types of compounds normally metabolized by the liver which accumulate in the blood in cirrhosis: ammonia, mercaptans, short-chain fatty acids and false neurotransmitter amines. Blood ammonia levels show the closest correlation with mental impairment, which tends to occur with blood levels above $3 \mu g/ml$. Glutamine, a metabolite of ammonia shows elevated levels in cerebrospinal fluid in encephalopathic patients.

The naked eye appearance of the brain in subjects with hepatic encephalopathy is often normal. Microscopically, there are characteristic changes: an alteration in the appearance of astrocytes and microcavitation and neuronal necrosis in the cerebral cortex. The astrocyte changes are discussed in Chapter 13. The changes in the cerebral cortex take the form of patchy laminar or pseudo-laminar necrosis with loss of neurons particularly in the deep layers of the cortex (Fig. 14.6). The microcavitation is often well seen at the junction between cortex and white matter and is due to focal oedema (Fig. 14.7). It may also be seen in the basal ganglia and cerebellum.

Wilson's disease (inherited hepatolenticular degeneration) tends to present either in children with clinical features of liver disease, or in adults with neurological symptoms of an extrapyramidal movement disorder. However, it occasionally presents with psychosis or dementia. It is an autosomal recessive disease of copper metabolism diagnosed by finding a low blood caeruloplasmin level, high tissue and urine copper levels and a

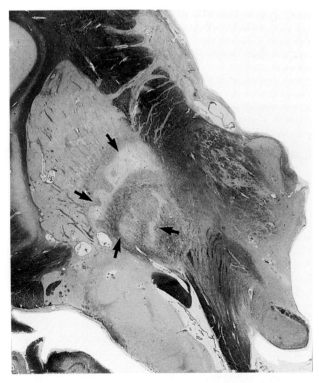

Fig. 14.3. Low power view of myelin stained section of the basal ganglia region from a case of carbon monoxide poisoning. Foci of necrosis in the globus pallidus appear pale (arrows).

Keyser–Fleischer ring in the iris. It produces a cirrhotic liver and changes in the brain which predominantly affect the basal ganglia (Duchen & Jacobs, 1992). The putamen and caudate nuclei show a brown discolouration and shrinkage and the putamen may show cystic degeneration visible in brain slices. Microscopic examin-ation shows changes that are maximal in the putamen, consisting of foci of neuronal loss and a prominence of astrocytes which resemble the type 2 astrocytes of acquired hepatic encephalopathy described in Chapter 13 (Fig. 13.4). There are also occasional, larger, multi-nucleated glial cells (Alzheimer type 1 glia). The large

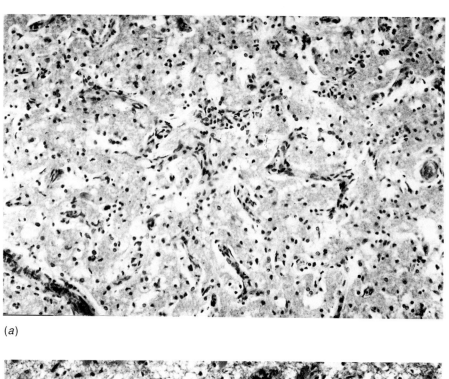

(a)

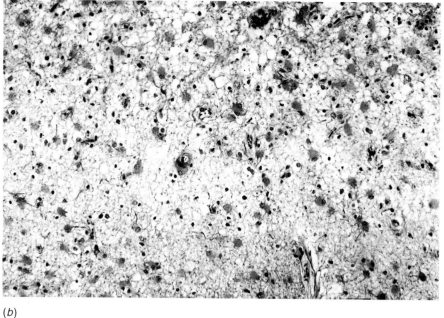

(b)

Fig. 14.4. (a) Proliferation of capillaries surrounded by macrophages, microglial cells and macroglia but no surviving neurons in cortex following hypoxia. (b) shows astrocytic reaction at a slightly later stage. Haematoxylin and eosin stain.

Table 14.2. *Possible causes of dementia in patients with chronic renal failure (after Cummings & Benson, 1992)*

Chronic renal failure only
Uraemic encephalopathy
Electrolyte imbalance
Anaemia
Hypertensive encephalopathy or cerebrovascular disease
(Chapter 5)
Drug accumulation
CNS effects of underlying cause of renal failure e.g. SLE
Chronic renal failure with dialysis
Dialysis dementia (see Aluminium)
Subdural haematoma (Chapter 19)
Emboli from shunt (Chapter 5)
Vitamin deficiency
Chronic renal failure with transplantation
Steroid psychosis
Progresive multifocal leukoencephalopathy (Chapter 17)
Lymphoma (Chapter 19)
Chronic glial nodule meningoencephalitis (e.g. due to CMV)
(Chapter 19)

necrotic foci show cystic degeneration with macrophage infiltration. The cytoplasm of the macrophages contains neutral fat, stainable in frozen sections with oil Red O or Sudan black stains, and iron. Petechial haemorrhages or their sequelae, perivascular macrophages containing iron, and perivascular fibrosis, are common, and capillary endothelial cells appear unduly prominent and swollen. Perivascular and parenchymal deposits of copper may be demonstrable with rhodanine or rubeanic acid stains. Other sites, besides the putamen, that are liable to be affected are the globus pallidus, thalamus and subthalamic nucleus. *Opalski cells* may be found occasionally, scattered in these regions. These are large cells with rounded cytoplasmic outline, granular cytoplasm, which is sometimes also vacuolated, and a small, darkly staining nucleus. The cerebellar dentate nuclei and cerebral cortex may additionally show foci of neuron loss. These changes may be considerably muted in patients treated long term with penicillamine.

PANCREATIC DISORDERS

Recurrent episodes of severe hypoglycaemia sufficient to cause structural damage to the brain are most often associated with excess insulin secretion by an islet cell tumour of the pancreas. This can cause progressive or episodic memory disturbance and personality change with aggression, apathy and emotional lability. In contrast, episodes of hypoglycaemia in diabetics only exceptionally are severe enough to produce structural damage to the brain and this is, as likely as not, after intentional overdose of insulin.

Severe hypoglycaemia produces changes in the central nervous system that closely mirror those due to severe anoxia, though with some differences of emphasis (Adams & Graham, 1992). If damage is widespread, and occurred more than a few months before death, there

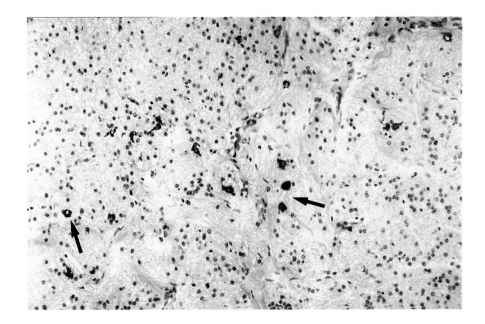

Fig. 14.5. Late effects of hypoxia on cerebral cortex. The tissue is intensely gliotic (small nuclei) but contains a few residual calcified, dead, neuronal remnants (arrows). Haematoxylin and eosin stain.

may be severe cerebral cortical atrophy. Pyramidal cortical neurons at the depths of sulci are particularly liable to be lost (Fig. 14.8), usually in a patchy distribution, with the temporal neocortex and striatum and the outer cortical laminae bearing the brunt of the damage. In contrast, Purkinje cells in the cerebellum and pyra-

midal neurons in the hippocampus are relatively spared. As with hypoxia, in the acute stage, the affected neurons show shrinkage and eosinophilia while, at a later stage, loss of neurons, microglial activation, astrocytosis and vascular capillary proliferation mark the sites of damage. Diffuse demyelination has also been described.

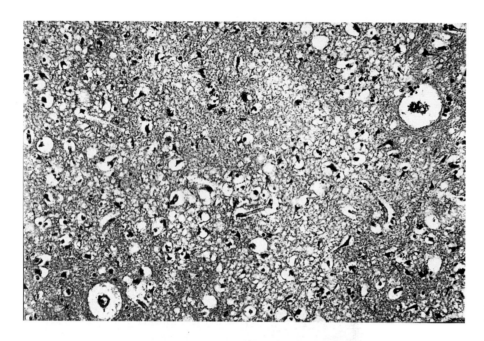

Fig. 14.6. Acute neuronal necrosis with shrinkage in large cortical pyramid cells in hepatic encephalopathy. Haematoxylin and eosin stain.

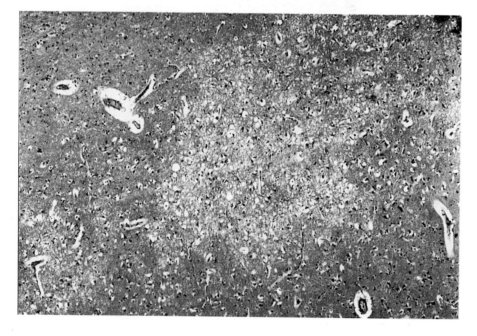

Fig. 14.7. Focus of microvacuolation of deep cerebral cortex in hepatic encephalopathy.

VITAMIN B$_{12}$ AND FOLATE DEFICIENCIES

Neurological manifestations of vitamin B$_{12}$ deficiency include dementia as well as peripheral neuropathy, myelopathy and optic neuropathy (Pallis & Lewis, 1974; Jacobs & Le Quesne, 1992). In man, vitamin B$_{12}$ deficiency is usually due to pernicious anaemia in which there is lack of production of intrinsic factor, a glycoprotein required for vitamin B$_{12}$ to bind to in order to be absorbed. The main cerebral manifestations are slowed mental reactions, confusion, memory defect and depression. These may show fluctuation in severity and can precede any haematological evidence of vitamin B$_{12}$ deficiency. Vitamin B$_{12}$ deficiency is present when the serum level is less than 100 pg per ml.

The cerebral and, better known and more common, spinal cord ('subacute combined degeneration') lesions of vitamin B$_{12}$ deficiency are similar and affect white matter. The cerebral lesions may not be detectable with the naked eye, but are seen in sections of the deep cerebral white matter. They have been described in only a relatively small number of cases. There is patchy but widespread loss of myelin, characteristically perivascular in distribution, with swelling between the myelin lamellae of surviving myelin sheaths and preservation of axons. Degeneration of the myelin is accompanied by focal collections of lipid-containing macrophages and a mild astrocytic reaction.

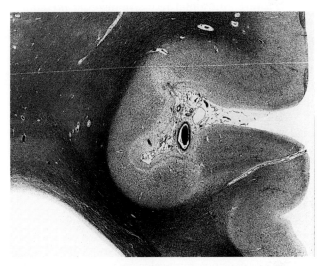

Fig. 14.8. Low power view of cerebral cortex from a patient who suffered an episode of severe hypoglycaemia. There is laminar necrosis affecting the cortex near the depth of the sulcus. Luxol fast blue/cresyl violet stain.

The spinal cord lesions commence at the thoracic level and chiefly affect the posterior and lateral white matter columns. From the thoracic level, they may spread upwards and downwards and into the anterior white columns. As in the cerebrum, there is demyelination, with a bubbly or honeycombed appearance to those myelin sheaths that remain. Axonal degeneration may occur in severe or long-standing cases.

Folate deficiency

Folate deficiency is present when the serum level is less than 2 μg per ml. In-born errors of folate metabolism can closely mimic the neurological manifestations of vitamin B$_{12}$ deficiency. Folate and vitamin B$_{12}$ both participate in the same sequence of biochemical reactions central to methyl group metabolism. Dietary folate deficiency much more frequently causes haematological than neurological disturbances, and its causal relationship with neurological disease is controversial. However, psychiatric disturbance in the elderly has been associated with folate depletion (Girdwood, 1968).

Pathogenesis of vitamin B$_{12}$ and folate nervous system lesions

A deficiency of methyl group metabolism is thought to be important in the pathogenesis of neurological disease due to vitamin B$_{12}$ and folate deficiencies. Methyl groups are needed for normal cell membrane stability and for the biosynthesis of choline, an important constituent of myelin. Vitamin B$_{12}$ is an essential co-factor for two enzymes involved in methyl group metabolism: methylmalonyl CoA mutase and methionine synthetase. The latter enzyme is also folate dependent.

PORPHYRIA

Porphyrias are genetic disorders in which there is over-production and excretion of porphyrins and their precursors. Neurological manifestations occur in the dominantly inherited acute intermittent, variegate and coproporphyria forms. No specific changes have been described in the brain, although there are commonly multiple foci of softening in the cerebrum, the origin of which has generally been considered to be ischaemia (Duchen & Jacobs, 1992). There is also a 'dying back' peripheral neuropathy with distal axonal degeneration and loss of and chromatolysis in anterior horn cells. In addition, posterior column axons are lost.

ALEXANDER'S DISEASE

This rare disease usually presents in infancy or childhood. A rare case has been described in a 39 year-old with mental retardation, ataxia, dysarthria and dementia (Walls et al., 1984). The brain in Alexander's disease may be somewhat enlarged, and the white matter is soft, discoloured and jelly-like. Microscopy shows demyelination and rarefaction of white matter with little or no sparing of subcortical fibres. The distinctive feature of the condition is the presence of vast numbers of Rosenthal fibres, condensations of astrocytic glial fibres, many of them arranged around blood vessels.

ADULT POLYGLUCOSAN BODY DISEASE (LAFORA DISEASE)

This is a rare autosomal recessive disease with onset of symptoms usually in the second decade (Gray et al., 1988). Presentation is most frequently with generalized seizures and myoclonus followed by dementia. Macroscopically, the brain shows only mild cerebral atrophy. Microscopically, there is an abundance of concentric inclusions occurring in neuronal cytoplasm, axons, dendrites and lying free in the neuropil of the brain. These bodies, which closely resemble corpora amylacea, are most numerous in the thalamus, globus pallidus, substantia nigra, superior olives, brain stem reticular formation, lateral geniculate bodies, dentate nuclei and pre- and post-central cortical gyri. The inclusions are stained intensely by PAS and by stains for acid muco-polysaccharides. They appear basophilic with haematoxylin and eosin stain. Outside the brain, they are found in skeletal muscle and liver. Biopsy of these tissues can enable a diagnosis to be made. The biochemical basis of the disease has not been elucidated.

KUF'S DISEASE (ADULT ONSET NEURONAL CEROID LIPOFUSCINOSIS)

Kuf's disease is the adult form of neuronal ceroid lipofuscinosis. Most cases are inherited recessively. It presents in early adult life with dementia, behavioural change and sometimes with violent psychosis. Motor disturbance, myoclonus, facial dyskinesia and ataxia may also be present. Diagnosis depends on finding the characteristic curvilinear or finger-print inclusions interspersed with eosinophilic granules in brain neurons (Lake, 1992). Unlike juvenile forms of neuronal ceroid lipofuscinosis, there is no retinal degeneration, and no storage of abnormal material outside the brain. Macroscopically, the brain at autopsy appears atrophic and the leptomeninges thickened. The cerebral cortex is narrowed, and the white matter abnormally firm and gliotic. Microscopic sections show some neuron loss, reactive gliosis and microglial activation. Some surviving neur-

ons contain prominent granular material with histochemical characteristics of lipfuscin, PAS-positive and sudan black-positive with strong autofluorescence. The stored material contains a proteolipid that consitutes subunit C of the mitochondrial ATP synthase.

CEREBROTENDINOUS XANTHOMATOSIS

This is an autosomal recessive condition in which there is a deficiency of liver mitochrondrial 26-hydroxylase deficiency which causes decreased bile acid formation and increased levels of bile acid intermediates including the high density lipoprotein cholestanol in serum and tissues (Bjorkhem & Skrede, 1990). Xanthones form in tendons, cataracts occur and deposits of cholesterol in brain lead to dementia, ataxia, long tract signs and pseudobulbar palsy. Neurological manifestations commence usually in the second and third decade, and progress to death in the fourth or fifth decades. The diagnosis can be made by demonstrating high levels of cholestanol in serum or tissues. The cholesterol deposits in brain discolour the white matter and lead to formation of cholesterol clefts in microscopic sections of white matter. These may be accompanied by a local foreign body giant cell reaction.

POLYCYSTIC LIPOMEMBRANOUS OSTEODYSPLASIA WITH SCLEROSING LEUKOENCEPHALOPATHY

This is a rare autosomal recessive disorder presenting with bone pain due to cysts and pathological fractures in early adult life. This symptom can be overlooked. Dementia and focal neurological symptoms develop in the fourth decade and lead to death usually in the fifth decade. The neurological deterioration is due to gliosis in subcortical white matter sometimes with calcification in vessel walls (Sourander, 1970). The diagnosis can be made on biopsies of bone and skin, which contain characteristic folding and wrinkling of the cell membranes of fat cells (Bird et al., 1983).

HYPOCALCAEMIA WITH CALCIFICATION OF THE BASAL GANGLIA

Dementia may be seen in hypoparathyroidism and other conditions causing hypocalcaemia. Extrapyramidal symptoms are also sometimes present. Increased amounts of calcium are found predominantly in the basal ganglia, internal capsule, lateral thalamic nuclei and dentate nuclei of the cerebellum (Fig. 14.9) (Oppenheimer & Esiri, 1992). The cerebral and cerebellar cortex may also be affected. The calcium deposits are detected as grittiness on slicing the brain. Microscopically, they are found in the walls of capillaries as calcospherites, and as more diffuse deposits or in the walls of larger vessels (Fig. 14.10). There is attenuation of adjacent neuropil but little astrocytic or microglial cell reaction.

NEURONAL INTRANUCLEAR INCLUSION DISEASE

This is a progressive neurological disease of unknown cause in which large numbers of eosinophilic intranuclear inclusion bodies (Marinesco bodies) are found in neurons and glia of the central and autonomic nervous systems. Children or adults may be affected. Adults present with dementia and a movement disorder resembling Huntington's chorea. Death usually occurs 5–20 years later.

The intranuclear inclusions are 3–13 μm across, eosinophilic, sharply demarcated and surrounded by a clear halo. They may be most easily found in astrocytes. They may show autofluorescence but do not stain with PAS, Sudan black or silver stain and they are immunoreactive for ubiquitin but negative for actin, microtubule and neurofilament antigens (Munoz-Garcia & Ludwin, 1986). Ultrastructurally, the bodies are not

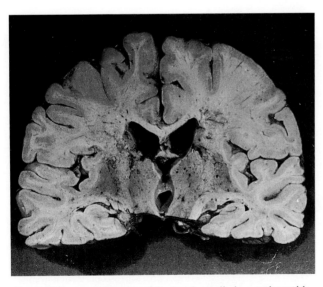

Fig. 14.9. Heavy calcification of the basal ganglia in a patient with progressive dementia. Coronal slice showing disrupted tissue in basal ganglia, and thalamus.

membrane bound and consist of material containing 8.5–9.5 nm diameter filaments (Haltia et al., 1984; Weidenheim & Dickson, 1995).

ADRENOLEUKODYSTROPHY

This is a sex-linked disorder due to deficiency of a peroxisomal enzyme, lignoceroyl CoA synthetase which is needed for the beta oxidation of very long-chain fatty acids (Naidu & Moser, 1990). Most cases present in childhood but a few present later with a progressive spastic paraparesis (myelopathy), peripheral neuropathy or dementia. Mild symptoms may be displayed in carrier females. Addison's disease is clinically evident in only 20% of sufferers at the time of neurological presentation. Diagnosis can be made by estimation of very long-chain fatty acids in serum.

At autopsy, the brain appears normal or mildly atrophic to external examination but on slicing shows marked, diffuse abnormality of the white matter which appears discoloured and gliotic (Fig. 14.11).

Microscopy shows diffuse demyelination of cerebral white matter with relative sparing of axons, and marked reactive astrocytosis (Fig. 14.12), macrophage and microglial cell activation and, in areas of active demyelination, neutral fat in phagocytes and an intense perivascular lymphocytic infiltrate (Griffin et al., 1985). Areas of chronic demyelination show loss of oligodendrocytes. In the spinal cord there is loss of fibres in pyramidal tracts and, sometimes loss of fibres in posterior columns also. Ultrastructurally, macrophages in affected cerebral white matter and peripheral nerves, and cortical cells of the adrenal gland show typical trilaminar inclusions. The adrenal glands typically show atrophy of the cortex but occasionally display a reactive hyperplasia. At the light microscope level, adrenal cortical cells show a fibrillary, striated appearance of the cytoplasm which is characteristic of the disease.

GM$_1$ AND GM$_2$ GANGLIOSIDOSIS

There is a rare adult form of GM$_1$ gangliosidosis, an autosomal recessive disease which presents in adults with dementia, dysarthria, gait disturbance and limb rigidity (Nakano et al., 1985). At autopsy the brain may appear macroscopically normal but microscopy shows ballooned neurons with pale cytoplasm and eccentrically placed nuclei (Fig. 14.13). Similar swollen neurons are present in myenteric and submucosal plexuses of the gut. The condition is due to deficiency of the lysosomal enzyme β galactosidase which may be assayed in white blood cells, cultured fibroblasts or, for pre-natal diagnosis, amniotic fluid cells. Ultrastructural appearances are similar to those in GM_2 gangliosidosis.

An adult form of the autosomal recessive storage disorder, *GM$_2$ gangliosidosis* is seen almost exclusively in Ashkenazi Jews. It is due to partial (<15% of normal) deficiency of the lysosomal enzyme hexosaminidase A (Argov & Navon, 1984). In addition to dementia there are likely to be upper and lower motor neuron manifestations and cerebellar ataxia and psychosis. Macroscopically, the brain shows loss of the normally clear distinction between grey and white matter but may be otherwise unremarkable. Microscopically, there are swollen, ballooned neurons similar to those seen in GM_1, gangliosidosis. These are present in sensory and autonomic ganglia as well as in the brain. The cytoplasm appears pale and foamy and contains excess PAS-positive, Sudan black-positive stored material, and excess acid phosphatase activity. Ultrastructurally, the stored material consists of close-packed membrane-bound lysosomal structures filled with concentric lamellae. Diagnosis can be made by assaying hexosaminidase A in white blood cells or cultured fibroblasts.

GAUCHER'S DISEASE, TYPE 1

Type 1 Gaucher's disease is an autosomal recessive disease, in adults presenting with dementia and psychosis. Some also suffer from seizures of myoclonic or generalized type and supranuclear gaze palsy (Neil, Glew & Peters, 1979). They are also likely to have splenomegaly, thrombocytopenia, and bone pain and erosion. Characteristic foam cells can be found in the bone marrow, and a diagnosis can be made by assaying for the enzyme that is deficient in this condition, β-glucocerebrosidase in white blood cells. Macroscopically, the brain appears normal at autopsy, but microscopically, collections of Gaucher's cells can be found in cerebral cortex, basal ganglia, brain stem and cerebellum. These are large macrophages measuring 20–100 μm across, some of them multinucleated. They contain coarsely fibrillary or striated cytoplasm and an eccentrically placed nucleus. Material stored in the cytoplasm is PAS positive and Sudan black negative. Acid phosphatase activity is excessive in the cytoplasm of these cells. Ultrastructurally, they contain twisted tubular cytoplasmic inclusions.

NIEMANN–PICK DISEASE

Niemann–Pick disease is an autosomal recessive disease in which there is accumulation of sphingomyelin due to a deficiency of sphingomyelinase or deficient cholesterol esterification. Cases with partial deficiencies can present as young adults with dementia and ataxia together with variable enlargement of liver and spleen (Fink *et al.*, 1989). The brain may show slight atrophy and firmness

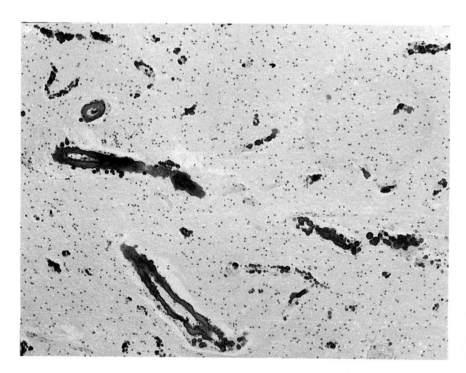

Fig. 14.10. Microscopic section from the case shown in Fig. 14.9 showing calcification in vessel walls and parenchyma.

of the white matter macroscopically. Neurons and glial cells in a widespread distribution show ballooned swollen cytoplasm and there is infiltration of the brain, particularly white matter, by large foamy, macrophages 20–90 μm across. Similar foamy macrophages infiltrate other organs and bone marrow. These macrophages contain either sphingomyelin, which gives a positive reaction in fresh cytostat sections with Sudan black and ferric haematoxylin, or material that is only weakly Sudan black positive. The deposits are also PAS positive and, in group 1 cases that lack sphingomyelinase, show red birefringence under polarized light after Sudan black staining. Acid phosphatase reaction is strongly positive around the foamy vacuoles. By electron microscopy the inclusions consist of loosely arranged lipid lamellae

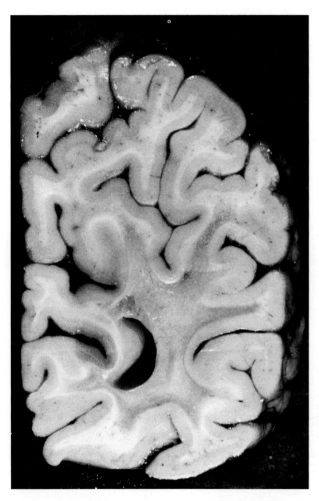

Fig. 14.11. Adrenoleukodystrophy. Appearance of diffusely discoloured and gliotic cerebral white matter.

contained in membrane-bound vacuoles. In group 2 cases, these are accompanied by dense osmiophilic inclusions.

MUCOPOLYSACCHARIDOSIS TYPE IIIB (SAN-FILIPPO'S DISEASE)

This is another autosomal recessive disease presenting usually in childhood with coarse features, organomegaly and dementia. Some cases have had onset of dementia in the third and fourth decades. (Van Schrojenstein – De Valk & Van de Kamp, 1987). Macroscopically, the brain may appear normal, but perivascular spaces may be unusually prominent in brain slices. These spaces are the site of leaking out of highly water-soluble acid mucopolysaccharides from perivascular macrophages. The material can be demonstrated in snap frozen fresh cryostat sections using a metachromatic stain. Sections of the brain may show, in addition to the perivascular macrophages, some neuronal swelling in cerebral cortex, hippocampus, basal ganglia and thalamus. The stored neuronal material is not mucopolysaccharide but gangliosides, and is Sudan black positive, Luxol fast blue positive and PAS positive. In some cases peripheral as well as central neurons contain this stored material. Ultrastructurally, the perivascular macrophages contain numerous empty cytoplasmic vacuoles with a few membrane fragments, while neurons contain gangliosides resembling material seen in the gangliosidoses (see above).

MITOCHONDRIAL DISORDERS

Mitochondrial cytopathies (encephalomyopathies)

There are three relatively well-defined neurological syndromes associated with primary abnormalities of mitochrondrial structure, function and DNA, that have been described from many centres worldwide: the Kearns–Sayre syndrome (KSS), myoclonic epilepsy with ragged red fibres (MERRF) and mitochondrial myopathy, encephalopathy, lactic acidosis and stroke-like episodes (MELAS). A syndrome of neuropathy, ataxia, retinitis pigmentosa and dementia (NARP) has also been described but seems much less common (Holt et al., 1990). All these syndromes are rare and present in childhood or early adult life. Dementia may be a feature of any of them though, except for NARP, is usually a relatively minor one (DiMauro et al., 1985; Petty, Harding & Morgan-Hughes, 1986). An abnormally elevated serum lactate concentration at rest or after exercise and skeletal muscle ragged red fibres can be found in KSS, MERRF and MELAS, but neither of these features is essential for diagnosis. Abnormal mitochondria have been demonstrated in brain in a few cases, for example, in the cells of the cerebellar cortex and dentate nuclei in MERRF (Fukuhara, 1991).

The mitochondrial cytopathies MERRF, MELAS and NARP are maternally transmitted. KSS is characteristically sporadic. Abnormalities of mitochondrial DNA (point mutations or deletions) have been demon-

strated for all these syndromes (mitochondrial DNA is of course supplied to offspring solely from the mother). Mitochondrial DNA codes for some of the polypeptides of the electron transport chain (the remainder being coded for by nuclear DNA) and codes for the specific mitochondrial ribosomal and transfer RNAs. Biochemical defects of mitochondrial metabolism involving respiratory chain enzyme defects have been demonstrated frequently in tissues from patients with mitochondrial

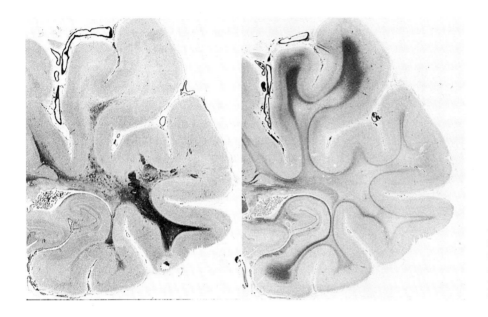

Fig. 14.12. Adrenoleukodystrophy. Adjacent sections of temporal lobe stained for myelin (*right*) and gliosis (*left*). There is diffuse demyelination and gliosis which is particularly prominent in middle and inferior temporal gyri white matter.

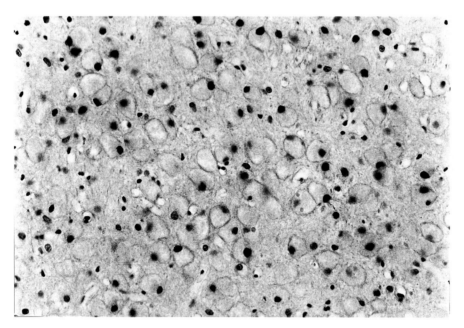

Fig. 14.13. GM$_1$ gangliosidosis. Ballooned pontine nuclei neurons. PAS stain.

cytopathies, but the relationship between an individual enzyme defect and the mode of clinical presentation is not entirely clear. Two factors are thought to account for the phenotypic variability. The first is that point mutations can be in genes coding for mitochondrial tRNAs (e.g. MELAS, MERRF) (Shoffner, 1991) and large deletions (as in KSS) lead to a lack of tRNAs required for translation, causing variably impaired mitochondrial respiratory chain protein synthesis (DiMauro *et al.*, 1991). Secondly, tissues containing mitochondrial DNA mutations usually also contain some normal mitochondrial DNA as well (i.e. they are heteroplasmic), and the proportions of the two vary from one tissue to another (Shanske *et al.*, 1990; Ponzetto *et al.*, 1990). The expression of the abnormal biochemical phenotype is a function of the proportion of mutant mitochondrial DNA. The manner in which these diseases arise and progress remains obscure, but is the subject of much continuing research. Apart from the abnormal brain mitochondria, not found in all cases, in neurons or endothelial and vascular muscle cells (Adachi *et al.*, 1973; Ohama *et al.*, 1987; Ihara *et al.*, 1989), there are no specific changes in the brain, but a number of different pathological changes have been found. Thus, MERRF has features of a system degeneration with cerebellar gliosis, neuronal loss in the dentate nucleus and atrophy of the inferior olives (Berkovic *et al.*, 1989; Fukuhara, 1991). In MELAS, lesions resembling cerebral infarcts may be found together with mineral deposits, neuronal degeneration and status

spongiosus particularly of grey matter. Changes in the CNS in KSS include status spongiosus of white matter, neuronal degeneration, astrocytosis and in some cases demyelination (Sparaco *et al.*, 1993). Samples of skeletal muscle frequently show the characteristic ragged red fibres – so named for the red reaction with a trichrome stain of the abnormally large clusters of mitochondria that accumulate in some muscle fibres. These same fibres show an excess of histochemically demonstrated mitochondrial enzymes succinic dehydrogenase and nicotinic acid dehydrogenase (Fig. 14.14). With electron microscopy, they show enlarged and structurally abnormal mitochondria containing 'parking lot' inclusions or concentric cristae (Fig. 14.15). Absence of ragged red fibres in muscle of some patients with genetically confirmed diagnoses may result from differences in levels of mutant mitochondrial DNA in the CNS and muscle or effects of variable genetic or environmental backgrounds.

LEIGH'S ENCEPHALOPATHY

This rare, often familial, condition usually presents in infancy or childhood but occasionally in adults. A wide variety of neurological symptoms and signs can occur, and these may include cognitive impairment, though hypotonia and respiratory disturbances are more prominent. At autopsy, the brain usually appears externally unremarkable, but multiple small foci of softening and brown discolouration may be visible in slices of the

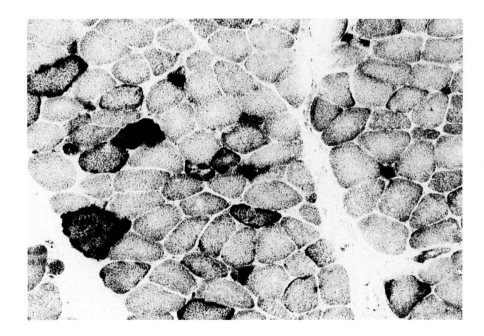

Fig. 14.14. 'Ragged red' muscle fibres in mitochondrial cytopathy. Excessive reaction product for the mitochondrial enzyme succinic dehydrogenase in some of the fibres.

fixed brain stem and basal ganglia. In histological sections microscopic foci of grey matter necrosis, sometimes with cyst formation, macrophage infiltration, capillary proliferation and pericapillary haemorrhages with, in chronic lesions, pericapillary fibrosis, are characteristic findings. The foci resemble areas of damage in Wernicke's encephalopathy (Chapter 13), but they spare the mamillary bodies and are found particularly as symmetrical foci in the brain stem (Fig. 14.16) and lack evidence of haemorrhage (Cavanagh & Harding, 1994). Lesions can be widespread with involvement of cerebral and cerebellar cortex, deep cerebral grey matter and spinal cord.

The aetiology of Leigh's encephalopathy seems to be heterogeneous with different mechanisms demonstrated in individual cases. The commonest defects described are in two mitochondrial enzymes: the pyruvate dehy-

drogenase complex (De Vivo *et al.*, 1978; Kretzschmar *et al.*, 1986) and cytochrome C oxidase (Willems *et al.*, 1977; Van Coster *et al.*, 1991). Occasional cases are said to resemble cases of mitochondrial cytopathy and have ragged red skeletal muscle fibres (Crosby & Chou, 1974; Egger *et al.*, 1982).

METACHROMATIC LEUKODYSTROPHY

Metachromatic leukodystrophy is an autosomal recessive disorder due to deficiency of the lysosomal enzyme arylsulphatase A. Most cases present in infancy or childhood but, in a few, the presentation is in adult life with personality change, psychosis or cognitive deficit (Waltz, Harik & Kaufman, 1987). At autopsy examination the brain may appear externally normal or show only slight atrophy. On slicing there is discolouration and undue firmness of the white matter, occasionally

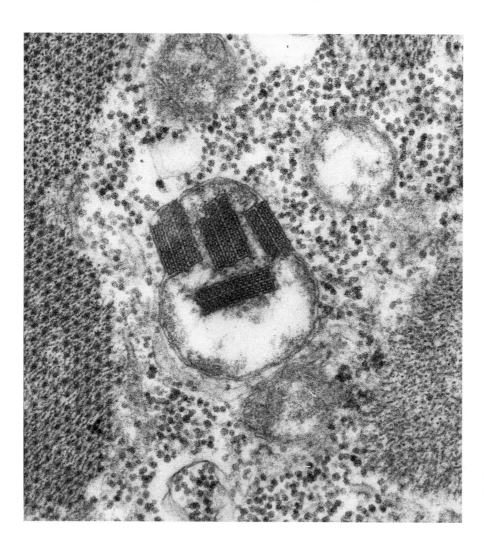

Fig. 14.15. Enlarged abnormal mitochondrion containing paracrystalline inclusions in mitochondrial myopathy. Uranyl acetate and lead citrate stain.

with cavitations in the region of the lentiform nuclei and internal capsules. On microscopy there is loss of myelin with relative sparing of axons and diffuse gliosis. The white matter is also infiltrated with macrophages which, in fresh cryostat sections, can be seen to contain meta-chromatic cytoplasmic granules (Fig. 14.17). Similar stored granules are found in some neurons in the basal ganglia, brain stem and cerebellum, but not usually in the cerebral cortex or peripheral ganglionic neurons. In paraffin sections the macrophages have PAS-positive cytoplasm, but many of the metachromatic granules are lost. Oligodendrocytes in affected white matter are reduced in number. The stored material in the metachro-matic granules consists ultrastructurally of stacks of membranous discs, concentric or radial lamellae, paired membranes or zebra bodies. Diagnosis of the condition during life can be made by assaying the enzyme arylsul-phatase A in blood leukocytes or cultured fibroblasts.

FABRY'S DISEASE

This is a sex-linked disorder due to deficiency of alpha galactosidase, another lysosomal enzyme. Psychosis and cognitive change occasionally develop in early adult life (Kaye *et al.*, 1988). More common features are pain in the extremities, angiokeratomas of the trunk and cor-

neal or lens opacities. Later features are cardiac disease, renal failure and strokes. These are associated with widespread deposits of trihexosylceramide, particularly in vascular endothelial and smooth muscle cells. In fresh frozen cryostat sections the stored material is PAS positive, Sudan black positive and birefringent. Acid phosphatase activity in swollen, affected cells is strongly positive. Stored material is also present in swollen neurons in the amygdala, hypothalamus, brain stem and intermediolateral column neurons of the spinal cord, and in sensory and autonomic ganglia. The brain may also show multiple infarcts of varying age related to the vascular pathology. Peripheral nerves may show loss of small diameter myelinated fibres. Stored material is also present in perineurial and endoneurial cells of peripheral nerves. On electron microscopy the stored material consists of densely stacked lamellae and occasional tubular inclusions. The deficiency of alpha galactosidase can be demonstrated in cultured fibroblasts.

KRABBE'S DISEASE (GLOBOID CELL LEUKODYSTROPHY)

This is an autosomal recessive disorder due to reduced activity of the lysosomal enzyme galactocerebroside beta galactosidase. Most cases present in infancy or

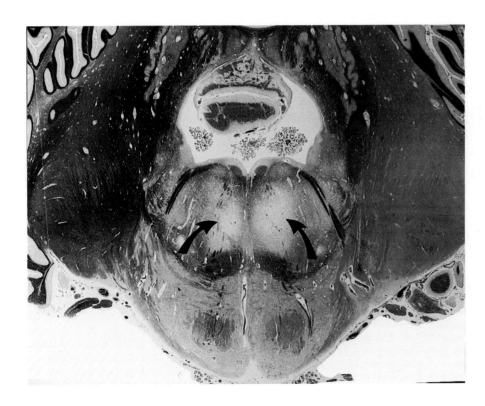

Fig. 14.16. Symmetrical foci of rarefaction (arrows) in the tegmentum of the pons in Leigh's encephalopathy. Myelin stain.

childhood. Occasional cases with onset in adult life have been described (Volk & Adachi, 1970). In these cases there were motor symptoms followed by dementia. The brain may be atrophied and shows discolouration and firmness of the white matter with, microscopically severe myelin loss, astrocytic gliosis and prominent collections of enlarged macrophages including multi-nucleated cells, but little or no neutral fat. Axons are relatively spared. Oligodendrocytes are reduced in number. The enlarged macrophages (globoid cells) are found chiefly in perivascular spaces and measure up to 50 μm across (Fig. 14.18). They contain stored material which, in fresh frozen sections, is PAS-positive, weakly sudanophilic, not metachromatic and strongly reactive for acid phosphatase. The stored material consists ultrastructurally of straight or curved tubular inclusions. Neurons do not contain stored material but neuronal loss may be seen particularly in the dentate nuclei, among Purkinje cells and in the inferior olives. Peripheral nerves show segmental demyelination and increased acid phosphatase in endoneurial cells but no globoid cells. Assay for the deficient enzyme can be carried out on white blood cells.

EFFECTS OF DRUGS
Altered cognitive function is extremely common as a side effect of many therapeutic and recreational drugs. In the vast majority of cases it is short lived and reversible when the drug is withdrawn. However, with persistent use there are some drugs that may lead to more longer-lasting effects on memory and intellect. Most produce no defined structural pathology but there is increasing evidence from sensitive imaging techniques that some produce structural changes. In a small number of cases neuropathological changes have been described at autopsy. These are outlined below. For details the papers referred to should be consulted, and the chapter on toxins by Jacobs and Le Quesne in Greenfield's *Neuropathology*, 5th edition 1992, is recommended.

Amphotericin B
This antifungal agent, when used intravenously, has been associated with severe neurological disturbances including dementia and akinetic mutism. Autopsy studies have described a diffuse cerebral leukoencephalopathy (Ellis *et al.*, 1982; Devinsky *et al.*, 1987). This encephalopathy has been reproduced in dogs.

Cyclosporin
Complications of the use of this drug for immunosuppression for organ transplantation include an encephalopathy with neuropsychiatric symptoms. The chief

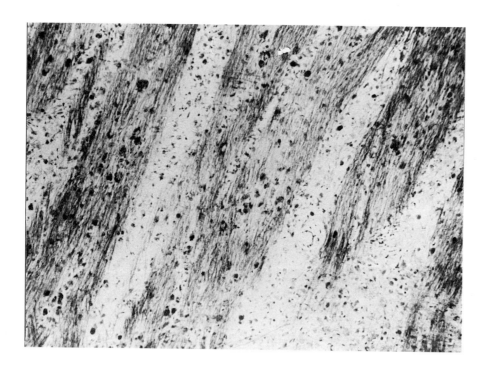

Fig. 14.17. Metachromatic leukodystrophy. Partially demyelinated pontine axonal bundles and irregular groups of macrophages containing darkly staining granular material which in frozen sections, can be seen to be metachromatic. Luxol fast blue/cresyl violet stain.

pathological findings in the few cases reported has been diffuse cerebral oedema (Jacobs & Le Quesne, 1992).

Methotrexate and other cancer chemotherapy

Methotrexate is a folic acid antagonist used in the treatment of leukaemia and some solid cancers. It may be given intravenously or intrathecally in combination with cranial and spinal irradiation for the treatment or prevention of central nervous system tumour invasion. This combination, or methotrexate used alone in high dosage, may be neurotoxic and give rise to an encephalopathy with confusion, ataxia and occasionally fits. This can be fatal. Autopsies have shown extensive damage to white matter with multifocal demyelination and necrosis in the centrum ovale (Fig. 14.19). Areas of necrosis are surrounded by oedema with sparse macrophages and astrocytosis (Fig. 14.20). Oligodendrocytes are reduced in number. Axons as well as myelin are severely damaged (Rubinstein et al., 1975; Price & Jamieson, 1975).

Similar effects on cerebral white matter to those attributed to methotrexate have also been described with the use, alone or in combination with radiotherapy, of other anti-cancer drugs 1,3-Bis-(2-chloroethyl)-1 nitroso urea (BCNU), cisplatin, cytosine arabinoside and thio-TEPA (Burger et al., 1981; Glass et al., 1986; Lee, Nauert & Glass, 1986).

Recreational drug abuse

Widespread cerebral dysfunction including cognitive impairment has been described in abusers of recreational drugs, opiates, amphetamines, etc. In some cases, strokes have occurred in association with the development of a necrotizing angiitis (Citron et al., 1970). In association with cocaine abuse, strokes due to cerebral haemorrhage or, less commonly, cerebral infarction have been described (Kaye & Fainstat, 1987; Klonoff, Andrews & Obana, 1989). In some of these cases, cerebral haemorrhage has been due to rupture of a berry aneurysm. Since cocaine causes vasoconstriction and raised blood pressure, some strokes of this type may be due to pre-existing lesions which are provoked to bleed by these well known effects of cocaine. In a few cases, a cerebral vasculitis has been associated with cocaine, as with other recreational drug abuse (Krendel et al., 1990). These complications may be associated with any route of cocaine administration (see Chapter 5).

Heroin, in addition to its association with the development of cerebral vasculitis and strokes, has also been implicated, after inhalation, in the development of a

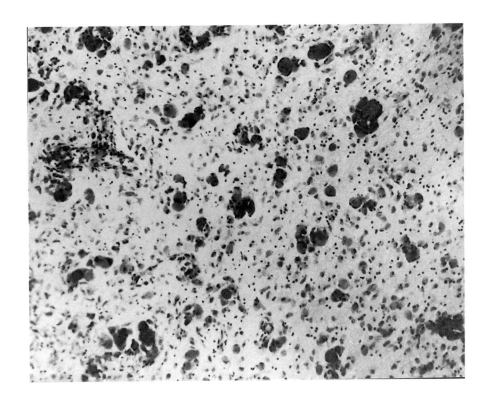

Fig. 14.18. Krabbe's leukodystrophy. Large 'globoid' macrophages containing PAS-positive material. PAS stain.

leukoencephalopathy. This produces a neurological syndrome in which ataxia rather than cognitive decline predominates. Its cause is uncertain, but it has been speculated that a contaminating neurotoxic agent is involved (Wolters *et al.*, 1982).

EFFECTS OF ENVIRONMENTAL TOXINS

Toxic effects of heavy metals on the nervous system have been recognized for many years. More recently, neuro-toxicological effects of organic compounds, many of them solvents, have been described. Many of these substances affect peripheral nerves, but some affect higher intellectual functions. Acute exposure is liable to cause confusion, drowsiness and coma, but more chronic exposure may lead to progressive dementia. In the case of some substances, for example, cadmium (Hart, Rose & Hamer, 1989), psychological impairment follow-

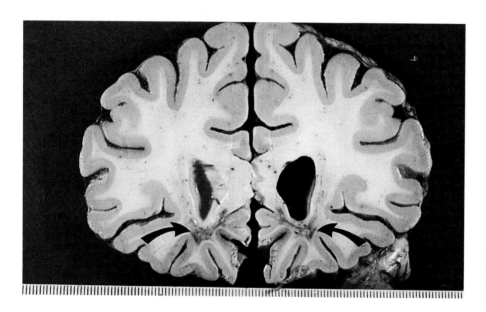

Fig. 14.19. Coronal slice across the frontal lobes in a case of methotrexate toxicity. The white matter inferior to the frontal horns of the ventricles is necrotic (arrows).

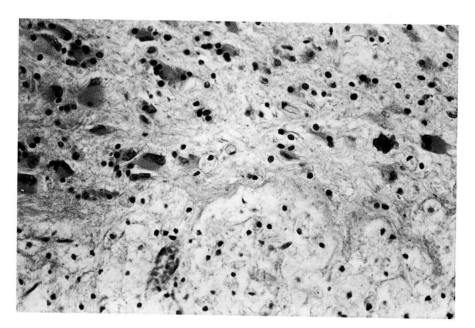

Fig. 14.20. Methotrexate toxicity. Oedema, swelling of oligodendrocytes (bottom) and reactive astrocytosis (above) in frontal lobe white matter,

ing excess exposure has been documented clinically but neuropathological studies are lacking. Those substances for which neuropathological changes have been described following excess exposure are summarized below.

Aluminium

The neurotoxic effects for humans of aluminium are a controversial subject with a large literature. Undoubted neurotoxicity of aluminium was demonstrated as long ago as 1897 by Dollken and more recently by Klatzo, Wisniewski & Streicher (1965) who showed that structures resembling neurofibrillary tangles were produced in rabbits after intracerebral injection of aluminium salts. This observation provoked interest in the possibility that aluminium toxicity might have a role in the aetiology of Alzheimer's disease, although enthusiasm for this idea was somewhat muted by ultrastructural studies that showed that the tangles formed in neurons after aluminium injection in animals were not formed of paired helical filaments as in Alzheimer's disease, but of straight 12 nm diameter filaments (Wisniewski & Soifer, 1979). Biochemically they also differ from the tangles of Alzheimer's disease being composed predominantly of neurofilaments and not tau protein as in Alzheimer's disease. However, interest in the potential toxicity of aluminium for humans was fuelled by the discovery that an encephalopathy that developed in some subjects undergoing renal dialysis for renal failure was attributable to high levels of aluminium in the dialysate water (Rozas, Port & Easterling, 1978; Alfrey, Legendre & Kaehny, 1976). The neuropathology of this encephalopathy, in which symptoms of dementia were prominent, was not that of Alzheimer's disease and consisted only of non-specific astrocytic and other reactive changes, principally in white matter (Alfrey et al., 1976; Burks et al., 1976). Nevertheless, further analysis of the aluminium content of brain in cases of Alzheimer's disease continued to point to possible excess amounts of aluminium there, though whether this had a primary role in the development of the disease or accumulated secondarily was hard to resolve. Furthermore, there has been difficulty in obtaining independent verification of some of these findings. Thus, while Crapper et al. (1976) reported excess amounts of aluminium in many regions of brain from subjects with Alzheimer's disease, McDermott et al. (1979) were unable to confirm this finding. Several studies have described aluminium and silicon in the cores of argyrophilic plaques in Alzheimer's disease (Perry & Perry, 1985; Candy et al., 1986), but this was not confirmed in more recent studies (Jacobs et al., 1989; Chafi et al., 1991; Landsberg, McDonald & Watt, 1992). However, reports of increased amounts of aluminium in neurofibrillary tangles have also been reported (Perl & Brody, 1980; Good et al., 1992; Lovell, Ehmann & Markesberg, 1993) and have not been questioned. Finally, there are epidemiological studies that have examined the relation of heavy exposure to aluminium by inhalation or ingestion (chiefly in medicinal antacid preparations) to mental impairment, and of levels of aluminium in water supplies to the prevalence of clinical dementia. These studies were reviewed by Doll (1993) who concluded that, while there was some evidence for neurotoxicity of aluminium in humans, there was not sufficient evidence at present to indicate that aluminium is the cause of Alzheimer's or any other specific dementing disease.

Bismuth salts

These salts, used medicinally for gastrointestinal disorders, have led to the development of an encephalopathy manifested by psychiatric symptoms, confusion, myoclonus and gait disturbance. Occasional epidemics of intoxication with bismuth salts have occurred. Pathological studies in fatal cases have shown necrotic lesions in the hippocampus and loss of Purkinje cells and basal ganglia neurons (Liessens et al., 1978).

Domoic acid

This is an excitatory amino acid present in seaweed. An acute toxic encephalopathy, due to eating mussels contaminated with the substance, has been reported from Canada (Perl et al., 1990; Teitelbaum et al., 1990). Acute neurological symptoms included headache, seizures, hemiparesis, ophthalmoplegia, loss of short term memory, agitation and coma. Follow-up of survivors showed a significant persisting memory deficit 12 months later. Neuropathological examination in four patients dying seven days to three months after ingestion of the toxin showed degeneration in the hippocampus and amygdala with lesser changes in subfrontal cortex, insula, nucleus accumbens, dorsal medial thalamus, claustrum and brainstem motor nuclei (Teitelbaum et al., 1990).

Ethylene oxide

This substance is used to sterilize heat-sensitive materials in industry. Industrial workers have occasionally suffered acute or chronic intoxication. Cognitive impairment, together with clumsiness, falls and irritability, has been described in chronic intoxication (Crystal et al.,

1988). Neuropathological studies of the CNS have not been described but peripheral neuropathy with axonal degeneration may also occur.

Lead

Acute lead intoxication is liable to cause an encephalopathy but chronic poisoning more commonly causes a peripheral neuropathy. In chronic encephalopathy, which occasionally occurs, there are changes to the cerebrovascular microvasculature, as in acute intoxication. Endothelial cell swelling, capillary obliteration and diffuse cerebral oedema occur. In *organic lead* toxicity, mainly resulting from repeated petrol sniffing, there are symptoms of sleep disturbance, psychosis and intense fear. The lead content of serum and brain is high and neuropathological case reports describe cerebellar atrophy and loss of hippocampal neurons (Valpey *et al.*, 1978).

Mercury

Inorganic mercury poisoning can cause psychological disturbances including dementia, followed by tremor. The cause of the psychological manifestations is not known but loss of cerebellar granule cells has been described (Davis *et al.*, 1974).

Methyl bromide

Methyl bromide is an odourless gas in use as a fumigant, a refrigerant and, until the early 1980s, in fire extinguishers. It has neurotoxic effects and has produced an acute encephalopathy with irrational behaviour, head-

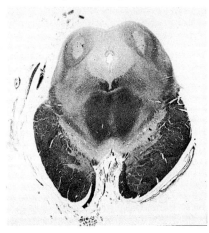

Fig. 14.21. Case of methyl bromide intoxication dying 30 days after onset of symptoms. There are symmetrical foci of necrosis in the inferior corpora quadrigemina. (Courtesy Dr M. V. Squier and with permission of Blackwell Science, publishers of *Neuropathol Appl Neurobiol*)

aches, nausea, disturbances of vision and speech, and coma. It may also cause mucosal irritation, skin blistering, pulmonary oedema and renal damage. Two cases dying 24 hours and 30 days, respectively, after acute intoxication had bilateral Wernicke-like lesions in inferior colliculi and mamilliary bodies (Fig. 14.21), demyelination in nerve roots of the cauda equina and cell loss in dorsal root ganglia. The peripheral neuropathy may have resulted from chronic exposure (Franken, 1959; Squier, Thompson & Rajagopolan, 1992). In another case (Roche *et al.*, 1958) and, in the case described by Franken (1959), there was cell loss in the dentate nuclei of the cerebellum.

Toluene

Some excess exposure to toluene can occur as a result of solvent abuse. Cognitive symptoms are among a wide variety of neurological abnormalities that can occur. Cerebellar ataxia is often also prominent. There is one case report of a fatal case with pathology (Rosenberg *et al.*, 1988) in which ill-defined myelin pallor was described. More recently the pathology in three cases of solvent vapour abuse was described (Kornfeld *et al.*, 1994). There was diffuse demyelination with accumulation of PAS-positive, but not foamy, macrophages. Chronic exposure to only mildly raised levels of toluene in an industrial setting has led to demonstrable impairment of neurobehavioural performance (Foo, Jeyaratnam & Koh, 1990).

Trimethyl tin

Compounds of trimethyl tin are produced as biproducts in the manufacture of dimethyl tin chloride, used as a stabilizer of plastics and for surface strengthening of glass. Occasionally, industrial workers have been exposed to excess amounts. Their symptoms have included psychological disturbance, confusion, ataxia, hearing loss and epilepsy. Post-mortem examination of one case showed abnormal neurons in the amygdala, temporal cortex, basal ganglia and pons, with cytoplasmic swelling, eccentric nuclei, loss of Nissl substance and cytoplasmic inclusions (Besser *et al.*, 1987).

REFERENCES

Adachi M, Toric J, Volk BW, Briet P, Wolintz A, Schneck L (1973) Electron microscopic and enzyme histochemical studies of cerebellum, ocular and skeletal muscles in chronic progressive ophthalmoplegia with cerebellar ataxia. *Acta Neuropathol* 23: 300–12.

Adams JH, Duchen LW (eds) (1992) *Greenfield's Neuropathology*. 5th edn, Arnold, London.

Adams JH, Graham D (1992) Hypoxia and vascular disorders. In Adams JH, Duchen LW (eds) *Greenfield's Neuropathology*. 5th edn, Arnold, London, pp 153–268.

Alfrey AC, Legendre G-R, Kaehny WD (1976) The dialysis encephalopathy syndrome: possible aluminium intoxication. *New Engl J Med* 294: 184–8.

Argov Z, Navon R (1984) Clinical and genetic variations in a syndrome of adult GM_2 gangliosidosis resulting from hexosaminidase A deficiency. *Ann Neurol* 16: 14–20.

Berkovic SF, Carpenter S, Evans A, Karpati G, Shoubridge EA, Andermann F, Meyer E, Tyler J, Diksic M, Arnold D, Wolfe LS, Andermann E, Hakim AM (1989) Myoclonus epilepsy and ragged red fibres (MERFF). *Brain* 112: 1231–60.

Besser R, Kramer G, Thümler R, Bohl J, Gutmann L, Hopf HC (1987) Acute trimethyl tin limbic-cerebellar syndrome. *Neurology* 37: 945–50.

Bird TD, Koerker RM, Leaird BJ, Vlcek BW, Thorning DR (1983) Lipomembranous polycystic osteodysplasia (brain, bone and fat disease): a genetic cause of presenile dementia. *Neurology* 33: 81–6.

Bjorkhem I, Skrede S (1990) Cerebrotendinous xanthomatosis. In Scriver CR, Beaudet AL, Sly WS, Valle D (eds) *The Metabolic Basis of Inherited Disease*. McGraw-Hill, NY, Chapter 51.

Burger PC, Kamenar E, Schold SC, Fay JW, Phillips GL, Herzig GP (1981) Encephalomyelopathy following high-dose BCNU therapy. *Cancer* 48: 1318–27.

Burks JS, Alfrey AC, Huddlestone J, Norenberg MD, Lewin E (1976) A fatal encephalopathy in chronic haemodialysis patients. *Lancet* i: 764–68.

Candy JM, Oakley AE, Klinowski J *et al* (1986) Aluminosilicates and senile plaque formation in Alzheimer's disease. *Lancet* i: 354–7.

Cavanagh JB, Harding BN (1994) Pathogenic factors underlying the lesions in Leigh's disease. *Brain* 117: 1357–76.

Chafi AH, Hauw J-J, Rancurel G, Berry JP, Galle C (1991) Absence of aluminium in Alzheimer's disease brain tissue: electron microprobe and ion microprobe studies. *Neurosci Lett* 123: 61–4.

Citron P, Halpern M, McCarron M, Lundberg GD, McCormick R, Pincus IJ, Tatter D, Haverback BJ (1970) Necrotising angiitis associated with drug abuse. *New Engl J Med* 283: 1003–11.

Coker SB (1991) The diagnosis of childhood neurodegenerative disorders presenting as dementia in adults. *Neurology* 41: 794–8.

Crapper DR, Krishnan SS, Quittkat S (1976) Aluminium, neurofibrillary degeneration and Alzheimer's disease. *Brain* 99: 67–80.

Crosby TW, Chou SM (1974) 'Ragged red' fibers in Leigh's disease. *Neurology* 24: 49–54.

Crystal HA, Schaumberg HH, Grober E, Fuld PA, Lipton RB (1988) Cognitive impairment and sensory loss associated with low-level ethylene oxide exposure. *Neurology* 38: 567–9.

Cummings JL, Benson DF (1984) *Dementia – A Clinical Approach*. Butterworth Heinemann, Boston 2nd edn.

Davis LE, Wands JR, Weiss SA, Price DL, Girling EF (1974) Central nervous system intoxication from mercurous chloride laxatives. *Arch Neurol* 30: 428–31.

Davis RL, Robertson DM (1996) *Textbook of Neuropathology*. 3rd edn, Williams and Wilkins, Baltimore.

Devinsky O, Lemann W, Evans AC, Moeller JR, Rottenberg DA (1987) Akinetic mutism in a bone marrow transplant recipient following total body irradiation and amphotericin B chemoprophylaxis. A positron emission tomographic and neuropathologic study. *Arch Neurol* 44: 414–17.

De Vivo DC, Haymond MW, Obert KA, Nelson JS, Pagliara AS (1979) Defective activation of the pyruvate dehydrogenase complex in subacute necrotizing encephalomyelopathy (Leigh's disease). *Ann Neurol* 6: 483–4.

DiMauro S, Bonilla E, Zeviani M, Nakagawa M, De Vivo D (1985) Mitochondrial myopathies. *Ann Neurol* 17: 521–8.

DiMauro S, Moraes CT, Shanske S, Lombes A, Nakase H, Mita S, Tritschler HJ, Bonilla E, Miranda AF, Schon EA (1991) Mitochondrial encephalomyopathies: biochemical approach. *Rev Neurol* 147: 443–9.

Doll R (1993) Review: Alzheimer's disease and environmental aluminium. *Age and Ageing* 22: 138–53.

Dollken A (1897) Ueber die Wirkung des Aluminium mit besonderer Besueecksichtigung der durch das Aluminium verursachten Läsionen im Zentralenervensystem. *Arch Exp Pathol Pharmacol* 40: 98–120.

Duchen LW, Jacobs JM (1992) Nutritional deficiencies and metabolic disorders. In Adams JH, Duchen LW (eds) *Greenfield's Neuropathology*. 5th edn, Arnold, London, pp 811–80.

Egger J, Wynne-Williams CJE, Erdohazi M (1982) Mitochondrial cytopathy or Leigh's syndrome? Mitochondrial abnormalities in spongiform encephalopathies. *Neuropediatrics* 13: 219–24.

Ellis WG, Bencken E, Le Couteur RA, Barbano JR, Woolfe BM, Jennings MB (1982) Leucoencephalopathy in patients treated with amphotericin B methylester. *J Inf Dis* 146: 125–37.

Fink JK, Filling-Katz MR, Sokol J, Cogan DG, Pikus A, Sonier B, Soong B, Pentcher PG, Comly ME, Brady RO, Barton NW (1989) Clinical spectrum of Niemann–Pick disease type C. *Neurology* 39: 1040–9.

Foo SC, Jeyaratnam J, Koh D (1990) Chronic neurobehavioural effects of toluene. *Br J Ind Med* 47: 480–4.

Franken L (1959) Étude anatomique d'un cas d'intoxication par le bromure de méthyle. *Acta Neurol Belgi* 59: 375–83.

Fukuhara N (1991) MERRF: a clinicopathological study. Relationship between myoclonus epilepsies and mitochondrial myopathies. *Rev Neurol* 147: 476–9.

Girdwood RH (1968) Abnormalities of vitamin B_{12} and folic acid metabolism – their influence on the nervous system. *Proc Nutrit Soc* 27: 101–7.

Glass JP, Lee YY, Burner J, Fields WS (1986) Treatment related leukoencephalopathy: a study of 3 cases and literature review. *Medicine* 65: 154–62.

Good PF, Perl DP, Bierer LM, Schmeidler J (1992) Selective accumulation of aluminium and iron in the neurofibrillary tangles of Alzheimer's disease: a laser microprobe (LAMMA) study. *Ann Neurol* 31: 286–92.

Gray F, Gherardi R, Marshall A, Janota I, Poirier J (1988) Adult polyglucosan body disease. *J Neuropathol Exp Neurol* 47: 459–74.

Griffin DE, Moser HW, Mendoza Q, Moench T, O'Toole S, Moser AB (1985) Identification of cells in the nervous system of patients with adrenoleukodystrophy. *Ann Neurol* 18: 660–4.

Haltia M, Somer H, Palo J, Johnson WG (1984) Neuronal intranuclear inclusion disease in identical twins. *Ann Neurol* 15: 316–21.

Hart RP, Rose CS, Hamer RM (1989) Neuropsychological effects of occupational exposure to cadmium. *J Clin Exp Neuropsychol* 11: 933–43.

Holt IJ, Harding AE, Petty RK, Morgan-Hughes JA (1990) A new mitochondrial disease associated with mitochondrial DNA heteroplasmy. *Am J Hum Genet* 46: 428–33.

Ihara Y, Namba R, Kuroda S, Sato T, Shirabe T (1989) Mitochondrial encephalomyopathy (MELAS): pathological study and successful therapy with coenzyme Q10 and idebenone. *J Neurol Sci* 90: 263–71.

Jacobs JM, Le Quesne PM (1992) Toxic disorders. In Adams JH, Duchen LW (eds) *Greenfield's Neuropathology*. 5th edn, Arnold, London, pp 881–7.

Jacobs RW, Duong T, Jones RE, Trapp GA, Scheibel AB (1989) A re-examination of aluminium in Alzheimer's disease analysis by energy dispersive X-ray microprobe and flameless atomic absorption spectrophotometry. *Can J Neurol Sci* 16: 498–503.

Kaye BR, Fainstat M (1987) Cerebral vasculitis associated with cocaine abuse. *JAMA* 258: 2104–6.

Kaye EM, Kolodny EH, Logigian EL, Ullman MD (1988) Nervous system involvement in Fabry's disease: clinical and biochemical correlation. *Ann Neurol* 23: 505–9.

Klatzo I, Wisniewski H, Streicher E (1965) Experimental production of neurofibrillary pathology. 1. Light microscopic observations. *J Neuropathol Exp Neurol* 24: 187–99.

Klonoff DC, Andrews BJ, Obana WG (1989) Stroke associated with cocaine abuse. *Arch Neurol* 46: 989–93.

Kornfeld M, Moser AB, Moser HW, Kleinschmidt-De Masters, Nolte K, Phelps A (1994) Solvent vapor abuse leukoencephalopathy. Comparison to adrenoleukodystrophy. *J Neuropathol Exp Neurol* 53: 389–98.

Krendal DA, Ditter SM, Frankel MR, Ross WK (1990)

Biopsy-proven vasculitis associated with cocaine abuse. *Neurology* 40: 1092–4.

Kretzschmar HA, De Armond SJ, Koch TK, Patel MS, Newth CJL, Schmidt KA, Packman S. (1986) Pyruvate dehydrogenase complex deficiency as the etiology of Leigh's disease. *Pediatrics* 79: 370–3.

Lake BD (1992) Lysosomal and peroxisomal disorders. In Adams JH, Duchen LW (eds) *Greenfield's, Neuropathology* 5th edn, Arnold, London, pp 709–810.

Landsberg JP, McDonald B, Watt F (1992) Absence of aluminium in neuritic plaque cores in Alzheimer's disease. *Nature* 360: 65–7.

Lapresle J, Fardeau M (1966) Les Leucoencéphalopathies de l'intoxication oxycarbonée. Etude de seize observations anatomoclinique. *Acta Neuropathol* 6: 327–48.

Lee Y-Y, Nauert C, Glass JP (1986) Treatment-related white matter changes in cancer patients. *Cancer* 27: 1473–82.

Liessens Jl, Monstrey J, Van den Eeckhout E, Djudzman R, Martin JJ (1978) Bismuth encephalopathy. A clinical and anatomopathological report of one case. *Acta Neurol Belg* 78: 301–9.

Lovell MA, Ehmann WD, Markesbery WR (1993) Laser microprobe analysis of brain aluminium in Alzheimer's disease. *Ann Neurol* 33: 36–42.

McDermott JR, Smith AI, Iqbal K *et al* (1979) Brain aluminium in aging and Alzheimer's disease. *Neurology* 29: 809–14.

Munoz-Garcia D, Ludwin SK (1986) Adult-onset neuronal intranuclear hyaline inclusion disease. *Neurology* 36: 785–90.

Naidu S, Moser HW (1990) Peroxisomal disorder. *Neurol Clin* 8: 507–19.

Nakano T, Ikeda S, Condo K, Yanagisawa N, Tsujis S (1985) Adult GM_1 gangliosidosis: clinical patterns and rectal biopsy. *Neurology* 35: 875–80.

Neil JF, Glew RH, Peters SP (1979) Familial psychosis and diverse neurologic abnormalities in adult onset Gaucher's disease. *Arch Neurol* 36: 95–9.

Ohama E, Ohara S, Ikuta F, Tanaka K, Nishizawa M, Miyatake T (1987) Mitochondrial angiopathy in cerebral blood vessels of mitochondrial encephalomyopathy. *Acta Neuropathol* 74: 226–33.

Oppenheimer DR, Esiri MM (1992) Diseases of the basal ganglia, cerebellum and motor neurons. In Adams JH, Duchen LW (eds) *Greenfield's Neuropathology*. 5th edn, Arnold, London, pp 988–1045.

Pallis & Lewis (1974) *The Neurology of Gastrointestinal Disease*. Walton JN (ed) Saunders, London.

Perl DP, Brody AR (1980) Alzheimer's disease: X-ray spectrographic evidence of aluminium accumulation in neurofibrillary tangle-bearing neurons. *Science* 208: 297–9.

Perl TM, Bedard L, Kosatsky T, Hockin JC, Todd ECD, Remis RS (1990) An outbreak of toxic encephalopathy caused by eating mussels contaminated with domoic acid. *N Engl J Med* 322: 1775–80.

Perry EK, Perry RH (1985) New insights into the nature of senile (Alzheimer-type) plaques. *Trends Neurosci* 8: 301–3.

Petty RKH, Harding AE, Morgan-Hughes JA (1986) The clinical features of mitochondrial myopathy. *Brain* 109: 915–38.

Ponzetto C, Bresolin N, Bordoni A, Moggio M, Meola G, Bet L, Prelle A, Scarlato G (1990) Kearns-Sayre syndrome: different amounts of deleted mitochondrial DNA are present in several autopic tissues. *J Neurol Sci* 96: 207–10.

Price RA, Jamieson PA (1975) The central nervous system in childhood leukaemia II. Subacute leucoencephalopathy. *Cancer* 35: 306–18.

Roche L, Colin M, Tommasi M, Lejeune E (1958) Intoxication mortelle par le bromure de methyle. *Ann Med Leg* 38: 364–72.

Rosenberg NL, Kleinschmidt-De Masters BK, Davis KA, Dreisbach JN, Holmes JT, Filley CM (1988) Toluene abuse causes diffuse central nervous system white matter changes. *Ann Neurol* 23: 611–14.

Rozas VV, Port PK, Easterling RE (1978) An outbreak of dialysis dementia due to aluminium in the dialysate. *J Dialysis* 2: 459–70.

Rubinstein LJ, Herman MM, Long TF, Wilbur JR (1975) Disseminated necrotizing leucoencephalopathy: a complication of treated central nervous system leukemia and lymphoma. *Cancer* 35: 291–305.

Shanske S, Morales CT, Lombes A, Miranda AF, Bonilla E, Levis P, Whelan MA, Ellsworth CA, DiMauro S (1990) Widespread tissue distribution of mitochondrial DNA-deletions in Kearns–Sayre syndrome. *Neurology* 40: 24–8.

Shoffner JM (1991) MERFF: a model disease for understanding the principles of mitochondrial genetics. *Rev Neurol* 147: 431–5.

Sourander P (1970) A new entity of phacomatosis B brain lesions (sclerosing leucoencephalopathy). *Acta Pathol Microbiol Scand Suppl* vol 215 Sect A and B; 44.

Sparaco M, Borilla E, DiMauro S, Powers JM (1993) Neuropathology of mitochondrial encephalomyopathies due to mitochondrial DNA defects. *J Neuropath Exp Neurol* 52: 1–10.

Squier MV, Thompson J, Rajagopolan (1992) Case report: neuropathology of methyl bromide intoxication. *Neuropathol Appl Neurobiol* 18: 579–84.

Teitelbaum JS, Zatorre RJ, Carpenter S, Gendron D, Evans AC, Gjedde A, Cashman NR (1990) Neurologic sequelae of domoic acid intoxication due to the ingestion of contaminated mussels. *N Eng J Med* 322: 1781–7.

Valpey R, Sumi M, Copass MK, Goble GJ (1978) Acute and chronic progressive encephalopathy due to gasoline sniffing. *Neurology* 28: 507–10.

Van Coster R, Lombes A, De Vivo DC, Chi TL, Dodson WE, Rothman S, Orrechio EJ, Grover W, Berry GT, Schwartz JF, Habib A, DiMauro S (1991) Cytochrome C oxidase-associated Leigh syndrome: phenotypic features and pathogenetic speculations. *J Neurol Sci* 104: 97–111.

Van Schrojenstein – De Valk HMJ, Van De Kamp JJP (1987) Follow-up on seven adult patients with mild San filippo disease. *Am J Med Genet* 28: 125–30.

Volk B, Adachi M (1970) Diffuse cerebral sclerosis. In Vinken PJ, Bruyn GW (eds) *Handbook of Clinical Neurology* Vol 10, Elsevier, NY, pp 67–93.

Walls TJ, Jones RA, Cartlidge NEF, Saunders M (1984) Alexander's disease with Rosenthal fibre formation in an adult. *J Neurol Neurosurg Psychiat* 47: 399–403.

Walters E Ch, van Wijngaarden GK, Stam FC *et al* (1982) Leukoencephalopathy after inhaling heroin pyrolysate. *Lancet* ii: 1233–7.

Waltz G, Harik SI, Kaufman B (1987) Adult metachromatic leukodystrophy. *Arch Neurol* 44: 225–7.

Weidenheim KM, Dickson DW (1995) Intranuclear inclusion bodies in an elderly demented woman: a form of intranuclear inclusion body disease. *Clin Neuropathol* 14: 93–9.

Willems JL, Monnens LAH, Trijbels JMF, Veerkamp JH, Meyer AEFH, van Dam K, van Haelst U (1977) Leigh's encephalomyelopathy in a patient with cytochrome C oxidase deficiency in muscle tissue. *Pediatrics* 60: 850–7.

Wisniewski HM, Soifer D (1979) Neurofibrillary pathology: current status and research perspectives. *Mech Aging Dev* 9: 119–42.

Wolters ECh, van Wijngaarden GK, Stam FC, Rengelink H, Lousberg RJ, Schipper ME, Verbeeten B (1982) Leucoencephalopathy after inhaling heroin pyrolysate. *Lancet* ii: 1233–7.

CHAPTER FIFTEEN

Hydrocephalus and dementia

M. M. Esiri

Introduction
Cerebrospinal fluid hydrodynamics and normal pressure hydrocephalus
Classification, prevalence, natural history and clinical features of NPH
Neuropathological findings in NPH
Recommended procedure for diagnosis of NPH

INTRODUCTION

The ancient term hydrocephalus refers to an excessive accumulation of fluid (water) inside the head. It is most readily detected in infants and children with congenital hydrocephalus, since its existence before the skull sutures are closed causes the formation of an enlarged head. Such children have long been recognized commonly to have mental impairment, manifest as mental retardation, although the extent of this is very variable. Morgagni (1769) first described hydrocephalus due to enlarged cerebral ventricles in an adult without head enlargement. If this condition develops insidiously during adult life, dementia is an almost invariable accompaniment, though not the only one. More familiarly hydrocephalus in adults develops acutely or subacutely and presents with symptoms of raised intracranial pressure: headache, vomiting and drowsiness. However, in this chapter we are concerned with chronic hydrocephalus in adults, a condition in which symptoms and signs of raised intracranial pressure are commonly clinically absent and in which the cerebrospinal fluid (CSF) pressure is often normal when measured randomly, hence the commonly used term, *normal pressure hydrocephalus* (*NPH*). The recognition of this condition, and the realization that it is responsible for some cases of progressive dementia in adults are recent (Riddoch, 1936; Foltz & Ward, 1956; McHugh, 1964; Hakim & Adams 1965; Adams *et al.*, 1965). Cases of NPH, some of which respond well to a shunting procedure, are to be distinguished from cases of dementia due to neurodegenerative diseases in which the ventricles dilate as a consequence of cerebral atrophy (*hydrocephalus ex vacuo*). It should be noted that making this distinction

can be difficult, and therefore neurodegenerative diseases need to be excluded when a case of possible NPH is being examined neuropathologically. As outlined below, the pathophysiology of NPH is still only poorly understood (Cummings & Benson, 1992; Pickard, 1991).

CEREBROSPINAL FLUID HYDRODYNAMICS AND NORMAL PRESSURE HYDROCEPHALUS

Anatomical and physiological studies in the first half of this century established the basic features of CSF hydrodynamics (for recent reviews, see Davson *et al.*, 1987; Herndon & Brumback 1989; Rosenberg, 1990). The CSF is (for the most part) secreted by an energy-requiring active transport process in the choroid plexus, portions of which are found throughout the ventricular system. The fluid so formed fills the ventricles and subarachnoid space. CSF is produced normally in man at a steady rate of 0.35 ml/min or 500 ml/day (Cutler *et al.*, 1968). Its rate of production does not appear to be altered as a result of CSF pressure changes or hydrocephalus (Lorenzo, Page & Watters, 1970; Lorenzo & Bresnan, 1973). The fluid circulates predominantly from lateral to third and fourth ventricles from where it escapes into the cisterna magna and the rest of the subarachnoid space through the foramina of Luschka and Magendie (Fig. 15.1). Once in the subarachnoid space it either seeps downwards around the spinal cord or flows up over the cerebral hemispheres to be absorbed principally into the superior sagittal sinus at specialized projections of the arachnoid membrane into the sinus, the arachnoid granulations, or pacchionian villi (Fig. 15.2). Some of the fluid around the spinal cord may be absorbed into veins at this level but absorption of most of the CSF takes place under the influence of the pressure gradient between CSF and venous blood within the sinuses.

Since the rate of CSF formation does not appear to vary, and hydrocephalus requires that the volume of CSF be increased, almost all forms of hydrocephalus must be attributed to reduced absorption. (Only exceptionally is increased CSF production thought to be responsible for hydrocephalus; in rare cases of choroid plexus papilloma or when CSF protein is excessively high.) The most obvious reason for reduced CSF absorption is a gross mechanical obstruction to CSF circulation, and in some cases of acute or subacute hydrocephalus such an obstruction can readily be found (Table 15.1). The increased volume of CSF retained by the ventricles is under increased pressure in these circumstances, and the ventricular dilatation is due to the increased pressure of CSF inside the ventricles. If the obstruction is relieved, the ventricles resume a normal or only marginally increased size because of a natural modest elasticity of the cerebral tissues. While pressure is high and access of CSF to the superior sagittal sinus prevented, new channels of absorption are probably opened up within periventricular white matter allowing the situation to stabilize at least temporarily.

The problem in NPH is to understand how the ventricles become dilated in the absence of persistently raised ventricular pressure, as apparently occurs. Sometimes it is reasonable to postulate that there may have been an episode of raised pressure at the commencement of the process. For example, there may have been a subarachnoid haemorrhage long before which resulted in transient hydrocephalus, a complication known to occur in most patients in the first few days after such a haemorrhage though it is only severe in some 20% of cases and needs surgical relief in only 7% (Pickard, 1984). With the establishment of alternative forms of CSF absorption the intraventricular pressure usually drops, but the ventricles can remain enlarged. Once slightly enlarged, they remain more susceptible than normal to further enlargement with mild pressure elevations, just as a balloon is easier to blow up once a small initial expansion has taken place. However, many cases of NPH have no history of a relevant antecedent event such as subarachnoid haemorrhage and no clinical symptoms suggestive of raised pressure, so that the impetus for ventricular enlargement in such cases remains a mystery.

Despite normal random CSF pressure readings in

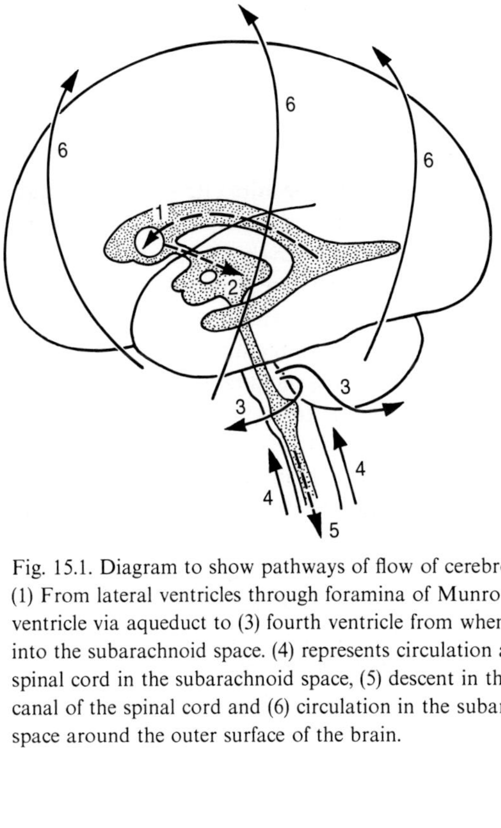

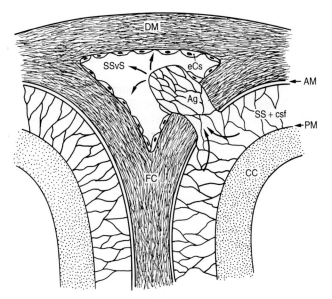

Fig. 15.1. Diagram to show pathways of flow of cerebrospinal fluid. (1) From lateral ventricles through foramina of Munro to (2) third ventricle via aqueduct to (3) fourth ventricle from whence it escapes into the subarachnoid space. (4) represents circulation around the spinal cord in the subarachnoid space, (5) descent in the central canal of the spinal cord and (6) circulation in the subarachnoid space around the outer surface of the brain.

Fig. 15.2. Diagram to show the manner of cerebrospinal fluid (csf) reabsorption via the arachnoid granulations (Ag) into the superior sagittal venous sinus (SSvS). DM: dura mater, FC: falx, PM: pia mater, AM: arachnoid mater, SS: subarachnoid space, CC: cerebral cortex, eCs: endothelial cell.

Table 15.1. *Causes of obstructive hydrocephalus after Cummings & Benson* (1992)

Non-communicating	Communicating
Aqueduct stenosis	*Post-haemorrhagic*
Congenital	
Inflammatory	*Post-traumatic*
Haemorrhagic	
Intraventricular obstructive lesion	*Post-infectious*
Tumours	
meningiomas	*Post-craniotomy*
papillomas	
ependymomas	*Idiopathic*
vascular malformations	*Neoplastic*
carcinomas	sagittal sinus meningioma
lymphomas	carcinomatosis of
craniopharyngiomas	leptomeninges
pituitary adenomas	lymphomatosis
Compressive lesions	tentorial tumour
Gliomas	
Other tumours as above	*Basilar impression*
Colloid cysts	
Haemorrhagic obstruction	*Ectatic basilar artery*
Obstruction of outlet foramina	
Posterior fossa neoplasms	
Posterior fossa vascular malformations	
Inflammatory processes in basilar cisterns	
Dandy–Walker malformation	
Arnold–Chiari malformation	
Arachnoid cysts	
Haemorrhagic obstruction	

patients clinically diagnosed as suffering from NPH, careful long-term monitoring of CSF pressure in series of such patients who respond favourably later to a shunting procedure has shown that they have mean pressure readings in the upper range of normal and they show spontaneous, short-lived periodic waves of elevated pressure (for review see Pickard, 1991). Thus, they are suffering from *intermittently raised*, rather than *normal* pressure hydrocephalus. The cause of these episodes of intermittent, mildly raised, pressure is not clear, but it is reasonable to consider that they play a part in the development of NPH.

CLASSIFICATION, PREVALENCE, NATURAL HISTORY AND CLINICAL FEATURES OF NPH

Two groups of patients with NPH can be identified clinically: those in which the disorder is *secondary* to previous intracranial disease or injury (the majority) and those without, in whom it is *idiopathic* (the minority). Katzman (1977) assembled from the literature 914 cases, 314 of them idiopathic and the remainder secondary. Among the latter the most common antecedent events were subarachnoid haemorrhage and head injury, followed by aqueduct stenosis, meningitis, previous craniotomy, obstructive lesions in the third or fourth ventricles and basilar artery ectasia. Rare causes were other tumours such as pituitary adenomas, basilar impression and syringomyelia (Table 15.2).

The prevalence of NPH in the community is unknown, but among patients presenting to neurologists with dementia, some 5% have been diagnosed as suffering from this condition (Marsden & Harrison, 1972; Katzman, 1977; Smith & Kiloh, 1981). Most cases have been diagnosed in the sixth and seventh decades. Cases above the age of 80 are rare, but it is possible that some of

Table 15.2. *Causes of NPH in 914 cases assembled by Katzman (1977)*

Subarachnoid haemorrhage	315
Head injury	102
Aqueduct stenosis	34
Meningitis	34
Post-craniotomy	43
Obstructive lesions of the fourth ventricle	21
Tumours obstructing the third ventricle	26
Basilar artery ectasia or aneurysm	11
Other tumours, including pituitary adenoma	7
Basilar impression with or without Paget's disease	4
Syringomyelia	1
'Encephalopathy', 'encephalitis'	2
Idiopathic (unknown)	314
associated with:	
Parkinson's disease	15
Alzheimer's disease	7
Cerebrovascular disease	4
Huntington's chorea	2
Chronic epilepsy	2

the apparent fall-off of cases over the age of 70 reflects the greater reluctance of clinicians to carry out detailed investigation in older patients.

NPH is characterized clinically by three main features which classically develop in sequence: gait disturbance, dementia and incontinence. It is very unlikely that a case of progressive dementia will be due to NPH unless the dementia develops alongside, if it does not follow, gait disturbance. Incontinence usually develops later. The symptoms are attributed to the expanded lateral ventricles stretching long descending fibres of the medially placed corticospinal motor fibres controlling the legs (gait disturbance) and fibres from the medial frontal lobe controlling the sphincters (urinary incontinence), with, in addition, stretching of callosal and ipsilateral cortico-cortical fibres (dementia). Reduced periventricular blood flow, possibly caused by hydrocephalic compression, is also likely to lead to a 'misery perfusion' state sufficient to cause periventricular axonal dysfunction (Vanneste, 1994). The gait disturbance, which may be difficult to define and highly variable, may be associated with spasticity or with features mimicking parkinsonism. Although problems with balance are often prominent, cerebellar ataxia is not present.

The mental symptoms are those thought by some (Benson & Cummings, 1990) to reflect subcortical rather than cortical dysfunction: slowing up of thought processes, vagueness, reduced interest and drive and reduced powers of abstract thought and concentration. Memory disturbance and disorientation are, however, uncommon. The triad of symptoms that is thought to characterize NPH, dementia, gait disturbance and incontinence, is not pathognomic for NPH; similar features may be seen in some cases of Parkinson's disease with dementia, Alzheimer's disease, multi-infarct dementia, after head injury, in multiple sclerosis, hypothyroidism, drug toxicity, Pick's disease and progressive supranuclear palsy (Fisher, 1977; Katzman, 1977; Pickard, 1991).

The widespread availability of CT scanning has greatly facilitated investigation of cases of NPH. Before it became available, pneumoencephalography was required to display the state of the ventricles and intracranial subarachnoid space, a tedious procedure that was sometimes associated with clinical deterioration in the patient. In NPH the CT scan characteristically displays greatly enlarged lateral ventricles and periventricular white matter low density together with at least partially obliterated superficial cerebral sulci. It may also show an obstructive lesion responsible for the condition. However, the features are not specific and some cases show wide cortical sulci and can be impossible to distinguish from hydrocephalus *ex vacuo*. MRI findings in NPH have yet to be described.

NEUROPATHOLOGICAL FINDINGS IN NPH

There have been remarkably few neuropathological studies of NPH published. Few centres see large numbers of such cases, and some of those cases that are diagnosed post-mortem have inadequate clinical documentation. There is also a problem in defining the idiopathic condition neuropathologically other than by exclusion of other neuropathology associated with dementia in a case with well preserved cerebral cortex and marked ventricular dilatation. Moreover, what constitutes 'marked' ventricular dilatation is generally not precisely defined, since measurement of ventricular volume post mortem is not readily accomplished. Ventricular dilatation is, in any event, a not uncommon incidental finding in clinically undemented elderly subjects, so that without a good clinical history its significance may be easily dismissed (Messert, Wannamaker & Dudley, 1972). Some clinically diagnosed cases have clear-cut evidence of communicating hydrocephalus with marked leptomeningeal thickening. Others, including some which have been demonstrated to benefit from a shunt,

Table 15.3. *Details of 14 cases of normal pressure hydrocephalus examined necropathologically at Oxford, 1971–91*

Case	Sex/age	Clinical features	Pathological findings	Brain wt
1	M 66	History of two brain stem strokes several years before death. Then had become 'forgetful' with an unsteady gait.	Gross hydrocephalus, thickened leptomeninges, old infarcts at right occipital pole, adjacent to right thalamus, in left occipital white matter and in the pons. No Alzheimer-type pathology or other dementing illness pathology.	1471 g
2	M 76	Loss of consciousness after head injury 30 years before death following which he had slurred speech and unsteady gait. Developed mild dementia during the last few years of his life.	Gross hydrocephalus with a brain that appeared swollen externally. Arachnoid cyst in posterior fossa containing clear cerebrospinal fluid on right with brain stem slightly shifted to the left. Syringobulbia.	1767 g
3	M 79	History of dementia, gait disturbance and Paget's disease. Details not available.	Basilar impression of skull with Paget's disease. External appearance of the brain unremarkable. Marked hydrocephalus. No Alzheimer-type pathology or other dementing illness pathology.	N/A
4	M 53	History of progressive dementia, clinically diagnosed as Alzheimer's disease.	Moderately thickened leptomeninges. Gross hydrocephalus. Moderate numbers of plaques in many areas of cortex and rare neurofibrillary tangles, limited to the hippocampus and parahippocampal gyrus (features not sufficient to diagnose Alzheimer's disease). No other dementing illness pathology.	N/A
5	M 77	Five year history of dementia and 3 year history of temporal lobe epilepsy. Increased limb tone and spasticity.	Gross enlargement of lateral ventricles, and compression of third ventricle by suprasellar non-functioning pituitary adenoma. No Alzheimer's disease or other dementing illness pathology.	
6	M 65	One year history of dementia and abnormal behaviour.	Gross hydrocephalus, normal leptomeninges. No Alzheimer's disease or other dementing illness pathology.	1490 g
7	M 75	Two year history of progressive dementia and incontinence. Previous history of high alcohol intake.	Gross hydrocephalus. Mild generalized cerebral atrophy. Few widespread plaques and no neurofibrillary tangles interpreted as insufficient to diagnose Alzheimer's disease. No other dementing illness pathology.	1230 g
8	F 67	Several months' history of progresive dementia and unsteadiness.	Slight generalized cerebral atrophy and slight leptomeningeal thickening. Gross hydrocephalus. No Alzheimer's disease or other dementing illness pathology.	1200 g
9	M 81	Severe head injury 12 years before death, with subdural and extradural haemorrhage. From 9 years before death, occasional incontinence and 4 years before death onset of difficulty walking and episodes of confusion and aggression, progressing to frank dementia. Able to walk only with two assistants, gait broad based.	Five burr holes, taut subdural membrane over right frontal lobe with calcification. A few old contusional scars and an old right frontal pole infarct. Gross hydrocephalus. No Alzheimer's disease pathology or other dementing illness pathology.	1300 g

Table 15.3. (*cont.*)

Case	Sex/age	Clinical features	Pathological findings	Brain wt
10	M 80	Three-year history of hesitant gait and frequent falls, 18 month history of incontinence, weak legs and some 'blackouts'. One-year history of mild dementia. Spastic, bilateral weakness on examination, oral kinesis and tremor of right hand. Found to be anaemic with subacute myelo-monocytic leukaemia.	Thickened leptomeninges and gross hydrocephalus with no cerebral atrophy. Small old infarct in head of left caudate nucleus. No Alzheimer's disease pathology or other dementing illness pathology.	1350 g
11	M 55	Many years' history of treated hypertension. One year's history of being withdrawn, slovenly, confused and incontinent. On examination, lower limbs spastic. First encephalogram showed communicating hydrocephalus and a shunt was inserted in the right lateral ventricle. Post-operative intracerebral haemorrhage occurred followed by death on the second post-operative day.	Three right-sided burr holes. Massive right intracerebral haemorrhage in white matter and lentiform nucleus. Acute posterior cerebral artery territory infarction secondary to uncal herniation. Gross dilatation of left lateral ventricle. Old softening with residual haemosiderin deposition in left caudate nucleus and dorsal thalamus.	1490 g
12	M 79	Five year history of increasing immobility and double incontinence. Previous excessive alcohol intake. Eighteen months' history of progressive dementia and aggressive behaviour.	Gross hydrocephalus. Old small, left cerebellar infarct. Rare neurofibrillary tangles confined to the hippocampus and a few plaques in all cortical areas, insufficient to diagnose Alzheimer's disease. No other dementing illness pathology.	1330 g
13	M 81	Six months' history of difficulty walking and 'drop attacks', followed by incontinence and mild confusion. On examination he had a staggering gait, brisk reflexes but downgoing plantar responses. Died shortly after.	Gyri at vertex clearly flattened, but leptomeninges normal. Severely stenosed left vertebral artery but no infarcts seen. Gross hydrocephalus. No Alzheimer's disease or other dementing illness pathology.	1510 g
14	F 70	History extending back several years of schizphrenia, falls and incontinence. Diagnosis of NPH made elsewhere. Four months before death examination showed dementia and Parkinsonian features, the latter considered to be drug induced.	Slight generalized atrophy, leptomeninges normal. Gross hydrocephalus, multiple small old infarcts in deep grey and cerebral white matter. Severe arteriolar sclerosis. Fresh almond-sized haemorrhage in left thalamus.	1151 g

have been shown after death to have changes of Alzheimer's disease or multiple small infarcts with apparently normal leptomeninges or leptomeningeal thickening (DeLand *et al.*, 1972; Vessal, Sperber & James, 1974; Earnest *et al.*, 1974; Koto *et al.*, 1977; Di Rocco *et al.*, 1977; Katzman *et al.*, 1977; Akai *et al.*, 1987; Derouesne *et al.*, 1987; Newton, Pickard & Weller, 1989). A few cases of AD are known to have severe ventricular dilatation (Tomlinson, Blessed & Roth, 1970) and these may have been mistaken for cases of NPH. However, a few cases of AD with not necessarily severe cortical pathology may show a marked degree of amyloid deposition in leptomeningeal blood vessel walls. This predisposes the vessels to leak and cause multiple small,

and occasionally larger, subarachnoid haemorrhages which could, at least potentially, result in a non-communicating hydrocephalus, although such cases do not appear to have been reported. It would be of interest to know if ventricular size in AD is larger in those cases with severe amyloid angiopathy than in other cases. Some cases with multiple deep infarcts may likewise have been diagnosed mistakenly as NPH, since the infarcts might be expected to have interrupted the same long fibres that are affected in NPH, thus giving rise to similar symptomology, while the cerebral atrophy that results gives rise to the ventricular dilatation. However, cases with multiple deep infarcts that have responded to shunting may be true cases of NPH precipitated by blood from partly haemorrhagic infarcts lying close to the lateral or third ventricles reaching the CSF and clogging up the subarachnoid space intermittently.

Our own experience of the neuropathology of NPH amounts to 14 cases so diagnosed at post mortem examination over a 20-year period in which a total number of approximately 500 cases of dementia were examined neuropathologically (Table 15.3). Cases of NPH therefore constituted 2.8% of the total. Most cases were not clinically diagnosed as NPH, but in all of them there was a history of dementia. There was a predominance of males and the average age was 72 years. In most cases a history of gait disturbance, albeit ill defined, was present. The neuropathological findings, apart from

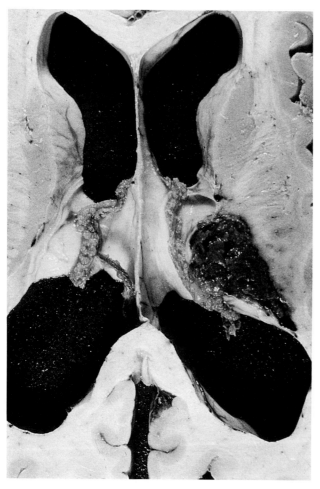

Fig. 15.3. Case of normal pressure hydrocephalus (case 14) with small organizing right thalamic haemorrhage lying close to the ventricular system.

severe hydrocephalus, were variable. One had a non-communicating hydrocephalus caused by obstruction by a pituitary adenoma. All the other cases had a communicating hydrocephalus. This was associated with pronounced leptomeningeal thickening in the subarachnoid space over the cerebral convexities, but without any inflammation or evidence of old haemorrhage, in three cases. One of these cases also had an old infarct in the caudate nucleus and another moderate numbers of argyrophilic plaques insufficient to diagnose Alzheimer's disease. In five cases there were deep vascular lesions, the majority old, small, white or deep grey matter infarcts. However, almost all these lesions contained some haemosiderin, indicating previous haemorrhage and, in one case, a small thalamic haemorrhage was present extending to the wall of the third ventricle in addition to old deep grey and white matter softenings (Fig. 15.3).

At post-mortem examination the brain weights in our cases of NPH averaged 1379 grams, with a range of 1151–1767 grams that is well within the normal range. Externally the cerebral cortex usually appeared normal or slightly flattened. In only three cases was there mild atrophy. The leptomeninges were normal, minimally or more markedly thickened. After fixation coronal slicing revealed brains with marked dilatation of the lateral ventricles and third ventricle, sometimes with fenestration of the septum. The corpus callosum appeared of normal or only slightly reduced width. (The stretching that the corpus callosum undergoes make it appear slightly narrowed.) (Fig. 15.4). Obstructive lesions or vascular softenings were present in some cases (Figs. 15.5 and 15.6). In microscopic sections of the deep cerebral white matter the myelin staining usually appeared normal, but in some cases it appeared diffusely pale and fibre densities in silver stains, attenuated. The ependymal lining of the lateral ventricles was fragmented and the subependymal tissue variably gliotic. In cases with thickened meninges there was dense acellular collagen deposition, without inflammatory change. In some cases there was haemosiderin deposition. Arachnoid granulations invaginating the sagittal sinus appeared normal or fibrotic.

In the hindbrain the fourth ventricle may or may not appear enlarged (even in communicating hydrocephalus, the fourth ventricle is not invariably enlarged because more pressure is required to dilate it than to dilate the already larger lateral ventricles and third ventricle with which it communicates).

RECOMMENDED PROCEDURE FOR DIAGNOSIS OF NPH

The diagnosis of NPH should be considered if the clinical features are consistent (and in any case of dementia if clinical details are scanty or non-existent) if the brain at autopsy appears normal or slightly *swollen* externally and the ventricles are markedly enlarged in the absence of significant atrophy. Marked leptomeningeal thickening in the presence of the above features further strengthens the case as does the finding of gross obstructive lesions along cerebrospinal fluid pathways. Arteries at the base of the brain should be examined

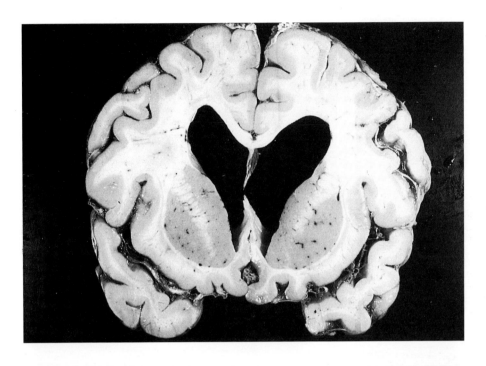

Fig. 15.4. Normal pressure hydrocephalus (case 13). Coronal slice across frontal and anterior temporal lobes. Frontal horns of the ventricles are markedly enlarged, the corpus callosum appears slightly narrow because of stretching and the cerebral cortex appears relatively well preserved and sulci narrow (compare with Fig. 3.6(e) in which the degree of ventriculation dilatation is comparable but the cortex is much more atrophic).

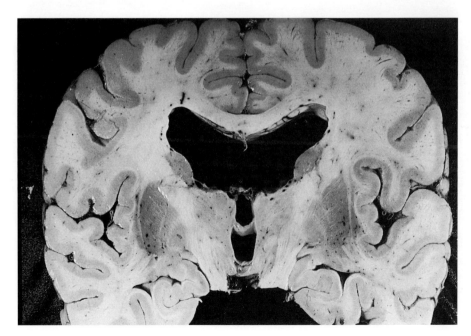

Fig. 15.5. Normal pressure hydrocephalus (case 2) due to an arachnoid cyst in the posterior fossa preventing normal outlet of cerebrospinal fluid from the fourth ventricle. Note enlarged third and lateral ventricles, relatively well-preserved corpus callosum and cerebral cortex and absence of a septum.

carefully for aneurysms and a search made for rusty discolouration of the leptomeninges which would suggest previous subarachnoid haemorrhage. A careful search should be made for old or fresh vascular lesions in the brain particularly in deep white matter and basal ganglia.

Sections should be examined of any focal lesions found and of periventricular white matter and

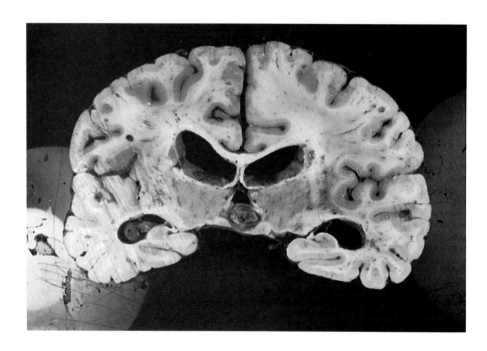

Fig. 15.6. Obstructive hydrocephalus due to non-functioning pituitary tumour in the third ventricle. The inferior horns of the lateral ventricles are particularly enlarged in this case (case 5).

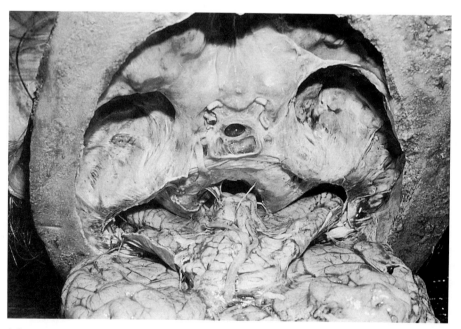

(a)

Fig. 15.7. Paget's disease with dementia due to hydrocephalus (case 3). (a) View of the inside of the skull during removal of the brain showing greatly thickened skull and compressed hindbrain. (b) Flattened cerebellum and slightly enlarged fourth ventricle. (c) Coronal slice through the cerebrum showing enlarged third and lateral ventricles and dorso-ventral compression of the hemispheres by excessive growth of the base of the skull.

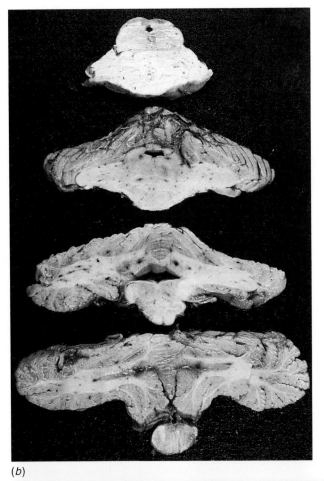

(b)

Fig. 15.7 (cont.)

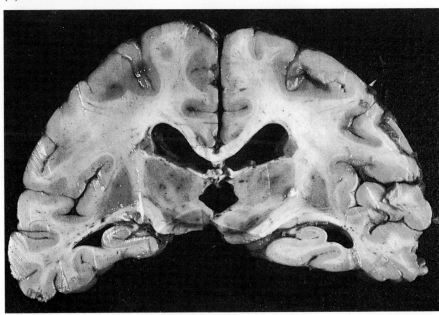

(c)

leptomeninges. Because NPH and Alzheimer's disease may co-exist it is also necessary to examine silver-stained sections of hippocampus and neocortex for features of Alzheimer's disease (Chapter 4a). A Congo red stain will reveal the extent of amyloid deposition in leptomeningeal vessels. In addition, since the features of gait disturbance and dementia occur in other neuro-degenerative diseases, these should also be excluded by examining sections of the substantia nigra, which will show cell loss and Lewy bodies if Parkinson's disease is present (Chapter 6) and cell loss and neurofibrillary tangles if progressive supranuclear palsy is present (Chapter 10). The pons and dentate nuclei of the cerebellum should also be examined, and will show loss of cells and presence of Lewy bodies in the locus ceruleus in Parkinson's disease and cell loss and neurofibrillary tangles in pontine tegmentum with cell loss in the dentate nuclei in progressive supranuclear palsy. Old head injury, multiple sclerosis and Pick's disease, which also enter into the differential diagnosis clinically, should have become apparent from the naked eye appearance of the brain.

REFERENCES

Adams RD, Fisher CM, Hakim S, Ojemann R, Sweet W (1965) Symptomatic occult hydrocephalus with 'normal' cerebrospinal fluid pressure: a treatable syndrome. *New Engl J Med* 273: 117.

Akai K, Uchigasaki S, Tanaka U, Komatsu A (1987) Normal pressure hydrocephalus. A neuropathological study. *Acta Pathol Jpn* 37: 97–110.

Benson DF, Cummings JL (1990) *Subcortical Dementia.* Oxford University Press.

Cummings JL, Benson DF (1992) Hydrocephalic dementia: Chapter 7 in *Dementia: A Clinical Approach.* Butterworths, Boston, 2nd ed, pp 213–36.

Cutler RWP, Page L, Galicich J, Watters GV (1968) Formation and absorption of cerebrospinal fluid in man. *Brain* 91: 707–20.

Davson H *et al* (eds) (1987) *Physiology and Pathophysiology of the Cerebrospinal Fluid.* Churchill Livingstone.

DeLand FH, James AE Jr, Ladd DJ, Konigsmark BW (1972) Normal pressure hydrocephalus: a histologic study. *Am J Clin Pathol* 58: 58–63.

Derouesne C, Gray F, Escourolle R, Lastaigne P (1987) 'Expanding cerebral lacunae' in a hypertensive patient with normal pressure hydrocephalus. *Neuropathol Appl Neurobiol* 13: 309–20.

Di Rocco C, Di Trapani G, Maira G, Bentivoglis M, Macchi G, Rossi GF (1977) Anatomo-clinical correlations in normotensive hydrocephalus. *J Neurol Sci* 33: 437–52.

Earnest MP, Fahn S, Karp JH, Rowland LP (1974) Normal pressure hydrocephalus and hypertensive vascular disease. *Arch Neurol* 31: 262–6.

Fisher CM (1977) The clinical picture in occult hydrocephalus. *Clin Neurosurg* 24: 270–84.

Fisher CM (1982) Hydrocephalus as a cause of gait disturbance in the elderly. *Neurology* 32: 1358–63.

Foltz EL, Ward AA (1956) Communicating hydrocephalus from subarachnoid bleeding. *J Neurosurg* 13: 546–66.

Hakim S, Adams RD (1965) The special clinical problem of symptomatic hydrocephalus with normal cerebrospinal fluid pressure. *J Neurol Sci* 2: 307–27.

Herndon RM, Brumback RA (eds) (1989) *The Cerebrospinal Fluid.* Academic Press, NY.

Katzman R (1977) Normal pressure hydrocephalus Chapter 4 In Wells CE (ed) *Dementia* 2nd edn. FA Davis, Philadelphia, pp 69–92.

Koto A, Rosenberg G, Zingesser IH, Horoupian D, Katzman R (1977) Syndrome of normal pressure hydrocephalus: possible relation to hypertensive and arteriosclerotic vasculopathy. *J Neurol Neurosurg Psychiat* 40: 73–9.

Lorenzo AV, Bresnan MJ (1973) Deficit in cerebrospinal fluid absorption in patients with symptoms of normal pressure hydrocephalus. *Dev Med Child Neurol Suppl* 29: 35–41.

Lorenzo AV, Page LK, Watters GV (1970) Relationship between cerebrospinal fluid formation, absorption and pressure in human hydrocephalus. *Brain* 93: 679–92.

McHugh PR (1964) Occult hydrocephalus. *Quart J Med* 33: 297–308.

Marsden CD, Harrison MJG (1972) Presenile dementia. *Letter Br Med J* 3: 50.

Messert B, Wannamaker B, Dudley A (1972) Reevaluation of the size of the lateral ventricles of the brain. *Neurology* 24: 941–51.

Morgagni GB (1769) *The Seats and Causes of Diseases Investigated by Anatomy.* Alexander B Trans. Miller and Caddell, London.

Newton H, Pickard JD, Weller RO (1989) Normal pressure hydrocephalus and cerebrovascular disease: findings of post mortem. *J Neurol Neurosurg Psychiat* 52: 804.

Pickard JD (1984) Early post-haemorrhagic hydrocephalus. *Br Med J* 289: 569–70.

Pickard JD (1991) Normal pressure hydrocephalus. In Swash M, Oxbury JO (eds) *Clinical Neurology.* Churchill Livingstone, Edinburgh, pp 151–64.

Riddoch G (1936) Progressive dementia without headache or changes in the optic disc, due to tumours of the third ventricle. *Brain* 59: 225–33.

Rosenberg GA (1990) *Brain Fluids and Metabolism.* Oxford University Press.

Smith SS, Kiloh LG (1981) The investigation of dementia: results of 200 consecutive admissions. *Lancet* ii: 824–7.

Tomlinson BE, Blessed G, Roth M (1970) Observations on the brains of demented old people. *J Neurol Sci* 11: 205–42.

Vanneste JAL (1994) Three decades of normal pressure hydrocephalus: are we wiser now? *J Neurol Neurosurg Psychiat* 57: 1021–5.

Vessal K, Sperber EE, James AE Jr (1974) Chronic communicating hydrocephalus with normal CSF pressures: a cisternographic-pathologic correlation. *Ann Radiol* (Paris) 17: 785–93.

CHAPTER SIXTEEN

Head injury and dementia

C. J. Bruton

Dementia pugilistica
Memory loss and dementia: boxing, acute head injury and Alzheimer's disease

The long-stay wards of mental hospitals provide asylum for many brain-damaged individuals. A few of these have become demented following a severe head injury; a few more became demented following a long career as a boxer. This chapter considers the relationship between head injury and dementia as it is seen by a neuropathologist working in a psychiatric hospital. This means, in part, that it examines an insidious occupational disorder that affects the nervous system of some boxers, often late in their careers, or sometimes years after they have retired from the sport. It is the description of a neurological and psychiatric disorder originally called the 'punch drunk' state (Martland, 1928), but renamed 'Dementia Pugilistica' by Millspaugh (1937) to avoid a pejorative reference to alcohol intoxication and to provide 'a distinctive term for a definite condition'. This chapter does not concern the sudden, fatal, 'single blow' head injury seen rarely in the boxing ring but it does attempt to compare the late effects of boxing with the neuropsychiatric and the neuropathological features of the type of dementia that occurs occasionally in the long-term survivors of severe 'non-boxing' head injuries.

DEMENTIA PUGILISTICA

The punch drunk state, described lucidly by Martland more than 60 years ago, was already known to fight fans and promoters who referred to affected boxers as 'slug nutty', 'goofy' or 'cuckoo'. Fighters of the slugging type who had little or no boxing skills, or second rate boxers used as sparring partners were thought most vulnerable. However, Martland considered that almost 50% of fighters would, if 'they stayed at the game long enough', develop the disease in a mild or a severe form. Martland, a pathologist interested in head injury and a boxing enthusiast, wrote objectively about the sport at a time

when boxing was largely untroubled by medical or administrative interference. He did not have the opportunity to examine a boxer's brain but considered that the punch drunk state was likely to be caused by the formation of multiple concussion haemorrhages in the deeper portions of the cerebrum as a direct result of repeated blows to the head. He interviewed and examined five affected boxers and noted the similarity between the punch drunk state and other neurological conditions such as the juvenile or the pre senile form of Parkinson's disease, the late effects of epidemic encephalitis or the effects of cerebral syphilis. A slight dragging of one leg, or a mild unsteadiness of gait that rarely affected a boxer's ability to fight, characterized the early symptoms. In Martland's experience, 'many cases remain mild in nature and do not progress beyond that point. In others, a very distinct dragging of the leg may develop and with this there is a general slowing in muscular movements, a peculiar mental attitude characterized by hesitancy of speech, tremors of the hands and nodding movements of the head necessitating withdrawal from the ring. Later, in severe cases, there may develop a peculiar tilting of the head, a marked dragging of one or both legs, a staggering, propulsive gait with the facial characteristics of the parkinsonian syndrome, tremors, vertigo and deafness. Finally, mental deterioration may set in necessitating commitment to an asylum.'

Martland discussed the legitimate doubts that might be raised by implying a causal connection between a career as a professional boxer and the development of a progressive extrapyramidal syndrome resembling paralysis agitans and considered that only the careful collection of data would definitely establish the existence of the syndrome. His forecast was realized, clinically, some 40 years later with the publication of a large study of ex-professional boxers (Roberts, 1969), although in the intervening decades there had been much comment on the condition in both the lay and the medical press (see Roberts, 1969; Corsellis, Bruton & Freeman-Browne, 1973 and Corsellis, 1989 for detailed refs.). Alarmed by the continued reports of possible brain damage in boxers, the Royal College of Physicians in London had set up a committee to report on the medical aspects of boxing. In 1967, they asked Roberts to interview and examine a randomly selected sample (1.5%) of all 16781 professional boxers who registered with the British Boxing Board of Control from its formation in 1929 until 1955. Roberts did not include boxers registered from 1956 onwards as he considered that they might have still been active in a professional career and less inclined to co-operate. Using classical neurological examination techniques combined with an electroencephalogram and a series of simple psychometric tests of intellectual function, Roberts found that 37 (17%) of 224 ex-boxers had clinically demonstrable lesions of the central nervous system. These followed a relatively stereotyped pattern with a variable degree of disturbed function affecting the cerebellar, pyramidal and the extrapyramidal systems. The mildest cases showed dysarthria with or without disequilibrium and evidence of asymmetrical pyramidal disease. The most severe cases had a severely disabling ataxia, disequilibrium, spasticity or rigidity and a striatal tremor associated with varying degrees of dementia. Only two of the 224 ex-boxers had disturbances of intellectual function that required long term hospital care; both these had paranoid psychoses. Nevertheless, minor degrees of intellectual function, particularly of memory were seen in several others. Roberts analysed the occurrence of neurological symptoms in terms of age and occupational exposure. He found that the occurrence of encephalopathy increased significantly with the number of professional fights and the length of a boxer's career. He found, however, that there was little evidence to support the progressive deterioration of clinical symptoms other than that conceivably attributable to normal ageing except one patient who had a cerebellar and dementing syndrome and three patients who had extrapyramidal signs.

Robert's study, published 25 years ago, remains the only large scale investigation of the prevalence of dementia pugilistica; more recent investigations have employed neuroimaging and sophisticated neuropsychometric testing procedures as well as neurological examination. Casson et al. (1984) studied 18 boxers (13

professionals and five amateurs) aged under 60 years who had no known history of neurological or psychiatric illness. Fifteen of these individuals had fought after 1960 and all the retired boxers were still associated with the sport. Three boxers showed evidence of disorientation, confusion and memory loss; one boxer had dysarthria and nystagmus while the fifth showed impairment of memory without disorientation. McLatchie et al. (1987) examined 20 active amateur fighters aged from 18 to 49 years who had, respectively, fought between four and 200 bouts. They found minor neurological abnormalities in seven boxers; the most severe of these included an extensor plantar response or an impairment of rapid alternating movements of the forearms and hands. Nevertheless, the presence of an abnormal neurological sign correlated significantly with an increasing number of fights. In a neuropsychological study, Brooks et al. (1987) examined 29 amateur boxers and 19 male controls matched for age, ethnicity and education. Within the boxing group, they used variables such as the number of knockouts or the number of bouts to detect possible changes in cognitive performance. None of these variables was a significant predictor of lower cognitive function and the boxers showed no significant evidence of impaired performance. Murelius and Haglund (1991) studied 50 former amateur boxers and 50 normal controls. A significant reduction in 'finger tapping' ability that correlated with the length of the boxing career and the number of bouts was the only difference attributable to boxing found between the two groups. Heilbronner, Henry & Carson-Brewer (1991) assessed 23 amateur boxers immediately before and after an amateur boxing event. These authors noted that the four boxers with the most extensive fight histories displayed slower dominant hand tapping speed after their bout. In the group as a whole, the boxers showed enhanced motor abilities but deficiency in verbal memory after boxing compared with their pre fight performance.

A collective evaluation of these recent investigations suggests that the fully fledged features of dementia pugilistica are nowadays rarely visible inside or outside the boxing ring. However, less severe forms of the disorder undoubtedly still exist. Neuropsychometric testing may be the most sensitive means to detect subtle neurological deficits in amateur boxers. Neuroimaging and clinically detectable abnormalities seem to occur almost exclusively in ex-professional boxers or in amateur boxers who have had a long boxing career and very many bouts.

The first neuropathological report on the late effects

of boxing was by Brandenburg and Hallervorden in 1954. This concerned an amateur boxer who had been a German middleweight champion. He boxed for 11 years and retired aged 38 years. After retirement his speech gradually became vague and he was forgetful and excitable. Parkinsonism and dementia developed in the year before his death at 51 years. The brain showed evidence of Alzheimer's disease with amyloid vascular change; the case was considered one of post-traumatic dementia. Grahmann and Ule (1957) published the post-mortem findings on a professional 'booth fighter' who retired, aged 25 years, when he had become 'soft'. Ten years later he developed attacks in which his left leg 'twitched'. Gradually his mental condition deteriorated, he spoke and moved slowly and he developed parkinsonism more marked on the left than the right. On naked-eye examination, the brain was atrophic with enlarged lateral ventricles and a sizeable cavum septum pellucidum. Histologically the brain showed neurofibril-

lary tangles scattered through the cortex and the brain stem. Senile plaques were not seen. Mawdsley and Ferguson (1963) and Ferguson and Mawdsley (1965) described the presence of a large cavum septum pellucidum with fenestrated walls in the brains of four ex-boxers. They confirmed the air encephalography appearances of septal abnormalities described in professional boxers by Spillane (1962). In 1967, Constantinidis and Tissot examined the brain of an ex-professional boxer who had been European Champion. His boxing career spanned seven years until he retired, aged 24 years, when he had developed a weakness of the left leg and some mental deterioration. The following year he developed parkinsonism and his intellect, memory and his behaviour deteriorated insidiously. He died aged 58 years. The brain was moderately atrophied and a septal cavum with fenestrations was noted. In addition, the substantia nigra was totally devoid of pigment and neurofibrillary tangles were seen in large numbers in the medial tem-

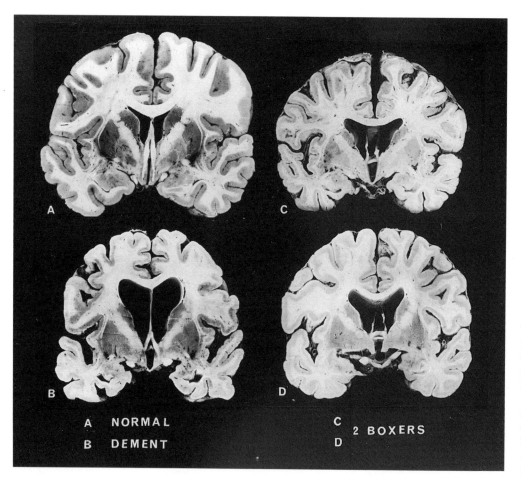

A NORMAL
B DEMENT

C
D 2 BOXERS

Fig. 16.1. A coronal slice from each of four brains to illustrate the septum pellucidum in punch drunk boxers. (× 0.25)

A. Shows a normal septum pellucidum separating the anterior horns of the lateral ventricles.

B. Septum pellucidum in a demented individual. The brain is atrophic. The lateral ventricles are greatly enlarged. The septum is narrowed and stretched but remains intact.

C,D. The characteristic appearances of the septum in punch drunk boxers. The septal leaves are widely separated and torn.

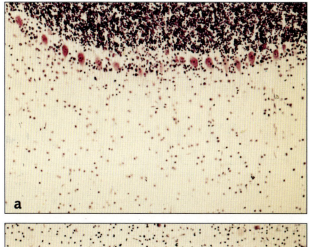

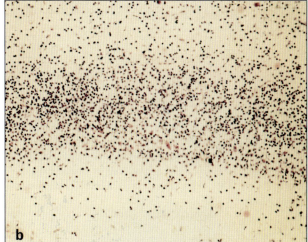

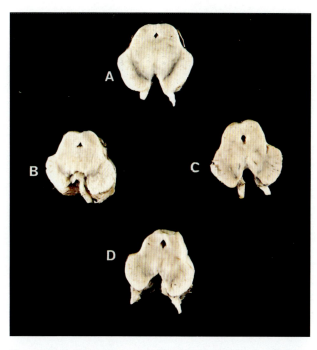

Fig. 16.5.(a). Nissl stain of cerebellum from a normal elderly male. The Purkinje cells, granule cells and molecular layer are intact. (b). Nissl stain from a scarred area of a boxer's cerebellum. There is a complete loss of Purkinje cells and some proliferation of the Bergmann glia.

Fig. 16.7.(a). Transverse cut through the mid-brain of an elderly male non-boxer to show the normal pigmentation of the substantia nigra ($\times$ 0.75). (b) (c) and (d). The substantia nigra of three punch drunk boxers. Some pigment is still visible in (b) but (c) and (d) are almost totally devoid of pigmentation ($\times$ 0.75).

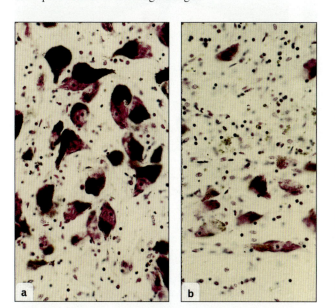

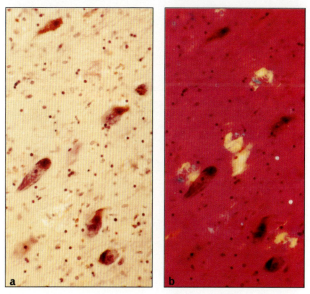

Fig. 16.8. Higher power view of pigmented nerve cells in substantia nigra (Nissl $\times$ 250). (a). Shows the nigra of a normal elderly male. (b). Shows loss on pigmented cells, free-lying pigment and glial proliferation in a punch drunk boxer's nigra.

Fig. 16.9.(a). Congo red and haematoxylin stained section of a boxer's mid-brain showing a few shrunken pigmented nerve cells and the faint remnants of several more degenerated neurons. (b). The same field under polarized light. Doubly refractile neurofibrillary tangles can be seen particularly in places where the degenerated neurons are visible in (a) ($\times$ 220).

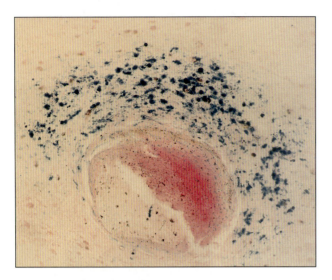

Fig. 16.10. Perivascular deposits of iron stained blue by Perl's ferrocyanide method (×100).

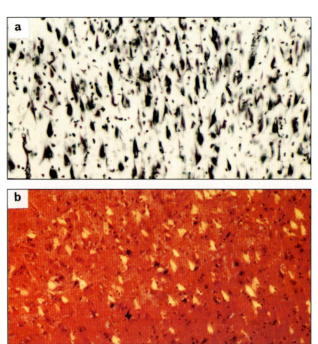

Fig. 16.11.(*a*). Alzheimer's neurofibrillary tangles affecting most neurons in the parahippocampal gyrus of a punch drunk boxer. Note the absence of senile plaques. von Braunmühl's silver stain (× 100). (*b*). Same area stained by Congo red under polarized light. The doubly refractile neurofibrillary tangles are clearly visible (× 100).

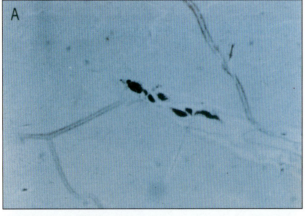

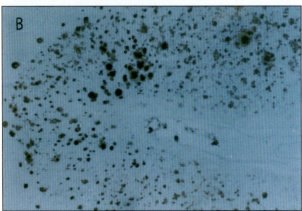

Fig. 16.12. Extensive immunoreactive plaque-like deposits of β-amyloid in cerebral cortex of punch drunk boxer. (*a*). Before and (*b*). after pre-treatment with formic acid (×50).

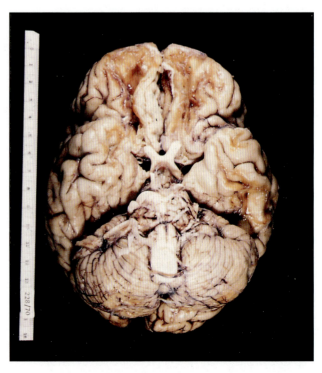

Fig. 16.13. Inferior surface of brain showing extensive bilateral orbito-frontal and temporal lobe scarring that are the hallmark of many severe non-missile head injuries.

poral grey matter and in the substantia nigra. Six years later, Corsellis and his colleagues (1973) refined the concept of dementia pugilistica when they examined the lives and the brains of 15 ex-boxers, 12 professionals and three amateurs, who had fought between 1900 and 1940. These boxers included two world and six national champions; 11 of the 15 were considered 'punch-drunk' and five ended their days in a mental hospital. The professional career of the world and national champions had been followed in the boxing press; detailed fight records were available in seven cases and the number of professional bouts ranged between 300 and 700; some boxers had averaged more than one fight per week. The mean age at death was 69 years. These individuals gave Corsellis and his co-workers a chance to assess some of the most severely affected cases of dementia pugilistica. Neuropathological examination showed a characteristic

pattern of damage in at least two thirds of the brains. The specific abnormalities, which involved the septal regions, the cerebellum, the mid-brain and the cerebral hemispheres will be considered in detail.

Abnormalities of the septum pellucidum

Two thin sheets of nervous tissue, which stretch between the undersurface of the corpus callosum and the dorsal surface of the fornix, make up the septum pellucidum. Normally, the two sheets fuse to give the appearance of a thin single membrane (Fig. 16.1a). Nevertheless in some individuals (see Schwidde, 1952 for details) they separate anteriorly to form a small closed space known as a 'cavum septi pellucidi'; more posteriorly, a similar interseptal space is known as the cavum Vergae. In atrophic brains where there is considerable enlargement of the lateral ventricles, the septum frequently becomes

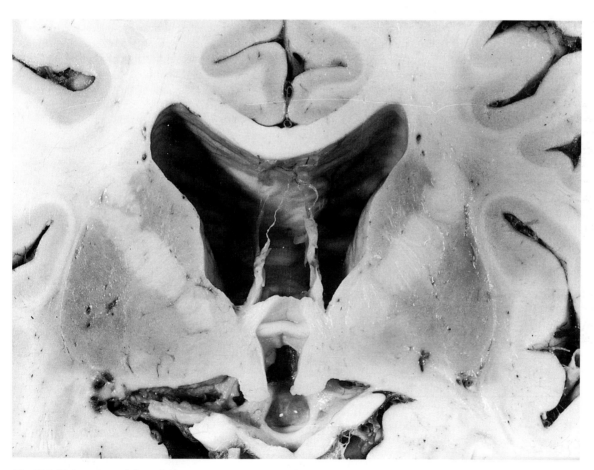

Fig. 16.2. Higher powered view of a boxers septum. The septal leaves are widely separated forming a large cavum. Only a few strands of tissue remain. (× 2.5)

stretched and narrowed (Fig. 16.1b). The situation in dementia pugilistica is, however, visibly different. The two leaves of the septum are separated forming a cavum which may be as much as 10 mm wide. In addition, the septal leaves are almost always torn (Figs. 16.1c & d & 2). The relationship between a career in boxing and the development of a fenestrated septal cavum was investigated by Corsellis et al. (1973) who examined the brains of 500 individuals, 200 men and 300 women, in the same way as those of the 13 boxers (Fig. 16.3). Twenty-five of the control brains had come from a general hospital. The rest were from patients who had died in a psychiatric hospital; cases with cerebral degenerative disorders were represented in large numbers. A torn septal cavum was seen in 77% of the boxers but in only 3% of non boxers; the average width of the boxers' cavum was three times that in the 'non-boxing' controls. In control patients, neither the sex of the patient, the age at death, the psychiatric diagnosis, the size of the lateral ventricles nor the presence of previous surgery such as a leucotomy appeared to influence the presence of a septal cavum. Nevertheless, five of the 15 non-boxing controls who had a torn septal cavum had firm clinical or neuropathological evidence of a past head injury. From this data, Corsellis and his colleagues concluded that the presence of a fenestrated cavum septum pellucidum was seldom likely to be found in any individual who had not suffered a head injury; furthermore, the presence of a large, widely separated, fenestrated cavum strongly suggested a history of repeated cerebral trauma. Their conclusion has since been supported by several neuroimaging studies in which septal abnormalities have been found in many professional boxers (Casson et al., 1984; Jordan & Zimmerman, 1988) yet are rarely seen in amateur fighters (McLatchie et al., 1987; Murelius & Haglund, 1991). Another example of a 'boxers' cavum' was described in the brain of a woman who had been battered repeatedly, for more than 35 years, by her husband (Roberts et al., 1990b). This unfortunate woman also had the classical 'boxing' stigmata known as 'cauliflower ears'.

The cause of the septal damage in boxers is uncertain. Nevertheless, a common-sense view of the possible mechanisms would include a mixture of the shearing stresses produced by swirling movements of the brain within the skull combined with the pulsation of fluid pressure waves generated within the ventricular system that result from repetitive 'small force' blows to the head. A detailed analysis of these mechanisms has been published recently by the British Medical Association (1993).

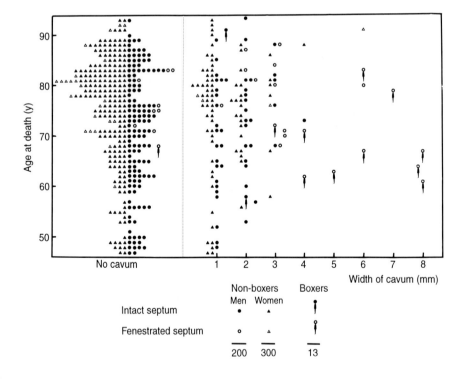

Fig. 16.3. The incidence of fenestrated and non-fenestrated septal cava in the brains of 500 non-boxers and 13 boxers tabulated according to age at death. (Reproduced with permission of the editor and publishers of *Psychological Medicine*.)

Cerebellar damage

The clinical picture of the punch drunk syndrome often suggests an involvement of the cerebellar pathways, yet the early neuropathological studies rarely mentioned the presence of cerebellar damage. Brandenburg and Hallervorden (1954) noted scattered loss and degeneration of Purkinje cells, while Grahmann and Ule (1957) and Payne (1968) mentioned localized folial atrophy. Corsellis et al. (1973), however, described the presence of well defined cortical scars on the inferior surface of both lateral cerebellar lobes in 10 of their 15 boxers. The scarring was most marked in the tonsillar region in the folia around the groove formed by the sloping edge of the foramen magnum. In the scarred areas the molecular layer of the cortex was narrowed and gliosed (Fig. 16.4). The digital white matter of the affected folia was also gliosed and often partly demyelinated. Purkinje cell loss was marked and there was usually some loss of granule cells (Fig. 16.5a & b; see colour plate). In 11 of the boxers, the degree of cerebellar damage was further assessed by measuring the mean distance between each Purkinje cell. The results were compared with the normal range found in 11 non boxing age-and-sex matched controls. The loss of Purkinje cells frequently spread diffusely beyond the limits of the visible, cortical scar and involved much of the ventral cerebellum (Fig. 16.6). The dorsal surface of the cerebellum was usually spared.

There is no direct evidence of the mechanism of the cerebellar damage seen in boxers. Nevertheless, cerebellar damage has been reported in acute head injuries and its pathogenesis has been discussed by Lindenberg and Freytag (1960). These authors described 'tonsillar herniation contusions' following a single blow head injury. They considered that the contusions had been produced when the brain had been forced 'toward and into the only emergency exit of the skull, the foramen magnum'. The present author has seen similar cerebellar tonsil scars in two individuals who had died shortly after a parachute accident. It seems likely that a comparable, but much less violent, mechanism is likely to produce the focal tonsillar scars in boxers.

Degeneration of the substantia nigra

Martland (1928), noted that the symptoms of the punch drunk state closely resembled those of the juvenile and the pre senile forms of paralysis agitans. Roberts (1969), found that parkinsonism had been described in almost 50% of cases of dementia pugilistica published before his clinical report. He went on to conclude that the extrapyramidal features of parkinsonism were an integral part of the neuropsychiatric syndrome seen in the more severely affected punch drunk boxers. Neuropathologically, the hallmark of parkinsonism is degeneration and loss of the pigmented nerve cells in the substantia nigra

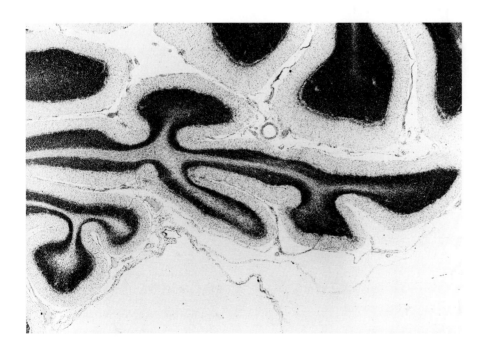

Fig. 16.4. Low power view of cerebellar folia in the tonsillar region of a boxer's cerebellum. The molecular layer of the scarred cortex is narrowed and intensely gliosed.

of the midbrain. Brandenberg and Hallervorden (1954) described degeneration of pigmented nerve cells and widespread neurofibrillary tangles in the substantia nigra in their case of dementia pugilistica. They considered the neuronal loss was less than that usually seen in post-encephalitic parkinsonism. Grahmann and Ule (1957) and Constantinidis and Tissot (1967) described a similar picture. A parkinsonian syndrome was described in the hospital records of four of the 15 cases reported by Corsellis and co-workers in 1973. In several others, the description of the boxers' movements in later life suggested that a degree of the syndrome had developed. On neuropathological examination, the authors noted gross lack of nigral pigment in the four cases diagnosed clinically (Fig. 16.7a–d; see colour plate); seven more of the remaining 11 were materially affected. The histological lesion, at its most severe, showed almost complete loss of pigmented nerve cells while many remaining ones showed neurofibrillary change (Fig. 16.8a & b and Fig. 16.9a & b; see colour plate). In less affected cases, there was a tendency to spare the medial nuclear groups whereas the intermediate and lateral groups were more damaged. The pigmented neurons of the locus ceruleus were similarly involved. Lewy bodies were, however, absent and the histology resembled that seen in postencephalitic parkinsonism rather than that of paralysis agitans (Oppenheimer & Esiri, 1992).

The precise relationship between trauma and parkinsonism is obscure. Specific mention of degenerating pigmented nerve cells has not featured in reports of mid brain damage seen in the survivors of an acute single blow head injury (Tomlinson, 1970; Adams, 1992). There is no doubt, however, that the repeated minor head injury seen in boxers may be followed, not infrequently, by the symptoms of parkinsonism which may deteriorate progressively as the years pass by (Roberts, 1969).

Involvement of the cerebral hemispheres

Contusions and haemorrhage in the grey and the white matter of the brain play an integral part in the pathogenesis of acute non boxing head injury (Adams, 1992). Such lesions have also been found in the brains of boxers who die suddenly during a boxing contest (Unterharnscheidt, 1970). Martland (1928) considered that similar pathology might be responsible for the symptoms of the punch drunk syndrome. He thought that single or multiple blows to the jaw and the head would produce multiple 'concussion haemorrhages' on the surface and in the deeper parts of the brain. Obviously, over a period of years, such lesions would either disappear or would show up only as focal scarring. Payne (1968) examined the brains of six professional boxers and noted small foci of degeneration scattered throughout the cerebral and the cerebellar grey and white matter. He considered that these lesions were compatible with previous cerebral injury. In contrast, Corsellis *et al.* (1973) identified rusty staining of the orbito-temporal cortical surface in only two of the 15 boxers' brains. Furthermore, micro-scars were not found in the cerebral cortex or the deeper grey and white matter unless vascular degeneration was

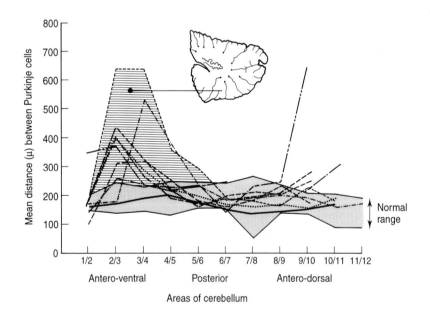

Fig. 16.6. Mean distance between Purkinje cells in the cerebellum of 11 boxers and 11 normal controls. The Purkinje cell loss is most marked in the tonsillar area of the cerebellum.

present to a degree which would at least throw doubt on the nature of their source. Nevertheless, in a subsequent analysis of the same material, Adams and Bruton (1989) used Perls' ferrocyanide method for iron and detected evidence of previous perivascular haemorrhage and/or meningeal siderosis (Fig. 16.10; see colour plate) in 77% of the ex-boxers compared with 11% of 94 age-and-sex matched non boxer controls. Adams and Bruton concluded that the degree of cerebral damage, as measured by the amount of free-lying haemosiderin, was minor and almost certainly could not have accounted for the extensive symptoms that characterize the punch drunk state.

More relevant, perhaps, to the signs and to the symptoms of dementia pugilistica is the occurrence of Alzheimer's neurofibrillary tangles found in nerve cells of the cerebral cortex and brainstem of many punch drunk boxers. Neurofibrillary tangles are present in small numbers of neurons in many elderly people but they almost always accompany senile plaques. The degree of plaque and tangle formation varies with age, but they occur together at their most extreme in individuals who have Alzheimer's disease. In contrast there are other, much rarer, conditions in which neurofibrillary change occurs in the complete or almost complete absence of senile plaques. These include the parkinsonism–dementia complex of Guam, a rare familial dementia with psychosis and degeneration of the amygdala, postencephalitic parkinsonism, progressive supranuclear palsy and some rare forms of chronic encephalitis (for review, see Sumi et al., 1992; Oppenheimer & Esiri, 1992). In Alzheimer's disease the brunt of the neurofibrillary tangle formation occurs in nerve cells in the medial temporal grey matter; the neurons in the diencephalic and periventricular regions are much less affected. In the rarer disorders the distribution of neurofibrillary tangles falls much less on the cerebral hemispheres than on the neuronal groups in the midbrain, pons and medulla. Neurofibrillary tangles in the boxers examined by Corsellis et al. (1973) were, however, distributed diffusely throughout both the cerebral cortex and the brainstem, although they were undoubtedly most prominent in the medial temporal grey matter (Fig. 16.11; see colour plate). Furthermore, the tangles, which were morphologically and immunohistochemically identical to those in Alzheimer's disease (Wisniewski et al., 1976; Roberts, 1988), were found in the complete or almost complete absence of senile plaques. The curious deficiency of senile plaques in the presence of large numbers of neurofibrillary tangles was also noted in the

boxers examined by Grahmann and Ule (1957) and by Constantinidis and Tissot (1967), although the brain of the punch drunk boxer described by Brandenberg and Hallervorden (1954) showed the typical features of Alzheimer's disease and was characterized by numerous neurofibrillary tangles in the presence of many senile plaques and amyloid vascular disease.

Senile plaques and neurofibrillary tangles have, until recently, almost always been identified by the use of silver stains or by Congo red preparations. The development of a specific antibody to the β-protein component of the senile plaque core (Allsop et al., 1986) has led to renewed interest in the detailed composition of senile plaques and also to the decision to reinvestigate the brains of punch drunk boxers. In 1990, Roberts, Allsop and Bruton examined the brains of 20 ex-boxers along with the brains from normal elderly individuals and Alzheimer's disease controls; their cases included 14 of the 15 individuals originally examined by Corsellis et al. Using the Congo red technique and conventional silver stains, 13 of the 20 boxers brains were found to contain numerous neurofibrillary tangles yet only three showed significant numbers of senile plaques. However, when stained for β-amyloid protein, 19 of the 20 brains showed extensive immunoreactive plaque-like deposits throughout the cerebral cortex (Fig. 16.12a & b; see colour plate). The degree and the distribution of the diffuse β-amyloid plaques in the boxers' brains resembled that found both in the 'control' cases of Alzheimer's disease and in an unusual case of 'premature Alzheimer's disease' which had followed a severe non boxing head injury (Clinton, Ambler & Roberts, 1991; Rudelli et al., 1982). The intriguing similarity between the neuropathology of dementia pugilistica, acute head injury and Alzheimer's disease has resurrected previous claims that head injury may precipitate some cases of Alzheimer's disease (Claude & Cuel, 1939; Corsellis & Brierley, 1959; Hollander & Strich, 1970). The evidence for these claims is discussed below.

MEMORY LOSS AND DEMENTIA: BOXING, ACUTE HEAD INJURY AND ALZHEIMER'S DISEASE

Disorders of memory, particularly of recent memory, are thought to result from disturbances centred on the limbic areas of the brain. The neural pathways that appear most directly concerned are those in the medial temporal grey matter including the hippocampus. These areas project via the fornix to the mamillary bodies and link to the thalami and to the septal regions (see

Corsellis, 1970; Amaral & Insausti, 1990 for detailed refs.). Many punch drunk boxers begin to show a degree of memory impairment towards the end of their boxing career; in a few cases the memory disorder merges imperceptibly into a state of dementia. Eleven of the 15 boxers examined, neuropathologically, by Corsellis *et al.* (1973) had documented clinical evidence of memory loss and in all these, the neurons of the medial temporal lobes of both cerebral hemispheres were riddled with more neurofibrillary tangles than anywhere else in the brain. Partly because of this degeneration, the loss of nerve cells also tended to be more severe in these medial temporal areas. In contrast, the limbic areas of the four remaining boxers, whose memories were reputedly unaffected, showed little or no evidence of neurofibrillary tangle formation and no evidence of cortical nerve cell loss. The presence and the anatomical distribution of neurofibrillary degeneration in the brains of punch drunk boxers led, not unreasonably, to the belief that the formation of tangles was intimately connected with the memory loss and dementia. Strong evidence has also been produced to indicate that the degree and distribution of neurofibrillary degeneration is closely connected with the degree of dementia seen in individuals who have Alzheimer's disease (Tomlinson, Blessed & Roth, 1970; Wilcock & Esiri, 1982; Tomlinson, 1992 for review). Alzheimer's disease is, however, additionally characterized by the presence of numerous argentophilic senile plaques; these degenerative structures have similarly been found to correlate with the symptoms of dementia (Tomlinson *et al.*, 1970). Furthermore, some authors consider that Alzheimer's disease may be diagnosed, in elderly subjects at least, by the presence of senile plaques in the complete absence of neurofibrillary tangles (Khachaturian, 1985; Terry, De Teresa & Hansen, 1987; Katzman *et al.*, 1988). The fact that the brains of many intellectually normal elderly people contain large numbers of senile plaques and few, or no, tangles (Tomlinson, 1972, 1980; Katzman *et al.*, 1988) has inclined others, including the present author, to take issue with these latter views. Nevertheless, the relationship between senile plaques, tangles and dementia remains a matter of debate not lessened by the detection of β-amyloid plaque-like deposits in the cortex of patients with Alzheimer's disease, in demented boxers and in individuals who die following an acute head injury. In a recent study, Roberts and his colleagues (1994) found plaque-like deposits of β/A4-amyloid protein in the cerebral cortex of 30% of 152 acute head injury cases aged between eight weeks and 85 years who died between four

hours and two and a half years after a severe head injury. The increasing age of the victim at the time of the head injury appeared to accentuate the amount of β-amyloid deposition. Furthermore, the immunoreactivity of the β/A4-amyloid precursor protein was increased in the perikarya of neurons near the β/A4-amyloid deposits. The quantity of β/A4-amyloid protein in the cortex of the head injury patients was less than that seen in cases of Alzheimer's disease but appreciably more than that found in normal controls of the same age. Roberts and co-workers discussed the genetic evidence (Hardy, 1992) that over expression or altered metabolism of β-amyloid precursor protein may be associated with familial forms of Alzheimer's disease and the epidemiological evidence (Mortimer *et al.*, 1991) that a previous history of head injury is the most consistent environmental factor associated with sporadic cases. They concluded their discussion with the following hypothesis: first, that an increased expression of β-amyloid precursor protein is part of an acute phase response to nerve cell injury in the human brain; second, that the extensive over expression of β/A4-amyloid precursor protein can lead to the deposition of β/A4-amyloid protein and the initiation of an Alzheimer's disease-type process within days of a head injury and third, that cerebral trauma may be an important aetiological factor in Alzheimer's disease.

Although attractive, their hypothesis does not, at present, address the crucial relationship between plaques and tangles and the undeniable association of tangles with the clinical symptoms of dementia. Nor does it explain why many elderly people function quite normally when their brains are riddled with senile plaques. However, it does merit further neuropathological examination of the evidence that links, directly, an acute head injury with a histologically indistinguishable dementing illness from that seen in Alzheimer's disease. Surprisingly, perhaps, there have been no more than a handful of cases suggesting such a link. Claude and Cuel (1939) described a woman aged 50 years who was knocked down by a car and suffered 'a brief loss of consciousness'. During the following months she became dull and apathetic. Within a year, her memory and her sense of orientation had noticeably deteriorated; after four years she had become completely demented and was admitted to an asylum. She died seven years after the initial head injury; her brain showed the typical appearances of Alzheimer's disease. In 1959, Corsellis and Brierley published the history of a man aged 50 years who injured his head in a road traffic accident. He was knocked unconscious, sustained a small scalp laceration and superficial bruises but was discharged from casualty 'no serious injury' having been detected. Within a few days, however, he began to complain of lack of concentration and an inability to work. He had frequent headaches, a muddled head and within three months complained bitterly that his memory had begun to fail. During the following year he was examined on several occasions concerning an insurance claim for damages which had been made after the accident. He was thought to have suffered 'considerable organic brain damage'. After four years he was severely demented and had been admitted to a psychiatric hospital. His speech was slurred and there were both coarse tremor and cogwheel rigidity of all four limbs. When he died, five years after the head injury, his brain showed a massive accumulation of typical senile plaques and neurofibrillary tangles throughout the cerebral cortex. An occasional plaque was seen in the deep grey matter and the pons. No plaques were seen in the midbrain and the medulla. At sub-cortical levels, neurofibrillary tangles were seen in some pigmented nerve cells in the substantia nigra and the locus ceruleus. Hollander and Strich (1970), detailed the history of a woman aged 69 years who fell and injured her head. She recovered consciousness in about half an hour but was confused. Within a short time she could answer questions rationally but had no recollection of the accident. The only abnormal neurological sign was defective upward and outwards gaze of the left eye. One week later she became unconscious for 40 hours. Bilateral frontal burr holes were performed and some clear fluid, under tension, was released on the left. She recovered consciousness after the surgery, but was then, 10 days after the head injury, unequivocally demented. She was disoriented, restless, facile, behaved inappropriately and her memory was poor. She was transferred to a mental hospital where she died three years later. Her brain showed numerous senile plaques, neurofibrillary tangles and extensive congophilic angiopathy in all cortical areas. There was congophilic angiopathy in the meninges over both hemispheres and widespread loss of myelin in both frontal lobes.

The three cases described above are similar in that they each involve a middle-aged individual who suffered a relatively minor head injury that was followed within days or weeks by the onset of a progressive, fatal, Alzheimer-type dementia. The case described by Hollander and Strich was complicated by neurosurgery performed to relieve raised intracranial pressure and the patient described by Corsellis and Brierley developed dysarthria and extrapyramidal signs in addition to the

dementia. Nevertheless, these reports represent almost the only neuropathological evidence to suggest that Alzheimer's disease may follow immediately in the wake of a single episode of cerebral trauma. The patient described by Rudelli et al. (1982) and subsequently examined by Clinton et al. (1991) is different but important in several respects. These authors described the neuropathological findings of a steelworker aged 22 years who was involved in a road traffic accident. He sustained a skull fracture and a left temporal haematoma which was evacuated surgically. He left hospital four weeks later with severe dysphasia, anterograde and retrograde amnesia, impaired judgement, impaired mentation and with personality change. His symptoms improved slowly during the next two years, helped by intensive speech therapy and re-education of basic learning skills. He returned to work as a caretaker and remained at work for five years until he began to develop progressive behavioural disturbances, episodes of incontinence and an occasional tremor of both hands. His impulsive outbursts continued for the next two years; they resulted in separation from his family and loss of his job. He was finally readmitted to hospital 13 years after the original head injury. His speech had reduced to single words and phrases. He stood with difficulty and walked with the aid of two people. He had extensive myoclonic jerking of the trunk and limbs. Tendon reflexes were increased; plantar responses were flexor. A CT scan showed moderate cerebral atrophy. He became bedridden and deteriorated progressively until his death 16 years after the road traffic accident. At post-mortem, the brain showed naked eye evidence of the severe head injury with 'contre-coup' scarring and extensive cortical destruction of the left and right frontal and temporal lobes. Histological examination showed that most of the temporal cortex was gliosed and necrotic, with remnants of gliotic cortex overlying extensive demyelination of the temporal white matter. In addition, many senile plaques and widespread neurofibrillary tangle formation characteristic of Alzheimer's disease were seen in all the remaining cortical areas.

The initial post-traumatic sequelae found in the young steelworker were obviously the direct result of brain damage caused at the time of the head injury; similar extensive bilateral contusions involving both the frontal and the anterior temporal lobes are the hallmark of many severe non-missile head injuries (Adams, 1992) (Fig. 16.13; see colour plate). Such injuries are likely to be followed by persisting cognitive impairment of a degree proportional to the amount of brain damage incurred (for review see Lishman, 1987) although the precise pathogenesis of this damage is controversial (Adams, 1992). In extreme cases, where head injury victims have remained in an almost decerebrate state for months or years, Strich (1969) and McLellan et al. (1986) emphasized the importance of diffuse axonal injury produced at the time of initial impact. However, Jellinger (1977) and Peters and Rothemunde (1977) considered that brain stem damage and secondary phenomena such as brain swelling, circulatory disturbances or hypoxia were of greater relevance. After closed head injury the impairment of intellect is usually global, affecting a wide range of cognitive functions together. Marked post-traumatic dementia is often accompanied by hemiparesis or quadriparesis; less severe damage is frequently associated with dysarthria, incontinence and apathy which may give rise, subsequently, to emotional lability or episodes of aggression. The chance of intellectual impairment increases with the age of the individual at the time of injury and also if the dominant hemisphere is more severely damaged (Lishman, 1987). Nevertheless, the normal clinical course is one of gradual improvement; a profound and enduring dementia is rare even after injuries of considerable severity. Miller and Stern (1965) followed up 100 consecutive severe head injuries, on average 11 years after the episode of trauma. One-half of the individuals had received closed head injuries, the other half had compound fractures of the skull. Only ten individuals showed evidence of a persistent dementia and of these, only five were unemployed. Roberts (1979), paid particular attention to the question of progressive post-traumatic dementia in his follow-up study of 331 civilians who had survived very severe head injuries. Each of his subjects had suffered either post-traumatic amnesia or coma for at least one week following an acute non missile head injury; they were re-examined from 3 years to 25 years later using standard neurological and psychometric tests. Roberts used the term 'fronto-limbic dementia' to describe the commonest form of post-traumatic personality change seen in some of the most physically disabled patients. This was characterized by a combination of disabling euphoria, disinhibition or anergia, associated with loss of memory and with outbursts of ungovernable rage. From his sample, Roberts identified 31 patients in whom there was evidence of progressive deterioration in intellectual function, personality, behaviour or neural disability. In ten of these patients (3% of the sample) the possibility was raised of a progressive dementia. He took into account associated factors such as age, alcoholism, epilepsy and hydrocephalus and considered that there was little unequivocal evidence to support the notion that a single head injury could set in train a progressive dementing process. In the light of these clinical studies, the outcome observed in Rudelli and co-workers' patient is very unusual. Similarly unusual is the detailed neuropathological examination of the brain of any patient who has developed dementia following a severe 'single blow' head injury. Strich (1956) found diffuse degeneration of the cerebral white matter in five individuals who survived, in an almost decerebrate state, for five to 15 months after a closed head injury. Four of the five were below 45 years old at the time of injury. Despite extensive histological investigation, which included several different silver stains, no evidence of plaque or tangle formation was mentioned. Other neuropathological reports have been reviewed by Adams (1992). None of these refers to the unexpected occurrence of large numbers of plaques or tangles.

The neuropathological link, therefore, between Alzheimer's disease and cerebral trauma rests, at present, with a handful of interesting case reports from single blow head injuries plus the two cases of dementia pugilistica (the boxer reported by Brandeberg and Hallevorden (1954) and Case No. 13 reported by Corsellis et al. (1973)) whose brains showed numerous senile plaques in addition to widespread neurofibrillary tangles. The presence of numerous β-amyloid deposits in the cerebral cortex of ex-boxers (Roberts, Allsop & Bruton, 1990a) and patients dying from acute head injury (Roberts et al., 1994) provides fascinating indirect evidence but will be pertinent only when the relationship between β-amyloid deposits and senile plaques has been established.

REFERENCES

Adams CWM, Bruton CJ (1989) The cerebral vasculature in dementia pugilistica. *J Neurol, Neurosurg, Psychiat* 52: 600–4.

Adams JH (1992) Head injury. *Greenfield's Neuropathology*, 5th edn, ed. J. H. Adams & L. W. Duchen, Chapter 3, pp 106–152. London: Edward Arnold.

Allsop D, Landon M, Kidd M, Lowe JS, Reynolds GP, Gardner A (1986) Monoclonal antibodies raised against a subsequence of senile plaque core protein react with plaque cores, plaque periphery and cerebrovascular amyloid in Alzheimer's disease. *Neurosci Lett* 68: 252–6.

Amaral DG, Insausti R (1990) Hippocampal formation. In Paxinos, G (ed) *The Human Nervous System*, Academic Press, San Diego USA; Ch 21, pp 711–755.

Brandenburg W, Hallervorden J (1954) Dementia pugilistica mit anatomischem Befund. *Virchow's Arch path Anat Physiol klin Med* 325: 680–709.

British Medical Association (1993) The Boxing Debate.

Brooks N, Kupshik G, Wilson L, Galbraith S, Ward R (1987) A neuropsychological study of active amateur boxers. *J Neurol, Neurosurg Psychiat* 50: 997–1000.

Casson IR, Siegel O, Sham R, Campbell EA, Tarlan M, DiDomenico A (1984) Brain damage in modern boxers. *J Am Med Assn* 251: 2663–7.

Claude H, Cuel J (1939) Démence pré-sénile post-traumatique après fracture du crâne; considérations medico-légales. *Ann Méd Lég* 19: 173–84.

Clinton J, Ambler MW, Roberts GW (1991) Post traumatic Alzheimer's Disease: Preponderance of a single plaque type. *Neuropath Appl Neurobiol* 17: 69–74.

Constantinidis J, Tissot R (1967) Lésions neurofibrillaires d'Alzheimer généralisées sans plaques séniles. *Arch Suis Neurol, Nurochir Psychiat* 100: 117–30.

Corsellis JAN (1970) The pathological anatomy of the temporal lobe with special reference to the limbic areas. In Harding Price J (ed) *Modern Trends in Psychological Medicine*, Butterworths, UK, Vol. 2, Chap. 12, pp 296–325.

Corsellis JAN (1989) The boxer and his brain. *Br Med J* 298: 105–9.

Corsellis JAN, Brierley JB (1959) Observations on the pathology of insidious dementia following head injury. *J Ment Sci* 105: 714–20.

Corsellis JAN, Bruton CJ, Freeman-Browne D (1973) The aftermath of boxing. *Psychol Med* 3: 270–303.

Ferguson FR, Mawdsley C (1965) Chronic encephalopathy in boxers. *8th International Congress of Neurology, Vienna*, Wiener Medizinische Akademie, Vienna, Vol 1, pp 81–4.

Grahmann H, Ule G (1957) Beitrag zur Kenntnis der chronischen cerebralen Krankheitsbilder bei Boxern. *Psychiat Neurol* 134: 261–83.

Hardy J (1992) Framing β-amyloid. *Nat Genet* 1: 233–4.

Heilbronner RL, Henry GK, Carson-Brewer M (1991) Neuropsychologic test performance in amateur boxers. *Am J Sports Med* 19: 376–80.

Hollander D, Strich S (1970) Atypical Alzheimer's disease with congophilic angiopathy presenting with dementia of acute onset. In: *Alzheimer's Disease and Related Conditions*, Wolstenholme GE, O'Connor M (eds), London: Churchill (Ciba Foundation Symposium), London, pp 105–35.

Jellinger K (1977) Pathology and pathogenesis of apallic syndromes following closed head injuries. In Ore GD, Gerstenbrand F, Lucking CH, Peters G, Peters UH (eds), *The Apallic Syndrome*, Springer Verlag, Berlin, pp 88–103.

Jordan BD, Zimmerman RD (1988) Magnetic resonance imaging in amateur boxers. *Arch Neurol* 45: 1207–8.

Katzman R, Terry R, DeTeresa R, Brown T, Davies P, Fuld P, Renbing X, Peck A (1988) Clinical, pathological, and neurochemical changes in dementia: a subgroup with preserved mental status and numerous neocortical plaques. *Ann Neurol* 23: 138–44.

Khachaturian ZS (1985) Diagnosis of Alzheimer's disease. *Arch Neurol* 42: 1097–105.

Lindenberg R, Freytag E (1960) The mechanism of cerebral contusions. *Arch Path* 69: 440–69.

Lishman WA (1987) *Organic Psychiatry*. Blackwell, Oxford.

McLatchie G, Brooks N, Galbraith S, Hutchison JSF, Wilson L, Melville I, Teasdale E (1987) Clinical neurological examination, neuropsychology, electroencephalography and computed tomographic head scanning in active amateur boxers. *J Neurol Neurosurg Psychiat* 50: 96–9.

McLellan DR, Adams JH, Graham DI, Kerr AE, Teasdale GM (1986) In Papo I, Cohadon F, Massaroti M (eds) *Le Coma Traumatique*, Liviana Editrice, Padova, pp 165–85.

Martland HS (1928) Punch drunk. *J Am Med Ass* 91: 1103–7.

Mawdsley C, Ferguson FR (1963) Neruological disease in boxers. *Lancet* ii: 795–801.

Miller H, Stern G (1965) The long-term prognosis of severe head injury. *Lancet* i: 225–9.

Millspaugh JA (1937) Dementia pugilistica. *US Nav Med Bull* 35: 297–303.

Mortimer JA, va Duijn CM, Chandra V, Fratiglioni L, Graves AB, Heyman A, Jorm AF, Kokmen E, Kondo K, Rocca WA, Shalat SL, Sioninen H, Hofman A (1991) Head injury as a risk factor for Alzheimer's disease: a collaborative re-analysis of case-control studies. *Int J Epidemiol* 20: S28.

Murelius O, Haglund Y (1991) Does Swedish amateur boxing lead to chronic brain damage? 4. A retrospective neuropsychological study. *Acta Neurol Scand* 83: 9–13.

Oppenheimer DR, Esiri MM (1992) Disease of the basal ganglia, cerebellum and motor neurons. In Adams JH, Duchen LW (eds) *Greenfield's Neuropathology*, London, Edward Arnold, 5th edn, Chapter 15, pp 988–1045.

Payne EE (1968) Brains of Boxers. *Neurochir* 11: 173–88.

Peters G, Rothemund E (1977) Neuropathology of the traumatic appalic syndrome. In Ore GD, Gerstenbrand F, Lucking CH, Peters G, Peters UH (eds), *The Apallic Syndrome*, Springer-Verlag, Berlin, pp 78–87.

Roberts AH (1969) *Brain Damage in Boxers. A Study of Prevalence of Traumatic Encephalopathy among Ex-professional Boxers*. Pitman, London.

Roberts AH (1979) *Severe Accidental Head Injury. An Assessment of Long-term Prognosis*. MacMillan Press, London.

Roberts GW (1988) Immunocytochemistry of neurofibrillary tangles in dementia pugilistica and Alzheimer's disease: evidence for common genesis. *Lancet* 332: 1456–8.

Roberts GW, Allsop D, Bruton CJ (1990a) The occult aftermath of boxing. *J Neurol, Neurosurg, Psychiat* 53: 373–8.

Roberts GW, Whitwell HL, Acland PR, Bruton CJ (1990b) Dementia in a punch-drunk wife. *Lancet* 335: 918–19.

Roberts GW, Gentleman SM, Lynch A, Graham DI (1991) βA-4 amyloid protein deposition in the brain after head injury. *Lancet* 338: 1422–3.

Roberts GW, Gentleman SM, Lynch A, Murray L, Landon M,

Graham DI (1994) β-Amyloid protein deposition in the brain following severe head injury: implications for the pathogenesis of Alzheimer's Disease. *J Neurol Neurosurg, Psychiat* 57: 419–25.

Rudelli R, Strom JO, Welch PT, Ambler MW (1982) Postraumatic premature Alzheimer's disease: neuropathologic findings and pathogenetic considerations. *Arch Neurol* 39: 570–5.

Spillane JD (1962) Five boxers. *Br Med J* 2: 1205–10.

Schwidde JT (1952) Incidence of cavum septi pellucidi and cavum vergae in 1,032 human brains. *AMA Arch Neurol Psychiat* 60: 625–32.

Strich SJ (1956) Diffuse degeneration of the cerebral white matter in severe dementia following head injury. *J Neurol, Neurosurg, Psychiat* 19: 163–85.

Strich SJ (1969) The pathology of brain damage due to blunt head injuries. In Walker AE, Caveness WF, Critchley M (eds) *The Late Effects of Head Injury*, Thomas, Springfield IL, pp 501–24.

Strich SJ (1970) Lesions in the cerebral hemispheres after blunt head injury. In Sevitt S, Stoner HB, *The Pathology of Trauma, J Clin Path* (*Lond*), 23, Suppl. (Roy Coll Path), 4, pp 166–71.

Sumi SM, Bird TD, Nochlin D, Raskin MA (1992) Familial presenile dementia with psychosis associated with cortical neurofibrillary tangles and degeneration of the amygdala. *Neurology* 42: 120–7.

Terry RD, DeTeresa R, Hansen LA (1987) Neocortical cell counts in normal human adult aging. *Ann Neurol* 21: 530–9.

Tomlinson BE (1970) Brain-stem lesions after head injury. *J Clin Path* 23: 154–65.

Tomlinson BE (1972) Morphological brain changes in non-demented old people. In von Praag HM, Kalverboer AF (eds), *Aging of the Central Nervous System*, DeErvon F. Bohn, New York, pp 37–57.

Tomlinson BE (1980) The structural and quantitative aspects of the dementias. In Roberts PJ (ed.) *Biochemistry of Dementia*, Wiley, Chichester, pp 15–52.

Tomlinson BE (1992) Ageing and the dementias. In Hume Adams J, Duchen LW, *Greenfield's Neuropathology*, Edward Arnold, London, 5th edn. Chap. 20, pp 1284–410.

Tomlinson BE, Blessed G, Roth M (1970) Observations on the brains of demented old people. *J Neurol Sci* 11: 205–42.

Unterharnscheidt F (1970) About boxing: review of historical and medical aspects. *Texas Rep Biol Med* 98: 421–95.

Wilcock GK, Esiri MM (1982) Plaques, tangles and dementia: a quantitative study. *J Neurol Sci* 56: 343–56.

Wisniewski HM, Narang HK, Corsellis JAN, Terry RD (1976) Ultrastructural Studies of the neuropil and neurofibrillary tangles in Alzheimer's disease and post-traumatic dementia. *J Neuropath Exp Neurol* 35: 367.

CHAPTER SEVENTEEN

Infectious diseases causing dementia

F. Scaravilli and M. J. G. Harrison

Introduction
Herpes simplex encephalitis
Subacute sclerosing panencephalitis (SSPE)
Progressive multifocal leukoencephalopathy (PML)
Encephalitis lethargica and post-encephalitic parkinsonism
The acquired immune deficiency syndrome (AIDS)
Neurosyphilis

INTRODUCTION

The possibility that some forms of dementia could be due to an infective agent, and that they might therefore be treatable, became clear with the discovery that penicillin was effective in cerebral syphilis. The experience of the epidemic of encephalitis lethargica, and now of HIV infection, has also made clear that a wide spectrum of psychiatric manifestations, including dementia, can be due to organic brain disease. The phenomenology of the dementia appears to differ only slightly between infective and other aetiologies, though the tempo varies a lot. Patients with progressive multifocal leukoencephalopathy (PML) or AIDS dementia may show very rapid cognitive decline as may those with Creutzfeldt–Jakob disease in contrast with the natural history of Huntington's or Alzheimer's disease. Perhaps the very rapidity of the process hides any subtle differences in psychopathology.

It is in the infective causes of dementia that the relative roles of cell loss, inflammatory cell proliferation, cytokines and neurotransmitters in the aetiology of cognitive and behavioural change is most intensely under study. The new tools of genetics, immunology and virology are being brought to bear on these conditions, and the coming decade promises much in the understanding of these dementias. The chapter reviews the clinical and neuropathological features of the most important examples as a back drop to those anticipated advances.

HERPES SIMPLEX ENCEPHALITIS

Herpes simplex is the commonest cause of fatal encephalitis and many hundreds of cases are seen in western countries each year. The virus (HSV) is an enveloped organism 120 nm in diameter with a DNA genome of the molecular weight of approximately 96×10^6 Daltons (Roizman & Batterson, 1985). Two types of HSV are described (Dowdle et al., 1967; Plummer, 1964), which differ on biological, biochemical and immunological grounds: type 1, representing the commonest cause of encephalitis, is acquired during early childhood and is associated with ocular and oral lesions; type 2 can also cause encephalitis, is associated with sexual activity and produces genital disease.

Both types are acquired via mucosal contacts; following a primary infection in the throat and mouth (type 1) or in the genital region (type 2), the virus reaches, through the peripheral nerves (Rawls, 1985), the regional sensory ganglia, where it remains latent (Blyth & Hill, 1984). The mechanisms of latency, which have not been completely clarified, are discussed by Esiri and Kennedy (1992). Once reactivated by various stimuli, which include sunlight, stress, fever, trauma and X-rays (Wildy et al., 1984; Kennedy, 1984), the virus travels back to the corresponding dermatome, using axonal transport, and produces a localized disease. In immunocompetent individuals this remains circumscribed and resolves within 1–2 weeks; in immunocompromised or otherwise debilitated patients it becomes a more severe and generalized problem. Of the two immunological mechanisms, the humoral and cellular, the former is probably not essential for the maintenance of latency (Sekizawa *et al.*, 1980). On the other hand, cell-mediated immunity plays a role in both infection and recurrence (Wildy *et al.*, 1982).

HSV encephalitis affects all sections of the adult community and all ages. It is estimated to affect 1 in 250 000 to 1 in 500 000 of the population every year. Most victims have previously been well, and the prevalence of a history of recurrent herpetic skin lesion (herpes labialis) is probably no greater than in the general public. One in 100–200 000 pregnancies is complicated by foetal or newborn infection, which is nearly always symptomatic and frequently lethal. Intrauterine infection may give rise to microcephaly or hydraencephaly. In disseminated post-partum infection, most often seen at 9–10 days, liver and adrenal involvement is usual. In the latter situation, 60–70% have associated encephalitis. Isolated HSV encephalitis presents somewhat later, at 16–17 days, and probably reflects the modifying effect of transplacental maternal antibodies. However, it still carries a high mortality and may be followed by microcephaly and spastic quadriplegia.

Both primary and recurrent infection can give rise to HSV encephalitis; primary infection probably accounts for one-third of cases and most of these are under 18 years of age. The acute disease may present with confusion, disorientation and bizarre behaviour, suggesting an acute dementing illness and long-term survivors frequently show evidence of memory impairment, personality change or frank dementia (Oxbury & MacCallum, 1973; Hierons, Janota & Corsellis, 1978).

The clinical presentation reflects the focal nature of the parenchymatous infection. Thus, the familiar mental state and conscious level changes of encephalitis, in general, are compounded by the features of frontal, temporal or brain stem infection. Hemiparesis, dysphasia, visual field loss or cranial nerve signs were recorded in 96 of 113 biopsy proven cases (Whiteley *et al.*, 1982). The other 17 cases had behavioural changes and evidence of localized CNS involvement on neuroimaging. The commonest clinical findings were headache, fever, personality changes, seizures, hemiparesis and ataxia, all of which affected more than 50% of victims.

The cerebrospinal fluid virtually always has a pleocytosis which often includes erythrocytes as well as white cells. Leukocyte counts of $10–1000/mm^3$ are seen. Hypoglycorrachia would suggest an alternative diagnosis. EEG may be helpful and the predilection for the temporal lobes seen in HSV encephalitis can be seen in the occurrence of focal repetitive complexes. The complexes (Fig. 17.1) are of simple morphology and independent on the two sides; they are not uniformly encountered and are not necessarily detected at presentation. Serial records may be necessary. The complexes may precede flattening of the record due to necrosis. The sensitivity of EEGs in the diagnosis of HSV encephalities has been estimated at 84%, but the specificity in the NIAID studies (Whiteley *et al.*, 1982) was only 32.5%. Localization to the temporal lobes may be seen on CT (Fig. 17.2) and nucleotide (Fig. 17.3) scans. MRI is more sensitive, and bilateral high signal in the temporal lobes with some swelling is very suggestive of the diagnosis. However, none of these tests is sufficiently diagnostic, and proof of the diagnosis has traditionally depended on brain biopsy (Soong *et al.*, 1991). Series of biopsy proven cases

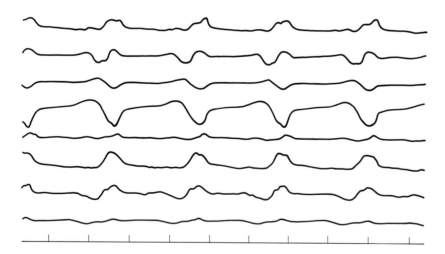

Fig. 17.1. EEG showing repetitive simple complexes over both temporal lobes (upper 4 channels from right, lower 4 from left) in a case of necrotic Herpes simplex encephalitis.

reveal the alternative conditions that can be confused clinically with HSV encephalitis (Whiteley *et al.*, 1982): commonest are tumours of the temporal lobe, vascular disease and other infections including tuberculosis, bac-

terial abscesses and other virus diseases. The continued need for histological proof of the diagnosis is, however, challenged by two developments: first, rapid identification of herpes virus in CSF has become possible by the

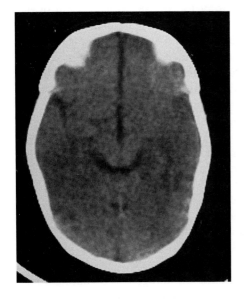
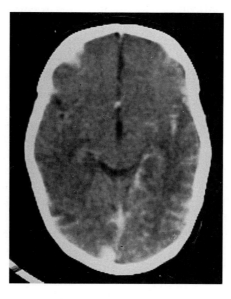

Fig. 17.2. CT showing low density changes in the temporal lobes due to Herpes simplex cephalitis. Post-contrast (right) there is enhancement, particularly on the right side. (Courtesy of Dr B. Kendall.)

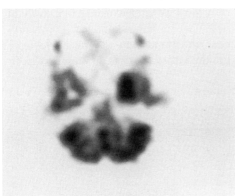
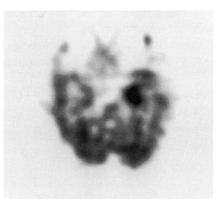

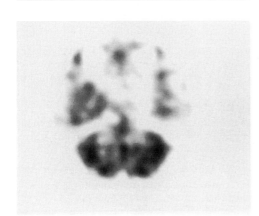
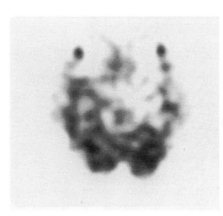

Fig. 17.3. HMPAO radionuclide scan showing increased perfusion in the right temporal lobe in a case of Herpes simplex encephalitis at 6 days (upper 2 slices), which became an area of low uptake (lower slices) at 60 days.

polymerase chain reaction (PCR) (Rowley *et al.*, 1990); secondly, successful antiviral treatment is now available with an agent of low toxicity, so that it may be prescribed without proof of the diagnosis (Sawyer & Ellner, 1988).

Treatment involves the use of acyclovir, which is phosphorylated by virus-encoded thymidine kinase in infected cells to an active anti-DNA metabolite. Relapses have occurred (see below), so the treatment period is now considered to be 21 rather than 10 days (Van Landigham, Marsteller & Ross, 1988). Despite treatment, survival may still be complicated by cognitive impairment with difficulties in new learning of verbal and visual material (Gordon *et al.*, 1990), even when the bedside assessment is unrevealing.

Neuropathology

The characteristic morphological features of HSV encephalitis are associated with type 1 virus. They consist of bilateral, though often asymmetrical, brain swelling and necrosis, particularly severe in the region of the temporal lobes and insulae (Fig. 17.4) and sometimes accompanied by haemorrhage. The involvement of hippocampus, amygdaloid nucleus, the parahippocampal, fusiform and inferior and middle temporal gyri, of the posterior orbital cortex, and the cingulate gyrus is responsible for the name 'limbic' given to this form of encephalitis. The lesions decrease in severity in the brain stem and spinal cord. In infants below the age of 1 year

and, occasionally, in adults, the softening tends to be more widespread, involving most of the brain. Although the grey matter is affected primarily, the process extends to the adjacent white matter which undergoes the same type of degenerative changes. The brain swelling produces compression of the ventricles, herniation of the hippocampi and downward displacement of the brain stem: in cases with asymmetrical swelling, a shift of the midline structures may take place.

On histological examination, necrotic changes may be most severe in the subpial areas and follow a perivascular course in the deeper laminae; however, there is considerable variation in severity and, in many areas, the whole thickness of the cortex, as well as the white matter, may be involved. There is extensive infiltration by macrophages, and small haemorrhages originating from the perivascular spaces are seen. In areas of rarefaction necrosis, very little or no cell reaction is present. Intranuclear eosinophilic inclusions (Cowdry type A) are found in neurons and oligodendrocytes (Fig. 17.5); however, according to Esiri and Kennedy (1992), they are neither a common feature nor easy to detect and the best way to visualize the antigen is by immunohistochemical techniques. Viral antigen remains detectable in brain tissue only for 3 weeks, according to a study of 29 cases by Esiri (1982*a*). Vascular damage with thrombi has been observed and there may also be necrosis or infiltration by inflammatory cells of the vessel walls. In

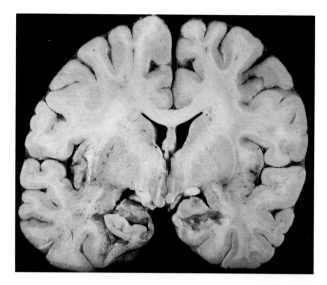

Fig. 17.4. Coronal section of the brain of a patient who died during the acute stage of Herpes simplex encephalitis. Both temporal lobes and the lower parts of the insulae are necrotic.

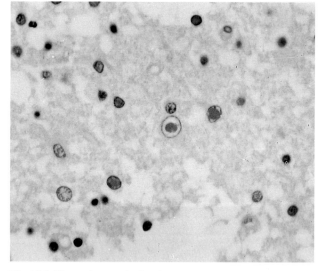

Fig. 17.5. Photomicrograph showing type A intranuclear inclusion bodies in neurons and glial cells of a case of Herpes simplex encephalitis. (H&E ×480)

less severely affected regions, foci of neuronophagia and microglial nodules can be seen (Fig. 17.6). The inflammatory process extends to the meninges which appear infiltrated by macrophages, lymphocytes and plasma cells. The white matter adjacent to the involved cortex may show widespread myelin loss and perivascular lymphocytic infiltration.

The brains of patients who have survived the acute encephalitis for months or years show shrinkage and cystic changes of the affected areas (Fig. 17.7) as well as degeneration in the brain stem and spinal cord containing the descending tracts originating from the necrotic cortical areas.

The discussion of the possible role of HSV2 as a cause of subacute encephalitis is appropriate in this chapter, since a prolonged and discrete illness may be associated with declining mental functions. Indeed, HSV2 is responsible for an aseptic meningitis following outbreaks of genital infection in immunocompetent people. The illness follows the cutaneous lesions by 3–12 days, is self-limited, and is accompanied by fever, headache, vomiting, photophobia and nuchal rigidity resulting from viraemia (Craig & Nahmias, 1973). Furthermore, Oommen, Johnson and Ray (1982) described a single case and reviewed four patients previously reported; four of these presented with psychosis whilst in one (case 1 in Brenneman et al., 1988 (see Oommen et al., 1982))

the symptoms were neurological. Patients 1 and 3 were immunosuppressed and, in them, the disease was fatal; pregnancy in patient 4 made her more susceptible to the virus (Young et al., 1976, in Oommen). All cases showed direct or indirect evidence of HSV2 in brain or CSF. Pathological changes in the personal case included perivascular lymphocytic infiltration of the subarachnoid spaces of the temporal lobe.

Subacute encephalitis has also been sporadically described with HSV1 infection: the two patients reported by Sage, Weinstein & Miller (1985) suffered from a slowly progressive disease; in one of them the virus was isolated from the brain biopsy taken only a few days before death; in the other, a 76 year-old woman, the disorder was characterized by gradual mental retardation, and virus was grown in several CSF specimens. In the case reported by Milstein and Biggs (1977), an 8 year-old boy suffered two episodes of neurological impairment. A brain biopsy showed evidence of an encephalitic process and anti-HSV antibodies were found in the serum.

Systemic treatment with early antiviral drugs adenine arabinoside (ara-A) or cytosine arabinoside (ara-C) considerably decreased the mortality of HSV encephalitis; however, recurrences of the process have also been described (Davis & McLaren, 1983; Dix et al., 1983). Histological examination of brain tissue, removed in

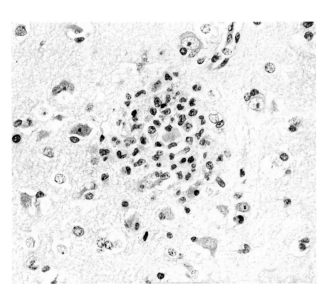

Fig. 17.6. A microglial nodule in an area of the brain less severely affected by the encephalitic process surrounds a necrotic nerve cell. (H&E × 300)

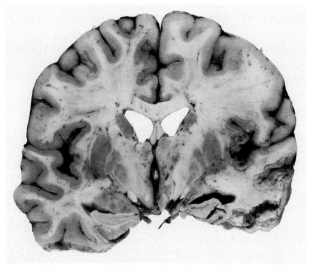

Fig. 17.7. Coronal section of the brain of a patient who survived several weeks the acute encephalitic episode. Complete necrosis of the affected area is associated with shrinkage and disintegration of the tissue.

the late states of the illness, showed non-specific inflammatory changes and no inclusion bodies. In both cases the virus was isolated from the brain biopsy. The pathogenesis of these recurrences has been discussed by Davis and McLaren (1983) who offer evidence in favour of both a reactivation of the virus and an active encephalitis. A third possibility is suggested by the finding in the case described by Koenig et al. (1979): whilst reactivation of HSV was not demonstrated, the perivascular demyelination and inflammatory infiltration suggested a post-infectious process, similar to that occurring in EAE.

The natural course and morphological appearances of HSV encephalitis seem to be modified by immunosuppression: Cappel and Klastersky (1973) described aseptic meningitis due to HSV1 in a leukaemic patient. HSV1 has been found in the brain of a patient with cardiac transplant (Hotson & Pedley, 1976) and in that of AIDS patients (Laskin, Stahl-Bayliss & Morgello, 1987: Pepose et al., 1984), but only as an incidental finding. The scarcity of reports has led to the suggestion that patients with advanced AIDS may be incapable of mounting an immune reaction sufficient to cause the typical acute necrotising encephalitis (Levy, Bredeson & Rosenblum, 1985). Indeed, experimental evidence lends some support to this view (Townsend & Baringer, 1979). In a personal AIDS-related case (Tan et al., 1993), however, the severe necrotic inflammatory response to HSV1 does not support the extrapolation of these experimental results to AIDS patients. Nevertheless, this case was also atypical, since intranuclear inclusion bodies were not only present at post-mortem, but extremely numerous, although the patient died 4 weeks after the onset of the disease and had received antiviral treatment for 3 weeks.

Pathogenesis

The localization of the pathological changes to the limbic system in HSV1 encephalitis has raised a number of speculations regarding the pathogenesis of this disease. Johnson and Mims (1968) suggested the olfactory route through the cribriform plate, but spread along nerves has also been demonstrated (Wildy, 1967; Kristensson et al., 1978). A systematic study of the olfactory tract was undertaken by Dinn (1979, 1980) and Esiri (1982a). Virus was found in all cases examined by the former but only in 9/15 by the latter. Esiri (1982a,b) concludes that, in some cases with negative findings in the olfactory tract, the encephalitis may originate from virus latent in the brain. An alternative hypothesis has

been presented by Damasio and Van Hoesen (1985): the localization to the limbic system could be due to a special affinity of the virus for this region of the adult brain.

SUBACUTE SCLEROSING PANENCEPHALITIS (SSPE)

SSPE was first described by Dawson, and the condition became known as subacute inclusion body encephalitis (Dawson, 1933). The present-day name was developed also to encompass cases described by Pette and Döring in 1939 and van Bogaert in 1945 under different designations. For a time it was thought that this dementing illness of adolescence was due to Herpes simplex, but in the 1960s a link with measles was demonstrated (Bouteille et al., 1965; Legg, 1967; see aetiopathogenesis). SSPE follows childhood acute measles by a number of years (5–10), but affects only 0.1 to 5 per million of the population. This incidence is falling as measles vaccination becomes more widespread (Editorial, 1990). High levels of measles antibodies are characteristic of the disease in both serum and CSF. The site of the reservoir of infection during the long latency before neurological signs become apparent is not entirely clear, but Brown and co-workers (1989) found some autopsy evidence of virus in lymphoid tissue.

The condition affects children and adolescents and occasionally young adults. Boys are more affected than girls (2–3 to 1). Acute measles before the age of 2 years appears to carry the greatest risk of latent infection and subsequent SSPE and 90% of cases are between 4 and 16 years of age at presentation. The disease tends to go through a series of stages (Jabour et al., 1969): initially there are behavioural changes, and subtle cognitive impairment becomes obvious. The patient becomes irritable and forgetful with an adverse effect on school performances. Disobedience, temper tantrums and even psychotic features may be seen (Duncan et al., 1989). The differential diagnosis includes adjustment disorders and depression and, in the absence of neurological signs, this diagnosis is not usually thought of. In the second stage, more focal functional deficits emerge, such as disturbances of writing, visuospatial orientation, apraxias and agnosias. There is no fever, neck stiffness or evidence of systemic disorder. Tumours and demyelinating disease may be mimicked, but the development of myoclonus at this stage is highly suggestive of SSPE. The jerks initially affect the head and upper limbs; they are repetitive with a frequency of one every 5 to 15 seconds and tend to consist of a flexion movement or a drop of the outstretched hands. With further progression, involuntary movements of a dystonic nature, ataxia and progressive dementia are seen. Chorioretinitis which can also be an early feature, and cortical blindness may lead to visual loss. In the third stage, spasticity increases and dementia is masked by impairment of consciousness. The terminal stage consists of decerebrate rigidity and coma. Death is usually due to pneumonia. The time scale of the illness is highly variable (Risk & Haddad, 1979). Thus, on one hand, 40% are dead within a year and some cases run an aggressive acute course with raised intracranial pressure, but, on the other, almost a half may show improvements or plateaux and some patients may survive the first attack for several years. The average half-life in Risk and Haddad's large series (1979) from the Middle East was 1.8 years.

The diagnosis tends to depend clinically on the recognition of the onset of myoclonus, which leads to definitive investigations. The CSF reveals an elevated protein due to the presence of locally synthesized IgG and oligoclonal bands are present on electrophoresis.

The measles complement fixing antibody is raised to 1/16 to 1/64. Serum antibody titres may be as high as 1/5000.

The EEG is frequently diagnostic, though it may be normal at the early stage of subtle behavioural change. Later, from stage two onwards, it is characterized by the presence of repetitive complexes. These may occur without clinical myoclonus, but coincide with any such movements that are visible. The complexes (Fig. 17.8) consist of 2 to 4 hertz high amplitude delta waves occurring bilaterally and synchronously every 5 to 7 seconds. The rest of the record may show slow wave and spike foci commonly in the frontal lobes (Markland & Panszi, 1975). Patients with much seizure activity may not show the repetitive discharges until they are given an injection of diazepam or a recording is made during sleep. CT scans are initially normal but go on to show atrophy and low density in the white matter (Fig. 17.9). MRI is more revealing with high signal on T2 weighted images in the white and deep grey matter. PET scans, in one case, suggested that some areas were the site of

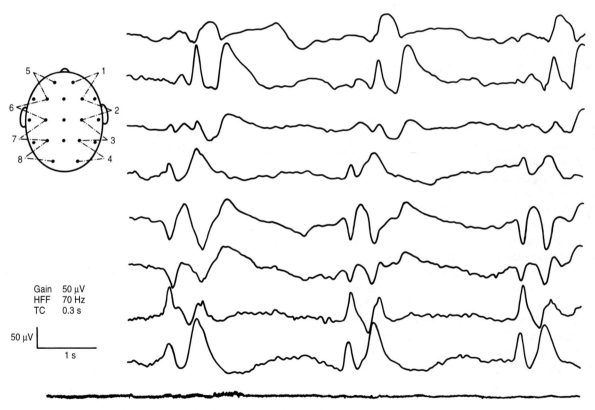

Fig. 17.8. EEG from a child with SSPE, showing characteristic repetitive complexes.

hypermetabolism due to the encephalitis, perhaps in relation to the myoclonic jerks (Huber *et al.*, 1989). There is no proven treatment. Various forms of immunotherapy have been tried including transfusion of compatible lymphocytes from an unaffected identical twin (Bakheit & Behan, 1991), all to no avail. Anti-viral agents have been claimed to affect individual patients, but the variable natural history and possibility of spontaneous partial recoveries and plateaux makes these uncontrolled observations impossible to assess.

Neuropathology

Both macro- and microscopic appearances of the nervous system in SSPE reflect the variable duration of the illness. In cases of short duration, the surface of the brain may appear macroscopically normal, whilst coronal slices show, at times, grey discolouration and granular appearance of the white matter. In cases with long duration, brains show various degrees of atrophy and increased consistency, with thickening of the leptomeninges and widening of the sulci. Reduction of brain tissue results in dilatation of the ventricular system (Fig. 17.10). Focal areas of softening can also be seen, particularly in the fronto-temporal regions; in some chronic cases, the white matter looks moth eaten, with spotty grey discolouration.

On microscopic examination, the inflammatory reaction, which involves both grey and white matter, varies from heavy in cases of short duration to discrete in the more chronic (Fig. 17.11). It consists of lymphocytes, plasma cells, histiocytes and macrophages, and is particularly obvious in the leptomeninges and perivascular spaces. Another histological feature of SSPE, nerve cell loss, may be so severe as to produce ulegyria or induce spongiform cortical changes. Cell loss is widespread, but is particularly severe in the cerebral cortex, thalamus, striatum and pallidus and, in cases of short duration, it may appear as foci of neuronophagia (Esiri & Kennedy, 1992); it becomes less pronounced in the brain stem, whilst the cerebellum is relatively spared, and the spinal cord is rarely involved. The latter, however, can be the site of secondary degeneration. Hyperplasia of both astrocytes and cells of the microglia/macrophage group is seen both in grey and white matter and, in the latter, it is more severe than the myelin loss. In the cortex, microglial cells may appear as rod cells with their long axis perpendicular to the surface of the brain.

Inclusion bodies are the most characteristic feature.

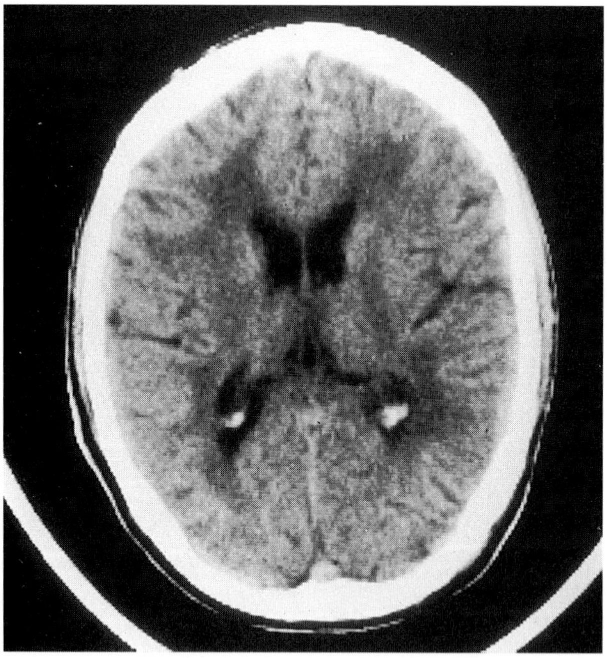

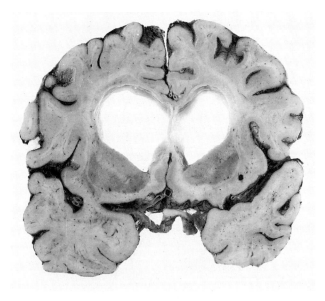

Fig. 17.9. CT scan from a child with SSPE, showing marked low density changes in the hemispheric white matter, especially in the periventricular regions.

Fig. 17.10. Coronal section of the brain of a patient with SSPE who survived for several years after the first episode. Note the extreme reduction in volume especially of the white matter and the considerable dilatation of the lateral ventricles.

They are homogeneous, round or oval structures 3–10 μm in diameter within the nuclei of neurons (Fig. 17.12), oligodendrocytes and, occasionally, astrocytes. They fill completely the nucleus, whose chromatin appears as a thin rim or small clumps lined by the nuclear membrane. Haloes separating the inclusion from the membrane are seldom seen. Leestma (1985) mentions the presence of inclusions also in the cytoplasm. With the electron microscope, inclusions appear to contain tangles of tubular structures with outside and inside diameters of 17 and 7 nm, respectively. The appearances are those of nucleocapsides of paramyxovirus. Antibo-

dies directed against measles virus confirm this aetiology. Indeed, in a study of six patients, who had survived from weeks to several years, Esiri *et al.* (1981) found that, in all of them, the antibody could visualize the virus; the authors point out, however, that the shorter the duration of the illness, the more numerous were the inclusions. Furthermore, the antigen was widely distributed, except in the cerebellum in which it could not be found.

Although the average survival time in SSPE is 1–2 years, patients who have survived for longer periods have been described. The cases with survival longer than 5 years have been reviewed by Dumas *et al.* (1980);

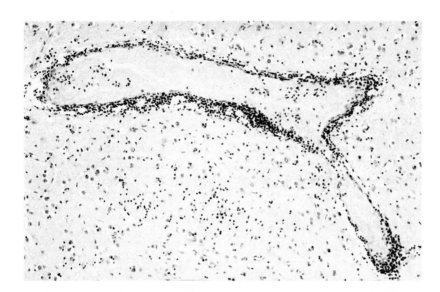

Fig. 17.11. Photomicrograph of the white matter in a case of SSPE. There is a discrete lymphocytic cuffing around a vein in the white matter. The surrounding parenchyma shows reactive gliosis. (H&E × 120)

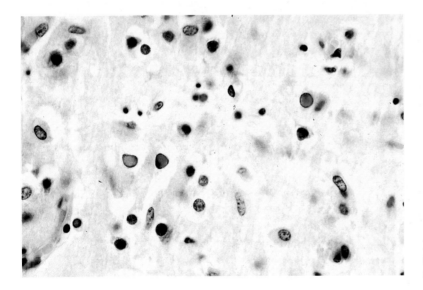

Fig. 17.12. Photomicrograph showing type A intranuclear inclusion bodies in the cortical grey matter in a case of SSPE. (H&E × 480)

moreover, Cobb and Morgan-Hughes (1968) and Cobb (1966) reported three additional patients who survived between 6 and 14 years. In all the cases with long survival, nerve cell loss is extreme, the white matter is thin and gliosis intense. On the other hand, inflammatory changes are scanty and, as in the cases described by Gutewa and Osetowska (1961), Himmelhoch et al. (1970) and Cobb, Marshall and Scaravilli (1984), inclusions are not seen. In addition, chronic cases may show the presence of neurofibrillary tangles (Fig. 17.13), of the type seen in Alzheimer's dementia. The first description of these changes is that of Malamud, Haymaker and Pinkerton (1950). In the patient reported by Cobb et al. (1984), who survived 14 years, tangles consisted of paired helical filaments 20 nm wide, with regular constrictions occurring every 70 nm. Mandybur et al. (1977) insist on the non-specificity of these findings; furthermore, although in the majority of the cases they are associated with long survivals, they have also been described in patients who have survived 12 months or less (Corsellis, 1951; Krücke, 1957; Bornstein et al., 1961; Case Report Mass. Gen. Hosp. 1986).

Aetio-pathogenesis

The finding by Bouteille et al. (1965) that inclusion bodies in SSPE contain nucleocapsides of paramyxovirus; by Connolly et al. (1967) of high titres of measles antibody in serum and CSF of patients; and, eventually, the isolation of the virus from culture of

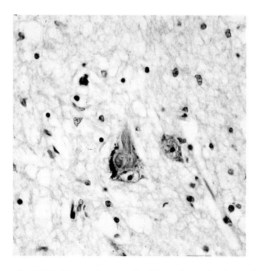

Fig. 17.13. Photomicrograph of the substantia nigra of a patient who survived for 14 years after the first episode of SSPE. A neuron contains neurofibrillary tangles. (H&E ×480)

brain tissue (Horta-Barbosa et al., 1969; Payne, Baublis & Itabashi, 1969) confirmed that measles virus is implicated in SSPE. It is now believed that the cerebral disease, which is considered a slow virus infection, is due to measles virus with defective M-protein persisting in the brain after an incomplete immune reaction.

Various theories have been put forward to explain the pathogenesis of this disorder: for one of them, which implies the involvement of a different strain of virus, there is, to date, no evidence (Choppin, 1981); the role of defective immune response is contradicted by evidence of production of IgG and IgM and of an adequate cell immunity (Agnarsdottir, 1977). However, in patients with SSPE, there is deficiency of antibody to virus protein M, necessary for the release of free measles virus (Hall, Lamb & Choppin, 1979). To date, however, both the long latency and the slow evolution of the disease have not received a satisfactory explanation.

PROGRESSIVE MULTIFOCAL LEUKOENCEPHALOPATHY (PML)

In 1958 Åstrom, Mancall and Richardson described three cases of an unusual demyelinating disease affecting particularly the posterior parts of the cerebral hemispheres. Two of the patients had leukaemia, the third Hodgkin's disease. The clinical picture was of dementia, with speech and pyramidal tract dysfunction. The CSF remained normal. The course was relentlessly progressive with death within 2 to 6 months. From the literature, they found another five cases, including examples in which the underlying disease was sarcoidosis and tuberculosis. In 1959, Cavanagh et al. suggested that the role of immunosuppression was critical and that a virus was probably responsible. Indeed, in 1965, Silverman and Rubinstein and ZuRhein and Chou observed that the intranuclear inclusions of the enlarged oligodendrocytes contained icosahedral particles, 39 nm in diameter, interpreted by the latter as papova virus, similar to the SV-40. Subsequently, Padgett et al. (1971) succeeded in cultivating the virus from a patient with PML. This non-enveloped, double-stranded DNA organism was called JC by the initials of the original patient's name.

Antibodies to JC are present in approximately 70% of the population, although people living in remote areas of the world tend to be free from the infection (Brown, Tsai & Gajdusek, 1975). By the age of six, 50% of the children have seroconverted and by middle adulthood 80–90% of the population have been infected. The virus persists in the kidneys and reaches the nervous system, probably via the blood stream. Houff et al. (1988) have demonstrated its presence in B lymphocytes of the marrow and spleen in cases of PML.

In the nervous system the virus exists as unintegrated forms of DNA sequences within oligodendrocytes, astrocytes and, possibly, in endothelial cells (Dorries, Johnson & ter Muelen, 1979) of the brain and other organs in patients with PML (Grinnel, Padgett & Walker, 1983a). JC viral genomes vary in different PML patients (Grinnell, Padgett & Walker, 1983b; Martin & Foster, 1984; Martin et al., 1985) as well as in the same patient, raising the question of whether the neurological illness is produced by a virus resident in the kidneys and reactivated by immunosuppression or by an exogenous strain (Dix & Bredesen, 1988).

Although the vast majority of cases of PML are produced by JC virus, SV-40 was isolated in two patients and it is estimated that 2–4% of the population have antibodies to SV-40. To date, however, there are no cases produced by this virus in HIV-positive patients. PML usually occurs in immunocompromised individuals (Brook & Walker, 1984), and cases have been reported in immunosuppressed monkeys (Gribble et al., 1975). However, in a small number of patients, no underlying immunosuppression could be found (Silverman & Rubinstein, 1965; Fermaglich, Hardman & Earle, 1969; Bolton & Rozdilsky, 1971).

The clinical presentation reflects the progressively enlarging demyelinating lesions; thus insidious, but progressive limb weakness or visual field defect is common, as is subcortical dysphasia, ataxia and eventually dementia. Features typical of mass lesions, like headache, are conspicuously rare, as are those implying grey matter involvement such as seizures. However, in AIDS, grey matter involvement is rather more noticeable than is traditionally encountered in the other risk groups. Thus Gerstmann syndrome, prosopagnosia, apraxia, unilateral neglect and spatial disorientation have all been documented in proven HIV cases. Focal presentations are very much the rule, though occasional cases show a rapid dementing illness in which focal problems develop secondarily. Most cases are eventually demented. The distinction from AIDS dementia in AIDS-related cases depends on focal signs and the result of investigations. The CSF is normal, except sometimes in AIDS-related cases when there may be elevated protein and pleocytosis due to HIV, not PML. EEGs show non-specific slow wave abnormalities related to the underlying white matter lesion(s) (Fig. 17.14). CT scans reveal non-enhancing hypodense white matter lesions that show no mass effect. They may be single or multiple and may affect cerebral hemispheres, the cerebellum or the brain stem. The parieto-occipital area is particularly likely to be affected. Magnetic resonance imaging is even more sensitive to the demyelination with low density on T1 and hyperdensity on T2 weighted images, again lacking mass effect (Fig. 17.15). The

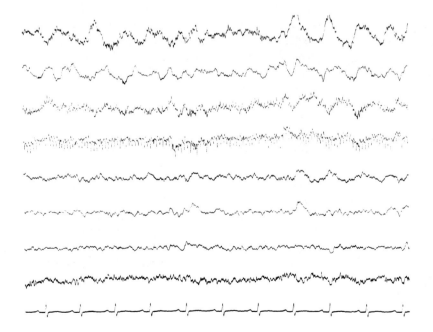

Fig. 17.14. EEG from a patient with progressive hemiparesis due to PML. There is a striking slow wave abnormality over the affected side (upper 2 channels), but the features are non-specific.

abnormal areas are homogeneous, but have indistinct margins and fail to enhance.

The clinical course usually consists of relentless progression with death between 10 days and 18 months; there have, however, been exceptions, even in HIV-related cases. In non-AIDS cases, recovery may attend improvement in the immune status of the patient, e.g. on stopping immunosuppressive treatment or in patients whose sarcoidosis responds to treatment. In AIDS patients, prolonged survival has been described (Berger & Mucke, 1988) for up to 30 months and this may relate to a more inflammatory histological picture. The average prognosis is more likely 4 months. Some patients have appeared to fluctuate spontaneously or in response to systemic factors, including antiviral therapy aimed at the HIV (Conway, Halliday & Brunham, 1990). Anecdotal accounts have reported a variety of attempts to treat PML with such agents as α-interferon, acyclovir, radiotherapy and steroids. The only agent with any real suggestion of efficacy is cytarabine and this is now the subject of a randomized trial (Portegies *et al.*, 1991).

Neuropathology

Macroscopically, the brain may show no changes or some cortical atrophy; however, in AIDS-related cases it is not uncommon to see a variable degree of swelling with flattening of the gyri; the leptomeninges remain invariably thin and transparent. On brain sections, the most obvious abnormality is the presence of white–grey or yellow foci of variable size, involving the cerebral (Fig. 17.16) and cerebellar white matter as well as the brain stem. Their consistency is soft and, on occasion, even semi-liquid. When, as in AIDS patients, death has occurred for other causes, an early, asymptomatic stage of the disorder may occasionally be observed: it consists of multiple small grey plaque-like lesions at the border between white and cortical grey matter, often impinging on the latter (Fig. 17.17).

Lesions appear as foci, in places confluent, of myelin loss and presence of foamy macrophages and a small

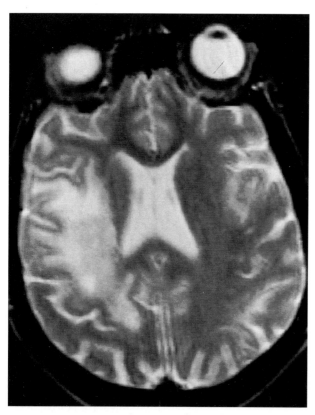

Fig. 17.15. MRI. T2 weighted image showing non-enhancing high signal area without mass effect in the white matter in a biopsy proven case of PML.

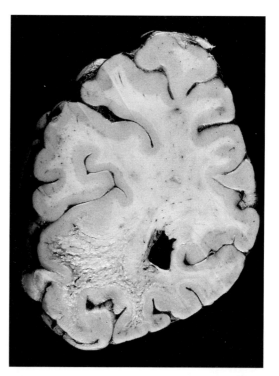

Fig. 17.16. Coronal section of the left occipital lobe in a case of PML. The white matter lateral to the ventricle, including the inferior part of the optic radiations, is necrotic.

number of lymphocytes, usually surrounding blood vessels. A florid astrocytic reaction is present and many of these cells show large, pleomorphic and hyperchromatic nuclei and abundant cytoplasm (Fig. 17.18). A number of oligodendrocytes contain greatly enlarged nuclei, some of which have an homogeneous amphophilic inclusion which displaces the chromatin towards the periphery (Fig. 17.19). In very extensive lesions their centre is poorly cellular with virtually no inclusion-bearing cells. Although histological changes are typically described in the white matter, it is not unusual that the adjacent grey matter be also involved.

The typical papova virus can usually be demonstrated in nuclei of oligodendrocytes (Fig. 17.20(a)) and, less frequently, in astrocytic processes. The virus consists of round and rod-shaped particles, 45 μm in diameter whose development within host cells has been described by Baker and Rayment (1987) and, in PML patients, by Scaravilli et al. (1989). However, an equally reliable and much faster method of diagnosis is the use of in situ hybridization techniques (Fig. 17.20(b)).

Since the outbreak of AIDS, PML has become a more common disease: indeed in large series, the incidence varies from 2 (Petito et al., 1986) and 5% (Budka et al., 1987; Vinters, Tomyiasu & Anders, 1989) to 7% (Lang et al., 1989). In the brains examined in London the incidence was 6%. The latter figures compare with 8% observed by Hooper, Pruitt and Rubin (1982) in immunocompromised HIV-negative patients. An association between PML and HIV encephalitis is not an uncommon finding and Orenstein and Jannotta (1988) suggested a synergistic action of the two viruses.

ENCEPHALITIS LETHARGICA AND POST-ENCEPHALITIC PARKINSONISM

During the epidemic of encephalitis lethargica in 1918 and 1920, a large number of patients developed mental symptoms due to the acute inflammatory changes in the brain. This clear-cut association of psychopathology with an organic brain disease had a major influence on psychiatric thinking. In the acute stages patients, after a flu-like prodrome, developed drowsiness or somnolence, perhaps with mild meningism. Brain stem involvement was often striking with pupillary abnormalities, eye movement disorders and mixed pyramidal and cerebellar signs. Other patients developed movement disorders such as chorea, often in association with agitated, restless behaviour. After this acute period which might last a few days, reversal of sleep rhythm was common. One paediatric unit had to reverse its day/night schedule to accommodate this reversed sleep pattern of its inmates, allowing them to sleep by day and play by night. Some patients became acutely parkinsonian or catatonic, when a severely demented state might be wrongly diagnosed.

The most dramatic chronic sequela of this encephalitis was a condition characterized by parkinsonism accompanied by oculogyric crises and compulsive thoughts and repetitive tic-like motor acts. Respiratory tics were particularly common. Pupillary changes and difficulty with accommodation and convergence were common ocular signs. One-third of the patients died during the acute stages; one third survived with sequelae, whilst another third recovered completely (Yahr, 1978).

The mental state in the aftermath of encephalitis lethargica more often resembled schizophrenia than dementia, but some patients were slow and apathetic. Many children became restless and excitable. Personality and behavioural changes probably far outnumbered examples of cognitive decline. The very varied clinical picture in both the acute and in the post-encephalitic stage presumably reflected the varied regional severity of inflammation and cell loss seen pathologically. Although the epidemic is over, rare cases in recent times have been thought to represent the same condition (Espir & Spalding, 1956).

Intellectual impairment has also been documented albeit rarely after a variety of other encephalitides (Bailey & Baker, 1958; Herzon, Shelton & Bruyn, 1957).

The aetiological agent of this disease, probably a

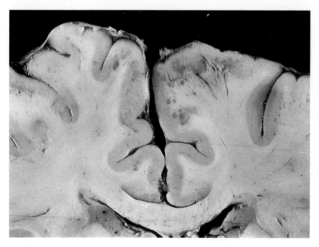

Fig. 17.17. Coronal section of the brain showing early PML lesions; these consist of multiple small foci of grey discolouration at the edge between cortex and white matter.

virus, has never been isolated; however, it was proven that it could pass through filters and that the disease could be transmitted to monkeys by injecting brain tissue from affected subjects (von Economo, 1931). The simultaneous occurrence of the swine influenza and encephalitis lethargica led some to consider the latter as due to the former (Ravenholt & Foege, 1982); however, as von Economo pointed out, half of his cases had occurred before the pandemic of influenza. Furthermore, the isolation in 1931 and the characterization of the properties of the virus of influenza strengthened the opinion that influenza and encephalitis could not be produced by the same agent.

Neuropathology

The neuropathological features of the acute stages of the encephalitis are based on the descriptions given by Buzzard and Greenfield (1919) and von Economo (1931). The cortical grey matter, basal ganglia, periaqueductal grey matter appear congested; histologically, vessels cuffed with lymphocytes and plasma cells are seen predominantly in the brain stem (tegmentum and substantia nigra), but also in the regions mentioned above and in the brain stem. Nerve cells, in particular those of the substantia nigra and oculomotor nuclei, show signs of degeneration and, in patients dying during the subacute stage, the disappearance of the pig-

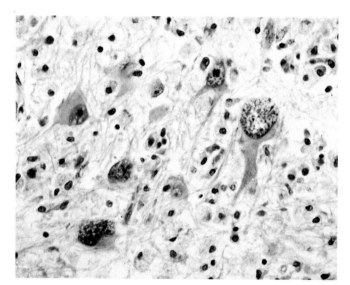

Fig. 17.18. Photomicrograph showing a number of atypical astrocytes with bizarre hyperchromatic nuclei in a case of PML. (H&E × 300)

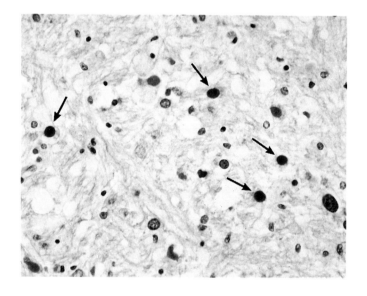

Fig. 17.19. In PML the nuclei of many oligodendrocytes are enlarged and contain amphophilic inclusions. (H&E × 480)

mented nuclei is marked by the presence of free melanin pigment.

In post-encephalitic parkinsonism, which may follow the acute disease after an interval of time varying from months to years, lesions have similar distribution; in the substantia nigra, cell loss is usually severe and uniformly distributed, sometimes complete, with extracellular pigment and reactive gliosis; the reticular midbrain formation may be so severely involved that the resulting atrophy may become macroscopically obvious. Similar changes in other nuclei of the brain stem vary from case to case and may be asymmetrical: the locus coeruleus,

the dorsal nucleus of the vagus, the reticular formation of the pons and medulla, nuclei of the 3rd, 4th, 6th and 12th cranial nerves may be specially involved, whilst the cerebellum and spinal cord are usually unaffected.

A characteristic feature of post-encephalitic parkinsonism is the presence, within surviving neurons, of neurofibrillary tangles. Their number varies considerably, but they are almost always present, whilst perivascular infiltrates of mononuclear cells are only occasionally seen. Tangles were described by Hallervorden (1935) and von Braunmühl (1949). On light microscopy, they consist of interweaving bundles of filaments within

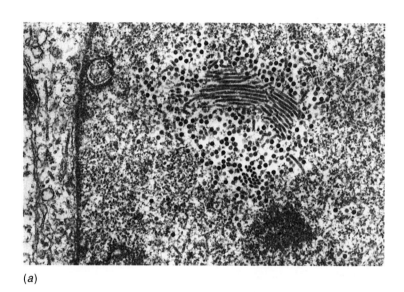

(a)

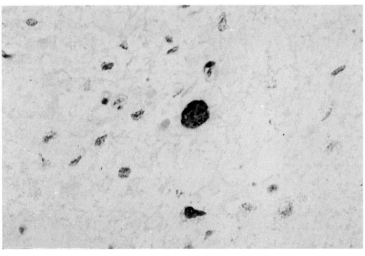

(b)

Fig. 17.20. (a) Electronmicrograph showing round and elongated viral particles in the nucleus of an oligodendrocyte in a case of PML. (× 36 000).
(b) Photomicrograph of an oligodendrocyte in a case of PML; the virus has been visualized by *in situ hybridization method* using a probe for papova virus. (× 480)

the nerve cell cytoplasm (Fig. 17.21(*a*)). They are weakly impregnated by silver methods and are Congo red positive; in the brain stem, cells containing tangles are ballooned; those in the cortex tend to assume a fusiform shape. In both cases the cell containing the fibrillary material may disappear and the latter may be its only remaining component. Ultrastructurally, fibrils consist of paired helical filaments 10 nm in diameter (Wisniewski, Terry & Hirano, 1970) arranged in bundles. Straight filaments, 15 nm in diameter, have also been described, but only in the locus coeruleus (Ishii & Nakamura, 1981). Immunohistochemistry has shown that they share the same antigenic properties of normal filaments but, in addition, are also visualized by antibodies to the filaments found in Alzheimer's disease (Fig. 17.21(*b*)) (Yen *et al.*, 1986).

THE ACQUIRED IMMUNODEFICIENCY SYNDROME (AIDS)

In the first review of the neurological manifestations of the emerging AIDS epidemic, Snider *et al.* (1983) described 18 patients with an encephalitic illness characterized by an onset with cognitive changes accompanied by malaise, lethargy, loss of libido and social withdrawal. Most progressed to severe dementia with confusion, incontinence, paraparesis and coma. The demonstration of microglial nodules in the central nervous system (CNS), some containing inclusions of cytomegalovirus (CMV), supported the hypothesis of an opportunistic infection as the cause of the neuro-psychiatric syndrome. The identification of the human immunodeficiency virus (HIV-1) by Barré-Sinoussi *et al.* (1983) was followed by its demonstration within the CNS by Shaw *et al.* (1985). HIV, and the other virus associated with AIDS (HIV-2) are RNA organisms belonging to the lentivirus group of the retrovirus family (Weiss, 1985). Like all retroviruses, their genome is encoded in single-stranded RNA and is replicated through the generation of a proviral DNA mediated by the action of the retroviral enzyme RNA-directed DNA polymerase (reverse transcriptase). The importance of HIV as a pathogen for the nervous system was suggested when some AIDS patients, suffering from the form of dementia described above, were found to have higher levels of HIV nucleic acid in the CNS than in lymphoid organs. This led Shaw *et al.* (1985) to propose the brain as the reservoir of HIV and that the virus should be considered neurotropic. It soon became recognized that the HIV-related encephalitis was a common form of neurological morbidity in AIDS; its incidence has been reported as affecting from 8 to 66% of the patients, depending on the referral population studied. Community-based estimates are of the order of 10% (Levy *et al.*, 1985). The influential papers by Navia *et al.* (1986*a,b*) led

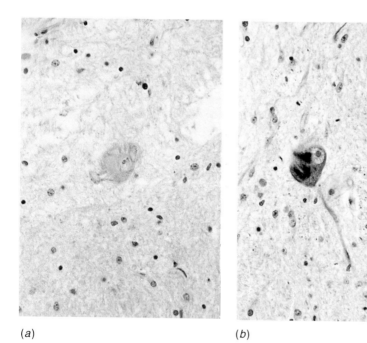

(*a*)   (*b*)

Fig. 17.21. (*a*) Photomicrograph of the midbrain in a case of post-encephalitic parkinsonism showing a nerve cell containing neurofibrillary tangles. (H&E × 300) (*b*) Immunohistochemical techniques using an antibody to phosphorilated filaments shows staining of the tangles. (× 300)

to the concept of an AIDS dementia complex. Although it usually occurs in the late stages of the disease, in 3–5% of the patients dementia may precede the onset of opportunistic infection and tumours (Levy & Bredesen, 1988; Navia *et al.*, 1986*c*; Harrison & McArthur, 1996).

It was hypothesized that variable combinations of cognitive impairment, motor disability and behavioural disturbance were all manifestations of the direct effects of the virus in the brain and were commonly related to encephalitis. The early pathological material revealed, however, that some demented patients showed little encephalitis, and not all patients with encephalitis had been noted to be impaired in life. Diagnostic criteria have been proposed (Nomenclature, 1991) to enable the relative contributions of dementia, motor and behavioural abnormalities to be documented. They also highlight the importance in all cases of excluding the confounding effects of depression, psychological stress, drug therapy, systemic illness and opportunistic infections or tumours of the CNS. Subtle difficulties with cognitive tasks not interfering with normal daily life are separately defined as it is not yet known whether such findings are predictive of functionally important deficits.

Early symptoms consist of forgetfulness and difficulty with concentration, loss of libido and interest in hobbies. Friends and partners report shifts in personality with apathy and social withdrawal and blunting of emotional responsiveness. Some patients develop seizures. Drowsiness is not usual and is more likely along with headache, when comparable changes in mental state turn out to be due to intracranial infection or lymphoma. The differential diagnosis in the early stages includes the effect of bereavement, anxiety, sensitivity to medication, recreational drugs and toxic confusional states, for example those accompanying the hypoxia of pneumonia. It has been suggested that subtle signs, such as the errors made in a task involving anti-saccadic eye movements, along with slowness in repetitive hand movements and slight unsteadiness of gait may be the first signs of the dementing process. However, these soft signs are difficult to interpret in patients who may be febrile or cachectic, and the results of their performance in prospective studies are awaited.

Later, the presence of overt dementia is clear and often accompanied by definite neurological signs, with primitive reflexes, bilateral spasticity, ataxia and bilateral extensor plantar responses. Nevertheless the role of AIDS-related myelopathy in some of these limb findings is often difficult to determine. Whilst most affected patients show the apathetic 'subcortical' type of dementia, some do show dysphasia and apraxia and others have a psychotic or manic state.

Electroencephalograms show slowing of dominant frequencies (Fig. 17.22), a sensitive but totally nonspecific finding. The CSF often shows pleocytosis and increase in protein, but differs in no way from that of patients at the same stage of immunodeficiency whose nervous system appears unaffected. CT scans may show atrophy and are necessary to exclude rival diagnoses (Harrison & McAllister, 1991). MRI is particularly

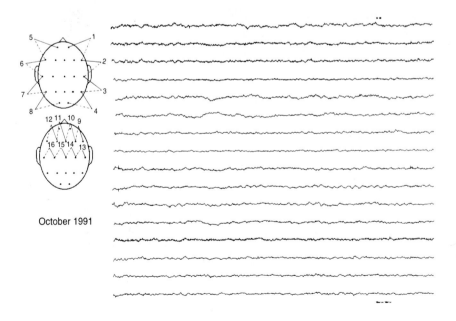

October 1991

Fig. 17.22. EEG showing diffuse slow wave disturbance in a case of HIV dementia.

useful in this context, often revealing changes in the white matter consisting of the hyperdensity of T2 weighted images (Fig. 17.23) of a patchy nature, which are thought to represent the imaging equivalent of myelin pallor in the leukodystrophic type of pathology sometimes encountered. MRI, like CT, also shows atrophy in many cases (Fig. 17.24). Unfortunately, however, clinico-pathological studies are few, and this area has not been completely elucidated.

The prognosis is variable. Whilst some patients progress rapidly to a mute, decerebrate, demented state, others show an apparent plateau, maintaining a moderate level of dementia for many months before dying of opportunistic infections. Most demented patients have well-developed immunodeficiency and have an AIDS-defining illness, such as pneumocystis pneumonia, months or years earlier; in a few cases, however, dementia is the first clinical sign of their immune status. The fact that all demented patients have at least laboratory evidence of immune deficiency and that no dementia can be detected

in asymptomatic HIV-positive individuals (McAllister *et al.*, 1992) suggests strongly that the dementia is a result of the effect of latent HIV invasion of the brain only when immune surveillance is lost (see also below).

Neuropathology

In most of the cases, macroscopic changes in the brains of patients with dementia are absent or difficult to recognize. When present, they consist of softening and grey discolouration of the white matter of the centrum semiovale. Microscopically, the most typical feature, indeed the hallmark of HIV infection in the brain, is the multinucleated giant cell (MGCs) first described by Sharer *et al.* (1986) in the brains of HIV-positive children. They contain large numbers of nuclei, usually arranged at the periphery of the cell and their cytoplasm appears more densely stained at the centre and is vacuolated at the periphery. Their appearance, however, may vary from 'macrophage-like' with abundant cytoplasm (Fig. 17.25(*a*)), to much smaller 'microglia-like' cells

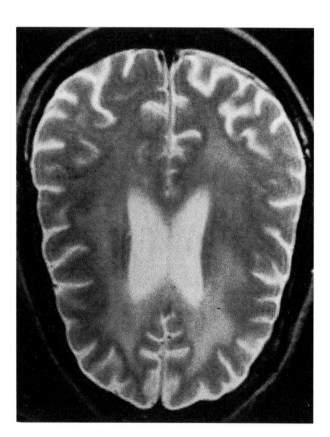

Fig. 17.23. MRI T2 weighted scan revealing high signal in the white matter associated with HIV dementia.

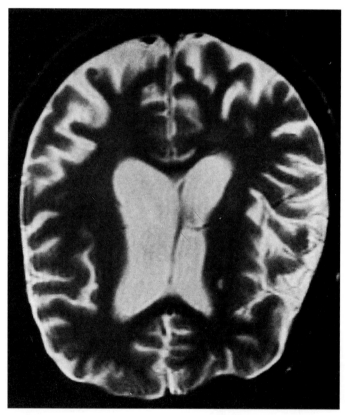

Fig. 17.24. MRI T2 weighted scan showing cerebral atrophy in an AIDS patient with enlarged ventricles and dilated sulci.

(Fig. 17.25(*b*)). MGCs represent syncytia of HIV-infected mononuclear cells and have the immunohistochemical properties of macrophages and the microglia (Budka, 1986, 1989; Budka *et al.*, 1987; Dickson, 1986; Gray *et al.*, 1987; Vazeux *et al.*, 1987; Esiri, 1993). The presence of HIV nucleic acids or protein within MGCs has been shown by various techniques (Fig. 17.26) (Koenig *et al.*, 1986; Sharer *et al.*, 1986; Wiley *et al.*, 1986; Pumarola-Sune *et al.*, 1987; Vazeux *et al.*, 1987) including electron microscopy (Budka *et al.*, 1987; Gray *et al.*, 1987; Meyenhofer *et al.*, 1987).

The demonstration that macrophages and MGCs are capable of HIV–RNA synthesis (Koenig *et al.*, 1986) supports the possibility that these cells may be the reservoir and the vehicle of spread of the virus.

The involvement of the white matter is another characteristic change and may produce two appearances (Budka *et al.*, 1987; Lang *et al.*, 1989; Budka *et al.*, 1991) which co-exist in one-third of the cases and probably represent extremes of a spectrum of HIV-induced changes. The first, the multifocal type, HIV-encephalitis (HIVE), previously called 'multifocal giant cell encepha-litis' (Budka, 1986; Budka *et al.*, 1987; Lang *et al.*, 1989), or subacute encephalitis (Gabuzda *et al.*, 1986), appears as multiple small lesions (Fig. 17.27) in which clusters of MGCs, rod cells and/or macrophages, reactive glial cells and few lymphocytes are disseminated in the white matter and are in places associated with small foci of necrosis. The other, the diffuse type or HIV-leukoen-cephalopathy (HIV-lep), also called 'progressive diffuse leukoencephalopathy' (Kleihues *et al.*, 1985), is charac-terized by diffuse and ill-defined white matter lesions (Fig. 17.28) in both cerebral and cerebellar hemispheres, usually not extending to the white matter of the gyri, corpus callosum, internal capsule, optic pathways and cerebellar peduncles. Myelin loss of variable severity is associated with proliferation of glial cells and/or perivascular infiltration by mononucleated and multi-nucleated cells (Budka *et al.*, 1987; Gray *et al.*, 1987; Lang *et al.*, 1989). Secondary degeneration of the cor-tico-spinal tracts is occasionally observed (Horoupian *et al.*, 1984; Dickson *et al.*, 1989).

The incidence of this form of HIV-related encepha-lopathy with MGCs in published studies varies from 1 in

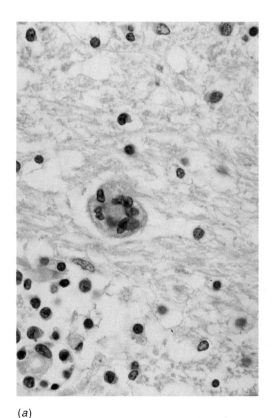

(*a*)

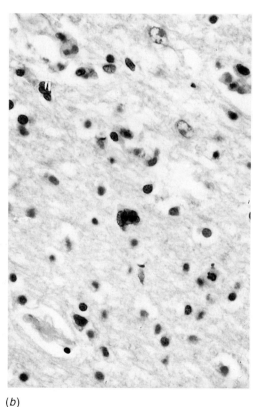

(*b*)

Fig. 17.25. (*a*) 'Macrophage-like' multinucleated giant cell (MGC) of HIV encephalitis; the central area of cytoplasm surrounded by nuclei is denser than the outer rim which appears vacuolated. (H&E × 480). (*b*) 'Microglia-like' MGC; this type is smaller than the previous one and shows clustered nuclei surrounded by scanty cytoplasm. (H&E × 480)

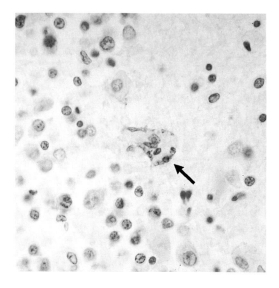

Fig. 17.26. Immunohistochemical method for HIV using p24 antibody reveals granular material within the cytoplasm of a MGC (arrow). (×480)

31 patients (Hénin *et al.*, 1987) to 15 (Lang *et al.*, 1989), 28 (Petito *et al.*, 1986) and 38% (Budka *et al.*, 1987); on the other hand, it is uncommon in haemophiliacs (Esiri *et al.*, 1989).

In addition to the white matter lesions, involvement of the cortical grey matter has also been described. Gliosis was described by de la Monte *et al.* (1987) in most of their cases; a diffuse poliodystrophy was reported in approximately 50 per cent of the brains by Budka *et al.* (1987), sometimes associated with gyral atrophy. On the other hand, MGCs and HIV antigens are much less commonly found in the cortex than in the subjacent white matter. A correlation between severity of cortical gliosis and severity of dementia was reported by Ciardi *et al.* (1990).

In addition, Wiley *et al.* (1990) reported cortical thinning and reduced number of nerve cells per unit area, particularly in the parietal lobe. Additional support to the theory of an involvement of the grey matter comes from work by Ketzler *et al.* (1990). These authors showed 18% reduction of neuronal density and decrease of the perikaryal volume fraction of 31%. These results were subsequently confirmed by Everall, Luthert & Lantos (1991, 1993) and Wiley *et al.* (1991*a*). In addition, the latter authors showed, by immunohistochemical methods, decreased density of synapses in the cortex as well as decreased dendritic branches as revealed by the Golgi method (Wiley *et al.*, 1991*b*).

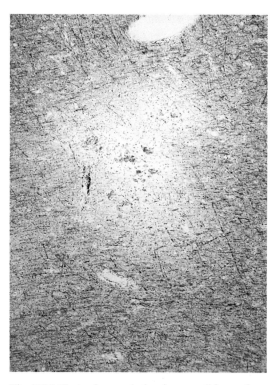

Fig. 17.27. Photomicrograph showing a small focus of demyelination surrounding a blood vessel. This appearance is characteristic of HIV encephalitis (HIVE). (LFB/cresyl violet ×40)

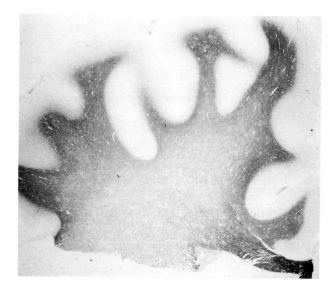

Fig. 17.28. HIV leukoencephalopathy (HIV-lep) is characterized by the presence of diffuse myelin pallor of the hemispheric white matter, with sparing of the gyri and corpus callosum. (LFB/cresyl violet)

A number of other morphological changes have been described in the nervous system in association with HIV. One of these, vacuolar myelopathy (VM), has no relevance in this chapter, since its clinical signs are spinal. The subject has been reviewed comprehensively by Petito (1993). However, vacuolar changes in the cerebral white matter, similar to VM, have been described by Schmidbauer et al. (1993). Their distribution mimics that of the extrapontine lesions in central pontine myelinolysis.

An aseptic meningitis may occur, in HIV-infected patients, at the time of seroconversion and is considered aetiologically related to the virus. It consists of a discrete infiltration of the leptomeninges by lymphocytes and a small number of macrophages.

A progressive encephalopathy has also been described in HIV-positive children (Epstein et al., 1985). Although usually normal at birth, their head circumference subsequently stops growing at a normal rate and a progressive neurological deterioration takes place, occasionally interrupted by short periods of remission. The main pathological changes in the brains of these children are: mineralization of blood vessels, present in 90% of the cases (Dickson et al., 1989); pallor and gliosis of the white matter, seen in 78%; the pallor has been interpreted by Sharer et al. (1990) as hypomyelination. Inflammation is found in 75% of the brains (Sharer et al., 1986) and includes lymphocytes, plasma and microglial cells, macrophages and, in 62% of the observations, MGCs (Sharer & Mintz, 1992). The neuropathology of AIDS in children is reviewed by Sharer & Mintz (1993).

Pathogenesis

The study of the pathogenetic mechanisms involved in the encephalopathy in AIDS must keep into account the observation that, in spite of the claims that HIV is neurotropic, microglia, macrophages and MGCs, but not neuroectodermal cells, are the only cells consistently infected in the CNS (Koenig et al., 1986; Stoler et al., 1986; Vazeux et al., 1987; Sidtis & Price, 1990; Esiri, 1993). Infected cells may contain between 500 and 1500 copies of HIV RNA, at least ten times the amount found in blood leukocytes (Harper et al., 1986). Whereas infected lymphocytes undergo cytolysis, infected monocytes are resistant to the cytopathic effect of the virus (Levy et al., 1985; Salahuddin et al., 1986). Also relevant is the mode and tempo of entry of HIV into the CNS. Among the various theories put forward, that of the 'Trojan horse' seems to gather most support: according to this theory, HIV is carried passively by T-lymphocytes and monocytes; whereas the former can enter and leave the brain, migration of blood monocytes is unidirectional (Meltzer et al., 1990). Support for an entry through the bloodstream comes from the observation that lesions of HIVE have an obvious perivascular location; moreover, Smith et al. (1990) have described abnormalities of the microvasculature also in HIV-lep. As for the time during the infection at which migration of these cells takes place, work by Carne et al. (1985), Cooper et al. (1985) and Goudsmit et al. (1986), showing that virus was present as early as at the time of seroconversion, has been confirmed by Sinclair, Gray and Scaravilli (1992). Using the polymerase chain reaction technique, the latter authors showed that brain tissue of an HIV-positive, non-AIDS, drug user who had died of an overdose contained HIV DNA provirus. These findings have subsequently been confirmed by An et al. (1996) in a larger cohort of patients.

If HIV were the cause of the cortical abnormalities described above, the virus would be expected to be present in this region. Indeed, the proposed haematogenous route of entry into the CNS (either by free virus (Wiley et al., 1986) or via latently infected peripheral blood mononuclear cells (Price et al., 1988; Haase, 1986), implies that HIV is present both in cortex and white matter. In contrast, viral antigens are more abundant in the latter (Budka, 1990; Kure et al., 1990). However, recent work, using separate samples of cortex and white matter, has shown not only that HIV proviral DNA can be repeatedly detected in the former, but also that there is a close correlation between the frequency of HIV provirus in the two regions of the same patient (Sinclair & Scaravilli, 1992). It is possible therefore that the difference between amounts of provirus and replication virus may be dependent on the tissue microenvironment. Indeed, in the rat brain, CD4 (the HIV binding molecule) is expressed consistently by microglial cells of the white, but only infrequently of the grey matter (Perry & Gordon, 1987). If a similar distribution of CD4 expressing cells exists in human brain, it may explain the difference in antigen distribution, since CD4-positive cells are permissive for HIV replication.

In spite of the large amount of clinico-pathological and experimental studies, the pathogenesis of the damage by HIV within the nervous system remains speculative.

Various possible mechanisms have been suggested to explain the loss of myelin; they include a shared antigenic polypeptide between the virus and the myelin, a 'bystander effect', the intervention of neurotoxins, enzymes, toxic oxygen metabolites, monokines including tumour necrosis factor, and block of neuronal receptors for neurotransmitters by HIV. The subject is discussed by Scaravilli *et al.* (1993).

Viral components have also been found to act as toxins to neuronal cell lines, neuronal tissue explants and the nervous system of animals (see Lipton, 1991). Included among these toxic factors are the viral proteins *gp120* (Brenneman *et al.*, 1988), and *tat* (Sabatier *et al.*, 1991), which may directly kill neurons through the agency of as yet unidentified factors, released from HIV infected macrophages (Giulian, Vaca & Noonan, 1990; Pulliam *et al.*, 1991). In addition, high levels of unintegrated proviral DNA, as detected in AIDS brains by Pang *et al.* (1990) and in animals (Robinson & Miles, 1985; Hoover *et al.*, 1987), are also associated with cytotoxicity. The above observations support the possibility that HIV is directly or indirectly neurotoxic *in vivo*; astrocytic and microglial cell reaction may be a consequence of neurotoxicity or be an independent reaction to the presence of HIV.

NEUROSYPHILIS
Dementia in association with syphilis occurs in the late stages of the infection (usually 10 or more years after the initial contact with the organism) and progresses to death in 2–10 years, unless antibiotic therapy is administered. Macroscopic changes in the brains of patients with this form of infection (general paralysis) consist of thickening of the leptomeninges, cortical atrophy and ventricular dilatation. The ependymal lining of the ventricles, particularly the fourth, is finely granular (granular ependymitis). Histologically, neuronal loss and atrophy are accompanied by perivascular aggregates of lymphocytes and plasma cells, astrocytic gliosis and presence of transformed microglia; these cells are hypertrophied and their elongated and slender nuclei extend perpendicularly to the pial surface (rod cells). They can be easily demonstrated by the Perl's method for iron. The presence of treponeme can be confirmed by the silver impregnation (Levaditi's) method.

Cases of neurosyphilis among HIV-positive individuals have been reported by Berger *et al.* (1984) who described a patient with meningo-encephalitis; by Johns, Tierney & Felstenstein (1987) who reported four cases (two meningo-vascular, one with acute meningitis and one asymptomatic). The patient published by Joyce, Haye & Ellis (1989) was a 21 year-old homosexual man who developed soreness of the right eye, photophobia and diminished visual acuity. Johns *et al.* (1987) suggest

that syphilis may show an aggressive behaviour in HIV-positive patients. Indeed, they believe that the immunosuppression induced by the virus may be worsened by the treponeme; alternatively, the meningitis which accompanies the brain invasion by either organism might facilitate the penetration of the other into the CNS.

However, the pathology of syphilis associated with AIDS is quite different from that seen in the pre-antibiotic era, probably because patients do not have a long survival time necessary to develop the classical features.

REFERENCES
Adle- Biasette H, Levy Y, Colombel M *et al* (1995) Neuronal apoptosis in HIV infection in adults. *Neuropathol Appl Neurobiol* 21: 218–27.

Agnarsdottir G (1977) Subacute sclerosing panencephalitis. In Waterson AP (ed) *Recent Advances in Clinical Virology* vol 1, Churchill Livingstone, Edinburgh, pp 21–49.

An SF, Ciardi A, Giometto B, Scaravilli T, Gray F, Scaravilli F (1996) Investigation on the expression of major histocompatibility complex class II and cytokines and detection of HIV-1 DNA within brains of asymptomatic and symptomatic HIV-1-positive patients. *Acta Neuropathol* 91: 494–503.

Åstrom KE, Mancall EL, Richardson EP (1958) Progressive multifocal leukoencephalopathy. A hitherto unrecognized complication of chronic lymphatic leukemia and Hodgkin's disease. *Brain* 81: 93–111.

Baker TS, Rayment I (1987) Parvoviridae. In Nermut MV and Steven AC (ed) *Animal Virus Structure; Perspectives in Medical Virology*. Elsevier, Amsterdam, pp 335–48.

Bailey P, Baker AB (1958) Sequelae of arthropod borne encephalitides. *Neurology* 8: 878–96.

Bakheit A, Behan PO (1991) Unsuccessful treatment of subacute sclerosing panencephalitis treated with transfusions of peripheral blood lymphocytes from an identical twin. *J Neurol Neurosurg Psychiat* 54: 377–8.

Barré-Sinoussi F, Nugeyre M, Daugut C *et al* (1983) Isolation of a T-lymphotropic retrovirus from a patient at risk for acquired immune deficiency syndrome. *Science* 220: 868–71.

Berger JR, Mucke L (1988) Prolonged survival and partial recovery in AIDS-associated progressive multifocal leukoencephalopathy. *Neurology* 38: 1060–5.

Berger JR, Moskowitz L, Fishl M *et al* (1984) The neurologic complications of AIDS: frequently the initial manifestation. *Neurology* 34 (suppl 1): 134–5.

Blyth WA, Hill TJ (1984) Establishment, maintenance and control of Herpes simplex virus (HSV) latency. In Rouse BT and Lopez C (eds) *Immunobiology of Herpes Simplex Virus Infection*, Boca Raton, Florida, pp 10–32.

Bolton CF, Rozdilsky B (1971) Primary progressive multifocal leukoencephalopathy. *Neurology* 21: 72–7.

Bornstein B, Sandbank U, Tamir M *et al* (1961) Subacute sclerosing leukoencephalitis with fulminating evolution. *Rev Neurol (Paris)* 105: 430–42.

Bouteille M, Fontaine C, Vedrenne C *et al* (1965) Sur un cas d'encéphalite subalguë à inclusions: étude anatomo-clinique et ultrastructurale. *Rev Neurol (Paris)* 113: 454–8.

Braunmühl A von (1949) Encephalitis epidemica und Synaresislehre. *Arch Psychiat Nervenkr* 181: 543–76.

Brenneman DE, Weatbrook GL, Fitzgerald SP *et al* (1988) Neuronal cell killing by the envelope protein of HIV and its prevention by vasoactive intestinal peptide. *Nature* 335: 639–42.

Brook BR, Walker DL (1984) Progressive multifocal leukoencephalopathy. *Neurol Clin* 2: 299–313.

Brosnan CF, Litwak MS, Schroeder CE, Selmaj K, Raine CS, Arezzo JC (1989) Preliminary studies of cytokine-induced functional effects on the visual pathways in the rabbit. *J Neuroimmunol* 25: 227–39.

Brown HR, Goller NL, Rudelli RD *et al* (1989) Postmortem detection of measles virus in non-neural tissues in subacute sclerosing panencephalitis. *Arch Neurol* 26: 263–8.

Brown P, Tsai T, Gajdusek DC (1975) Seroepidemiology of human papovaviruses. Discovery of virgin populations and some unusual patterns of antibody prevalence among remote peoples of the world. *Am J Epidemiol* 102: 331–40.

Budka H (1986) Multinucleated giant cells in brain: a hallmark of the acquired immune deficiency syndrome (AIDS). *Acta Neuropathol* 69: 253–8.

Budka H (1989) Human immunodeficiency virus (HIV)-induced disease of the central nervous system: pathology and implications for pathogenesis. *Acta Neuropathol* 77: 225–36.

Budka H (1990) Human immunodeficiency virus (HIV) envelope and core proteins in CNS tissues of patients with the acquired immune deficiency syndrome (AIDS). *Acta Neuropathol* 79: 611–19.

Budka H, Costanzi G, Cristina S *et al* (1987) Brain pathology induced by infection with the human immunodeficiency virus (HIV). *Acta Neuropathol* 75: 186–98.

Budka H, Wiley CE, Klihues P *et al* (1991) HIV associated disease of the nervous system: review and nomenclature and proposal for neuropathology-based terminology. *Brain Pathol* 1: 143–52.

Buzzard EF, Greenfield JG (1919) Lethargic encephalitis: its sequelae and morbid anatomy. *Brain* 42: 305–8.

Cappel R, Klastersky J (1973) Herpetic meningitis (type 1) in a case of acute leukemia. *Arch Neurol* 28: 415–16.

Carne CA, Tedder RS, Smith A *et al* (1985) Acute encephalopathy coincident with seroconversion for anti-HTLV-III. *Lancet* ii: 1206–8.

Case Report of the Massachusetts General Hospital (1986) Case 25-1986. *N Engl J Med* 314: 1689–700.

Cavanagh JB, Greenbaum D, Marshall AHE *et al* (1959) Cerebral demyelination associated with disorders of the reticuloendothelial system. *Lancet* ii: 524–9.

Choppin PW (1981) Measles virus and chronic neurological diseases. *Ann Neurol* 9: 17–20.

Ciardi A, Sinclair E, Scaravilli F *et al* (1990) Involvement of the cerebral cortex in HIV-encephalopathy. A morphological and immuno-histochemical study. *Acta Neuropathol* 81: 51–9.

Cobb WA (1966) The periodic events of subacute sclerosing leucoencephalitis. *Electroencephal Clin Neurophysiol* 21: 278–94.

Cobb WA, Marshall J, Scaravilli F (1984) Long survival in subacute sclerosing pancephalitis. *J Neurol Neurosurg Psychiat* 47: 176–83.

Cobb WA, Morgan-Hughes JA (1968) Non fatal subacute sclerosing panencephalitis. *J Neurol Neurosurg Psychiat* 31: 115–23.

Connolly JH, Allen IV, Hurwitz LJ *et al* (1967) Measles virus antibody and antigen in sub-acute sclerosing panencephalitis. *Lancet* i: 542–4.

Conway B, Halliday WC, Brunham RC (1990) Human immunodeficiency virus-associated progressive multifocal leukoencephalopathy: apparent response to 3-Azido-3-deoxythymidine. *Rev Infect Dis* 12: 479–82.

Cooper DA, Gold J, McLean P *et al* (1985) Acute AIDS retrovirus infection. Definition of a clinical illness associated with seroconversion. *Lancet* i: 537–40.

Corsellis JAN (1951) Subacute sclerosing leucoencephalitis: a clinical and pathologic report of two cases. *J Ment Sci* 97: 570–83.

Craig CP, Nahmias AJ (1973) Different patterns of neurological involvement with Herpes simplex virus type 1 and 2: Isolation of Herpes simplex virus type 2 from the buffy coat of two adults with meningitis. *J Infect Dis* 127: 365–72.

Damasio AR, Van Hoesen GW (1985) The limbic system and the localisation of Herpes simplex encephalitis. *J Neurol Neurosurg Psychiat* 48: 297–301.

Davis LE, McLaren LC (1983) Relapsing Herpes simplex encephalitis following antiviral therapy. *Ann Neurol* 13: 192–5.

Dawson JR (1933) Cellular inclusions in cerebral lesions of lethargic encephalitis. *Am J Pathol* 9: 7–16.

Dickson DW (1986) Multinucleated giant cells in acquired immunodeficiency syndrome encephalopathy: origin from endogenous microglia? *Arch Pathol Lab Med* 110: 967–8.

Dickson DW, Belman AL, Parky D *et al* (1989) Central nervous system pathology in pediatric AIDS: an autopsy study. *APMIS* 8 (suppl): 40–57.

Dinn JJ (1979) Distribution of Herpes simplex virus in acute necrotizing encephalitis. *J Pathol* 129: 135–8.

Dinn JJ (1980) Transolfactory spread of virus in Herpes simplex encephalitis. *Br Med J* 281: 1392.

Dix RD, Bredesen DE (1988) Opportunistic viral infections in acquired immunodeficiency syndrome. In Rosenblum ML, Levy RM and Bredesen DE (ed) *AIDS and the Nervous system* Rowen Press, New York, pp 221–61.

Dix RD, Baringer JR, Panitch HS et al (1983) Recurrent Herpes simplex encephalitis: recovery of virus after Ara-A treatment. Ann Neurol 13: 196–200.

Dorries K, Johnson RT, ter Meulen V (1979) Detection of polyoma virus DNA in PML-brain tissue by in situ hybridization. J Gen Virol 42: 49–57.

Dowdle WR, Nahmias AJ, Harwell RW et al (1967) Association of antigenic type of herpesvirus hominis with site of viral recovery. J Immunol 99: 974–80.

Dumas M, Girard PL, Gray F et al (1980) Rémission clinique et électroencéphalographique prolongée et totale puis décès au cours d'une panencéphalite subaiguë. Rev Neurol (Paris) 136: 165–83.

Duncan CM, Kent JNG, Harbord M et al (1989) Subacute sclerosing panencephalitis presenting as schizophreniform psychosis. Brit J Psychiat 155: 557–9.

Economo C von (1931) Encephalitis Lethargica: Its Sequelae and Treatment. Translated by KO Newman, Oxford University Press, London.

Editorial (1990) SSPE in the developing world. Lancet ii: 600.

Epstein LG, Sharer LR, Joshi VV et al (1985) Progressive encephalopathy in children with acquired immunodeficiency syndrome. Ann Neurol 17: 488–96.

Esiri MM (1982a) Herpes simplex encephalitis: an immunohistological study of the distribution of viral antigen within the brain. J Neurol Sci 54: 209–26.

Esiri MM (1982b) Viruses and Alzheimer's disease. J Neurol Neurosurg Psychiat 45: 759.

Esiri MM (1992) Role of macrophage in HIV encephalitis. In Scaravilli F (ed) The Neuropathology of HIV Infection. Springer-Verlag, London, p 235–50.

Esiri MM, Kennedy PGE (1992) Virus diseases. In Adams JH, Duchen LW (ed) Greenfield's Neuropathology. Edward Arnold, London, 334–99.

Esiri MM, Oppenheimer DR, Brownell B et al (1981) Distribution of measles antigen and immunoglobulin-containing cells in the CNS in subacute sclerosing panencephalitis (SSPE) and atypical measles encephalitis. J Neurol Sci 53: 29–43.

Esiri MM, Scaravilli F, Millard PR et al (1989) Neuropathology of HIV infection in haemophiliacs: comparative necropsy study. Br Med J 299: 1312–15.

Espir MLE, Spalding JMK (1956) Three recent cases of encephalitis lethargica. Br Med J 1: 1141–4.

Everall I, Luthert PJ, Lantos PL (1991) Neuronal loss in the frontal cortex in HIV infection. Lancet ii: 1119–21.

Everall I, Luthert PJ, Lantos PL (1993) A review of neuronal damage in human immunodeficiency virus infection: its assessment, possible mechanism and relationship to dementia. J Neuropathol Exp Neurol 52: 561–6.

Fermaglich J, Hardman JM, Earle KM (1969) Progressive multifocal leukoencephalopathy. Neurology 19: 287 (abstr).

Gabuzda DH, Ho DD, de la Monte SM et al (1986) Immunohistochemical identification of HTLV-III antigen in brains of patients with AIDS. Ann Neurol 20: 289–95.

Giulian D, Vaca K, Noonan CA (1990) Secretion of neurotoxins by mononuclear phagocytes infected with HIV-1. Science 250: 1593–96.

Gordon B, Selnes OA, Hart J et al (1990) Long term cognitive sequelae of acyclovir-treated Herpes simplex encephalitis. Arch Neurol 47: 646–7.

Goudsmit J, Wolters E, Bakker M et al (1986) Intrathecal synthesis of antibodies to HTLV- III in patients without AIDS or AIDS related complex. Br Med J 292: 1231–4.

Gray F, Gherardi R, Baudrimont M et al (1987) Leucoencephalopathy with multinucleated giant cells containing human immune deficiency virus-like particles and multiple opportunistic cerebral infections in one patient with AIDS. Acta Neuropathol 73: 99–104.

Gray F, Lescs M-C, Keohane C et al (1992) Early brain changes in HIV infection neuropathological study of 11 HIV seropositive, non-AIDS cases. Neuropathol Exp Neurol 51: 177–85.

Gribble DH, Haden CC, Schwartz LW et al (1975) Spontaneous progressive multifocal leukoencephalopathy (PML) in macaques. Nature 254: 602–4.

Grinnel BW, Padgett BL, Walker DL (1983a) Distribution of nonintegrated DNA from JC papovavirus in organs of patients with progressive multifocal leukoencephalopathy. J Infect Dis 147: 669–75.

Grinnell BW, Padgett BL, Walker DL (1983b) Comparison of infectious JC virus DNAs cloned from human brain. J Virol 45: 299–308.

Gutewa J, Osetowska E (1961) A chronic form of subacute encephalitis (a case with a history of 5 years). Clinical and pathological study. In van Bogaert L, Radermecker J, Hozay J, Lowenthal A (ed) (1969) Encephalitides, Proceedings of a Symposium, Antwerp Elsevier, Amsterdam, pp 384–404.

Haase AT (1986) Pathogenesis of lentivirus infections. Nature 322: 130–6.

Hahn RD, Webster B, Werckhardt G et al (1959) Penicillin treatment of general paralysis (dementia paralytica) Arch Neurol Psychiat 81: 557–90.

Hall WW, Lamb RA, Choppin PW (1979) Measles and SSPE virus proteins: lack of antibodies to the M protein in patients with subacute sclerosing panencephalitis. Proc Nat Acad Sci USA 76: 2047–51.

Hallervorden J (1935) Anatomische Untersuchungen zur Pathogenese des postencephalitischen Parkinsonismus. Deutsch Zeit Nervenheilk 136: 68–77.

Harper ME, Marselle LM, Gallo RC et al (1986) Expression of lymphocytes expressing human T-lymphotropic virus type II in lymph-nodes and peripheral blood from infected individuals by in situ hybridization. Proc Natl Acad Sci USA 83: 772–6.

Harrison MJG, MacAllister RH (1991) Neurological complications of HIV infection. In Infections of the Nervous System Lambert HP (ed) Edward Arnold, London, pp 343–60.

Harrison MJG, McArthur JC (1996) *Neurology and AIDS* Churchill Livingstone, London.

Hatch WC, Pousada E, Loser L, Rashbaum WK, Lyman WD (1994) Neural cell targets of human immunodeficiency virus type I in human fetal organotypic cultures. *AIDS Human Retroviruses* 10: 1597–607.

Hénin D, Duyckaerts C, Chaunu MP *et al* (1987) Etude neuropathologique de 31 cas de syndrome d'immunodépression acquise. *Rev Neurol (Paris)* 143: 631–42.

Herzon H, Shelton JT, Bruyn HB (1957) Sequelae of Western equine and other arthropod borne encephalitides. *Neurology* 7: 535–48.

Hierons R, Janota I, Corsellis JAN (1978) The late effects of necrotising encephalitis of the temporal lobes and limbic areas: a clinico-pathological study of 10 cases. *Psychol Med* 8: 21–42.

Himmelhoch J, Pincus J, Tucker G *et al* (1970) Sub-acute encephalitis: behavioural and neurological aspects. *Br J Psychiat* 116: 531–8.

Ho SS, Rota JR, Schooley RT *et al* (1985) Isolation of HTLV – III from cerebrospinal fluid and neural tissues of patients with neurological syndromes related to the acquired, immunodeficiency syndrom. *N Engl J Med* 313: 1493–7.

Hook EW, Marra CM (1992) Acquired syphilis in adults. *New Eng J Med* 326: 1060–9.

Hooper DC, Pruitt AA, Rubin RH (1982) Central nervous system infection in the chronically immunodepressed. *Medicine* 61: 166–88.

Hoover EA, Mullins JI, Quackenbush SL *et al* (1987) Experimental transmission and pathogenesis of immunodeficiency syndrome in cats. *Blood* 70: 1880–92.

Horoupian DS, Pick P, Spigland I *et al* (1984) Acquired immune deficiency syndrome and multiple tract degeneration in a homosexual man. *Ann Neurol* 15: 502–5.

Horta-Barbosa L, Fuccillo DA, Sever JL *et al* (1969) Subacute sclerosing panencephalitis: isolation of measles virus from a brain biopsy. *Nature* 221: 974.

Hotson JR, Pedley TA (1976) The neurological complications of cardiac transplantation. *Brain* 99: 673–94.

Houff SA, Major EO, Katz DA *et al* (1988) Involvement of JC-infected mononuclear cells from bone marrow and spleen in the pathogenesis of progressive multifocal leukoencephalopathy. *N Engl J Med* 318: 305.

Huber M, Herholz K, Pawlik G *et al* (1989) Cerebral glucose metabolism in the course of subacute sclerosing panencephalitis. *Arch Neurol* 46: 97–100.

Ishii T, Nakamura Y (1981) Distribution and ultrastructure of Alzheimer's neurofibrillary tangles in postencephalitic parkinsonism of Economo type. *Acta Neuropathol* 55: 59–62.

Jabour JT, Garcia JH, Lemmi H *et al* (1969) Subacute sclerosing panencephalitis, a multidisciplinary study of 8 cases. *JAMA* 297: 2248–54.

Johns DR, Tierney M, Felstenstein D (1987) Alteration in the natural history of neurosyphilis by concurrent infection with the human immunodeficiency virus. *N Engl J Med* 316: 1569–72.

Johnson RT, Mims CA (1968) Pathogenesis of viral infections of the nervous system. *N Engl J Med* 278: 23–30.

Joyce PW, Haye KR, Ellis ME (1989) Syphilitic retinitis in a homosexual man with concurrent HIV infection: case report. *J Neurol Neurosurg Psychiat* 65: 244–7.

Kennedy PGE (1984) Herpes simplex virus and the nervous system. *Postgrad Med J* 60: 253–9.

Ketzler S, Weis S, Haug H *et al* (1990) Loss of neurons in the frontal cortex in AIDS brains. *Acta Neuropathol* 80: 92–4.

Kleihues P, Lang W, Burger PC *et al* (1985) Progressive diffuse leukoencephalopathy in patients with acquired immune deficiency syndrome (AIDS). *Acta Neuropathol* 68: 333–9.

Koenig H, Rabinowitz SG, Day E *et al* (1979) Post-infectious encephalomyelitis after successful treatment of Herpes simplex encephalitis with adenine arabinoside. Ultrastructural observations. *N Engl J Med* 300: 1089–93.

Koenig S, Gendelman HE, Orenstein JM *et al* (1986) Detection of AIDS virus in macrophages in brain tissue from AIDS patients with encephalopathy. *Science* 233: 1089–93.

Kristensson K, Vahlne A, Persson LA *et al* (1978) Neural spread of Herpes simplex virus types 1 and 2 in mice after corneal or subcutaneous (foot-pad) inoculation. *J Neurol Sci* 35: 331–40.

Krücke W (1957) Über eine besondere Form der spontanen Encephalitis. *Nervenartz* 28: 289–301.

Kure K, Weidenheim KM, Lyman WD *et al* (1990) Morphology and distribution of HIV-1 gp41-positive microglia in subacute AIDS encephalitis. *Acta Neuropathol* 80: 393–400.

Lang W, Miklossy J, Deruaz JP *et al* (1989) Neuropathology of the acquired immune deficiency syndrome (AIDS): a report of 135 consecutive autopsy cases from Switzerland. *Acta Neuropathol* 77: 379–90.

Laskin OL, Stahl-Bayliss CM, Morgello S (1987) Concomitant Herpes simplex virus type 1 and cytomegalovirus ventriculoencephalitis in acquired immunodeficiency syndrome. *Arch Neurol* 44: 843–7.

Leestma JE (1985) Viral infections of the nervous system. In Davis RL, Robertson DN (ed) *Textbook of Neuropathology* Williams and Wilkins: Baltimore, p 747.

Legg NJ (1967) Virus antibodies in subacute sclerosing panencephalitis: a study of 22 cases. *Br Med J* iii: 350–2.

Levy RM, Bredesen DE (1988) Central nervous system dysfunction in acquired immunodeficiency syndrome. *J AIDS* 1: 41–64.

Levy RM, Bredesen DE, Rosenblum ML (1985) Neurological manifestations of the acquired immune deficiency syndrome (AIDS): experience at UCSF and review of the literature. *J Neurosurg* 62: 517–24.

Lipton SA (1991) HIV-related neurotoxicity. *Brain Pathol* 1: 193–99.

Lipton SA, Sucher NJ, Kaiser PK, Dreyer EB (1991) Synergistic effects of HIV coat protein and NMDA receptor-mediated neurotoxicity. *Neuron* 7: 111–18.

McAllister RH, Herns MV, Harrison MJG *et al* (1992) Neurological and neuropsychological performance in HIV seropositive asymptomatic individuals. *J Neurol Neurosurg Psychiat* 55: 143–8.

Malamud N, Haymaker W, Pinkerton H (1950) Inclusion encephalitis with a clinicopathologic report of three cases. *Am J Pathol* 26: 133–53.

Mandybur TI, Nagpaul AS, Pappas Z *et al* (1977) Alzheimer neurofibrillary change in subacute sclerosing panencephalitis. *Ann Neurol* 1: 103–7.

Markand O, Panszi JG (1975) The electroencephalogram in subacute sclerosing panencephalitis. *Arch Neurol* 32: 719–26.

Martin JD, Foster GC (1984) Multiple JC virus genomes from one patient. *J Gen Virol* 65: 1405–11.

Martin JD, King DM, Slauch JM *et al* (1985) Differences in regulatory sequence of naturally occurring JC virus variants. *J Virol* 53: 306–11.

Martiney JA, Litwak M, Berman JW, Arezzo JC, Brosnan CF (1990) Pathophysiologic effect of interleukin –1b in the rabbit retina. *Am J Pathol* 137: 1411–23.

Meltzer MS, Skillman DR, Gomatos PJ *et al* (1990) Role of mononuclear phagocytes in the pathogenesis of human immunodeficiency virus infection. *Ann Rev Immunol* 8: 169–94.

Merrill JE, Koyanagi Y, Zack J, Thomas L, Martin F, Chen IS (1992) Induction of interleukin-1 and tumour necrosis factor alpha in brain cultures by human immunodeficiency virus type 1. *J Virol* 66: 2217–25.

Meyenhofer MF, Epstein LG, Cho E-S *et al* (1987) Ultrastructural morphology and intracellular production of human immunodeficiency virus (HIV) in brain. *J Neuropathol Exp Neurol* 46: 474–84.

Miller F, Moskophidis M (1983) Estimation of the local production of antibodies to Treponema pallidum in the central nervous system of patients with neurosyphilis. *Br J Vener Dis* 59: 80–4.

Milstein JM, Biggs HE (1977) Recurrent encephalitis with elevated titers for Herpes simplex. *Arch Neurol* 34: 434–6.

Monte S de la, Ho DD, Schooley RT *et al* (1987) Subacute encephalomyelitis of AIDS and its relation to HTLV-III infection. *Neurology* 37: 562–9.

Nath A, Hartloper V, Furer M, Fowke KR (1995) Infection of human fetal astrocytes with HIV-I: viral tropism and the role of cell to cell contact in viral transmission. *J Neuropathol Exp Neurol* 54: 320–30.

Navia BA, Price RW (1987) The acquired immunodeficiency syndrome dementia complex as the presenting or sole manifestation of human immunodeficiency virus infection. *Arch Neurol* 44: 65–9.

Navia BA, Cho E-S, Petito CK *et al* (1986a) The AIDS dementia complex: II. Neuropathology. *Ann Neurol* 19: 525–35.

Navia BA, Jordan BD, Price RW *et al* (1986b) The AIDS dementia complex. I. Clinical features. *Ann Neurol* 19: 517–24.

Navia BA, Petito CK, Gold JWM *et al* (1986c) Cerebral toxoplasmosis complicating the acquired immune deficiency syndrome: clinical and neuropathological findings in 27 patients. *Ann Neurol* 19: 224–38.

Nomenclature and research case definitions for neurologic manifestations of human immunodeficiency virus-type 1 (HIV-1) infection (1991) *Neurology* 41: 778–85.

Oommen KJ, Johnson PC, Ray CG (1982) Herpes simplex type 2 virus encephalitis presenting as psychosis. *Am J Med* 73: 445–8.

Orenstein JM, Jannotta F (1988) Human immunodeficiency virus and papovavirus infections in acquired immunodeficiency syndrome. *Hum Pathol* 19: 350–61.

Oxbury JM, MacCallum FO (1973) Herpes simplex virus encephalitis: clinical features and residual damage. *Postgrad Med J* 49: 387–9.

Padgett BL, Walker DL, Zurhein GM *et al* (1971) Cultivation of papova-like virus from human brain with progressive multifocal leukoencephalopathy. *Lancet* i: 1257–60.

Pang S, Koyanagi Y, Miles S *et al* (1990) High levels of unintegrated HIV-1 DNA in brain tissue of AIDS dementia patients. *Nature*, 343: 85–9.

Panteleo G, Menzos S, Vaccarezza M *et al* (1995) Studies in subjects with long-term non-progressive human immunodeficiency virus infection. *N Engl J Med* 332: 209–16.

Payne FE, Baublis JV, Itabashi HH (1969) Isolation of measles virus from cell cultures of brain from a patient with subacute sclerosing panencephalitis. *N Engl J Med* 281: 585–9.

Pepose JS, Hilborne LH, Cancilla P *et al* (1984) Concurrent Herpes simplex and cytomegalovirus retinitis and encephalitis in the acquired immune deficiency syndrome (AIDS). *Ophthalmology* 91: 1669–77.

Perry VH, Gordon S (1987) Modulation of CD4 antigen on macrophages and microglia in rat brain. *J Exp Med* 166: 1138–43.

Petito CK (1993) Myelopathies. In *Neuropathology of HIV Infection* Scaravilli F (ed) Springer-Verlag: London, pp 187–99.

Petito CK, Cho E-S, Lemann W *et al* (1986) Neuropathology of acquired immunodeficiency syndrome (AIDS): an autopsy review. *J Neuropathol Exp Neurol* 45: 635–46.

Petito CK, Roberts B (1995) Evidence of apoptotic cell death in HIV encephalitis *Am J Path* 146: 1121–30.

Pette H, Döring G (1939) Über eine endemische panencephalitis vom charakter der encephalitis Japonica. *Deutsch Z Nervenheilkd* 149: 7–44.

Piatak M, Saag MS, Yang LC *et al* (1993) High levels of HIV-1 in plasma during all stages of infection determined by competitive PCR. *Science* 259: 1749–54.

Plummer G (1964) Serological comparison of the herpes viruses. *Br J Exp Pathol* 45: 135–41.

Portegies P, Algra PR, Hollak CE *et al* (1991) Response to

cytarabine in progressive multifocal leukoencephalopathy in AIDS. *Lancet* i: 680–1.

Price RW, Brew B, Sidtis *et al* (1988) The brain in AIDS: central nervous system HIV-1 infection and AIDS dementia complex. *Science* 239: 586–92.

Pulliam L, Herndier BG, Tang NM, McGrath MS (1991) Human immunodeficiency virus-infected macrophages produce soluble factors that cause histological and neurochemical alterations in cultured brains. *J Clin Inv* 87: 503–12.

Pumarola-Sune T, Navia BA, Cordon-Cardo C *et al* (1987) HIV antigen in the brain of patients with the AIDS dementia complex. *Ann Neurol* 21: 490–6.

Ravenholt RT, Foege WH (1982) 1918 influenza, encephalitis lethargica, Parkinsonism. *Lancet* ii: 860–4.

Rawls WE (1985) Herpes simplex virus. In: Fields BN, Knipe DM, Chanock RM *et al.* (ed) *Virology*. Raven Press, New York, 527–62.

Risk WS, Haddad FS (1979) The variable natural history of subacute sclerosing panencephalitis. *Arch Neurol* 36: 610–4.

Robinson HL, Miles BD (1985) Avian leukosis virus-induced osteoporosis in association with persistent synthesis of viral DNA. *Virology* 141: 130–43.

Roizman B, Batterson W (1985) Herpesviruses and their replication. In: Fields BN, Knipe DM, Chanock RM *et al.* (ed) *Virology*. Raven Press, New York, 497–526.

Rowley AH, Whitley RJ, Lakeman FD *et al* (1990) Rapid detection of Herpes simplex virus DNA in cerebrospinal fluid of patients with Herpes simplex encephalitis. *Lancet* 335: 440–1.

Sabatier J-M, Vives E, Mabrouk K *et al* (1991) Evidence for neurotoxic activity of *tat* from human immunodeficiency virus type 1. *J Virol* 65: 961–67.

Sage JI, Weinstein MP, Miller DC (1985) Chronic encephalitis possibly due to Herpes simplex virus: two cases. *Neurology* 35: 1470–2.

Saito Y, Sharer LR, Epstein LG *et al* (1994) Overexpression of nef as a marker of restricted HIV-infection of astrocytes in post mortem pediatric centred nervous tissues. *Neurology* 44: 474–81.

Salahuddin SZ, Lynfield R, Lowenthal DA *et al* (1986) Isolation of a new virus, HTLV, in patients with lymphoproliferative disorders. *Science* 234: 596–601.

Sawyer J, Ellner J (1988) To biopsy or not to biopsy in suspected Herpes simplex encephalitis. *Med Decision Making* 8: 95–101.

Scaravilli F (1992) Neuropathology of HIV-1 and HTLV-1 infection. In *Neurological Aspects of Human Retroviruses* Rudge P (ed) Balliere Clinical Neurology, Balliere Tindall, London, p 211–38.

Scaravilli F, Gray F, Mikol J *et al* (1993) Pathology of the nervous system. In *The Neuropathology of HIV Infection* Scaravilli F (ed) Springer-Verlag, London, p 99–169.

Scaravilli F, Ellis DS, Tovey G *et al* (1989) Unusual development of polyoma virus in the brains of two patients with the acquired immune deficiency syndrome (AIDS). *Neuropathol Appl Neurobiol* 15: 407–18.

Schmid P, Conrad A, Syndulko K *et al* (1994) Quantifying HIV-1 proviral DNA using the polymerase chain reaction on cerebrospinal fluid and blood of seropositive individuals with and without neurologic abnormalities. *J Acq Immunodef Synd* 777–88.

Schmidbauer M, Budka H, Okeda R *et al* (1990) Multifocal vacuolar leukoencephalopathy: a distinct HIV-associated lesion of the brain. *Neuropathol Appl Neurobiol* 16: 437–43.

Sekizawa T, Openshaw H, Wohlenberg C *et al* (1980) Latency of Herpes simplex virus in absence of neutralizing antibody: model for reactivation. *Science* 210: 1026–8.

Sharer LR, Dowling PC, Michaels J *et al* (1990) Spinal cord disease in children with HIV-1 infection: a combined molecular biological and neuropathological study. *Neuropathol Appl Neurobiol* 16: 317–31.

Sharer LR, Epstein LG, Cho E-S *et al* (1986) Pathologic features of AIDS encephalopathy in children: evidence for LAV/HTLV-III infection in brain. *Hum Pathol* 17: 271–84.

Sharer LR, Mintz M (1992) Neuropathology of AIDS in children. In *Neuropathology of HIV Infection* Scaravilli F (ed) Springer-Verlag: London, pp 201–14.

Shaw GM, Harper ME, Hahn BH *et al* (1985) HTLV-III infection in brains of children and adults with AIDS encephalopathy. *Science* 227: 177–82.

Sidtis JJ, Price RW (1990) Early HIV-1 infection and the AIDS dementia complex. *Neurology* 40: 323–6.

Sinclair E, Gray F, Ciardi A, Scaravilli F (1994) Immunohistochemical changes and PCR detection of HIV provirus DNA in brains of asymptomatic HIV-positive patients. *J Neuropathol Exp Neurol* 53: 43–50.

Snider WD, Simpson DM, Nielsen S *et al* (1983) Neurological complications of acquired immune deficiency syndrome analysis of 50 patients. *Ann Neurol* 14: 403–18.

Silverman L, Rubinstein LJ (1965) Electron microscopic observations on a case of progressive multifocal leukoencephalopathy. *Acta Neuropathol* 5: 215–24.

Sinclair E, Scaravilli F (1992) Detection of HIV proviral DNA in cortex and white matter of AIDS brains by non-isotopic polymerase chain reaction: correlation with diffuse poliodystrophy. *AIDS* 6: 925–32.

Sinclair E, Gray F, Scaravilli F (1992) PCR detection of HIV proviral DNA in the brain of an asymptomatic HIV-positive patient. *J Neurol* 239: 469–70.

Smith TW, De Girolami U, Hénin D *et al* (1990) Human immunodeficiency virus (HIV) leukoencephalopathy and the microcirculation. *J Neuropathol Exp Neurol* 49: 357–70.

Snider WD, Simpson DM, Nielsen S *et al* (1983) Neurological complications of acquired immunodeficiency syndrome: analysis of 50 patients. *Ann Neurol* 14: 403–18.

Soong S-J, Watson NE, Caddell GR *et al* (1991) Use of brain biopsy for diagnostic evaluation, of patients with suspected herpes simplex encephalitis: a statistical model and its clinical implications. *J Inf Dis* 163: 17–22.

Stoler MH, Eskin TA, Benn S *et al* (1986) Human T-cell lymphotrophic virus type III infection of the central nervous system. Preliminary *in situ* analysis. *JAMA* 256: 2360–4.

Tan SV, Guiloff RJ, Scaravilli F, Klapper PE, Cleator GM, GM, Gazzard BG (1993) Herpes Simplex type I encephalitis in acquired immunodeficiency syndrome. *Ann Neurol* 34: 619–22.

Tornatore C, Chandra R, Berger JR, Major ED (1994) HIV-1 infection of subcortical astrocytes in the pediatric central nervous system. *Neurology* 44: 481–7.

Townsend JJ, Baringer JR (1979) Morphology of central nervous system disease in immunosuppressed mice after peripheral herpes simplex virus inoculation. *Lab Invest* 40: 178–82.

Tramont EC (1991) Syphilis of the nervous system in *Infections of the central nervous system*. HP Lambert, DC Decker (eds) Philadelphia, pp 207–17.

Tyor WR, Glass JD, Griffin JW *et al* (1992) Cytokine expression in the brain during the acquired immunodeficiency syndrome, *Ann Neurol* 31: 349–60.

van Bogaert L (1945) Une leucoencéphalite sclérosante sub-aiguë. *J Neurol Neurosurg Psychiat* 8: 101–20.

Van Landingham KE, Marsteller HB, Ross GW (1988) Relapse of Herpes simplex encephalitis after conventional acyclovir therapy. *JAMA* 259: 1051–3.

Vazeux R, Brousse N, Jarry A *et al* (1987) AIDS subacute encephalitis. Identification of HIV-infected cells. *Am J Pathol* 126: 403–10.

Vinters HV, Tomyiasu U, Anders KH (1989) Neuropathologic complications of infection with the human immunodeficiency virus (HIV) *Adv AIDS Pathol* 1: 101–30.

Weiss RA (1985) Human T-cell retroviruses. In *RNA Tumour Viruses* Weiss RA (ed) Cold Spring Harbor, New York, pp 405–85.

Whiteley RJ, Soong S-J, Linneman C *et al* (1982) Herpes simplex encephalitis clinical assessment. *JAMA* 247: 317–20.

Wildy P (1967) The progression of herpes simplex virus to the central nervous system of the mouse. *J Hyg* 65: 173–92.

Wildy P, Field HJ, Nash AA (1982) Classic herpes latency revisited. In: Mahy BW, Minson AC, Darby GK (ed) *Virus Persistence*, Society for General Microbiology Symposium 33. Cambridge Univ Press, Cambridge, 133–68.

Wildy P *et al* (1984) Inhibition of herpes simplex virus multiplication by activated macrophages etc. *Infect Immunol*, 37: 40–5.

Wiley CA, Schrier RD, Nelson JA *et al* (1986) Cellular localization of human immunodeficiency virus infection within the brain of acquired immune deficiency syndrome patients. *Proc Natl Acad Sci USA* 87: 7089–93.

Wiley CA, Masliah E, Hansen L *et al* (1990) Cerebral cortical abnormalities in AIDS. *J Neuropathol Exp Neurol* 49: 350 (abstr).

Wiley CA, Masliah E, Morey M *et al* (1991a) Neocortical damage during HIV infection. *Ann Neurol* 29: 651–7.

Wiley CA, Ge N, Morey M *et al* (1991b) Golgi impregnation studies of dendritic pathology in HIV encephalitis. *J Neuropathol Exp Neurol* 50: 324 (Abstr).

Wisniewski H, Terry RD, Hirano A (1970) Neurofibrillary pathology. *J Neuropathol Exp Neurol* 29: 163–76.

Yahr MD (1978) Encephalitis lethargica (von Economo's disease, epidemic encephalitis). In Vinken PJ, Bruyn GW (ed) *Handbook of Clinical Neurology* North-Holland, Amsterdam, pp 451–7.

Yen SH, Dickson DW, Peterson C *et al* (1986) Cytoskeletal abnormalities in neuropathology. *Progr Neuropath* 6: 63–90.

ZuRhein GM, Chou SM (1965) Particles resembling papovaviruses in human cerebral demyelinating disease. *Science* 148: 1477–9.

CHAPTER EIGHTEEN

Schizophrenia and its dementia

P. J. Harrison

Macroscopic brain changes in schizophrenia
Microscopic brain changes in schizophrenia
The nature of the disease process: the neurodevelopmental model
The dementia of schizophrenia and its neuropathological basis
Suggestions for the neuropathological study of schizophrenia
Conclusions

Prior to the 1970s, a combination of methodological problems and neglect meant that virtually nothing was known of the cerebral substrate of schizophrenia. This culminated in the well-known remark that 'schizophrenia is the graveyard of neuropathologists' (Plum, 1972) and the disregard of earlier studies (Corsellis, 1976; Jellinger, 1985). Over the past 20 years, a resurgence of interest, and an improved quality of research, have resurrected the field to the point where we can now be confident that there is a neuropathology of schizophrenia, albeit one which remains poorly characterized.

This chapter reviews the evidence for structural brain changes in schizophrenia and their interpretation before addressing two specific issues. First, some studies have found evidence for neurodegenerative lesions in schizophrenia. It is important to determine if these represent part of the core pathology or whether, in line with the prevailing theory, they are superimposed upon a neurodevelopmental disease process. Secondly, cognitive impairment is present in some schizophrenics, and the question arises as to whether it is associated with a different neuropathological picture from that of schizophrenia itself.

MACROSCOPIC BRAIN CHANGES IN SCHIZOPHRENIA

Contemporary interest in the neuropathology of schizophrenia may be traced to the report of Johnstone and colleagues (1976) who demonstrated enlarged lateral ventricles in a group of chronic schizophrenics. Ventricular enlargement in schizophrenia has since become a highly robust finding, albeit one of small magnitude

(Daniel et al., 1991). It is accompanied by a loss of cortical grey matter (Zipursky et al., 1992). Post-mortem findings confirm ventricular enlargement and also show a slight shrinkage of the brain (< 5%) in terms of weight, length and cortical volume (Table 18.1).

A variety of data suggest that the changes may be greater in certain brain regions. Whilst these findings are less clear cut, it is noteworthy that structures within the temporal lobe, particularly the parahippocampal gyrus and hippocampus, are smaller in schizophrenics in most post-mortem series (Table 18.1), as they are in some imaging studies (e.g. Degreef et al., 1992a). Important supportive evidence comes from an MRI study of identical twins discordant for the disease, which found that the affected twin had smaller hippocampi than the unaffected twin (Suddath et al., 1990). It remains uncertain whether temporal lobe alterations account for, or are in addition to, the diffuse brain involvement indicated by ventricular dilatation and loss of cortical substance. Furthermore, some MRI data suggest that the predominant tissue reduction may occur in prefrontal regions (Andreasen et al., 1994), or is enhanced in association cortex (Schlaepfer et al., 1994). These findings require corroboration from post-mortem studies. A further complexity is that there may be an interaction between cerebral lateralization and the pathology of schizophrenia. This proposal arises from data indicating that changes are more pronounced in the left than the right hemisphere (Brown et al., 1986; Crow et al., 1989; Bogerts et al., 1990), and that normal brain asymmetries are lost in the disease (Bilder et al., 1994; Falkai et al., 1992, 1995a,b). However, other data do not provide

Table 18.1. *Macroscopic neuropathological findings in schizophrenia*[a]

Area	Alteration in schizophrenia	Positive reports	Negative reports
Brain weight	Decreased	Brown et al., 1986[c] Pakkenberg, 1987 Bruton et al., 1990	Heckers et al., 1991a
Cortical volume[b]	Decreased	Pakkenberg, 1987	Heckers et al., 1991a
Brain length	Decreased	Bruton et al., 1990	
Lateral ventricles[b]	Increased size	Brown et al., 1986 Pakkenberg, 1987 Crow et al., 1989 Bruton et al., 1990	
Medial temporal lobe[b,d]	Decreased size	Bogerts, Meertz & Schonfeldt-Busch, 1985 Brown et al., 1986 Falkai & Bogerts, 1986 Colter et al., 1987 Falkai et al., 1988 Jeste & Lohr, 1989 Altshuler et al., 1990 Bogerts et al., 1990	Heckers et al., 1990
Basal ganglia	Decreased size of globus pallidus	Bogerts et al., 1985	Bogerts et al., 1990 Heckers et al., 1991a
	Increased size of striatum[e]	Heckers et al., 1991a	
Corpus callosum	Abnormal size or shape	Rosenthal & Bigelow, 1972 Bigelow et al., 1983	
Mediodorsal thalamus	Decreased size	Pakkenberg, 1990	
Periventricular grey matter	Thinned	Lesch & Bogerts, 1984	
Substantia nigra (lateral)	Decreased volume	Bogerts et al., 1983	
Sylvian fissure	Shortened on left	Falkai et al., 1992	
Sulcogyral patterns	Abnormal	Jakob & Beckmann, 1986	Bruton et al., 1990

[a] The Table lists positive post-mortem findings identified by comparison with controls. For clarity, the Table does not indicate studies which found interactions with hemisphere or sex (see Falkai & Bogerts, 1994).

[b] Positive findings which are supported by imaging data. The other changes listed in the Table have either not been looked for in imaging studies or no consensus has emerged.

[c] Compare to affective disorder controls.

[d] Hippocampus, parahippocampal gyrus or parahippocampal white matter.

[e] Follow up imaging studies suggest that increased striatal volumes result from neuroleptic treatment (Chakos et al., 1994).

evidence for lateralized effects (see, for example, Weinberger et al., 1991; Flaum et al., 1995) and the matter remains controversial. Genetic (Crow et al., 1989) and other (Bracha, 1991; Roberts, 1991; Zaidel et al., 1995; Zaidel et al., 1997) hypotheses have been put forward to account for any association of schizophrenia with altered cerebral asymmetry which may exist.

In summary, schizophrenia is associated with a slight reduction in cortical volume which is most apparent in the temporal lobe and which may be more marked in the left hemisphere. Possible explanations for these findings are discussed below.

MICROSCOPIC BRAIN CHANGES IN SCHIZOPHRENIA

Stimulated by the discovery of reliable macroscopic brain changes in schizophrenia, histological studies of the disease have been rekindled. Many abnormalities have been reported, but few yet constitute wholly established findings (Table 18.2).

Table 18.2. *Histological findings in schizophrenia*[a]

Area	Alteration in schizophrenia	Positive reports	Negative reports
Entorhinal cortex /parahippocampal gyrus	Abnormal cytoarchitecture[b]	Jakob & Beckmann, 1986 Arnold *et al.*, 1991 Falkai & Bogerts, 1994	
	Decreased neuron number	Falkai *et al.*, 1988	
Hippocampus	Decreased pyramidal neuron number or density	Falkai & Bogerts, 1986 Jeste & Lohr, 1989	Heckers *et al.*, 1991*b* Benes *et al.*, 1991*b* Arnold *et al.*, 1995*a* Zaidel *et al.*, 1997
	Decreased pyramidal neuron size	Benes *et al.*, 1991*b* Arnold *et al.*, 1995*a* Zaidel *et al.*, 1996	Christison *et al.*, 1989
	Pyramidal neuron disarray	Kovelman & Scheibel, 1984 Conrad *et al.*, 1991	Christison *et al.*, 1989 Benes *et al.*, 1991*b* Arnold *et al.*, 1995*a* Zaidel *et al*, 1996
Cingulate gyrus (area 24)	Decreased interneuron density[d]	Benes *et al.*, 1986, 1991*a*	
	Increased vertical axon number	Benes *et al.*, 1987	
Frontal cortex (area 10)	Decreased interneuron density[d]	Benes *et al.*, 1986, 1991*a*	
	Increased pyramidal neuron density[d]	Benes *et al.*, 1991*a*	
Frontal cortex (area 9)	Increased neuron density	Selemon *et al.*, 1995	Akbarian *et al.*, 1995
	Decreased neuron size	Raikowska *et al.*, 1994	
Visual cortex (area 17)	Increased neuron density	Selemon *et al.*, 1995	
Prefrontal and temporal cortex	Altered location of NADPH-d neurons[e]	Akbarian *et al.*, 1993	
Mediodorsal thalamus	Decreased neuron number	Pakkenberg, 1990, 1993*a*	
Nucleus accumbens	Decreased neuron number	Pakkenberg, 1990, 1993*a*	
Substantia nigra (lateral)	Decreased neuron size	Bogerts *et al.*, 1983	
Septal nuclei	Swollen neurons with granular accumulations	Averback, 1981	
Mesopontine nuclei	Increased neuron number	Garcia-Rill *et al.*, 1995	

[a] Positive histopathological findings in schizophrenia compared with controls. Studies of gliosis are summarized in Table 18.3.
[b] Taking the form of abnormal or ectopic pre-α cell clusters, paucity of neurons in superficial laminae, or abnormal surface invaginations.
[c] Neuronal density selectively increased in right hippocampus.
[d] Changes limited to specific laminae.
[e] NADPH-d = nicotinamide-adenine dinucleotide phosphate-diaphorase.

Entorhinal cytoarchitectural abnormalities

In an influential paper, Jakob & Beckmann (1986) reported abnormalities in the anterior parahippocampal gyrus (entorhinal cortex), including aberrant pre-α cell clusters and a paucity of neurons in superficial laminae, especially on the left side. Similar cytoarchitectural findings have been reported in two additional series of brains, suggesting that they are robust (Arnold *et al.*, 1991; Falkai, Bogerts & Rozumek, 1988; Falkai & Bogerts, 1994). However, the cytoarchitecture of the entorhinal cortex, including the organization of the pre-α cell layer, is complex and variable (Insausti *et al.*, 1995). Thus, if the region differs in size or shape in schizophrenia (Table 18.1), the reported abnormalities may be confounded by having examined sections from different levels in cases and controls. Stereological stu-

Table 18.3. *Gliosis in schizophrenia[a]*

Author	Region	Number of cases/controls	Parameter measured	Technique	Finding in schizophrenia
Studies without neuropathological 'purification'					
Stevens (1982)	Multiple areas	25/20	Gliosis	Holzer stain	Increased
Bogerts et al. (1983)	Substantia nigra	6/6	Glial number	Nissl stain	Unchanged
Benes et al. (1986)	Frontal and cingulate cortex	10/10	Glial density	Nissl stain	Unchanged/decreased
Falkai & Bogerts (1986)[e]	Hippocampus	15/9	Glial number	Nissl stain	Unchanged/decreased
Owen et al. (1987)	Frontal and temporal cortex; hippocampus; amygdala; putamen; hypothalamus	39/44	MAO-B activity[b]	Enzyme assay	Unchanged/decreased
Falkai et al. (1988)[e]	Entorhinal cortex	15/9	Glial number	Nissl stain	Unchanged
Bruton et al. (1990)[f]	Cortex; periventricular region	48/56	Gliosis rating	Holzer stain	Increased
Casanova et al. (1990)	Dentate gyrus	6/7	Glial number	Holzer stain	Unchanged
Pakkenberg (1990)	Mediodorsal thalamus; ventral striatum; amygdala	12/12	Absolute glial number	Nissl stain; stereology	Unchanged/decreased
Karson et al. (1993)	Cortical areas, cerebellum, pontine tegmentum	4-12/3-10	GFAP[c]	Immunoblot	Unchanged
Studies with neuropathological 'purification'					
Roberts et al. (1986)[g]	Multiple	5/7	GFAP	Immunoreactivity	Unchanged
Roberts et al. (1987)	Temporal lobe	18/12	GFAP	Immunoreactivity	Unchanged
Stevens et al. (1988a)[g]	Caudate, cingulate white matter periventricular region	5/7	GFAP	Cell counts	Unchanged
Crow et al. (1989)[f]	Temporal, frontal and parietal cortex; hippocampus; amygdala and caudate	18/20	Gliosis	DBI[d] immuno-reactivity; Holzer stain	Unchanged
Benes et al. (1991a)	Prefrontal and cingulate cortex	18/12	Glial density	Nissl stain	Unchanged
Selemon et al. (1995)	Prefrontal and visual cortex	16/19	Glial density	Nissl stain	Unchanged

[a] The studies in the first half of Table 18.3 included all schizophrenics or had purely clinical criteria for exclusion (e.g. a history of cognitive impairment). The studies in the second half of Table 18.3 had neuropathological criteria for exclusion of brains (e.g. infarcts, Alzheimer's disease).

[b] MAO: monoamine oxidase. The β form of the enzyme is mainly glial.

[c] GFAP: glial fibrillary acidic protein, a glial marker.

[d] DBI: diazepam-binding inhibitor, a glial marker.

[e-g] Studies sharing the same superscript were carried out on the same brains.

dies of the entire parahippocampal region are needed to confirm the findings, given their potential importance (see below).

Neuronal size

Decreased hippocampal neuronal size is the other reasonably well replicated finding in schizophrenia (Benes, Sorensen & Bird, 1991b; Arnold et al., 1995a; Zaidel, Esiri & Harrison, 1996). The one apparently negative report was based upon measurement of only 12 neurons per hippocampus (Christison et al., 1989). Reduced neuronal size has also been reported in neocortical areas (Raikowska, Selemon & Goldman-Rakic, 1994), suggesting that it may be a widespread phenomenon. It is unlikely to be an artefact of treatment with antipsychotic drugs, since the studies found no association between neuronal size and degree of drug exposure, and cortical neuronal size in rats is unaffected by long-term haloperidol administration (Benes et al., 1985).

Neuronal density and number

In the hippocampus, initial studies suggested a reduced pyramidal neuron density in some subfields in schizophrenia (Falkai & Bogerts, 1986; Jeste & Lohr, 1989). However, two further studies were negative (Benes et al., 1991b; Arnold et al.,1995a) and an increased hippocampal neuron density has also been reported which is limited to the right side (Zaidel et al., 1997). A stereological count of hippocampal neuron number showed no differences between cases and controls (Heckers et al., 1991b). The data in neocortex are also conflicting (Benes, Davidson & Bird, 1986; Benes et al., 1991a; Akbarian et al., 1995: Selemon, Rajkowska & Goldman-Rakic, 1995; see Table 18.3). Overall, it is unclear whether there is any consistent pattern of neuronal density alteration in schizophrenia.

Neuronal disarray

Kovelman & Scheibel (1984) found pyramidal neurons in the left hippocampal formation to be arranged in an aberrant orientation in schizophrenia, especially anteriorly and at the borders of adjacent subfields. Although this group replicated their finding and showed it to be a bilateral phenomenon, four other groups have failed to do so (Table 18.2).

Subcortical cytoarchitectural findings

Pakkenberg (1990, 1993a) counted neurons in the mediodorsal thalamic nucleus, nucleus accumbens, ven-tral pallidum and basolateral amygdala and found reductions of 40–50% in the first two nuclei but not the latter two in schizophrenics. Histological changes have also been reported in septal nuclei (Averback, 1981), and an increase of mesopontine cholinergic neurons has been found (Garcia-Rill et al., 1995). No alterations in cell number have been found in the locus ceruleus (Lohr & Jeste, 1988; Garcia-Rill et al., 1995) or cerebellum (Lohr & Jeste, 1986).

Ultrastructural and synaptic alterations

There are few electron microscopy data in schizophrenia. The largest biopsy study examined tissue from Brodmann area 10 from five schizophrenics and reported several differences in neurons and oligodendrocytes compared to four neurosurgical controls (Miyakawa et al., 1972). The differences included hyperplastic endoplasmic reticulum and granular accumulations in myelinated fibres. Many synapses also appeared abnormal, particularly in terms of clustering of presynaptic vesicles, an observation repeated in an autopsy sample (Soustek, 1989). Interpretation of these data is confounded by potential peri-mortem artefacts and by the fact that synaptic morphology is affected by antipsychotic drugs in rats (Harrison, 1993) and in non-schizophrenic cases (Jellinger, 1977). An alternative approach to study synaptic involvement in schizophrenia is by the measurement of synaptic proteins such as synaptophysin. Recent data indicate that the abundance of synaptophysin is decreased in the medial temporal lobe (Eastwood & Harrison, 1995), suggestive of a reduced synaptic density in the disease.

Gliosis

The issue of whether gliosis is observed in schizophrenia has become critical because its absence, in the presence of macroscopic and cytoarchitectonic abnormalities, has been used to support a developmental as opposed to a degenerative disease process (see below). The data and their interpretation are complex, and gliosis has been called the 'most inscrutable lesion' of schizophrenia (Bruton et al., 1990).

Earlier reports suggested that gliosis, especially periventricularly, was common in schizophrenia (Nieto & Escobar, 1972; Fisman, 1975; Stevens, 1982). These were influential, arguably out of proportion to the data, as being indicative of a viral or inflammatory aetiology. In contrast, subsequent studies have cast considerable doubt on the presence of, and explanation for, gliosis in schizophrenia (Table 18.3). Indeed, with one partial and illuminating exception (Bruton *et al.*, 1990), none has found an excess of gliosis, defined in several ways, in schizophrenia. In their valuable prospective series, Bruton and colleagues found that the schizophrenic group overall did show an increased frequency of gliosis compared to the control group. However, they then divided their schizophrenic brains into those with and those without additional pathology (e.g. vascular disease, neurofibrillary tangles). In the 'purified' group, no gliosis was found in any area even though the core changes of brain shrinkage, shortening and ventricular enlargement were still present; gliosis was limited to those cases of schizophrenia where the additional pathology was observed. The cases in each subgroup did not differ clinically (Johnstone *et al.*, 1994). These data, together with the other studies listed in Table 18.3, imply strongly that gliosis in schizophrenia is an accompaniment of coincidental or superimposed pathological changes rather than being an inherent feature of the disease.

One caveat to this conclusion must be mentioned. Most contemporary studies of gliosis have used immunochemical or biochemical markers rather than traditional techniques such as the Holzer stain. The relative sensitivity and reliability of these methods for detecting chronic gliosis remain controversial (Stevens *et al.*, 1991), contributing to differences of opinion as to whether the many negative findings cited in Table 18.3 mean that gliosis has been entirely excluded from the core pathological phenotype of schizophrenia (Roberts, Bruton & Crow, 1988; Stevens, Casanova & Bigelow, 1988*b*). Moreover, the incidence of neurodegenerative lesions, including focal areas of gliosis, appears to be higher than expected, being present in approximately 50% of cases (Stevens, 1982; Jellinger, 1985, Bruton *et al.*, 1990). There are several possible explanations. Firstly, that there is a subtype of schizophrenia which *is* due to an inflammatory or neurodegenerative pathology (see Bruton, Stevens & Frith, 1994). Secondly, that the schizophrenic brain is more vulnerable to neurodegenerative processes, either as a result of the initial lesion, or secondary to institutionalization, medication, and so on. Thirdly, it may be an artefact of tissue collection. Brains from control subjects are easily obtained and may be discarded if there is a history of other medical conditions, head injury, or a prolonged terminal phase. In contrast, because of the difficulties of collection, brains from schizophrenics may not be subject to such rigorous assessment. Therefore, a higher proportion of schizophrenic brains used for research may have

non-specific focal pathologies arising from coincidental events during life.

THE NATURE OF THE DISEASE PROCESS: THE NEURODEVELOPMENTAL MODEL

The prevailing view of schizophrenia is one of a neurodevelopmental rather than a neurodegenerative disorder, whereby it results from an anomaly of brain maturation, probably occurring in late fetal or early post-natal life (Weinberger 1987, 1995; Roberts, 1991; Murray *et al.*, 1992). The delay between a putatively pre-natal disease process and the onset of symptoms in adulthood is accounted for by the intervening events of brain maturation such as synaptic pruning and myelination (Weinberger, 1987; Benes *et al.*, 1994; Walker, 1994).

The neurodevelopmental model is built on a combination of clinico-epidemiological and neuropathological foundations. The former come into three main categories. (1) The known environmental risk factors for the disease all relate to pre- or peri-natal events (such as maternal influenza, maternal malnutrition and birth complications; Waddington, 1993). (2) Schizophrenics have a high frequency of minor physical anomalies (Green *et al.*, 1989) and abnormal dermatoglyphics (Bracha *et al.*, 1991) which are both associated with intrauterine maldevelopment. (3) Pre-schizophrenic infants and children show an excess of neuromotor (Jones *et al.*, 1994, Walker, 1994) and behavioural (Done *et al.*, 1994; Jones *et al.*, 1994) abnormalities.

Several aspects of the structural imaging and neuropathological data have contributed to the establishment of the neurodevelopmental model. The demonstration that the structural pathology (decreased medial temporal lobe and increased lateral ventricular volumes) is present at or before the onset of symptoms or medication, and is essentially non-progressive thereafter (Degreef *et al.*, 1992*a*; Jaskiw *et al.*, 1994; Marsh *et al.*, 1994, but see DeLisi *et al.*, 1995), excludes the possibility that the brain changes are secondary to chronic disease or its treatment. It is also known that there is an increased incidence of schizophrenia-like illnesses associated with abnormalities usually considered developmental in origin, including cavum septum pellucidum (Degreef *et al.*, 1992*b*), temporal lobe epilepsy (Roberts *et al.*, 1990) and metachromatic leukodystrophy (Hyde, Ziegler & Weinberger, 1992).

More direct neuropathological support for the neurodevelopmental model comes from the histological data. Importantly, the absence of gliosis in schizophrenia

(Table 18.3) is taken to infer that the disease process cannot have been active for a considerable period before death, and is most likely to have occurred prior to the gliotic response to brain injury which begins near the end of the second trimester (Friede, 1989). Hence the importance of determining whether gliosis is or is not a cardinal feature of schizophrenia. However, an absence of gliosis should not be equated with proof that the disease process operated prenatally, since the onset, quantitative characteristics and permanence of gliosis in human brain are poorly understood and even the recognition of gliosis can be problematic (da Cunha et al., 1993). Furthermore, it is apparent in experimental animals that chronic gliosis is not a ubiquitous response to neural injury; its occurrence is dependent upon the timing, nature and site of the lesion (Anezaki et al., 1992; Norton et al., 1992; Kalman et al., 1993). Thus, an absence of detectable gliosis in schizophrenia does not of itself exclude the possibility that the pathogenic process continues well after the second trimester, nor that it might include a degenerative component. Nevertheless, the existing data are strongly supportive of a primarily neurodevelopmental pathology, especially when considered in conjunction with the presence of cytoarchitectural abnormalities (Table 18.2). In particular, the features in the entorhinal cortex appear dysplastic, reflecting disturbed neuronal migration or perhaps programmed cell death, in keeping with a late second trimester time of origin (Weinberger, 1995). This view is supported by data showing an aberrant distribution of subplate neurons in the cortex in schizophrenics (Akbarian et al., 1993, 1996).

THE DEMENTIA OF SCHIZOPHRENIA AND ITS NEUROPATHOLOGICAL BASIS

Having argued the case for a pathogenesis in which degenerative lesions in schizophrenia are secondary or artefactual, there is a further factor which complicates the issue: some schizophrenics are demented. It needs to be determined, therefore, whether the inclusion of cognitively impaired patients in neuropathological studies might confound the question of neurodegenerative changes in schizophrenia.

Establishing the relationship between dementia and schizophrenia has proved difficult both clinically and neuropathologically. Despite its original name of dementia praecox, dementia is not a diagnostic feature of schizophrenia. However, substantial cognitive impairment is present in a considerable proportion (perhaps 10–30%) of acute (Hoff et al., 1992) and chronic (John-stone et al., 1978; Davidson et al., 1995) cases. It may particularly affect semantic memory (McKenna, 1994) within the context of a widespread impairment (Blanchard & Neal, 1994). The deficits appear to be largely static rather than inexorably progressive (Goldberg et al., 1993; Heaton et al., 1994).

The neuropathology of dementia in schizophrenia has been approached in two ways. First, in terms of whether neurodegenerative lesions are commoner than expected in schizophrenics; this issue has already been discussed with regard to gliosis (Table 18.3). Secondly, whether schizophrenics with cognitive impairment have a different neuropathological picture to those without.

The frequency of Alzheimer's disease in schizophrenia

Three recent studies have specifically investigated the frequency of Alzheimer's disease in schizophrenia. In a review of 100 consecutive autopsies on psychiatric inpatients, 23 schizophrenics (mean age 79 years) were included, of whom 8 (34%) were found to have Alzheimer's disease (Buhl & Bojsen-Moller, 1988). Soustek (1989) reported that 22% of schizophrenics, out of a total of 225, had Alzheimer's disease, increasing to 61% of those aged over 70. In the largest series, Prohovnik and colleagues (1993) reviewed the neuropathological findings in 544 schizophrenics. The prevalence of Alzheimer's disease was 9% (< 65 years), 16% (65–74 years), 33% (75–84 years) and 45% (over 85 years); the overall frequency of Alzheimer's disease was 28%. Although no control groups were included in any of these studies, the figures for Alzheimer's disease are considerably higher than its age-specific prevalence determined from population surveys. The occurrence of Alzheimer's disease in schizophrenia can also be determined from data in three case-control series; in contrast to the above findings, none of these reports a clear excess of Alzheimer's disease neuropathology in their schizophrenic cases (Stevens, 1982; Jellinger, 1985; Bruton et al., 1990).

The neuropathological basis of dementia in schizophrenia

The specific neuropathological correlates of dementia in schizophrenia have only recently been sought. In the first series, 13 schizophrenics who had significant and well-characterized cognitive impairment underwent detailed neuropathological investigation. There was no evidence of Alzheimer's disease, or indeed any other neurodegenerative process, in excess of that found in an age-matched control group (Purohit et al., 1993; Haroutunian et al., 1994). An absence of neurodegenerative pathology has been reported in two further series, each containing ten elderly demented schizophrenics (Casanova *et al.*, 1993; Arnold, Franz & Trojanowski, 1994; Arnold *et al.*, 1994). No cell loss or senile plaque formation was reported in the nucleus basalis of Meynert in ten similar cases (El-Mallakh *et al.*, 1991). Furthermore, Johnstone *et al.* (1994) showed that schizophrenics with cognitive impairment had a similar frequency of Alzheimer's disease and other neurodegenerative disorders compared to those without such deficits.

It is difficult to reconcile the evidence from the preceding paragraphs: the first suggesting strongly that Alzheimer's disease pathology is common in schizophrenia, whereas the smaller but prospective and more rigorous recent studies find no evidence for any neurodegenerative disorder, even in schizophrenics with severe cognitive impairment. Certainly, the archival studies must be interpreted cautiously, given that neither schizophrenia nor Alzheimer's disease was diagnosed by contemporary criteria, a fact illustrated by re-analysis of the New York study which showed that up to 23% of the cases did not satisfy diagnostic criteria for Alzheimer's disease (Prohovnik *et al.*, 1993). Additionally, only 20% of schizophrenics dying came to autopsy in this survey, which may have led to ascertainment bias. As a further factor contributing to the apparent excess of Alzheimer-type pathology in schizophrenics it has been suggested that antipsychotic drugs promote neurofibrillary tangle formation (Wisniewski *et al.*, 1994). Even if an increased frequency of Alzheimer's disease were confirmed in schizophrenics, it is clear that their cognitive impairment is not attributable to Alzheimer's disease nor to any other recognized neurodegenerative process. Thus an alternative substrate for the dementia of schizophrenia must be sought.

SUGGESTIONS FOR THE NEUROPATHOLOGICAL STUDY OF SCHIZOPHRENIA

The neuropathology of schizophrenia is of a subtlety which requires that particular care is taken during the planning, execution and interpretation of research. Many shortcomings in this regard have been recognized (see Benes, 1988; Lantos, 1988; Casanova & Kleinman, 1990). They include the potential confounding effects of medication, mode of death and post-mortem interval, as well as the subsequent dissection, processing and storage of the brain. The rapid progress of the field in the past decade is attributable as much to better experimental design and greater attention to these variables as to the developments in technical and analytical methods. Nevertheless, difficulties remain and there is scope for further improvement.

Prior to any research investigation, brains should be investigated for the presence of neurodegenerative lesions; neuropathological examination may also reveal a neurological condition producing the phenotype of schizophrenia which went undiagnosed during life (Davison, 1983). Thereafter, brains with neurodegenerative abnormalities should either be excluded from research studies or else analysed as a separate subgroup. Researchers should also ensure that the criteria used for inclusion of brains in a study are the same for schizophrenics as for controls.

Three basic issues about the neuropathology of schizophrenia require clarification. First, little is known regarding whether any of the alterations reported here are specific to schizophrenia. Addressing this question requires the collection of cases of bipolar disorder (manic depression), schizoaffective disorder, and other related disorders to which schizophrenics can be compared. Inclusion of subjects in these other categories will also aid in the recognition of neuropathological changes resulting from medication, since many of them will have been treated with the same range of drugs. Secondly, it is unclear whether there are correlations between the clinical subsyndromes of schizophrenia (e.g. positive *vs.* negative or paranoid *vs.* hebephrenic subtypes) and the associated neuropathological profile, or whether all schizophrenics share a common pathology which differs only in severity (see Daniel *et al.*, 1991; Roberts & Bruton, 1990; Gur *et al.*, 1994). These issues of diagnostic specificity and pathological heterogeneity can best be addressed by prospective studies which permit detailed clinicopathological correlations (Arnold *et al.*, 1995*b*). Thirdly, the anatomical localization of the changes needs to be clarified (Shapiro, 1993). The putative existence of hemispheric differences indicates the need to specify which side of the brain is being studied, and to examine bilaterally wherever possible. Sampling of multiple brain areas defined using precise anatomical criteria is to be encouraged. Finally, there is a pressing need for attempts to replicate neuropathological findings in schizophrenia. The increasing collaboration between research laboratories in terms of the sharing of tissue and the standardization of protocols for handling, dissection and processing of material is a positive step in this direction.

CONCLUSIONS

It is certain that, as a group, schizophrenics have decreased cerebral volume and enlarged ventricles. These changes are small, but they are present at the onset of disease and show only minimal progression thereafter. Thus, there is a pathology which is not secondary to chronic disease or its treatment. A number of studies suggest that morphological changes are greatest in the medial temporal lobe and connected cortical regions. The histological features which are relatively well established comprise cytoarchitectural abnormalities in the entorhinal cortex and decreased cortical neuronal size, together with the negative findings regarding gliosis. These data have contributed significantly to the rediscovery of schizophrenia as a brain disorder and to the hypothesis that it is neurodevelopmental and not neurodegenerative in nature. The dementia of schizophrenia is not caused by Alzheimer's disease and it lacks a neuropathological explanation.

ACKNOWLEDGEMENTS

P.J.H. is a Wellcome Senior Research Fellow in Clinical Science. I thank the Stanley Foundation for additional research support.

REFERENCES

Akbarian S, Vinuela A, Kim JJ, Potkin S, Bunney WE Jr, Jones EG (1993) Distorted distribution of nicotinamide-adenine dinucleotide phosphate–diaphorase neurons in temporal lobe of schizophrenics implies anomalous cortical development. *Arch Gen Psychiat* 50: 178–87.

Akbarian S, Kim JJ, Potkin SG, Hagman JO, Tafazzoli A, Bunney WE Jr, Jones EG (1995) Gene expression for glutamic acid decarboxylase is reduced without loss of neurons in prefrontal cortex of schizophrenics. *Arch Gen Psychiat* 52: 258–66.

Akbarian S, Kim JJ, Potkin SG, Hetrick WP, Bunney WE Jr, Jones EG (1996) Maldistribution of interstitial neurons in prefrontal white matter of the brains of schizophrenic patients. *Arch Gen Psychiat* 53: 425–36.

Altshuler LL, Casanova MF, Goldberg TE, Kleinmann JE (1990) The hippocampus and parahippocampus in schizophrenic, suicide and control brains. *Arch Gen Psychiat* 47: 1029–34.

Andreasen NC, Flashman L, Flaum M, Arndt S. Swayze V II, O'Leary DS, Ehrhardt JC, Yoh WTC (1994) Regional brain abnormalities in schizophrenia measured with magnetic resonance imaging. *J Am Med Assoc* 272: 1763–9.

Anezaki T, Yanagisawa K, Takahashi H, Nakajima T, Miyashita K, Ishikawa A, Ikura F, Miyatake T (1992) Remote astrocytic response of prefrontal cortex is caused by lesions in the nucleus basalis of Meynert, but not in the ventral tegmental area. *Brain Res* 574: 63–9.

Arnold SE, Hyman BT, Van Hoesen GW, Damasio AR (1991) Some cytoarchitectonic abnormalities of the entorhinal cortex in schizophrenia. *Arch Gen Psychiat* 48: 625–32.

Arnold SE, Franz BR, Trojanowski JQ (1994) Elderly patients with schizophrenia exhibit infrequent neurodegenerative lesions. *Neurobiol Aging* 15: 299–303.

Arnold SE, Franz BR, Gur RC, Gur RE, Shapiro RM, Moberg PJ, Trojanowski JQ (1995a) Smaller neuronal size in schizophrenia in hippocampal subfields that mediate cortical-hippocampal interactions. *Am J Psychiat* 152: 738–48.

Arnold SE, Gur RE, Shapiro RM, Fisher KR, Moberg PJ, Gibney MR, Gur RC, Blackwell P, Trojanowski JQ (1995b) Prospective clinicopathologic studies of schizophrenia: accrual and assessment of patients. *Am J Psychiat* 152: 731–7.

Averback P (1981) Structural lesions of the brain in young schizophrenics. *Can J Neurol Sci* 8: 73–6.

Benes FM (1988) Post-mortem structural analyses of schizophrenics brain: study designs and the interpretation of data. *Psychiatr Dev* 3: 213–26.

Benes FM, Paskevich PA, Davidson J, Domesick VB (1985) Synaptic rearrangements in medial prefrontal cortex of haloperidol-treated rats. *Brain Res* 348: 15–20.

Benes FM, Davidson J, Bird ED (1986) Quantitative cytoarchitectural studies of the cerebral cortex of schizophrenics. *Arch Gen Psychiat* 43: 31–5.

Benes FM, Majocha R, Bird ED, Marotta CA (1987) Increased vertical axon numbers in cingulate cortex of schizophrenics. *Arch Gen Psychiat* 44: 1017–21.

Benes FM, McSparren J, Bird ED, SanGiovanni JP, Vincent SL (1991a) Deficits in small interneurons in prefrontal and cingulate cortices of schizophrenic and schizoaffective patients. *Arch Gen Psychiat* 48: 996–1001.

Benes FM, Sorensen I, Bird ED (1991b) Reduced neuronal size in posterior hippocampus of schizophrenic patients. *Schizophr Bull* 17: 597–608.

Benes FM, Turtle M, Khan Y, Farol P (1994) Myelination of a key relay zone in the hippocampal formation occurs in the human brain during childhood, adolescence, and adulthood. *Arch Gen Psychiat* 51: 477–84.

Bigelow LB, Nasrallah HA, Rauscher FP (1983) Corpus callosum thickness in chronic schizophrenia. *Br J Psychiat* 143: 284–7.

Bilder RM, Wu H, Bogerts B, Degreef G, Ashtari M, Alvir JMJ, Snyder PJ, Lieberman JA (1994) Absence of regional hemispheric volume asymmetries in first-episode schizophrenia. *Am J Psychiatr* 151: 1437–47.

Blanchard JJ, Neale JM (1994) The neuropsychological signature of schizophrenia: generalized or differential deficit? *Am J Psychiat* 151: 40–8.

Bogerts B, Häntsch J, Herzer M (1983) A morphometric study of dopamine-containing cell groups in the mesencephalon of normals, Parkinson patients, and schizophrenics. *Biol Psychiat* 18: 951–69.

Bogerts B, Meertz E, Schonfeldt-Busch R (1985) Basal ganglia and limbic system pathology in schizophrenia. *Arch Gen Psychiat* 42: 784–91.

Bogerts B, Falkai P, Haupts M, Greve B, Ernst S, Tapernon-Franz U, Heinzmann U (1990) Post-mortem volume measurements of limbic system and basal ganglia structures in chronic schizophrenia. *Schizophr Res* 3: 295–301.

Bracha HS (1991) Etiology of structural asymmetry in schizophrenia: an alternative hypothesis. *Schizophr Bull* 17: 551–3.

Bracha HS, Torrey EF, Bigelow LB, Lohr JB, Linnington BB (1991) Subtle signs of prenatal maldevelopment of the hand ectoderm in schizophrenia: a preliminary monozygotic twin study. *Biol Psychiat* 30: 717–25.

Brown R, Colter N, Corsellis JAN, Crow TJ, Frith CD, Jagoe R, Johnstone EC, Marsh L (1986) Postmortem evidence of structural brain changes in schizophrenia. *Arch Gen Psychiat* 43: 36–42.

Bruton CJ, Crow TJ, Frith CD, Johnstone EC, Owens DGC, Roberts GW (1990) Schizophrenia and the brain: a prospective clinico-neuropathological study. *Psychol Med* 20: 285–304.

Bruton CJ, Stevens J, Frith CD (1994) Epilepsy, psychosis, and schizophrenia: Clinical and neuropathological considerations. *Neurology* 44: 34–42.

Buhl L, Bojsen-Moller M (1988) Frequency of Alzheimer's disease in a postmortem study of psychiatric patients. *Dan Med Bull* 35: 288–90.

Casanova MF, Kleinman JE (1990) The neuropathology of schizophrenia: a critical assessment of research methodologies. *Biol Psychiat* 27: 353–62.

Casanova MF, Stevens JR, Kleinman JE (1990) Astrocytosis in the molecular layer of the dentate gyrus: a study in Alzheimer's disease and schizophrenia. *Psychiat Res: Neuroimaging* 35: 149–66.

Casanova MF, Carosella NW, Gold JM, Kleinman JE, Weinberger DR, Powers RE (1993) A topographical study of senile plaques and neurofibrillary tangles in the hippocampi of patients with Alzheimer's disease and cognitively impaired patients with schizophrenia. *Psychiat Res* 49: 41–62.

Chakos MH, Lieberman JA, Bilder RM, Borenstein M, Lerner G, Bogerts B, Wu H, Kinon B, Ashtari M (1994) Increase in caudate nuclei volumes of first-episode schizophrenic patients taking antipsychotic drugs. *Am J Psychiatr* 151: 1430–6.

Christison GW, Casanova MF, Weinberger DR, Rawlings R, Kleinman JE (1989) A quantitative investigation of hippocampal pyramidal cell size, shape, and variability of orientation in schizophrenia. *Arch Gen Psychiat* 46: 1027–32.

Colter N, Battal S, Crow TJ, Johnstone EC, Brown R, Bruton CJ (1987) White matter reduction in the parahippocampal gyrus of patients with schizophrenia. *Arch Gen Psychiat* 44: 1023.

Conrad AJ, Abebe T, Austin R, Forsythe S, Scheibel AB (1991) Hippocampal pyramidal cell disarray in schizophrenia as a bilateral phenomenon. *Arch Gen Psychiat* 48: 413–17.

Corsellis JAN (1976) Psychoses of obscure pathology. In Blackwood W, Corsellis JAN (eds). *Greenfield's Neuropathology*, 3rd edn. Edward Arnold: London, pp 903–15.

Crow TJ, Ball J, Bloom SR, Brown R, Bruton CJ, Colter N, Frith CD, Johnstone EC, Owens DGC, Roberts GW (1989) Schizophrenia as an anomaly of development of cerebral asymmetry. *Arch Gen Psychiat* 46: 1145–50.

da Cunha A, Jefferson JJ, Tyor WR, Glass JD, Jannotta FS, Vitkovic L (1993) Gliosis in human brain: relationship to size but not other properties of astrocytes. *Brain Res* 600: 161–5.

Daniel DG, Goldberg TE, Gibbons RD, Weinberger DR (1991) Lack of bimodal distribution of ventricular size in schizophrenia: a Gaussian mixture analysis of 1056 cases and controls. *Biol Psychiat* 30: 887–903.

Davidson M, Harvey PD, Powchik P, Parrella M, White L, Knobler HY, Losonczy MF, Keefe RSE, Katz S, Frecska E (1995) Severity of symptoms in chronically institutionalized geriatric schizophrenic patients. *Am J Psychiat* 152: 197–207.

Davison K (1983) Schizophrenia-like psychoses associated with organic cerebral disorders: a review. *Psychiatr Dev* 1: 1–34.

Degreef G, Ashtari M, Bogerts B, Bilder RM, Jody DN, Alvir JMJ, Lieberman JA (1992a) Volumes of ventricular system subdivisions measured from magnetic resonance images in first-episode schizophrenic patients. *Arch Gen Psychiat* 49: 531–7.

Degreef G, Bogerts B, Falkai P, Greve B, Lantos G, Ashtari M, Lieberman JA (1992b) Increased prevalence of the cavum septum pellucidum in MRI scans and post mortem brains of schizophrenic patients. *Psychiat Res* 45: 1–13.

DeLisi LE, Tew W, Xie S-H, Hoff AL, Sakuma M, Kushner M, Lee G, Shedlack K, Smith AM, Grimson R (1995) A prospective follow-up study of brain morphology and cognition in first-episode schizophrenic patients: preliminary findings. *Biol Psychiat* 38: 349–60.

Done D, Crow TJ, Johnstone E, Sacker A (1994) Childhood antecedents of schizophrenia and affective illness: social adjustment at ages 7 and 11. *BMJ* 309: 699–703.

Eastwood SL, Harrison PJ (1995) Decreased synaptophysin in the medial temporal lobe in schizophrenia demonstrated using immunoautoradiography. *Neuroscience* 69: 339–43.

El-Mallakh RS, Kirch DG, Shelton R, Fan K-J, Pezeshkpow G, Kanhouwa S, Wyatt RJ, Casanova JE (1991) The nucleus basalis of Meynert, senile plaques and intellectual impairment in schizophrenia. *J Neuropsychiat* 3: 383–6.

Falkai P, Bogerts B (1986) Cell loss in the hippocampus of schizophrenics. *Eur Arch Psychiatr Neurol Sci* 236: 154–61.

Falkai P, Bogerts B (1993) Brain development and schizophrenia. In Kerwin RW (ed). *Neurobiology and Psychiatry*, vol 2. Cambridge University Press, Cambridge, pp 43–70.

Falkai P, Bogerts B, Rozumek M (1988) Limbic pathology in schizophrenia: the entorhinal region – a morphometric study. *Biol Psychiat* 24: 515–21.

Falkai P, Bogerts B, Greve B, Pfeiffer U, Machus B, Folsch-Reetz B, Majtenyi C, Ovary I (1992) Loss of Sylvian fissure asymmetry in schizophrenia. A quantitative post-mortem study. *Schizophr Res* 7: 23–32.

Falkai P, Bogerts B, Schneider T, Greve B, Pfeiffer U, Pilz K, Gonsiorczyk C, Majtenyi C, Ovary O (1995a) Disturbed planum temporale asymmetry in schizophrenia. A quantitative post mortem study. *Schizophr Res* 14: 161–76.

Falkai P, Schneider T, Greve B, Klieser E, Bogerts B (1995b) Reduced frontal and occipital asymmetry on the CT-scans of schizophrenic patients. Its specificity and clinical significance. *J Neural Transm (Gen Sect)* 99: 63–77.

Fisman M (1975) The brain stem in psychosis. *Br J Psychiat* 126: 414–22.

Flaum M, Swayze VW II, O'Leary DS, Yuh WTC, Ehrhardt JC, Arndt SV, Andreasen NC (1995) Effects of diagnosis, laterality, and gender on brain morphology in schizophrenia. *Am J Psychiat* 152: 704–14.

Friede RL (1989) *Developmental Neuropathology*, 2nd edn. Springer, Berlin, pp 577.

Garcia-Rill E, Biedermann JA, Chambers T, Skinner RD, Mrak RE, Husain M, Karson CN (1995) Mesopontine neurons in schizophrenia. *Neuroscience* 66: 321–35.

Goldberg TE, Hyde TM, Kleinman JE, Weinberger DR (1993) Course of schizophrenia: neuropsychological evidence for a static encephalopathy. *Schizophr Bull* 19: 797–804.

Green MF, Satz P, Gaier DJ, Ganzell S, Kharabi F (1989) Minor physical anomalies in schizophrenia. *Schizophr Bull* 15: 91–9.

Gur RE, Mozley PD, Shtasel DL, Cannon TD, Gallacher F, Turetsky B, Grossman R, Gur RC (1994) Clinical subtypes of schizophrenia: Differences in brain and CSF volume. *Am J Psychiat* 151: 343–50.

Haroutunian V, Davidson M, Kanof PD, Perl DP, Powchik P, Losonczy M, McCrystal J, Purohit DP, Bierer LM, Davis KL (1994) Cortical cholinergic markers in schizophrenia. *Schizophr Res* 12: 137–44.

Harrison PJ (1993) Effects of neuroleptics on neuronal and synaptic structure. In Barnes TRE (ed) *Antipsychotic Drugs and their Side Effects*. Academic Press: London, pp 99–110.

Heaton R, Paulsen JS, McAdams LA, Kuck J, Zisook S, Braff D, Harris J, Jeste DV (1994) Neuropsychological deficits in schizophrenics. Relationship to age, chronicity and dementia. *Arch Gen Psychiat* 51: 469–76.

Heckers S, Heinsen H, Heinsen YC, Beckmann H (1990) Limbic structures and lateral ventricle in schizophrenia. *Arch Gen Psychiat* 47: 1016–22.

Heckers S, Heinsen H, Heinsen Y, Beckmann H (1991a) Cortex, white matter and basal ganglia in schizophrenia: a volumetric postmortem study. *Biol Psychiat* 29: 556–66.

Heckers S, Heinsen H, Geiger B, Beckmann H (1991b) Hip-pocampal neuron number in schizophrenia. *Arch Gen Psychiat* 48: 1002–8.

Hoff AL, Riordan H, O'Donnell DW, Morris L, DeLisi LE (1992) Neuropsychological functioning of first-episode schizophreniform patients. *Am J Psychiat* 149: 898–903.

Hyde TM, Ziegler JC, Weinberger DR (1992) Psychiatric disturbances in metachromatic leukodystrophy. *Arch Neurol* 49: 401–6.

Insausti R, Tunon T, Sobreviela T, Insausti AM, Gonzalo LM (1995) The human entorhinal cortex: a cytoarchitectonic analysis. *J Comp Neurol* 355: 171–98.

Jakob H, Beckmann H (1986) Prenatal developmental disturbances in the limbic allocortex in schizophrenics. *J Neural Transm* 65: 303–26.

Jaskiw GE, Juliano DM, Goldberg TE, Hertzman M, Urow-Hamell E, Weinberger DR (1994) Cerebral ventricular enlargement in schizophreniform disorder does not progress. A seven year follow up study. *Schizophr Res* 14: 23–8.

Jellinger K (1977) Neuropathologic findings after neuroleptic long term therapy. In Roizin L, Shiraki H, Grcevic N (eds). *Neurotoxicology*. Raven Press, New York, pp 25–42.

Jellinger K (1985) Neuromorphological background of pathochemical studies in major psychoses. In Beckmann H, Riederer P (eds). *Pathochemical Markers in Major Psychoses*. Springer: Berlin, Heidelberg, pp 1–23.

Jeste DV, Lohr JB (1989) Hippocampal pathologic findings in schizophrenia: a morphometric study. *Arch Gen Psychiat* 46: 1019–24.

Johnstone EC, Crow TJ, Frith CD, Husband J, Kreel L (1976) Cerebral ventricular size and cognitive impairment in chronic schizophrenia. *Lancet* ii: 924–6.

Johnstone EC, Crow TJ, Frith CED, Stevens M, Kreel L, Husband J (1978) The dementia of dementia praecox. *Acta Psychiat Scand* 57: 305–24.

Johnstone EC, Bruton CJ, Crow TJ, Frith CD, Owens DGC (1994) Clinical correlates of postmortem brain changes in schizophrenia: decreased brain weight and length correlate with indices of early impairment. *J Neurol Neurosurg Psychiat* 57: 474–9.

Jones P, Rodgers B, Murray R, Marmot M (1994) Child developmental risk factors for adult schizophrenia in the British 1946 birth cohort. *Lancet* 344: 1398–402.

Kalman M, Csillag A, Schleicher A, Rind C, Hajos F, Zilles K (1993) Long-term effects of anterograde degeneration on astroglial reaction in the rat geniculo-cortical system as revealed by computerized image analysis. *Anat Embryol* 187: 1–7.

Karson CN, Casanova MF, Kleinman JE, Griffin WST (1993) Choline acetyltransferase in schizophrenia. *Am J Psychiat* 150: 454–9.

Kovelman JA, Scheibel AB (1984) A neurohistological correlate of schizophrenia. *Biol Psychiat* 19: 1601–21.

Lantos PL (1988) The neuropathology of schizophrenia: a critical review of recent work. In Bebbington P, McGuffin P (eds). *Schizophrenia: The Major Issues*. Heinemann/Mental Health Foundation, London, pp 73–89.

Lesch A, Bogerts B (1984) The diencephalon in schizophrenia: evidence for reduced thickness of the periventricular grey matter. *Eur Arch Psychiatr Neurol Sci* 234: 212–19.

Lohr JB, Jeste DV (1986) Cerebellar pathology in schizophrenia? A neuronometric study. *Biol Psychiat* 21: 865–75.

Lohr JB, Jeste DV (1988) Locus ceruleus morphometry in aging and schizophrenia. *Acta Psychiatr Scand* 77: 689–97.

McKenna PJ (1994) *Schizophrenia and Related Syndromes*. Oxford, Oxford University Press.

Marsh L, Suddath RL, Higgins N, Weinberger DR (1994) Medial temporal lobe structures in schizophrenia: relationship of size to duration of illness. *Schizophr Res* 11: 225–38.

Miyakawa T, Sumiyoshi S, Deshimura M, Suzuki T, Tomonari H, Yasuoka F, Tatetsu S (1972) Electron microscopic study on schizophrenia: mechanism of pathological changes. *Acta Neuropathol (Berl)* 20: 67–77.

Murray RM, O'Callaghan E, Castle DJ, Lewis SW (1992) A neurodevelopmental approach to the classification of schizophrenia. *Schizophr Bull* 18: 319–32.

Nieto D, Escobar A (1972) Major psychoses. In Miniler J (ed). *Pathology of the Nervous System*, volume 3. McGraw Hill, New York, pp 2654–65.

Norton WT, Aquino DA, Hozumi I, Chiu F-C, Brosnan CF (1992) Quantitative aspects of reactive gliosis: a review. *Neurochem Res* 17: 877–85.

Owen F, Crow TJ, Frith CD, Johnson JA, Johnstone EC, Lofthouse R, Owens DGC, Poulter M (1987) Selective decreases in MAO-B activity in post-mortem brains from schizophrenic patients with type II syndrome. *Br J Psychiat* 151: 744–52.

Pakkenberg B (1987) Post-mortem study of chronic schizophrenic brains. *Br J Psychiat* 151: 744–52.

Pakkenberg B (1990) Pronounced reduction of total neuron number in mediodorsal thalamic nucleus and nucleus accumbens in schizophrenics. *Arch Gen Psychiat* 47: 1023–8.

Pakkenberg B (1993a) Leucotomized schizophrenics lose neurons in the mediodorsal thalamic nucleus. *Neuropathol Appl Neurobiol* 29: 373–80.

Pakkenberg B (1993b) Total nerve cell number in neocortex in chronic schizophrenics and controls estimated using optical dissectors. *Biol Psychiat* 34: 768–72.

Plum F (1972) Prospects for research on schizophrenia. 3. Neurophysiology, neuropathological findings. *Neurosci Res Program Bull* 10: 384–8.

Prohovnik I, Dwork AJ, Kaufman MA, Willson N (1993) Alzheimer-type neuropathology in elderly schizophrenia patients. *Schizophr Bull* 19: 805–16.

Purohit DP, Davidson M, Perl DP, Powchik P, Haroutunian VH, Bierer LM, McCrystal J, Losonczy M, Davis KL (1993) Severe cognitive impairment in elderly schizophrenic patients: a clinicopathological study. *Biol Psychiat* 33: 255–60.

Raikowska G, Selemon LD, Goldman-Rakic PS (1994) Reduc-

tion in neuronal size in prefrontal cortex of schizophrenics and Huntington patients. *Soc Neurosci Abstr* 20: 620.

Roberts GW (1991) Schizophrenia: a neuropathological perspective. *Br J Psychiat* 158: 8–17.

Roberts GW, Bruton CJ (1990) Notes from the graveyard: neuropathology and schizophrenia. *Neuropathol Appl Neurobiol* 16: 3–16.

Roberts GW, Done DJ, Bruton C, Crow TJ (1990) A 'mock-up' of schizophrenia: temporal lobe epilepsy and schizophrenia-like psychosis. *Biol Psychiat* 28: 127–43.

Roberts GW, Colter N, Lofthouse R, Bogerts B, Zech N, Crow TJ (1986) Gliosis in schizophrenia. *Biol. Psychiat* 21: 1043–50.

Roberts GW, Colter N, Lofthouse R, Johnstone EC, Crow TJ (1987) Is there gliosis in schizophrenia? Investigation of the temporal lobe. *Biol Psychiat* 22: 1459–68.

Roberts GW, Bruton CJ, Crow TJ (1988) Response: gliosis in schizophrenia. *Biol Psychiat* 24: 729–31.

Rosenthal R, Bigelow LR (1972) Quantitative brain measurements in chronic schizophrenia. *Br J Psychiat* 121: 259–64.

Schlaepfer TE, Harris GJ, Tien AY, Peng LW, Lee S, Federman EB, Chase GA, Barta PE, Pearlson GD (1994) Decreased regional cortical grey matter volume in schizophrenia. *Am J Psychiat* 151: 842–8.

Selemon LD, Rajkowska G, Goldman-Rakic PS (1995) Abnormally high neuronal density in the schizophrenic cortex. *Arch Gen Psychiat* 52: 805–18.

Shapiro RM (1993) Regional neuropathology in schizophrenia: Where are we? Where are we going? *Schizophr Res* 10: 187–239.

Soustek Z (1989) Ultrastructure of cortical synapses in the brain of schizophrenics. *Zentralbl Allg Pathol Pathol Anat* 135: 25–32.

Stevens CD, Altshuler LL, Bogerts B, Falkai P (1988a) Quantitative study of gliosis in schizophrenia and Huntington's chorea. *Biol Psychiat* 24: 697–700.

Stevens JR (1982) Neuropathology of schizophrenia. *Arch Gen Psychiat* 39: 1131–9.

Stevens JR, Casanova M, Bigelow L (1988b) Gliosis and schizophrenia. *Biol Psychiat* 24: 727–9.

Stevens JR, Casanova M, Poltorak M, Germain L, Buchan GC (1991) Comparison of immunocytochemical and Holzer's methods for detection of acute and chronic gliosis in human postmortem material. *J Neuropsychiat Clin Neurosci* 4: 168–73.

Suddath RL, Christison GW, Torrey EF, Casanova MF, Weinberger DR (1990) Anatomical abnormalities in the brains of monozygotic twins discordant for schizophrenia. *N Engl J Med* 322: 789–94.

Waddington J (1993) Schizophrenia: developmental neuroscience and pathobiology. *Lancet* 341: 531–5.

Walker, E (1994) Developmentally moderated expressions of the neuropathology underlying schizophrenia. *Schizophr Bull* 20: 453–80.

Weinberger DR (1987) Implications of normal brain development for the pathogenesis of schizophrenia. *Arch Gen Psychiat* 44: 660–9.

Weinberger DR (1995) Schizophrenia: from neuropathology to neurodevelopment. *Lancet* 346: 552–7.

Weinberger DR, Suddath RL, Casanova MF, Torrey EF, Kleinman JE (1991) Crow's 'lateralization hypothesis' for schizophrenia. *Arch Gen Psychiat* 48: 85–7.

Wisniewski HM, Constantinidis J, Wegiel J, Bobinski M, Tarnawski M (1994) Neurofibrillary pathology in brains of elderly schizophrenics treated with neuroleptics. *Alz Dis Assoc Disord* 8: 211–27.

Zaidel DW, Esiri MM, Eastwood SL, Harrison PJ (1995) Asymmetrical hippocampal circuitry and schizophrenia. *Lancet* 346: 656–7.

Zaidel DW, Esiri MM, Harrison PJ (1996) Neuronal size, shape and orientation in the normal left and right hippocampus are altered in schizophrenia. *Soc Neurosci Abstr* 22: 731.

Zaidel DW, Esiri MM, Harrison PJ (1997) The hippocampus in schizophrenia: lateralised increase in neuronal density and altered cytoarchitectural asymmetry. *Psychol Med* In Press.

Zipursky RB, Lim KO, Sullivan EV, Brown BW, Pfefferbaum A (1992) Widespread cerebral grey matter volume deficits in schizophrenia. *Arch Gen Psychiat* 49: 195–205.

CHAPTER NINETEEN

Other diseases that cause dementia

M. M. Esiri

Space-occupying lesions
Inflammatory conditions
Consequences of cerebral irradiation
Multiple sclerosis
Epilepsy
Superficial haemosiderosis of the central nervous system
Whipple's disease
Other obscure conditions

In this chapter we consider a number of diverse pathological conditions that may occasionally give rise to a clinical picture in which dementia predominates (Table 19.1). We illustrate the chapter with cases of this type from our own and our colleagues' experience. Other neurological features are also likely to be present at some stage in the course of these diseases. In some, perhaps most, such cases these other clinical features may have led to the correct diagnosis being established before clinical dementia develops, but in a few the diagnosis may be impossible to achieve before death. Therefore, a pathologist can expect to encounter these diseases occasionally among cases of dementia presenting at autopsy. Full treatment of pathological aspects of these diseases is beyond the scope of this chapter and for details a more general textbook of neuropathology should be consulted, e.g. *Greenfield's Neuropathology* (Adams & Duchen, 1992) or Davis and Robertson's *Textbook of Neuropathology* (1996).

SPACE-OCCUPYING LESIONS

Subdural haematoma

Subdural haematomas may produce symptoms of dementia that mimic those of Alzheimer's disease, vascular dementia or normal pressure hydrocephalus (Stuteville & Welch, 1958; Perlmutter & Gobles, 1961). Dementia may also develop in those operated on for subdural haematomas. Chronic subdural haematomas are particularly liable to present as dementia rather than with symptoms more suggestive of raised intracranial pressure. These may occur apparently spontaneously in the elderly, or after trivial head injury or complicate shunt insertions and other intracranial operations. However, as chronic subdural haematomas may occur as a consequence of cerebral atrophy, which produces a less good fit of the brain inside the skull, care should be taken in ascribing dementia to a small chronic subdural haematoma and a neurodegenerative condition should first be excluded, particularly if the brain is atrophic. Large, chronic unilateral or bilateral subdural haematomas may, however, be the only significant pathological findings in an elderly demented patient with a normal sized or slightly oedematous brain (Fig. 19.1). Subdural haematomas occur over the vertex and are immediately apparent when the top of the skull is removed and the dura opened. The chronic variety usually forms a part-membranous and part-fluid pad over the arachnoid from which it can be readily lifted away. Microscopically, the membranous component consists of a meshwork of thin walled sinusoidal capillaries from which blood continually seeps to maintain the chronic haematoma. Products of haemoglobin breakdown, together with macrophages and a few fibroblasts, fill the loose interstices between the vessels.

Intracranial neoplasms

A number of different types of intracranial neoplasm may produce a primarily dementing clinical picture. Some 5% of cases of dementia may be associated with

Table 19.1. *Diseases considered in this chapter that may rarely cause dementia as a predominating clinical feature*

Space-occupying lesions
1. Subdural haematoma
2. Intracranial neoplasms
   Gliomas
   Meningiomas

Inflammatory conditions
1. Sarcoidosis
2. Behcet's syndrome
3. Paraneoplastic syndrome (limbic encephalitis)
4. Glial nodule encephalitis
5. Other

Consequences of cerebral irradiation

Multiple sclerosis

Epilepsy

Superficial haemosiderosis of the central nervous system

Whipple's disease

Other obscure conditions
   Coeliac disease with dementia
   Multifocal leukoencephalopathy with calcification

such lesions that also produce raised intracranial pressure (Cummings & Benson, 1992; Lishman, 1987). Tumours may cause symptoms of dementia mainly by obstructing flow of cerebrospinal fluid and producing hydrocephalus (Chapter 15). This is particularly true of posterior fossa and midline tumours such as craniopharyngiomas or extrasellar pituitary adenomas, and carcinomatosis of the leptomeninges, which obstructs cerebrospinal fluid flow in the subarachnoid space. Other tumours produce dementia by interfering with widespread cerebral function, as may occur with *multiple small cerebral metastases* each of which may be surrounded by oedema (Fig. 19.2). Periventricular spread of carcinoma, glioma or lymphoma deposits may also present with memory disturbance by destroying the fimbriae or fornices and invading the corpus callosum (Fig. 19.3). This can occur either when the primary site of the tumour is in the fimbriae or fornices or by intra- or peri-ventricular spread. In such cases the affected parts may appear irregularly softened and necrotic but not necessarily grossly expanded. *Intravascular (angiotropic) lymphoma* is another rare cause of dementia, in this case producing its effect on higher brain functions by produc-

ing multiple ischaemic lesions (see Chapter 5).

Intrinsic gliomas, particularly those diffusely involving a cerebral hemisphere or the frontal lobes bilaterally, with extension through the corpus callosum, also occasionally produce dementia with few or no focal neurological signs or obvious headache (Fig. 19.4). Temporal lobe gliomas may similarly present in this way (Fig. 19.5). Low- or middle-grade astrocytomas are usually found to be the histological tumour cell type responsible, though there may be foci of frankly malignant astrocytoma or glioblastoma present by the time the patient dies. Gliomas arising close to the ventricular system and disseminating to other parts of the brain via cerebrospinal fluid pathways may also give rise to dementia. The presence of a glioma does not necessarily provide the entire explanation for a dementing illness.

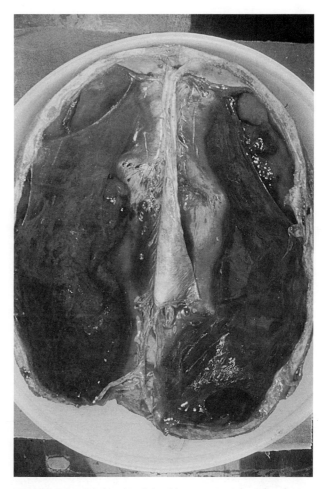

Fig. 19.1. Bilateral chronic subdural haematomas obscuring the cortical surfaces at the vertex.

We have seen two elderly demented subjects in whom Alzheimer's disease co-existed with malignant glioma; others are reported in the literature.

Extrinsic meningiomas, which predominantly compress rather than invade or infiltrate the brain, may present with dementia. Large, slowly growing, olfactory

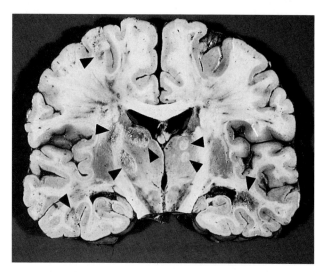

Fig. 19.2. Multiple bilateral small metastatic deposits from a primary lung carcinoma (arrow heads). In this case the deposits show little surrounding oedema or mass effect. There is no shift of midline structures as deposits on the two sides are evenly balanced.

groove meningiomas in the subfrontal region are particularly notorious in this respect (Fig. 19.6). Sphenoidal wing meningiomas abutting on the temporal lobe may do likewise. However, it is important to realize that careful clinicopathological correlation needs to be considered when an intracranial tumour is discovered in a demented subject. Small, benign meningiomas are unlikely to have caused dementia on their own and are more likely to be incidental findings. An elderly patient with a long history of progressive intracranial dementia, and even a large tumour at autopsy, may also have Alzheimer's disease. We have seen a large meningioma occurring in conjunction with severe pathological changes of Alzheimer's disease. Similarly, multiple cerebral metastases are unlikely to be the cause of long-standing dementia in an elderly patient and an additional neurodegenerative disease should be sought. On the other hand, in a younger patient with a short history of rapidly progressive dementia, multiple cerebral metastases may provide a convincing pathological explanation for the clinical picture. Likewise, a large, slowly growing frontal meningioma is an adequate explanation for dementia in a patient with clinical signs and symptoms referable predominantly to frontal lobe dysfunction. As with other forms of mixed pathology, the presence of a cerebral tumour on its own may not account for dementia, but may summate with a normally sub-clinical level of Alzheimer-type pathology to produce clinical dementia.

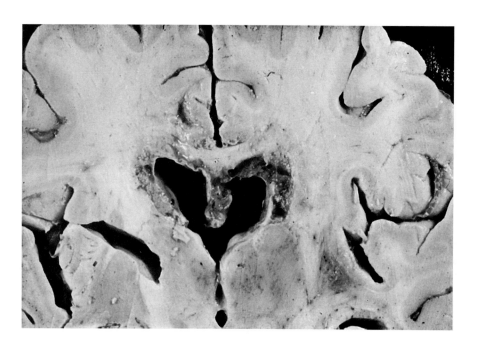

Fig. 19.3. Primary CNS lymphoma with periventricular spread causing necrosis of the fimbria, corpus callosum and caudate nuclei. White matter of the adjacent left cingulate gyrus is also affected.

INFLAMMATORY CONDITIONS

Sarcoidosis

This is a chronic granulomatous inflammatory condition of unknown aetiology in which the CNS may be involved on its own or together with systemic organs. Dementia may occasionally be a presenting symptom in this condition (Cordingley et al., 1981). It can produce mass lesions within the brain, chronic meningitic foci, arteritic damage or hydrocephalus and any combination of these pathological features (Figs. 19.7 and 19.8). These lesions should be sought in the leptomeninges and parenchyma of the cerebrum, cerebellum or brainstem. Vasculitic foci may be present in the same region. Macroscopically, there is usually some thickening and opacity of the leptomeninges and coronal slices may reveal hydrocephalus, possibly with grossly visible granulomas. The microscopic lesions resemble tuberculoid granulomata with multinucleated giant cells but caseation does not occur and no organisms can be demonstrated.

Behcet's syndrome

Clinical features of Behcet's syndrome are recurrent ulceration of the mouth and genitalia and iridocyclitis. Some cases develop neurological disease in addition, and symptoms may include dementia.

Neuropathological lesions of Behcet's syndrome consist of multiple, focal ill-defined areas of congestion and softening in the brain, particularly the upper brain stem, deep cerebral grey matter and internal capsules. The nature of these lesions is inflammatory and in some instances vasculitic. Affected tissues contain perivascu-

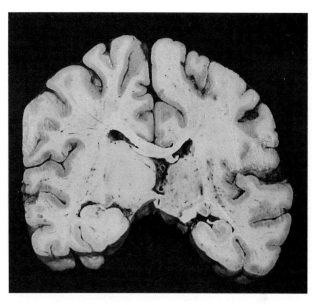

Fig. 19.4. Case of diffuse gliomatosis of the left cerebral hemisphere in which mental deterioration was the predominant feature. The diffuse neoplastic process affected astrocytes and caused enlargement particularly of the left thalamus and hippocampus.

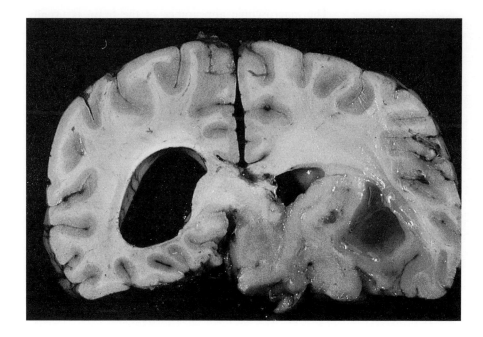

Fig. 19.5. Case of an anaplastic astrocytoma of the right temporal lobe in which the principal clinical features were dementia and epilepsy. There is a gelatinous, ill-defined tumour infiltrating the right inferior temporo-occipal region. Note also a marked bilateral hydrocephalus.

lar and parenchymal inflammatory cell infiltrates consisting predominantly of lymphocytes, and activated microglial cells, some of which form nodules. There is a more diffuse microglial and astrocyte reaction. Neuro-

nal or axonal loss is seen within the main foci of damage. The cause of the condition is unknown.

Paraneoplastic syndrome (limbic encephalitis)

Limbic encephalitis is one of a number of remote effects of carcinoma on the nervous system (Currie, 1992). It commonly presents with dementia, personality change and prominent memory disturbance. By far the most common associated neoplasm is small cell lung carcinoma, but many other forms of carcinoma have also been associated with it: breast and gynaecological cancer in women, renal carcinoma and a variety of lymphoreticular neoplasms. Although it is common for the carcinoma to be clinically occult and small in size occasionally, despite a careful search at autopsy, no tumour is discovered. Clinically, the disease usually runs a subacute or chronic course lasting one to two years, but some cases are fatal within a few months of onset. The changes in higher cerebral functions include prominent memory impairment, hallucinations, reduced alertness, anxiety, depression and global or patchy cognitive deficits. Commonly, there are other neurological manifestations including epilepsy, cerebellar ataxia, brain stem encephalitis, extrapyramidal movement disorder, myelopathy, radiculopathy or subacute sensory peripheral neuropathy. In rapidly progressive cases, the condition may be easily mistaken for spongiform encephalopathy clinically.

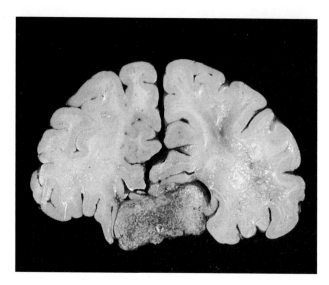

Fig. 19.6. Olfactory groove meningioma in an 84 year-old demented woman with no other dementing disease pathology. Note the severe longstanding white matter pathology on the right attributable to chronic oedema.

Neuropathology

The macroscopic appearance of the brain is usually within normal limits but there may be slight atrophy, particularly of the temporal lobes. It is necessary to take blocks for microscopic examination from a wide selection of brain regions: multiple areas of cortex, hippocampus basal ganglia, thalamus, brainstem, cerebellum, spinal cord, peripheral ganglia and nerves. Microscopically, there are perivascular mononuclear inflammatory cell infiltrates, microglial nodules, occasional neurophagia and reactive astrocytes. These are particularly prominent in the grey and white matter of the hippocampus and medial temporal lobe, though they are not necessarily confined to these regions (Fig. 19.9). The majority of the inflammatory cells are T-cells and macrophages. Deep grey matter of the basal ganglia, thalamus and brainstem are also liable to be affected. Neuron cell loss may also be prominent and out of proportion to the severity of the inflammatory cell reaction (Fig. 19.10). The cerebellum may also show severe pathology either in the form of severe Purkinje

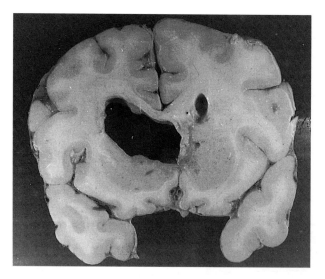

Fig. 19.7. Sarcoidosis of the CNS. Granulomatous lesions in periventricular tissues and subarachnoid space have caused hydrocephalus.

cell loss or with inflammatory cell changes in dentate nuclei and white matter, with severe loss of dentate nucleus neurons and Wallerian degeneration in the superior cerebellar peduncles. The spinal cord and peripheral nerve roots, sensory ganglia and nerve trunks may show further inflammatory changes, axonal damage and neuron loss.

Aetiology of paraneoplastic encephalitis
The most likely explanation for this condition is that it represents an autoimmune attack directed at antigens shared between the tumour cells and the nervous system. Such shared antigens have been demonstrated in small cell lung cancer, gynaecological cancers and cerebellar Purkinje cells (Anderson, Rosenblum & Posner, 1988;

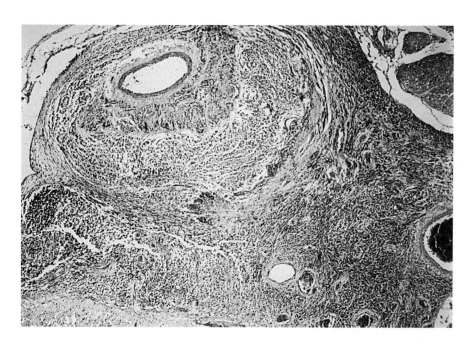

Fig. 19.8. Sarcoidosis of the CNS. Low power microscopy showing dense granulomatous inflammation surrounding a small artery in the subarachnoid space. Haematoxylin and eosin stain.

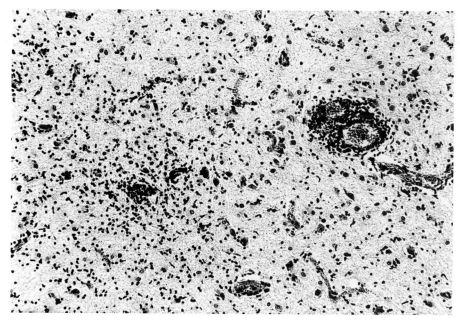

Fig. 19.9. Perivascular and more diffuse infiltrates of lymphocytes, macrophages and microglial cells in temporal lobe cortex from a case of paraneoplastic encephalitis. Haematoxylin and eosin stain.

Kornguth, 1989; Sakai *et al.*, 1991). As yet, there is little experimental evidence to support this hypothesis as it relates to cases of limbic encephalitis, but, in cases with predominantly cerebellar ataxia associated with gynaecological cancers, antineuronal antibodies have been demonstrated in serum and cerebrospinal fluid, and, in cases of peripheral neuropathy associated with small cell lung cancer, antibodies directed against a different neuronal protein have been detected in serum (Graus *et al.*, 1986; Graus, Cordon-Cardo & Posner, 1987). The neuronal proteins involved are not as yet fully characterized. The strongest evidence available to support an autoimmune aetiology for a paraneoplastic syndrome relates to the Lambert–Eaton myasthenic syndrome, a condition in which there is defective neuromuscular transmission at the neuromuscular junction associated with small cell lung cancer. In this condition, the clinical and neurophysiological features can be transferred to normal mice using the serum of affected patients and antibodies have been demonstrated to the voltage-gated calcium channels present both in the cell membranes of the small cell lung cancer tumour cells and in the pre-synaptic terminals of peripheral motor nerve fibres (Vincent, Lang & Newson-Davis, 1989). There is suggestive histopathological evidence of an enhanced local immune response to small cell lung cancer associated with the Lambert–Eaton myasthenic syndrome as compared to small cell lung cancer without the syndrome and small cell lung cancer associated with the Lambert–Eaton syndrome shows less expression of MHC

Class 1 antigens on the tumour cells than in control cases without the syndrome (Morris *et al.*, 1992).

An alternative hypothesis for the paraneoplastic syndrome, more widely supported previously than at present, is that it is associated with an unidentified virus infection. This was suggested by the pathological features which are consistent with those of a viral encephalitis. Whereas considerable evidence in favour of the autoimmune hypothesis has been forthcoming in recent years, no recent evidence supports this viral hypothesis.

Glial nodule encephalitis

Mention should be made for the sake of completeness of *glial nodule encephalitis*, a condition in which multiple microglial nodules, varying in frequency from rare to numerous, may be found predominantly in grey matter of the cerebral hemispheres. The condition is largely confined to immunosuppressed patients, and it is generally considered that most cases are due to cytomegalovirus (CMV) infection. Typical intranuclear inclusion bodies, immunocytochemical staining for CMV antigens, and *in situ* hybridization for CMV nucleic acid in occasional cells supports this view. Most cases do not show clinical symptoms but severe cases may be expected to show some decline of cognitive function (Booss & Esiri, 1986). Most cases occur in the context of AIDS and it may be expected that dementia in such cases can usually be attributed to other lesions, particularly those associated with local presence of HIV (Chapter 17), rather than to co-existing glial nodule encephalitis.

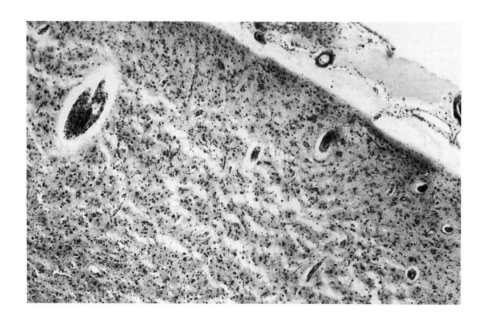

Fig. 19.10. Low power view of temporal lobe cortex from a case of paraneoplastic encephalitis associated with small cell lung carcinoma. There is severe loss of pyramidal neurons and reactive astrocytosis. Haematoxylin and eosin stain.

Other inflammatory conditions associated with dementia

Occasionally inflammatory brain disease of uncertain aetiology is held responsible for isolated cases of dementia complicating systemic immune-mediated diseases. An example is a reported case of dementia in which a 15-month dementing illness in a 56 year-old woman with Sjögren's syndrome was shown by brain biopsy to be associated with a meningoencephalitis. Treatment with corticosteroids produced resolution of the dementia (Caselli *et al.*, 1991). Another example is provided by the case of a 47 year-old male who developed cognitive impairment and a severe memory disorder in association with cat scratch disease (Revol *et al.*, 1992).

CONSEQUENCES OF CEREBRAL IRRADIATION

A variety of different forms of brain damage following cerebral irradiation have been described (Zeman & Samorajski, 1971; Burger *et al.*, 1981; Sheline, Wara & Smith, 1980; de Angelis, Delattre & Posner, 1989). These are uncommon and not always predictable, though they are more likely to occur with high dosages of radiation, or when radiation is combined with chemotherapy (see Chapter 14). They can occur over a long time interval following the radiation, from a few months to many years later, and their pathogenesis is poorly understood. The most common of these is a multifocal leukoencephalopathy that produces insidious but progressive personality change and intellectual decline over a period of months, though not all those who show CT evidence of lesions develop well-recognized symptoms. The pathology of this condition is described in Chapter 14. A second pattern of pathology consists of coagulation necrosis associated with fibrinoid necrosis of blood vessels (Fig. 19.11) in cerebral white matter. A third pathological change is multifocal, sharply demarcated pontine lesions in which there is myelin loss, focal axonal swelling with or without deposition of calcium salts and some relatively mild macrophage infiltration (Breuer, Blank & Schoene, 1978). These lesions resemble those described below (p. 410). Fourthly, and exceptionally, a form of focal neuronal gigantism has been described in the brain following irradiation (Lampert & Davis, 1964; Caccamo *et al.*, 1989). In this condition, developing 6 and 13 years after brain irradiation, there is marked thickening of affected gyri which may be visible to the naked eye, disorganization of cortical laminar architecture and the presence of large, abnormal neurons and telangiectatic blood vessels in the affected cortex.

MULTIPLE SCLEROSIS

Multiple sclerosis is a white matter demyelinating disease of unknown aetiology. It produces generally sharply demarcated, demyelinated foci, chiefly around veins and the ventricular system of the brain and in optic nerves and spinal cord. The clinical course is one of relapses and remissions, or of more consistent pro-

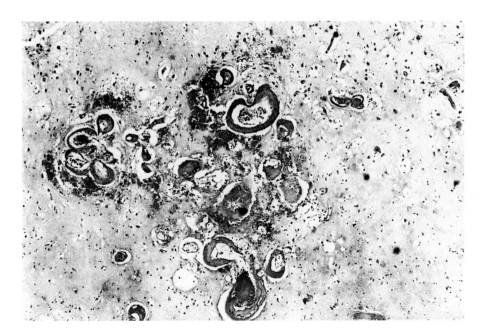

Fig. 19.11. Radiation necrosis with fibrinoid necrosis of temporal lobe vessels.

gression. Most patients develop their first symptoms between the ages of 20 and 40 years, and the average duration of the disease is at least 22 years. In most cases the diagnosis is made on clinical grounds and may be backed up by neuroimaging studies, neurophysiological evidence of slowed conduction velocities in the CNS or the finding of oligoclonal bands of immunoglobulin in cerebrospinal fluid. Occasionally, in clinically atypical cases, the diagnosis can only be made at autopsy. Dementia in clinically definite cases of multiple sclerosis is common. Various studies have found evidence of clinical dementia in 40–65% of patients with multiple sclerosis (Surridge, 1969; Rao *et al.*, 1991). Neuropsychological investigation reveals deficits in as many as 50% of patients who appear intellectually intact (Peyser *et al.*, 1980). Rarely, the clinical presentation and course of the disease are dominated by dementia (Bergin, 1957; Mendez & Frey, 1992; Fontaine *et al.*, 1994).

Neuropathology

To external appearance the brain may seem normal or slightly atrophic. Focal plaques of demyelination may be evident, however, on the ventral surface of the pons or the optic nerves may be diffusely grey and atrophic or show focally defined plaques of demyelination. In co-

ronal sections of the brain and transverse sections of the spinal cord, the plaques of demyelination are seen most easily in white matter where they form usually well-defined circular or more irregular patches of grey–brown discolouration measuring a few millimetres to two or three centimetres across (Fig. 19.12). Periventricular white matter is particularly likely to be affected with coalescing lesions liable to be found in the walls of any parts of the lateral ventricles. Blocks for microscopic examination should be taken from macroscopically affected regions. Frozen sections stained with oil red O are useful for assessing the age of lesions, old lesions

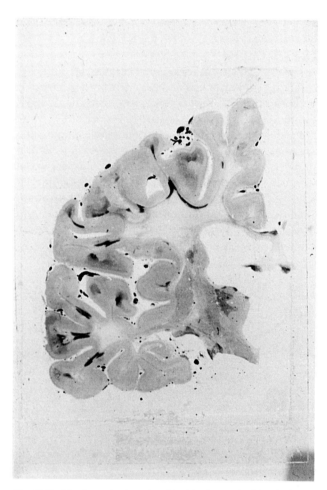

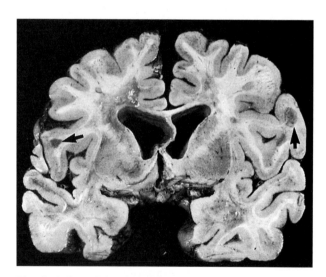

Fig. 19.12. Case of chronic multiple sclerosis with prominent symptoms of dementia. White matter of the centrum semiovale is extensively demyelinated as is the white matter of both temporal lobes. A few small discrete plaques in subcortical or cortical areas can also be seen (examples arrowed). Note considerable cortical atrophy, narrowing of the corpus callosum and enlargement of the lateral ventricles.

Fig. 19.13. Myelin-stained section (black) of a cerebral hemisphere section from a case of longstanding multiple sclerosis with severe dementia. Almost the entire cerebral white matter is demyelinated, with flecks of myelin remaining only in some immediately subcortical regions. Note severe enlargement of the lateral ventricle and thinning of the corpus callosum consequent upon accompanying Wallerian degeneration of axons.

containing little stainable fat but subacute ones containing an abundance of fat in lipid phagocytes. Microscopically, recently formed lesions also have a prominent inflammatory cell infiltrate consisting chiefly of T-cells, macrophages and plasma cells while old lesions are relatively acellular and gliotic. Occasionally, small, old plaques characteristic of multiple sclerosis are found at autopsy in patients with no neurological history, or only trivial symptoms of neurological disease in the distant past (Gilbert & Sadler, 1983). If such lesions are found in a patient with a history of severe, recent dementia, another disease, most commonly Alzheimer's disease, is likely to be also present, and appropriate microscopic examination for this should be undertaken. In such cases the mild multiple sclerosis lesions are likely to be an incidental finding.

Cases of multiple sclerosis with prominent dementia are likely to show at autopsy a predominance of cerebral demyelinated plaques and considerable cerebral atrophy consequent upon extensive periventricular and diffuse or frontal lobe cerebral white matter lesions (Fig. 19.13) (Bergin, 1957; Filley *et al.*, 1989; Mendez & Frey, 1992). Long-standing lesions show loss of axons, as well as complete loss of myelin in the central regions of the plaques. Demyelination of nerve fibres entering the corpus callosum and coursing through the centrum semiovale provide a reasonable explanation for symptoms of dementia in most cases of multiple sclerosis. Subcortical U-fibres are usually spared (Brownell & Hughes, 1962; Allen & Kirk, 1992). However, in a personally studied case in which the diagnosis was only made at autopsy and in which a nine-year progressive history was dominated by symptoms and signs of dementia with some spastic motor weakness, the cerebral lesions chiefly affected subcortical white matter.

Differential diagnosis

Other white matter lesions causing dementia need to be distinguished from those of multiple sclerosis. Usually, the clinical history makes the distinction clear, but there may be overlap clinically particularly with progressive multifocal leukoencephalopathy, diffuse ischaemic white matter damage of Binswanger type or due to vasculitis and with post-infectious leukoencephalitis (perivenous encephalitis) (Fig. 19.14). Rarely, the white matter lesions of Marchiafava Bignami disease, which are virtually confined to alcoholics, may also require distinction from multiple sclerosis. Pathologically, the lesions of multiple sclerosis can be distinguished from those of progressive multifocal leukoencephalopathy by

the absence of oligodendrocyte intranuclear inclusions and lack of detectable JC virus antigens or nucleic acid in multiple sclerosis and by the characteristic distribution of lesions particularly in optic nerves, periventricular regions and spinal cord in multiple sclerosis. The large, pleomorphic nuclei found in astrocytes in PML are also absent from the reactive astrocytes of MS plaques though, in both diseases, the astrocytes can be large and quite bizarre in appearance. Large lesions in PML are formed by the coalescence of multiple small lesions and this is usually evident in sections. Multiple sclerosis is most reliably distinguished from ischaemic lesions of white matter by comparing myelin and axonal

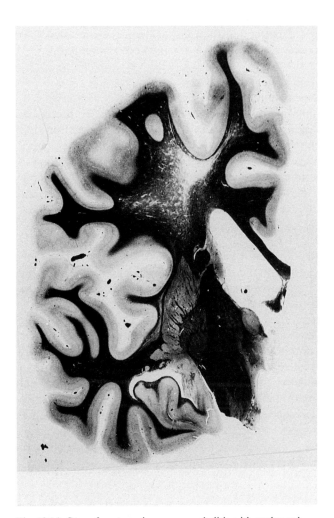

Fig. 19.14. Case of acute perivenous encephalitis with prolonged survival in a demented state. This myelin-stained section shows demyelinated lesions in the centrum semiovale. There is some confluence of the lesions but there remains an impression of a multifocal origin to the lesion.

stains. In multiple sclerosis lesions, most axons are preserved whereas in ischaemic lesions most are destroyed. It should be noted that some elements of vasculitis may be present within venular walls in multiple sclerosis, but this does not give rise to infarcts as does the vasculitis associated with collagen and other primarily vasculitic diseases. The clinical history in perivenous encephalitis is usually short and monophasic and presents more characteristically as an acute encephalopathy than dementia. Rare chronic cases do, however, occur (Fig. 19.14). Multiple sclerosis plaques differ from the foci of perivenous encephalitis in being more irregularly distributed and larger in size. In perivenous encephalitis, there are thin sleeves of demyelination around most small veins in the cerebral white matter, but they are such narrow zones that they are barely appreciable to naked eye examination.

Aetiology

The aetiology of multiple sclerosis is unknown. An immune reaction undoubtedly occurs in the acute lesions and is much less in evidence in the older ones, but the provoking antigen is unidentified. Local presence of a foreign antigen is suspected to trigger the formation of lesions. Others consider that there is no need to implicate local presence of a foreign antigen and suspect the disease to be autoimmune in origin.

EPILEPSY

Readily controlled, mild epilepsy is not usually associated with dementia unless the epilepsy is symptomatic of an underlying cerebral disease that also causes dementia (Table 19.2). However, severe intractable epilepsy *per se* can be associated with a deteriorating intellectual function. Those patients shown to have continuing epileptiform activity on the EEG despite treatment show more intellectual deterioration than otherwise matched patients who show little such EEG abnormality (Dobrill & Wilkins, 1976). In addition to this suggestive evidence that severe, repeated epileptic activity can itself cause intellectual deterioration, cognitive impairment is also a well-recognized side effect of excessive anticonvulsant medication.

Neuropathology

Mild epilepsy is rarely associated with structural neuropathological changes unless there is a focal lesion provoking the seizures, such as a small cortical glioma, arteriovenous malformation or cavernous angioma. Severe, long-standing epilepsy of the type which may be

Table 19.2. *Conditions commonly giving rise both to epilepsy (including myoclonic epilepsy) and dementia*

Alzheimer's disease (esp. late) (see Chapter 4)
Paraneoplastic syndrome (see this chapter)
Herpes simplex encephalitis (see Chapter 17)
Superficial haemosiderosis (see this chapter)
Kuf's disease (see Chapter 14)
Lafora body disease (see Chapter 14)
Mitochondrial cytopathies (see Chapter 14)
Polycystic lipomembraneous osteodysplasia with sclerosing encephalopathy (see Chapter 14)
Adrenoleukodystrophy (see Chapteer 14)
Gaucher's disease (see Chapter 14)
Leigh's encephalopathy (see Chapter 14)
Methotrexate toxicity (see Chapter 14)
Trimethyl tin toxicity (see Chapter 14)
Pick's disease (see Chapter 8)
Some neurodegenerative conditions (Chapter 10)
Familial oculomeningeal amyloidosis (see Chapter 11)
Post-head injury (see Chapter 16)
Ramsay Hunt syndrome (see this chapter)

associated with intellectual impairment may show characteristic neuropathological changes which are thought to result from the excessive electrical discharges that accompany the epilepsy. These pathological changes chiefly affect the cerebral cortex, hippocampus and cerebellum. The hippocampal lesion consists of neuron loss and gliosis largely confined to the CA1 sector of the pyramidal cell layer, the CA4 or end folium and the dentate fascia granule cell layer. Usually the hippocampus on one side only is affected and the structure may appear atrophied to naked eye examination with corresponding enlargement of the adjacent inferior horn of the ventricle (Fig. 19.15). This lesion is known as *Ammon's horn sclerosis*. Development of this lesion in the hippocampus may give rise to psychomotor epilepsy. There may also be secondary atrophy in the ipsilateral mamillary body with severe Ammon's horn sclerosis. In the cortex there may be patchy loss of pyramidal neurons particularly in the temporal lobes. If the epilepsy has developed early in life, the whole temporal lobe or even the whole cerebral hemisphere on one side may be small, and the contralateral cerebellar hemisphere also small.

The cerebellar lesion in epilepsy chiefly affects the cortical Purkinje cell layer where severe loss of Purkinje cells may be present together with reactive astrocytosis of the Purkinje cell or molecular layer of the cortex. Experimental evidence has shown that such a lesion can be caused by phenytoin intoxication, but it is not certain whether the anticonvulsant or the epilepsy itself is the principal factor in the development of epileptic cerebellar damage seen in humans (Jacobs & Le Quesne, 1992).

The fully developed Ammon's horn sclerosis and cerebral hemiatrophy with contralateral cerebellar atrophy are distinctive of severe epileptic brain damage.

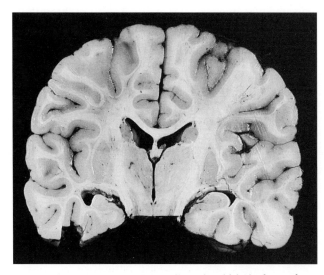

Fig. 19.15. Case of temporal lobe epilepsy in which the focus of damage is on the left side. The left hippocampus is atrophic and the inferior horn of the ventricle on the left is correspondingly dilated. (The defect in the left inferior temporal cortex is artefactual.)

Milder degrees of hippocampal damage affecting CA1 and CA4 but not the dentate fascia granule cells are less specific and resemble hippocampal damage seen in severe hypoxia.

The pathogenesis of hippocampal and cortical epileptic brain damage is thought to involve excessive release during the epileptic discharges of the excitotoxic neurotransmitter glutamate (Lothman, 1991). This excessive neurotransmitter release has the capacity to damage and ultimately destroy post synaptic neurons with glutamate receptors by causing excessive stimulation of receptors, opening of calcium-gated ion channels and the entry into the cells of excessive calcium.

Ramsay Hunt syndrome and Unverricht–Lundborg's syndrome

These two rare conditions combine myoclonic or generalized epilepsy and cerebellar ataxia with mild dementia as progressive neurodegenerations. In Unverricht–Lundborg syndrome (Baltic myoclonus) myoclonus is the presenting and predominant symptom while, in Ramsay Hunt syndrome, ataxia predominates. In Unverricht–Lundborg syndrome the main pathology is usually confined to loss of cerebellar Purkinje cells possibly with some additional degeneration in thalamic nuclei (Haltia, Kristensson & Sourander, 1969; Koskiniemi et al., 1974). In Ramsay Hunt syndrome, the pathology usually consists of degeneration of neurons in

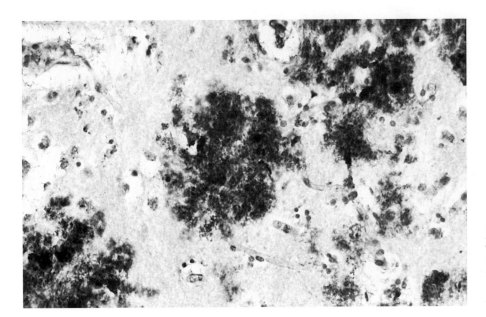

Fig. 19.16. Whipple's disease. Focus of macrophages containing granular PAS-positive cytoplasmic material with more finely granular PAS-positive staining in the surrounding neuropil. PAS stain.

the inferior olives and dentate nucleus (Roger, Soulayrol & Hassonn, 1968; Bird & Shaw, 1978; Gray *et al.*, 1986; Tassinari *et al.*, 1989). Some cases clinically diagnosed as Ramsay Hunt syndrome have been shown to have a mitochondrial cytopathy (MERRF) (Chapter 14), and there is a recent case described in which progressive dementia was associated with cerebral white matter demyelination in addition to the more typical pathology in dentate nuclei and inferior olives (Kobayashi *et al.*, 1994).

SUPERFICIAL HAEMOSIDEROSIS OF THE CENTRAL NERVOUS SYSTEM

Superficial haemosiderosis of the central nervous system is a condition associated with repeated subarachnoid haemorrhages. It is seen in a variety of spontaneously developing or iatrogenically induced lesions including hemispherectomy, arterial aneurysms, arteriovenous malformations and vascular tumours. A dementing syndrome may eventually evolve as a consequence of the repeated bleeding episodes. A component of the pathology in such cases is often hydrocephalus (Chapter 15). In

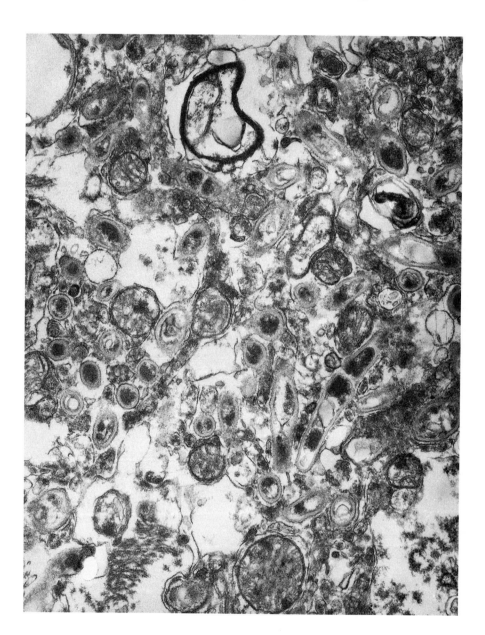

Fig. 19.17. Electron micrograph showing longitudinal and transverse sections across Whipple's disease organisms occupying the neuropil from a case of cerebral Whipples disease. Uranyl acetate and lead citrate stain.

addition, the cerebellar cortex appears to be damaged directly by the toxic effects of superficial deposits of iron-containing pigments with loss of the molecular layer and of Purkinje cells from exposed surfaces (Hughes & Oppenheimer, 1969).

WHIPPLE'S DISEASE

Whipple's disease is a rare condition due to chronic infection with a recently classified actinomycete (Relman *et al.*, 1992). It usually presents with clinical manifesta-

tions relating to small intestinal disease: malabsorption syndrome, weight loss and abdominal pain. However, neurological involvement also occurs and occasionally is seen on its own (Adams *et al.*, 1987; Fleming, Wiesner & Shorter, 1988). The organisms can be found in macrophages in affected organs, chiefly small intestinal mucosa, lymph nodes and brain.

Progressive dementia is a prominent clinical feature of central nervous system involvement with Whipple's disease. It may be accompanied by myoclonus, ataxia

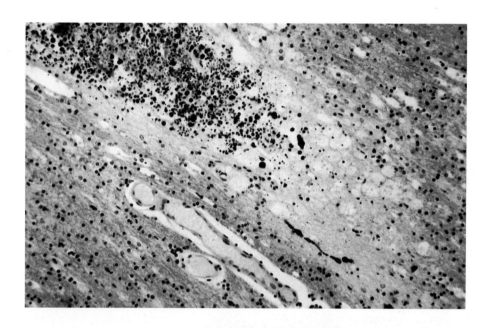

Fig. 19.18. Case of calcifying leukoencephalopathy. Focal necrosis in frontal lobe white matter with axonal spheroid formation and early calcification. There is some oedema in surrounding white matter. Haematoxylin and eosin stain.

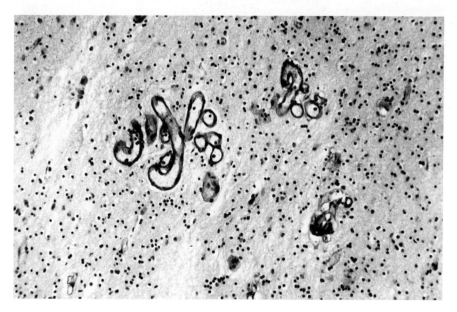

Fig. 19.19. Another case of calcifying leukoencephalopathy. This field illustrates two clusters of small, thin-walled vascular lumens perhaps representing abnormally tortuous vessels in temporal lobe white matter. Haematoxylin and eosin stain.

and signs and symptoms of brain stem dysfunction. Occasionally obstructive hydrocephalus develops. The pathology is usually centred on the diencephalon and upper brain stem, though lesions may also be widespread in the cerebrum. Small infarcts may be found in the cerebral cortex in association with leptomeningeal involvement. Lesions contain collections of PAS-positive macrophages (Fig. 19.16) together with a variable, sometimes inconspicuous, lymphocyte infiltrate. The organisms, which lie in macrophages or free in the neuropil, are 1.5–2.5 μm × 0.2 μm in size and are argyrophilic and gram-positive. Their bacterial form can be appreciated readily on ultrastructural examination (Fig. 19.17).

OTHER OBSCURE CONDITIONS

Coeliac disease with dementia

A number of differing neurological complications of coeliac disease have been described, including dementia of moderate or severe degree. In some cases dementia was the main complaint and gastrointestinal disturbances were mild (Collin et al., 1991). Some of the neurological complications of coeliac disease are attributable to vitamin E deficiency, but this is not known to give rise to dementia. The neuropathology of this condition is not described, but CT scans have been reported to show diffuse cerebral or cerebellar atrophy.

Multifocal leukoencephalopathy with calcification

A rare condition, in some cases associated with a predominantly dementing clinical disease, has been described in which foci of necrosis with calcification are found in the base of the pons and, in some cases, in cerebral white matter (Breuer et al., 1978; Vinters, Anders & Barach, 1987).

Most of the cases described in the literature have been immunodeficient at the time of onset of the disease, either because of an immunodeficiency disease such as AIDS, an inherited immunodeficiency or because they have been receiving chemotherapy for malignancies. However, other cases with very similar pathology have not had such antecedent history (Morris et al., 1995). The neurological disease lasts from a few months to a few years. Investigations are likely to reveal a mild cerebrospinal fluid pleocytosis or no abnormality. Focal calcification in the base of the pons may be identified on CT scan.

The neuropathological lesions may not be noticeable to the naked eye but consist of microscopic foci of cavitating necrosis with prominent calcification of degenerate axons in the same vicinity (Fig. 19.18). The surrounding neuropil is vacuolated. The pontine lesions mainly involve the pontocerebellar fibres and spare neighbouring neurons and corticospinal tracts. Inflammation is not conspicuous, organisms cannot be identified in the lesions, and vessels show non-specific but rather characteristic changes with clusters of thin-walled, possibly abnormally tortuous veins of uncertain pathogenic significance (Fig. 19.19), though fibrin thrombi may occasionally be seen within them. The cause of this condition is unknown. Some attention has been drawn in the literature to similarities to methotrexate toxicity, but not all patients have been on this or similar chemotherapy.

REFERENCES

Adams JH, Duchen LW (1992) Greenfield's Neuropathology. Arnold, London 5th edn.

Adams M, Rhyner PA, Day J, De Armond S, Smuckler EA (1987) Whipple's disease confined to the central nervous system. Ann Neurol 21: 104–8.

Allen IV, Kirk J (1992) Demyelinating diseases. In Adams JH, Duchen LW (eds) Greenfield's Neuropathology. Arnold, London 5th edn, pp 447–520.

Anderson NE, Rosenblum MK, Posner J (1988) Paraneoplastic cerebellar degeneration: clinical–immunological correlations. Ann Neurol 24: 559–67.

Bergin JD (1957) Rapidly progressing dementia in disseminated sclerosis. J Neurol Neurosurg Psychiat 20: 285–92.

Bird TD, Shaw CM (1978) Progressive myoclonus and epilepsy with dentato-rubral degeneration: a clinicopathological study of the Ramsay Hunt syndrome. J Neurol Neurosurg Psychiat 41: 140–9.

Booss J, Esiri MM (1986) Viral Encephalitis: Pathology, Diagnosis and Management. Blackwell Scientific Publications, Oxford.

Breuer AC, Blank NK, Schoene WC (1978) Multifocal pontine lesions in cancer patients treated with chemotherapy and CNS radiotherapy. Cancer 41: 2112–20.

Brownell B, Hughes JT (1962) The distribution of plaques in the cerebrum in multiple sclerosis. J Neurol Neurosurg Psychiat 25: 315–20.

Burger PC, Kamenar E, Schold SC, Fay JW, Phillips GL, Herzig GP (1981) Encephalomyelopathy following high dose BCNU therapy. Cancer 48: 1318–27.

Caccamo D, Herman MM, Urich H, Rubinstein LJ (1989) Focal neuronal gigantism and cerebral cortical thickening after therapeutic irradiation of the central nervous system. Arch Pathol Lab Med 113: 880–5.

Casselli RJ, Scheithauer BW, Bowles CA, Trenerry MR, Meyer

FB, Smiglelski JS, Rodriguez M (1991) The treatable dementia of Sjögren's syndrome. *Ann Neurol* 30: 98–101.

Collin P, Pirttila T, Nurmikko T, Somer H, Erita T, Keyriläinen O (1991) Celiac disease, brain atrophy and dementia. *Neurology* 41: 372–5.

Cordingley G, Navarro C, Bruse JCM, Healton EB (1981) Sarcoidosis presenting as senile dementia. *Neurology* 31: 1148–51.

Cummings JL, Benson DF (1992) Dementia: a clinical approach. 2nd edn Butterworth Heinemann, Boston.

Currie S (1992) Non-metastatic consequences of malignant disease. In Swash M, Oxbury J (eds) *Clinical Neurology*. Churchill, Livingstone, London, pp 1656–78.

Davis RL, Robertson DM (eds) (1996) *Textbook of Neuropathology*. Williams and Wilkins, Baltimore 3rd edn.

De Angelis LM, Delattre J-Y, Posner JB (1989) Radiation-induced dementia in patients cured of brain metastases. *Neurology* 39: 789–96.

Dobrill CB, Wilkins RJ (1976) Relationships between intelligence and electroencephalographic epileptiform activity in adult epileptics. *Neurology* 26: 525–31.

Dropcho EJ (1989) The remote effects of cancer on the nervous system. *Neurol Clin* 7: 579–603.

Filley CM, Heaton RK, Nelson LM, Burks JS, Franklin GM (1989) A comparison of dementia in Alzheimer's disease and multiple sclerosis. *Arch Neurol* 46: 157–61.

Fleming JL, Wiesner RH, Shorter RG (1988) Whipple's disease: clinical, biochemical and histopathologic features and assessment of treatment in 29 patients. *Mayo Clin Proc* 63: 539–51.

Fontaine B, Seilhean D, Tourbah A, Daumas-Duport C, Duyckaerts C, Benoit N, Devaux B, Hauw J-J, Ramcurel G, Lyon-Caen O (1994) Dementia in two histologically confirmed cases of multiple sclerosis: one case with isolated dementia and one case associated with psychiatric symptoms. *J Neurol Neurosurg Psychiat* 57: 353–9.

Gilbert JJ, Sadler M (1983) Unexpected multiple sclerosis. *Arch Neurol* 40: 533–6.

Graus F, Elkon KB, Cordon-Cardo C, Posner JB (1986) Sensory neuronopathy and small cell lung cancer: antineuronal antibody that also reacts with tumour. *Am J Med* 80: 45–52.

Graus F, Cordon-Cardo C, Posner JB (1987) Autoimmune pathogenesis of paraneoplastic neurological syndromes. *CRC Crit Dev Clin Neurobiol* 3: 245–99.

Gray F, Signoret JL, Colin R, Hauw JJ, Escourolle R, Lhermitte F (1986) Dyssynergie cérébelleuse myoclonique (Syndrome de Ramsay Hunt) et telangiectasies cérébelleuse. *Rev Neurol* 142: 29–33.

Haltia M, Kristensson K, Sourander P (1969) Neuropathological studies in three Scandinavian cases of progressive myoclonus epilepsy. *Acta Neurol Scand* 45: 63–77.

Hughes JT, Oppenheimer DR (1969) Superficial siderosis of the central nervous system. *Acta Neuropathol* 13: 56–74.

Jacobs JM, Le Quesne PM (1992) Toxic disorders. In Adam JH, Duchen LW (eds) *Greenfield's Neuropathology*. 5th edn. Arnold, London, pp 881–987.

Kobayashi K, Morikawa K, Fukutani Y, Miyazu K, Nakamura I, Yamaguchi N, Watanabe H (1994) Ramsay Hunt syndrome: progressive mental deterioration in association with unusual cerebral white matter change. *Clin Neuropathol* 13: 88–96.

Kornguth SE (1989) Neuronal proteins and paraneoplastic syndromes. *New Engl J Med* 321: 1607–8.

Koskiniemi M, Donner M, Majuri H, Haltia M, Norio R (1974) Progressive myoclonus epilepsy. A clinical and histopathological study. *Acta Neurol Scand* 50: 307–32.

Lampert PW, Davis RL (1964) Delayed effects of radiation on the human central nervous system: 'early' and 'late' reactions. *Neurology* 14: 912–17.

Lishman WA (1987) Organic Psychiatry. The psychological consequences of cerebral disorder. Blackwell Scientific Publications, Oxford.

Lothman EW (1991) Basic mechanisms of the epilepsies. *Curr Op Neurol Neurosurg* 4: 253–8.

Mendez MF, Frey WHII (1992) Multiple sclerosis dementia. *Neurology* 42: 696.

Morris CS, Esiri MM, Marx A, Newsom-Davis J (1992) Immunocytochemical characteristics of small cell lung carcinoma associated with the Lambert–Eaton myasthenic syndrome. *Am J Pathol* 140: 839–45.

Morris JH, McLean C, Rossi M, Esiri MM (1995) Multifocal calcifying leucoencephalopathy as a cause of progressive dementia: report of 4 cases. *Neuropathol Appl Neurobiol* 24: 441.

Perlmutter I, Gobles C (1961) Subdural haematoma in older patients. *JAMA* 176: 212–14.

Peyser JM, Edwards KR, Poser CM, Filskov SB (1980) Cognitive function in patients with multiple sclerosis. *Arch Neurol* 37: 577–9.

Rao SM, Leo GJ, Bernardin L, Unverzagt F (1991) Cognitive dysfunction in multiple sclerosis. 1 Frequency, patterns and prediction. *Neurology* 41: 685–91.

Relman DA, Schmidt TM, MacDermott RP, Falkow S (1992) Identification of the uncultured bacillus of Whipple's disease. *New Engl J Med* 327: 293–301.

Revol A, Vighetto A, Jouvet A, Aimard G, Trillet M (1992) Encephalitis in cat scratch disease with persistent dementia. *J Neurol Neurosurg Psychiat* 55: 133–5.

Roger J, Soulayrol R, Hassonn J (1968) La synnergie cérébelleuse myoclonique (syndrome de Ramsay-Hunt). *Rev Neurol* 119: 85–106.

Sakai K, Ogasawava T, Hirose G, Jaeckle KA, Greenlee JE (1991) Analysis of autoantibody binding to 52-kD paraneoplastic cerebellar degeneration-associated antigen expressed in recombinant proteins. *Ann Neurol* 33: 373–80.

Sheline GE, Wara WM, Smith V (1980) Therapeutic irradiation and brain injury. *Int J Radiat Oncol Biol Phys* 6: 1215–28.

Stuteville P, Welch K (1958) Subdural haematoma in the elderly person. *JAMA* 168: 1445–9.

Surridge D (1969) An investigation into some psychiatric aspects of multiple sclerosis. *Br J Psych* 115: 749–64.

Tassinari CA, Michelucci R, Genton P, Pellissier JF, Roger J (1989) Dyssynergia cerebellaris myoclonica (Ramsay Hunt syndrome): a condition unrelated to mitochondrial encephalomyopathies. *J Neurol Neurosurg Psychiat* 52: 262–5.

Vincent A, Lang B, Newsom-Davis J (1989) Autoimmunity to the voltage-gated calcium channel underlies the Lambert–Eaton myasthenic syndrome, a paraneoplastic disorder. *TINS* 12: 496–502.

Vinters HV, Anders KH, Barach P (1987) Focal pontine leukoencephalopathy in immunosuppressed patients. *Arch Pathol Lab Med* 111: 192–6.

Zeman W, Samorajski T (1971) Effects of irradiation on the nervous system. In Berdjis GG (ed) *Pathology of Irradiation*. Williams & Wilkins, Baltimore, pp 213–77.

Morphometric methods and dementia

J. M. Anderson

Introduction
Assessment of tissue volumes
Assessment of microscopical changes
Some practical aspects

INTRODUCTION

Many important observations on the histopathology of dementing illnesses have been based on measurements of the changes seen in brain slices or on microscopy. Morphometry is valuable because it provides objectivity and a much greater degree of precision than semi-quantitative visual grading. Especially when cellularity is to be judged, direct visual observation lacks discrimination and is inconsistent compared to measuring techniques. In addition, the numerical values obtained by morphometry give greater scope for statistical analysis. They also facilitate comparisons between different histological events or between histology and psychometric or neurochemical data.

Leading histological changes in the pathology of dementia include tissue atrophy, neuron loss and accumulation of various inclusions and aggregates. This Appendix therefore focuses on (a) methods for measuring the volume of the cranial cavity, the brain and its component parts and (b) methods for estimating the volume fraction or the numerical density of particulate structures in microscopical sections.

ASSESSMENT OF TISSUE VOLUMES

Whole brain

Brain weight or volume by itself is of limited value for estimating cerebral atrophy since the normal range for brain weight is very wide at all ages (Dekaban & Sadowsky, 1978). Large numbers of cases are required if meaningful differences are to be detected between study groups. In an individual case, little can be inferred about the degree of atrophic change from brain weight or volume alone; for example, after the loss of 20% of tissue

an atrophic brain which was 1500 g in health and is now reduced to 1200 g still falls within the normal adult range at all ages. Grading cerebral atrophy by visual appraisal of features such as widening of sulci or the size of the ventricular system has been attempted, but this subjective procedure has not proved sufficiently robust to elucidate the differences between the atrophy of Alzheimer's disease and that of normal old age.

Comparison must be made with cranial cavity volume for reliable data on cerebral atrophy in individuals or in small groups. This point was recognized by Reichard (1905), who devised a method for measuring the skull cavity with water; his technique depended on accurate cutting of the calvarium, precise plugging of the foramena with putty and repeated measurements. Reichard's method and other early methods involving the use of sand or millet seed were laborious and of doubtful accuracy. The balloon method introduced by Davis and Wright (1977) was therefore an important advance since it was easier to perform and reproducible; repeated measurements by the authors varied by less than 1%. More recently, Harper et al. (1984) have developed a technique for the production of a polyurethane cast of the cranial cavity. This procedure also is reproducible with a 2% error only. It has the advantage that a permanent record of the size and shape of the intracranial dimensions is obtained.

Since the cranial cavity volume does not alter with advancing age (Davis & Wright, 1977), the brain volume expressed as a percentage of cranial cavity gives an index of brain atrophy. Brain volume/cranial cavity volume % in both sexes remains at $92.2 \pm 1.6\%$ (SEM) until 55 years of age and thereafter declines to about 85% in persons over 80 years of age (Davis & Wright, 1977; Hubbard & Anderson, 1981).

Brain volume measurement

FROM BRAIN WEIGHT

For many studies, a sufficiently accurate estimate may be obtained by weighing the brain and dividing the weight in grams by the specific gravity to find the volume in ml. The mean specific gravity of unfixed human brain is 1.0376 with a very small age-related decrement in adult life (SG of brain $= 1.040 - [(4.87)10^{-5}.\text{age}]$, $p = 0.02$) (Davis & Wright, 1977). Even if the brain volume is measured directly this calculation provides a useful check on the result.

USING A DISPLACEMENT APPARATUS

The principle underlying this procedure is to place the brain in a container filled with isotonic saline and to measure the volume of the displaced saline. This can be done by means of an open container (such as a brain pot) fitted with an overflow spout; the container is filled with saline until the spout is overflowing; when the excess has been discharged the brain is gently placed in the reservoir with another container in position under the spout to collect the displaced fluid. The weight of the displaced saline divided by the specific gravity (1.005 for isotonic saline at 20 °C) gives the volume of the brain. Reading the volume of the fluid from graduations on a measuring cylinder is somewhat less precise than recording the weight.

An alternative method favoured by Davis and Wright (1977) and Harper *et al.* (1984) makes use of a glass or plastic desiccator jar. The procedure is as follows. First,

the two large parts of the desiccator are sealed together with grease, the jar is filled to the top with saline through the lid aperture and the ground glass attachments positioned in the aperture. The apparatus is then weighed (*a*). Secondly, the brain is weighed (*b*). Lastly, the brain is placed upside down in the bottom half of the jar, the lid positioned, saline added to the top as before and the weight of jar, brain and saline recorded (*c*). The weight of the saline displaced by the brain is given by $(a + b - c)$ and the volume of the brain is found by dividing this value by 1.005, the specific gravity of isotonic saline.

Cranial cavity measurement

THE BALLOON METHOD OF DAVIS AND WRIGHT (1977)

The aim is to fill the cranial cavity completely with a water-filled balloon and then record the weight of the water in the balloon. The arrangement of the apparatus is shown in Fig. A1.1. The items needed are a sphygmomanometer, a large glass jar with rubber bung, lengths of glass and rubber tubing, a screw clip, a quantity of large size, good quality party balloons and some lubricating jelly. A metal coronet clamp is required to hold the calvarium in place during the measurement.

The dura mater is removed from the calvarium, but only the tentorium cerebelli is removed from the floor of the skull. Two V-shaped apertures about 15 mm deep are cut into the margin of the skull cap, one laterally to take the tube from the water reservoir and another anteriorly to give a view of the balloon filling the cranial cavity. Any sharp bony spicules in the cut edge or in the floor of the skull are removed with bone shears. The

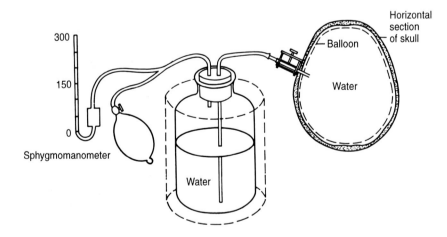

Fig. A1.1. Diagram of the apparatus for cranial cavity measurement by the balloon method. (Reproduced from *Neuropathology and Applied Neurobiology* **3**, 1977 with permission of Blackwell Scientific Publications, Oxford.)

balloon is tied to the tubing while filled with a small amount of water so as to avoid air bubbles, and its surface is lubricated. The tubing from the reservoir is filled with water and connected to the section carrying the screw clip. Balloon and adjacent tubing are placed in position as the calvarium is replaced; the clamp is then secured. The balloon is now filled with water by pumping the sphygmomanometer bulb until a pressure of 150 mm Hg is reached at which point the screw clip is tightened. The calvarium clamp is then released, the balloon carefully removed from the skull cavity, the water released into a container and weighed. The weight of water in grams is equal to the cranial cavity volume in millilitres.

THE POLYURETHANE CAST METHOD OF HARPER *ET AL.* (1984)

The materials needed for this technique are the reagents Daltolac GP8 and Supracec DND (ICI), a roll of polyethylene film, e.g. Cling Film (Boots) and a skull clamp. Apparatus to measure the volume of the cast is also required.

Most of the dura mater is left in position, but the tentorium cerebelli and falx cerebri are trimmed off. An opening about 10 mm wide is cut in the vertex of the skull to allow escape of air as the polyurethane foam expands. The cranial cavity surface is dried with paper towels and a wad of paper used to plug the foramen magnum. The interior of both portions of the skull are then lined with polyethylene film; it is important to exclude moisture from the polyurethane mixture, otherwise the foam remains soft and sticky. The film need not follow the contours of the skull exactly since the heat of the reaction and the expansion of the foam push the film into the crevices; the film is punctured opposite the vertex aperture. Equal quantities of the reagents are used. For a head of circumference 500 mm, 40 ml of each reagent is used and for every additional 10 mm of head circumference a further 1 ml of each reagent is added. Once the mixture is made it must be transferred to the base of the skull without delay. The head is held upright and the calvarium clamped in position. Excess foam protrudes through the aperture in the vertex. A rigid cast is formed in 5–10 minutes, and the required hardness can be judged from the overflow material. The cast remains deformable for up to 15 minutes, but it must not be left too long in the skull otherwise it will be difficult to remove. The cast is extracted by rotating the occipital lobes and posterior fossa contents upwards and backwards. The volume of the cast is found by displacement as described above.

Component parts of the brain

The method of choice for finding the volume of parts of the brain largely depends on the size of the component to be examined. The approach is different for a large structure such as the cerebral cortex than for smaller structures, for example, individual basal ganglia. In both instances, however, measurements are made of the area occupied by the structure in serial slices or sections taken at a fixed interval through the thickness of the structure and the volume is found by calculation from the areal measurements.

The easiest procedure for large structures is to measure the *area fraction* or *proportion* of the component in brain slices by point-counting. The proportion of points lying over a feature is equal to the area proportion, i.e. area of the structure divided by the area of the remainder of the brain slice.

$$P_{Pi} = \text{points over feature } i/\text{total points counted} = A_{Ai} \quad (1)$$

By the Delesse principle, the area proportion of a component as seen in the cut surfaces of a tissue is directly proportional to the volume proportion in the whole tissue. A mathematical proof of this is given by Weibel & Elias (1967).

$$A_{Ai} = V_{Vi} \quad (2)$$

The area/volume proportion multiplied by the volume of the entire specimen yields the absolute volume of the component.

$$V_{Vi}.(\text{total tissue volume}) = \text{absolute volume of } i \quad (3)$$

This method is best suited to structures which comprise 5% or more of the tissue volume. For structures smaller than 5% of the hemisphere volume it is more accurate to make *absolute area* measurements (mm^2) from each of the brain slices in which the structure appears. Very small structures obviously must be measured from microscopical sections. Again, the absolute area (mm^2) has to be recorded from each of several step sections. The volume is then found by integration of these areal values using Simpson's equation (see below).

Volume estimation by point-counting brain slices

Serial slices of brain at a regular interval are obtained. Since brain tissue is non-uniform in composition, slices through the full thickness of the structure of interest must be measured. If the initial cut is at random, this provides a stratified random sample which is the best type of sampling for anisotropic tissues (Aherne & Dunnill, 1982). The interval will often be 10 mm, since this is the thickness at which brain slices are cut by hand with a knife guide, but an interval down to 5 mm is possible if an electrical slicing machine is employed. Point-counting is then performed. This procedure is equivalent to dividing the tissue into many small squares and counting the number of squares corresponding to the various components.

A transparent point counting lattice is prepared from a cellulose acetate sheet marking the points with a waterproof pen; a sheet of graph paper placed under the acetate provides a guide. A lattice with points at the angles of equilateral triangles of side 10 mm is generally used (Fig. A1.2). This is laid over each slice at random thereby ensuring a stratified random sample at the counting stage also. One or both surfaces may be counted, depending on the size of count required for an acceptable standard error (see below). All the points lying over the brain slice are recorded, divided into the features of interest; a haematological tally counter is a convenient aid when counting. The number of points over cortex, white matter, etc. from all the slices are summed and expressed as a fraction of the total point count. These fractions multipled by the volume of the cerebrum gives the absolute volumes in ml.

Miller, Alston and Corsellis (1980) used an automatic image analyser as a point counter to determine total cerebral hemisphere grey and white matter volumes from serial slices. Grey matter colouration was enhanced by staining with a modification of Mulligan's method (1931).

Volume estimation using Simpson's rule

This method is applicable to brain slices if the feature of interest is relatively small yet easily seen in the gross specimen. Such features include the ventricular system and multiple lacunar infarcts, for example. For smaller structures, such as individual nuclei, microscopical step sections at a known interval through the structure are prepared. In practice this calls for serial sections with every nth section mounted and stained; perhaps every tenth section would be taken for very small nuclei, giving an interval of 0.1 mm, if the sections are 10 μm thick. For bigger nuclei n might be 20 or 25.

Working with brain slices, the first step is to make tracings on cellulose acetate sheets from each of the slices of the areas to be measured. The area of the feature is

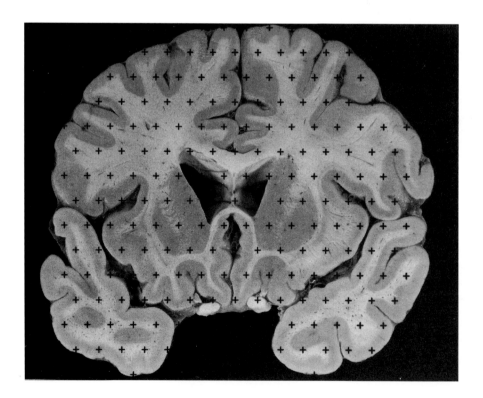

Fig. A1.2. Coronal slice of brain overlaid with a point-counting grid. The proportion of points over cerebral cortex, white matter, basal ganglia and ventricles, when summed for all the slices of the cerebrum, is equivalent to the volume proportions of these components.

then determined by point-counting, but on this occasion the number of points is used to calculate the actual area in each slice separately; to find this the point score is divided by the density of the points on the grid. For example, if the interval between the points is 5 mm, then 1 cm^2 will on average contain 4 points and dividing the point count by 4 will give the area of the structure in cm^2.

With microscopical sections there are several different ways to obtain area measurements. This can be done (a) at the microscope using a graticule in a measuring eyepiece; the graticule consists of a lattice of points or a net of lines, the intersections serving as points; (b) by projecting the image and drawing a tracing on paper or (c) by means of an interactive image analyser. The eyepiece graticule procedure involves point-counting and a similar calculation to that described above for brain slice tracings. Once a suitable magnification is chosen the interval between the points must be found using a stage micrometer. This device consists of a slide carrying an etched line 2 mm long divided into 10 μm intervals; the eyepiece grid is aligned with the micrometer and the length of the point interval read off. The point density of the grid can then be found (Fig. A1.3).

Tracings on paper can also be measured by point-counting using a lattice on transparent sheet as for brain slices. The tracing point score is divided (a) by the point density to find the area of the tracing in cm^2 and then (b) by the square of the linear magnification to obtain the

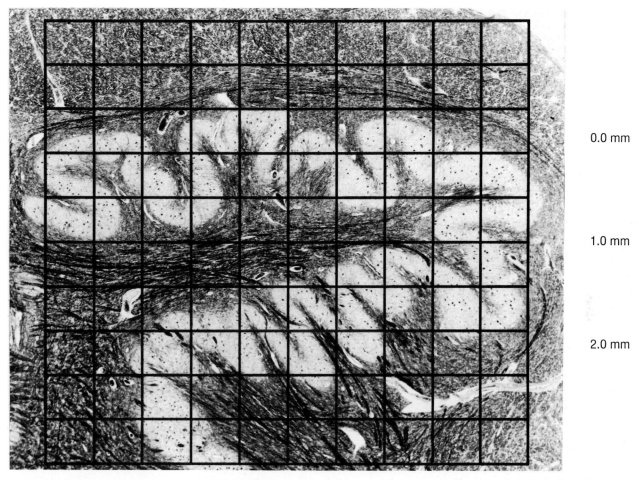

0.0 mm

1.0 mm

2.0 mm

Fig. A1.3. Section of the inferior olivary nucleus with lattice graticule superimposed. Comparison with a stage micrometer shows the intersections of the grid to be spaced at 0.425 mm giving a point density of 5.5/mm^2. Since 28 points fall over the grey matter of the nucleus, the area of this tissue in the grid field is 5.1 mm^2. For a complete measurement of the nucleus at this magnification three contiguous grid fields would be needed in each step section.

Table A1.1. *Measurement of cerebral ventricular volume from brain slices using Simpson's Rule*

Slice no.	Point score	Area (cm^2)	Slice no.	Point score	Area (cm^2)
0	0	0	1	6	1.5
2	21	5.25	3	23	5.75
4	21	5.25	5	23	5.75
6	25	6.25	7	24	6.0
8	23	5.75	9	22	5.5
10	22	5.5	11	30	7.5
12	41	10.25	13	41	10.25
14	32	8.0	15	19	4.75
16	13	3.25	17	0	0

On slicing the brain at a spacing of 0.7 cm, 16 slices contained parts of the ventricular system. Point counting was performed with a test grid of points spaced at 0.5 cm intervals.
The values for Simpson's equation are: $h = 0.7$;
$A_o + A_a = 0$; $4(A_1 + A_3 + ... A_{n-1}) = 188$;
$2(A_2 + A_4 + ... A_{n-2}) = 99$.
The volume of the ventricles is
$V = (0.33)(0.7)(0 + 188 + 99) = 67 \text{ cm}^3$.

actual area on the slide. Alternatively, a planimeter can be employed to give the tracing area. Many laboratories are now equipped with image analysis apparatus and when available this will be the instrument of choice for this work because of its speed and computing facilities. Interactive image analysers provide accurate area measurements of microscopic features by use of an electronic mouse to select the area required from a televized image.

Having obtained an area measurement for each slice or section the values are entered into Simpson's equation to calculate the volume:

$$V = \tfrac{1}{3}h\,[(A_o + A_n) + 4(A_1 + A_3 + ... A_{n-1}) + 2(A_2 + A_4 + ... A_{n-2})] \qquad (4)$$

The value h is the interval between the sections or the cut surfaces. A worked example is shown in Table A1.1.

ASSESSMENT OF MICROSCOPICAL CHANGES

Volume proportions
The point-counting procedure described above for estimating the volume proportion (V_V) of gross structures from brain slices is also applicable to microscopical sections. Measurement of V_V of a histological component can often be just as useful as a count (N_V) and may be easier to obtain.

At the microscope the measurement is obtained with an eyepiece graticule carrying either a lattice of points or a net of lines; a triangular array of points is the more efficient (Aherne & Dunnill, 1982). Starting at a random point at the edge of the structure of interest, the grid is counted over successive adjacent fields going over and back through the structure in rows or columns. This provides a stratified random sample. For example, cerebral cortex measurements would usually be taken in successive columns starting at a random field just beneath the pia mater and travelling through to the white matter to avoid a potential sampling error from the six variable layers of the cortex. The total points over each feature of interest are counted and divided by the total points for all the fields to find the area proportion (A_A) which, by the theorem of Delesse is equal to the volume proportion (V_V). Fields are counted until A_A does not change materially with the addition of further points. V_V can be converted into absolute volume (ml) by multiplying V_V by the volume of the gross structure.

Although a very large number of points must be counted when the component is proportionately small, the measurement is well suited to image analysers; these instruments derive their data from a television image consisting of at least 5×10^5 contiguous picture points per field and so a huge point score is soon achieved.

This technique is free of the problems of split cell error which complicates volumetric counts (N_V) (see below), but it is susceptible to another systematic error due to section thickness known as the Holmes effect (Holmes, 1927). In theory, A_A should be recorded from the surfaces of opaque tissue slices or from infinitely thin translucent sections. In practice, the profiles of many structures seen on microscopy are derived from rounded particles of finite thickness and so their images tend to be too large (Fig. A1.4). Fortunately, the Holmes effect can be disregarded in many studies provided section thickness is kept constant when test and control are affected equally. However, it can become important if the particles in the tissue change in size significantly under the conditions of the study or if precise volumetric data are required.

The additional measurements needed for correction are (i) section thickness t and (ii) mean particle diameter D from which the factor K is derived:

$$K = 1 + 3t/2D \qquad (5)$$

and the true volume proportion V_V is derived from the observed volume proportion V_{V0} by:

$$V_V = 1/K \ V_{V0} \qquad (6)$$

Particle numbers

Profile count or particle count?

The first choice of measurement for microscopical changes may be a count of cells, or perhaps a count of one of the abnormal deposits such as senile plaques, neurofibrillary tangles or Lewy bodies. Commonly, such a count is performed per unit area of the section. It must be appreciated that this is a profile count and not a particle count. The number of cellular profiles per area (N_A) of standard sections is considerably higher than the true number of cells per volume (N_V). Furthermore, there is usually no simple relationship between N_A and N_V because of variable size, shape and spatial orientation of particles. Accordingly, the percentage difference

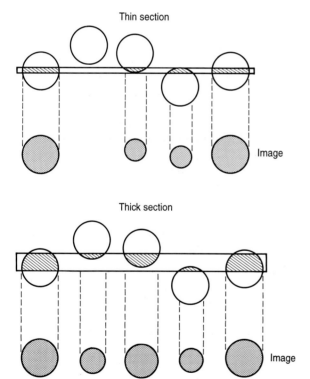

Fig. A1.4. The Holmes effect. Increased section thickness increases area proportion measurements since the number of fragments tends to be greater and so also is the mean size of the profiles.

in N_A under the conditions of a study is unlikely to equate exactly with the percentage change in N_V. Nevertheless, this type of count may be adequate if there is a substantial difference between test and control and if there is no change in the size of the particles in the condition studied. N_A might be considered reasonable for plaques and tangles, for example, and in most publications counts of plaques and tangles are indeed expressed as N_A. However, a more precise volumetric count (N_V) may sometimes reveal significant changes not apparent in a profile count. N_V is always required when microscopical data are to be integrated with gross measurements of tissue volume to allow for the effects of tissue atrophy on cell packing density.

Although the concept of N_V is readily understood, it can be a problematical measurement to perform for cells and other small particles. For larger particles, i.e. those of diameter greater than ten times section thickness, the measurements are reasonably straightforward, since the section can be considered infinitely thin and the third dimension ignored. However, when counting particles of diameter less than ten times section thickness tissue sections must be considered as slices of finite thickness and a correction for fragments employed. Over the past 50 years, a succession of methods have been developed to calculate V_V from two-dimensional sections based on assumptions about the geometrical shape of particles. A correction can be achieved easily if the particles are spherical, but if they are non-spherical and/or variable in size, the calculations are unwieldy. Estimation of N_V for neurons by counting all the ellipsoidal profiles of cell bodies is therefore fraught with difficulty. However, these problems can be minimized by counting nucleoli instead, which are single in most neurons (Konigsmark, 1970). Split cell error is then very much smaller and correction formulae for spheres can be applied. The correction proposed by Abercrombie (1946) is often used for counts of nucleoli. For a full account of traditional methods for obtaining volumetric counts of cells in nervous tissue, the reviews by Ebbesson and Tang (1965), Konigsmark (1970) and Aherne and Dunnill (1982) are recommended.

Recently, a new family of three-dimensional measuring techniques has been developed which will largely replace the older methods for measurements on cells since they are devoid of assumptions about particle shape, orientation or spatial distribution. These methods have been reviewed by Gundersen et al. (1988). They include a three-dimensional probe termed 'the disector' for recording N_V, introduced by Sterio (1984).

A volumetric method for large particles

Structures such as neuritic plaques, which are approximately spherical and mainly 50–300 μm in diameter, can be counted accurately in standard 5 μm sections using the method of Weibel & Gomez (1962). Placing a lattice of squares over the microscopical fields, two measurements are made: (i) the volume proportions (V_V) of the plaques from a point count covering the whole grid and (ii) the number of plaque profiles (N_A) within the grid, following the usual rule that plaques cutting the right and upper margins of the grid are counted while those cutting the left and lower margins are not; also, fused plaques would be counted separately. The grid is moved systematically through adjacent fields. A magnification of $\times$ 100 is suitable. When sufficient fields have been counted to yield a stable estimate for each of these values, N_V is obtained from the equation:

$$N_V = N_A{}^{3/2}/\beta\sqrt{V_V} \qquad (7)$$

in which β is a shape coefficient, relating particle volume to mean profile area. For spheres $\beta = 1.38$. Values for other shapes are listed by Weibel & Bolender (1975). If size distribution differences are thought to exist, then the distribution of plaque transection diameters should be obtained and a factor K calculated.

$$K = (D_3/D_1)^{3/2} \qquad (8)$$

where D_1 and D_3 are the first and third moments of the diameter distribution. The formula for N_V becomes:

$$N_V = KN_A{}^{3/2}/\beta\sqrt{V_V} \qquad (9)$$

Abercrombie's correction for small particles

The formula developed by Abercrombie (1946) is given here because it is easy to apply and has been very widely used. As shown in Fig. A1.5, any spherical particle lying with its centre between A and B will be represented in section CD. The formula to correct for fragments is then:

$$N_V = N_A.t/(t + 2r) \qquad (10)$$

in which t is the section thickness and r is the radius of the particle.

It can be seen that, for example, counts of nucleoli of radius 2 μm in a section of thickness 10 μm have a correction factor of 10/14 or 0.71. This formula has been criticized because it tends to over-correct, no account being taken of hidden fragments or fragments which are too thin to be visible. However, in most brain nuclei, the neurones are widely spaced so that there is no error from hidden fragments.

Ebbesson and Tang's method for small particles

More sophisticated split cell correction formulae have been devised which allow for visible fragments, fragments obscured behind larger cells and very thin fragments of insufficient optical density to be visible. These formulae depend on knowing not only (a) the mean radius of each of the different cell types in the tissue (b) the section thickness but also (c) the vertical thickness of the smallest visible fragment, a difficult measurement to obtain. Ebbesson and Tang (1965) pointed out that, by making counts from two serial sections of different thickness there is no need to measure mean cell size or the thickness of the smallest visible fragment. Since the number of fragments at the edges of a 10 μm section are the same as in a 20 μm section, subtraction of the two counts gives the number of whole particles per 10 μm thickness (Fig. A1.6). The formula is then simplified to:

$$N_{v(a-b)} = N_{Va} - N_{Vb} \qquad (11)$$

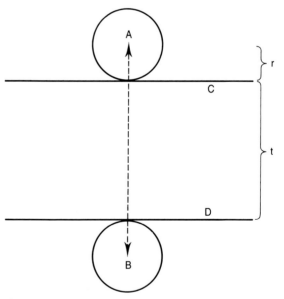

Fig. A1.5. Abercrombie's correction. The diagram shows two particles with their centres at A and B and just cut by section CD. All particles with centres between A and B will be included in the section although many of the profiles seen will be fragments. An estimate of the number of whole fragments in the section is given by multiplying the observed count by $(t/t + 2r)$.

in which N_{V_a} and N_{V_b} are the observed counts in sections of thickness a and b and $N_{V(a-b)}$ is the estimated count in thickness $(a - b)$.

The count can be made of the nucleoli or nuclei without greatly affecting the result. As before, a squared grid is employed and a succession of adjacent fields in columns or rows are observed. If a series of section pairs are counted and averaged, this reduces any error which may be due to variable section thickness. The disadvantage of this procedure is that it calls for accurate microtomy and for an instrument to check section thickness.

A three-dimensional probe for particle counts: the disector

A method for making counts of N_V in three dimensions has recently been introduced by Sterio (1984). This is now undoubtedly the method of choice for particle counting since it completely avoids split cell error, is independent of particle shape and unbiased by cell size. By this procedure, small and large cells are sampled with a uniform probability, in contrast to single section measurements in which large particles tend to be over-represented. The method is also very efficient. Braendgaard *et al.* (1989) have shown that, using the disector

procedure, it is possible to estimate accurately the total number of neurons in the human neocortex in less than half a day.

The disector probe consists of two parallel sections a known distance apart. Two physically separate sections can be used, but it is very much quicker to make observations in a single thick section at two planes of focus (the optical disector). A field within a counting frame is examined first in the upper or 'look-up' plane and then in the lower or 'reference' plane; cells are counted if they appear in the lower plane but not in the upper. Any such cell must begin in the sample volume enclosed by the two planes (Fig. A1.7). The number of cell 'tops' (Q^-) is summed from a succession of paired fields until about 100–200 have been counted and then N_V is calculated from:

$$N_V = \Sigma Q^- / \Sigma v(\text{dis}) \tag{12}$$

where $v(\text{dis})$ is the volume of the disector, i.e. the area of the frame multiplied by the depth of the second plane of focus of the optical disector.

Physically separate sections are probably easiest to examine in photomicrographs. Alternatively, two projection microscopes are required, aligning the sections so that the images of the parallel fields coincide. The optical disector is much more convenient; a 20–25 μm section is obtained of which a slice perhaps 10 μm deep is examined focusing down in 2 μm steps. For this procedure, a microscope must be modified by the addition of an electronic step motor which moves the stage in the z-axis by a known distance. Counts are made with high numerical aperture oil immersion lenses and matched

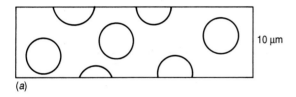

10 μm

(a)

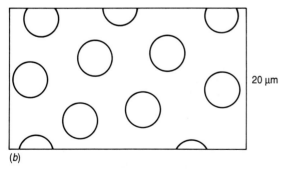

20 μm

(b)

Fig. A1.6. In sections of unequal thickness a thick section A contains more whole particles than a thin section B, but the number of fragments at the cut edges of the sections is closely similar. The difference in the counts is therefore equal to the number of whole particles per section thickness A–B.

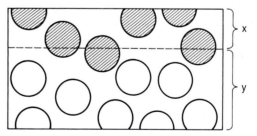

Fig. A1.7. The optical disector principle. In a thick section the uppermost plane of focus x is examined and the cells noted. A count is then made of previously invisible cells which come into focus on racking down into a lower (reference) plane y of known thickness. This volumetric count of cell 'tops' is unbiased by cell size or shape.

condenser to give the smallest possible focal depth. A detailed description of disector counts of large nuclei of the human brain and integration of these counts with gross measurements is given by Pakenberg and Gundersen (1988).

Particle sizes

Methods for measuring *mean size* of particles from single thin sections have similar problems to particle counts in that they are subject to bias due to simplifying assumptions about shape and orientation of the particles. Cell size can only be measured by these techniques if the shape is taken to be spherical or ellipsoidal. Calculation of the *size distribution* of a mixed population of cells from thin sections is even longer and more difficult since a solution has to be found from a complex mixture of profiles many of which are from the margins of the cells. A full discussion of this subject can be found in Aherne & Dunnill (1982).

Fortunately, many of the objects of interest in the brain are small enough to be contained wholly within a section. It is then possible to bring the equatorial plane of the cell or nucleus into focus for measurement; in the case of neurones this is usually assumed to be when the nucleolus is sharply outlined. The three-dimensional disector provides certain advantages for measurements of cellular dimensions. The disector selects a sample of cells which is unbiased by shape or size (Sterio, 1984) and in addition, when thick sections are used the equatorial profiles can be examined. Gundersen *et al.* (1988) recommend that the radius from a fixed point in the cell such as the nucleolus be used for cell size and describes a procedure for ensuring that the measurements are taken in an isotropic plane in a structurally orientated tissue like the cerebral cortex. They also suggest that a four-way record of radius be taken, finding that this gives an accuracy comparable with values obtained from three-dimensional reconstruction of cells from serial sections.

SOME PRACTICAL ASPECTS

In this section attention is drawn to some technical points to be considered when planning a morphometric study.

Tissue fixation and processing

Fixation in formalin causes brain weight to increase by 1–6% after 1–3 months (Dam, 1979), whereas fixation over years results in shrinkage. More pronounced shrinkage is caused by tissue processing; this varies with the processing schedule, but it can be as much as 50% by

volume during LVN embedding. Such shrinkage can greatly affect measurements of N_A and N_V and may therefore need correction, particularly if there is any reason to suppose that test and control might be affected differently.

A fixation shrinkage factor is obtained by recording the brain volume again after fixation and calculating the value f^3 = fresh volume/fixed volume. A processing factor is determined by finding the area of the fixed tissue block and then the area of the resulting section. One method is to draw tracings on cellulose acetate sheet and measure these by planimetry or point counting as described on page 415. The processing factor is given by p^2 = block area/section area from which p^3 is derived by cubing the square root of p^2; this calculation is used because the third dimension (depth of the block) cannot be measured easily after processing. The values f^3 and p^3 can then be used to convert the observed volumetric measurements into data referable to fresh tissue volume. Since there is considerable variation between cases, it is best to measure these effects in each brain.

If very small samples such as biopsies are being studied, it is not practicable to measure f^3 and p^3. Reliance must then be placed on careful standardization of laboratory procedures. Glycolmethacrylate embedding causes least shrinkage, and for this reason it is often preferred to paraffin wax or LVN for morphometric studies.

Selecting the sample

In any morphometric study, sampling requires careful consideration. This applies both to the selection of tissue blocks and to microscopic sections and fields. The aim is to measure no more than is necessary for accuracy while, at the same time, avoiding an unrepresentative sample. Since the central nervous system is composed of anisotropic tissue, a very small sample is unlikely to be representative and several pieces of tissue or sections at levels must be examined. The question is what is the most efficient procedure to adopt?

Completely random sampling of brain tissue has been shown to result in a greater coefficient of error than systematic sampling (Ebbesson & Tang, 1967, Konigsmark *et al.*, 1969). Accordingly, in most studies of the brain a systematic scheme is used although a starting point is chosen at random; this is referred to as stratified random sampling. For example, in sampling the cerebral cortex slices are made through the cerebrum starting at a random point, and the same number of blocks are taken from each slice following a set plan. Pakkenberg &

Gundersen (1988) have described an optimal sampling scheme for tissue blocks from large nuclei of the human brain. It is important to remember that increasing the number of blocks has a greater effect on reducing the variance of a measurement than increasing the number of sections or fields counted.

Stratified random sampling is also employed for the selection of microscopical fields. The procedure usually followed when measuring the cerebral cortex has been described on page 418. In selecting sections for a count of cells along the length of a small discrete nucleus, the first section is chosen at random and then every nth section is mounted and stained. The size of the period n is related to the number of cells in the nucleus. For a big nucleus such as the inferior olive, which has a population of 430 000 neurons, a standard error of 5% of the mean is obtained when $n = 100$ (Moatamed, 1966) whereas, for a smaller nucleus such as the sixth cranial nerve with 22 000 neurons, a period of $n = 10$ is required for the same degree of accuracy (Konigsmark et al., 1969). It is necessary to examine the structure of interest to see if it is homogenous; if not, sections must be taken along the full length in all cases or, failing that, the blocks must be taken consistently from the same point with reference to an anatomical landmark.

Provided the cellular density of a nucleus is consistent, the number of fields or sections needed for a count of N_V with a chosen standard error can be estimated by entering values from a small pilot study into De Hoff's (1967) formula:

$$n = [(200.Sx)/(y.\bar{x})]^2 \qquad (13)$$

in which y is the percentage error (usually taken as 5%), S_x is the standard deviation and $\bar{x}$ the mean of the pilot sample. For example, if the pilot mean $\pm$ SD is 20 ± 5, then 100 sections must be counted, but if the SD is 2.5 then 25 will suffice.

With regard to *estimates of A_A and V_V* by the point counting procedure, the standard error of the measurement is given by:

$$SE = \sqrt{P_P(100 - P_P)/T} \qquad (14)$$

in which P_p is the percentage of the test points over the feature of interest and T is the total point score. The percentage standard error is:

$$SE\% = SE \times 100/P_P \qquad (15)$$

The total number of points needed to give a SE% of 2.5–10% for components of different size is shown in Table A1.2.

Confirmation of the adequacy of sampling can obtained from an average summation graph constructed during the course of a count (Fig. A1.8). The cumulative mean value is calculated after each field (or section) is counted. The mean fluctuates initially, but eventually becomes steady when sufficient measurements have been made.

Table A1.2. *The relationship between the volume proportion of a feature, the total point count and the percentage standard error*

Volume proportion of feature of interest	Total point count required for % standard error at		
	2.5%	5%	10%
50%	1600	400	100
20%	6400	1600	400
10%	14 400	3600	900
5%	30 400	7600	1900
2.5%	62 400	15 600	3900

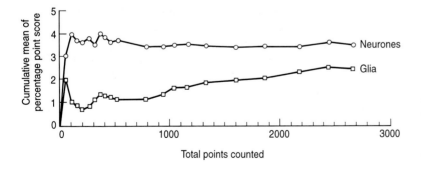

Fig. A1.8. Graph showing cumulative averages of area proportion measurements of cells in successive fields of the hippocampal formation. A steady value for neurones is achieved at a total count of 1000 points, but 2500 points must be counted to obtain an unvarying mean for glial cells. (Reproduced from *Theory and Practice of Histological Techniques* ed. J. D. Bancroft and A. Stevens, 3rd edition, 1990 with permission of Churchill Livingstone, Edinburgh.)

Section thickness and magnification

Section thickness has an important bearing on morphometric results. The optimal thickness depends on the counting method chosen. For A_A and V_V the sections should be as thin as possible to minimise the Holmes effect, whereas for N_V and cell size measurements thick sections are usually preferred. It is clearly important to maintain consistency and this is more likely if the same microtomist cuts all the sections using the same microtome. If a check on section thickness is desired this can be achieved with an interference microscope (Hale, 1958) or by means of the Surfometer, an instrument which records the contour of surfaces (Pearse & Marks, 1974). Magnification should be kept constant throughout a study, since higher magnification produces greater resolution and higher values (Ebbesson & Tang, 1965).

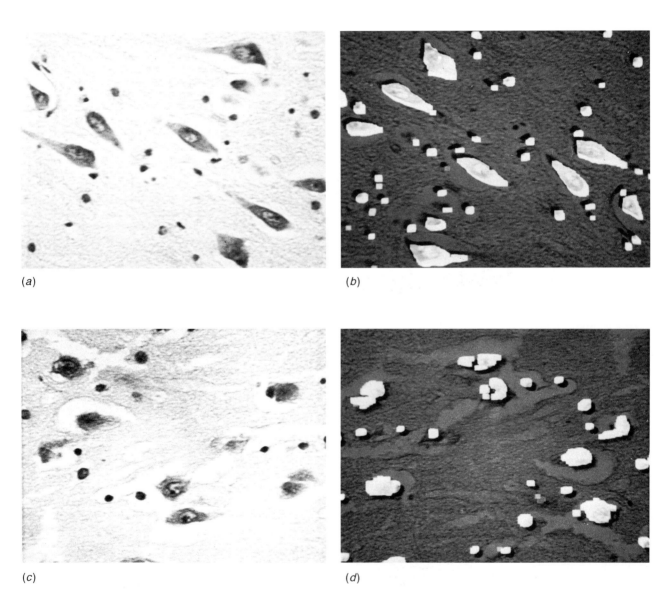

(a)

(b)

(c)

(d)

Fig. A1.9. Photographs of an automatic image analyser monitor showing the hippocampal formation directly ((a) and (c)) and in detection mode ((b) and (d)). A detection threshold which is suitable for brain collected 12 hours after death ((a) and (b)) results in a fragmented image of cells in brain tissue obtained 72 hours after death ((c) and (d)).

Post-mortem decay

Most work on dementia involves the study of necropsy material collected at varying times after death. Post-mortem autolysis results in the gradual lysis of nucleic acids which are the chief cellular compounds stained by dyes such as haemalum, cresyl violet and gallocyanin. The optical density of brain cells becomes reduced, and this effect pronounced when the interval between death and necropsy exceeds two days. This change is more noticeable when sections are thin. The image of neurones on an image analyser may be broken up and record as several small fragments (Fig. A1.9), so that it may be necessary to edit the image with the electronic light pen (Terry & Deteresa, 1982). Data on cell content should therefore be checked to see if there is any correlation with post-mortem interval. Allowance can be made for this by the statistical technique of multiple linear regression; this allows three or more variables to be analysed simultaneously and then for two to be compared while holding the other constant. For example, if cell content, age and post-mortem interval are the three variables, a three-way regression equation permits comparison of the average effect of age on cell content while post-mortem interval is kept constant (Anderson et al., 1983).

REFERENCES

Abercrombie M (1946) Estimation of nuclear population from microtome sections. *Anat Rec* 94: 239–47.

Anderson JM, Hubbard BM, Coghill GR, Slidders W (1983) The effect of advanced old age on the neurone content of the cerebral cortex. Observations with an automatic image analyser point counting method. *J Neurol Sci* 58: 233–44.

Aherne WA, Dunnill MS (1982) *Morphometry*. Arnold, London.

Braendgaard H, Evans SM, Howard CV, Gundersen HJG (1989) The total number of neurones in the human neocortex unbiasedly estimated using optical disectors. *J Microsc* 157: 285–304.

Dam AM (1979) Shrinkage of the brain during histological procedures with fixation in formaldehyde solutions of different concentrations. *J Hirnforsch* 20: 115–19.

Davis PJM, Wright EA (1977) A new method for measuring cranial cavity volume and its application to the assessment of cerebral atrophy at autopsy. *Neuropath Appl Neurobiol* 3: 341–58.

De Hoff RT (1967) Sampling of material and statistical analysis in quantitative stereology. In Elias H (ed) *Proceedings of the Second International Congress for Stereology*, Springer-Verlag, New York.

Dekaban AS, Sadowsky D (1978) Changes in brain weights during the span of human life. Relation of brain weights to body heights and body weights. *Ann Neurol* 4: 345–56.

Ebbesson SOE, Tang D (1965) A method for estimating the number of cells in histological sections. *J Roy Microscop* 84: 449–64.

Ebbesson SOE, Tang D (1967) A comparison of sampling procedures in a structured cell population. In Elias H (ed) *Proceedings of the Second International Congress on Stereology* Springer-Verlag, New York, pp 131–2.

Gundersen HJG, Bagger P, Bendtsen TF, Evans SM, Korbo L, Marcussen N, Moller A, Nielsen K, Nyengaard JR, Pakkenberg B, Sorensen FB, Vesterby A, West MJ (1988) The new stereological tools: disector, fractionator, nucleator and point sampled intercepts and their use in pathological research and diagnosis. *Acta Path Microbiol Immunol Scand* 96: 857–81.

Hale AJ (1958) *The Interference Microscope in Biological Research*. Livingstone, Edinburgh.

Harper C, Kril J, Raven D, Jones N (1984) Intracranial cavity volumes: a new method and its potential applications. *Neuropathol Appl Neurobiol* 10: 25–32.

Holmes AH (1927) *Petrographic Methods and Calculation* Murby & Co, London.

Hubbard BM, Anderson JM (1981) A quantitative study of cerebral atrophy in old age and senile dementia. *J Neurol Sci* 50: 135–45.

Konigsmark BW, Kalyanaraman UP, Corey P, Murphy EA (1969) An evaluation of techniques in neuronal population estimates: the sixth nerve nucleus. *Johns Hopkins Med J* 125: 146–58.

Konigsmark BW (1970) Methods for the counting of neurons. In *Contemporary Research Methods in Neuroanatomy*, Nauta WJH, Ebbesson SOE (eds) Springer-Verlag, New York, pp 315–34.

Miller AKH, Alston RL, Corsellis JAN (1980) Variations with age of the volumes of grey and white matter in the cerebral hemispheres of man: measurements with an image analyser. *Neuropathol Appl Neurobiol* 6: 119–32.

Moatamed F (1966) Cell frequencies in the human inferior olivary nuclear complex. *J Comp Neurol* 128: 109–16.

Mulligan JH (1931) A method for staining the brain for macroscopic study. *J Anat* 65: 468–72.

Pakkenberg B, Gundersen HJG (1988) Total number of neurones and glial cells in human brain nuclei estimated by the disector and the fractionator. *J Microsc* 150: 1–20.

Pearse AD, Marks R (1974) Measurement of section thickness in quantitative microscopy with special reference to enzyme histochemistry. *J Clin Path* 27: 615–18.

Reichard M (1905) Über die Bestimmung der Schadelkapazität an der Leiche. *Allg Zeit Psychiat* 62: 787–801.

Sterio DC (1984) The unbiased estimation of numbers and sizes of arbitrary particles using the disector. *J Microsc* 134: 127–36.

Terry RD, Deteresa R (1982) The importance of video editing

in automated image analysis in studies of the cerebral cortex. *J Neurol Sci* 53: 413–21.

Weibel ER, Bolender RP (1975) Stereological techniques for electron microscopic morphometry. In Hayat MA (ed) *Principles and Techniques of Electron Microscopy* Van Norstrand Reinhold, New York, pp 237–96.

Weibel ER, Elias H (1967) Introduction to stereological principles. In Weibel ER, Elias H, *Quantitative Methods in Morphology*, Springer-Verlag, Berlin, pp 89–98.

Weibel ER, Gomez DM (1962) A principle for counting tissue structures on random sections. *J Appl Physiol* 17: 343–8.

Addresses of dementia brain banks

M. M. Esiri and J. H. Morris

We list here the addresses of dementia brain banks in Australia, Canada, Europe and the USA of which we are aware. Users of this book may be interested in contacting banks as suppliers or users of material or for advice about setting up a brain bank. A few recent references on the setting-up and uses of dementia brain banks are also listed.

DEMENTIA BRAIN BANKS IN AUSTRALIA

Neuropathology Unit
Department of Pathology
University of Sydney
NSW 200 6
Professor Clive Harper
Telephone: 612-692-2414
Fax: 612-692-3429

Department of Pathology
University of Melbourne
Parkville
Victoria 3052
Professor Colin Masters
Telephone: 613-344-5867
Fix: 613-344-4004

DEMENTIA BRAIN BANKS IN CANADA

Kinsmen Laboratory of Neurological Research
The University of British Columbia
2255 Wesbrook Mall
Vancouver
British Columbia V6T 1Z3
Professor E McGeer
Telephone: 604-822-7377
Fax: 604-822-7086

Canadian Brain Tissue Bank at the Banting Institute
Room 127, 100 College St
Toronto
Ontario M5G 1L5
Dr T P Morley
Telephone: 416-977-3398

DEMENTIA BRAIN BANKS IN EUROPE

Neurological Tissue Bank
Servico de Neurologia
Hospital Clinico y Provincial
Villarroel 170
Barcelona 08036
SPAIN
Dr F F Cruz-Sánchez

Neuropathology Department
Radcliffe Infirmary
Oxford
UK
Dr J H Morris

Austro German Brain Bank
Department of Psychiatry
Clinical Chemistry
University of Würzburg
GERMANY
Dr W Gsell

Department of Neurology
Abt. für Neurologie
Universitätsklinikum
Rudolf Virchow
Augustenburger Platz 1
D-W-1000 Berlin 65
GERMANY
Dr K Jendroska

Laboratoire de Neuropathologie R Escorolle
INSERM U360
Hôpital de la Salpêtrière
47 Blvd de L'Hôpital
F-75651 Paris
Cedex 13
FRANCE
Dr C Duyckaerts

The Netherlands Brain Bank
Meiberdreof 33
1105 AZ Amsterdam
THE NETHERLANDS
Dr R Ravid

Parkinson's Disease Society Brain Bank
Institute of Neurology
1 Wakefield Street
London WC1N 1PJ
UK
Dr S Daniel

MRC Brain Bank
Department of Psychiatry
Addenbrookes Hospital
Cambridge CB2 2QQ
UK
Dr C Wischik

MRC Brain Bank
Neurochemical Pathology Unit
Newcastle General Hospital
Newcastle-upon-Tyne
NE4 6BE
UK
Professor J Edwardson

MRC Brain Bank for Research on Alzheimer's Disease
Institute of Psychiatry
Denmark Hill
London SE5 8AF
UK
Professor P Lantos

Dementia Brain Bank
University of Manchester
Department of Pathological Sciences
Manchester M13 9PT
UK
Dr D M A Mann

Brain Bank
Department of Pathology
Huddinge University Hospital
F42, S-141
86 Huddinge
SWEDEN
Dr I Alafuzoff

DEMENTIA BRAIN BANKS IN NORTH AMERICA
Institute for Biogerontological Research
PO Box 1278
Sun City AZ 85372
Arizona
Joseph Rogers PhD

Geriatric Neurobehavior and Alzheimer's Center
Rancho Los Amigos Medical Center
University of Southern California
12838 Erickson Avenue
Downey CA 902 42
California
Helena Chui MD

Neuropathology Autopsy Core
University of Southern California Medical Center
2011 Zonal Avenue
Los Angeles CA 90033
California
Carol A Miller MD

UCSD National Alzheimer's Disease Brain Bank
Department of Pathology
M-012, BSB Rm 1004
University of California
San Diego
La Jolla CA 92093
California
George G Glenner MD

National Neurological Research Bank
VA Wadsworth Medical Center
Wilshire and Sawtelle Blvds
Los Angeles CA 90073
California
Wallace W Tourtellotte MD PhD

Department of Neurosciences and Psychiatry
University of California
San Diego
La Jolla CA 92093
California
Robert D Terry MD
Lawrence Hansen MD

Department of Neurology
D4-5, University of Florida
1501 North West Nine Avenue
Miami FL 33101
Florida
Deborah C Mash PhD

Mayo Clinic Jacksonville
4500 San Pablo Road
Jacksonville FL 32224
Florida
Neill R Graff-Radford

Center for Alzheimer's Disease and Related Disorders
PO Box 19230
Southern Illinois School of Medicine
Springfield IL 62794-9230
Illinois
Robert G Struble PhD

Rush Presbyterian St Luke's Medical Center
Department of Pathology
1653 W Congress Parkway
Chicago IL 60612-3864
Illinois
Elizabeth J Cochran MD

Indiana University Medical Center
Division of Neuropathology
635 Barnhill Drive
MS A142, IN 46223
Indiana
Bernardino Ghetti MD

The University of Iowa
College of Medicine
Department of Anatomy
650 Newton Road
Iowa City IO 52242
Iowa
Antonio R Damasio MD PhD

Sanders-Brown Research Center on Aging
University of Kentucky
101 Sanders-Brown Building
Lexington KY 40536-0230
Kentucky
William R Markesbery MD

Brain Tissue Resource Center
McLean Hospital
115 Mill Street
Belmont MA 02178
Massachusetts
Edward D Bird MD

Center for Neurologic Diseases
Brigham & Women's Hospital
75 Francis Street
Boston MA 02115
Massachusetts
Dennis J Selkoe MD

Massachusetts General Hospital
Department of Neuropathology
Warren 321
Fruit Street
Boston MA 02114
Massachusetts
E Tessa Hedley-Whyte MD

University of Massachusetts Medical Center
Department of Neurology
55 Lave Avenue North
Worcester MA 01655
Massachusetts
James E Hamos PhD

Department of Neurology
Michigan Alzheimer's Disease Research Center
University of Michigan
1103 E Huron Street
Ann Arbor MI 48104-1687
Michigan
Anne B Young MD PhD

Alzheimer's Treatment & Research Center
St Paul-Ramsey Medical Center
640 Jackson Street
St Paul MN 55101
Minnesota
William H Frey II PhD

Department of Pathology
Mayo Clinic
200 First Street, SW
Rochester MN 55905
Minnesota
Joseph E Parisi MD

SLUMC/Alzheimer's Association Brain Bank
Dept of Psychiatry and Human Behavior
St Louis University Medical Center
1221 S Grand Blvd
St Louis MO 63104
Missouri
George T Grossberg MD

Department of Pathology
Box 8118
Washington University School of Medicine
660 South Euclid Avenue
St Louis MO 63110
Missouri
Daniel W McKeel Jr MD

Department of Pathology
UMKC Neurodegeneration Autopsy Program
Truman Medical Center
2301 Holmes Street
Kansas City MO 64108
Missouri
Joseph L Parker MD

Kathleen Price Bryan Brain Bank
Department of Pathology
Box 3712
Duke University Medical Center
Durham NC 27710
North Carolina
Barbara J Crain MD PhD

Department of Psychiatry
Mt Sinai School of Medicine
One Gustave L Levy Place
NY 10029-6571
New York
Kenneth L Davis MD

University of Rochester School of Medicine
Box 673
601 Elmwood Avenue
Rochester NY 14642
New York

Department of Pathology and Neuroscience
Albert Einstein College of Medicine
1300 Morris Park Avenue
Bronx NY 10461
New York
Peter Davies PhD

Alzheimer's Disease Research Center
Columbia University
630 West 168th Street
NY 10032
New York
James M Powers MD

Department of Pathology
New York University Medical Center
550 First Avenue
NY 10016
New York
Douglas C Miller MD PhD

Institute of Pathology
Case Western Reserve University
2085 Adelbert Road
Cleveland OH 44106
Ohio
Pierluigi Gambetti MD

Division of Neuropathology
Ohio State University College of Medicine
N-112B Upham Hall
473 W 12th Avenue
Columbus OH 43210
Ohio
Leopold Liss MD

Department of Pathology
University of Cincinnati College of Medicine
231 Bethesda Avenue
Cincinnati OH 45267-0524
Ohio
Frank P Zemlan PhD

Division of Neuropathology
Oregon Health Sciences University
3181 SW Sam Jackson Park Road
L113 Portland
OR 97201
Oregon
Melvyn J Ball MD

Alpers Neuropathology Laboratory
Department of Neurology
Thomas Jefferson University
130 South 9th Street
Suite 400
Philadelphia PA 19107
Pennsylvania
Patricio F Reyes MD

National Disease Research Interchange
2401 Walnut Street
Suite 408
Philadelphia PA 19103
Pennsylvania
Gayle Trofe

Western Psychiatric Institute and Clinic
3811 O'Hara Street, Room E-1230
Pittsburg PA 15213
Pennsylvania
George S Zubenko MD PhD

University of Tennessee Medical Center
1924 Alcoa Highway
Knoxville TN 37920
Tennessee
Robert C Switzer III PhD

206 Psychology Building
University of Texas at El Paso
El Paso TX 79968
Texas
Donald E Moss PhD

Department of Pathology
Baylor College of Medicine
Mail Station 205, Methodist Hospital
6565 Fannon, Houston, TX 77030
Texas
Joel B Kirkpatrick MD

Department of Pathology
Neuropathology Laboratory
University of Texas Southwestern Medical Center
5323 Harry Hines Blvd
Dallas TX 75235-9072
TEXAS
Charles L White III MD

Department of Pathology
SM-30
University of Washington
2707 NE Blakely Street, GG-19
Seattle WA 98195
Washington
Murray A Raskind MD

Zablocki VA Medical Center
Research Center 151
Milwaukee WI 53295
Wisconsin
Piero Antuono MD

REFERENCES

Bidaut-Russell M, Dowd DM, Grossberg GT, Zimmy GA (1991) Survey of US Alzheimer brain banks: a 1990 directory. *Alz Dis Assoc Dis* 5: 188–93.

Cruz-Sánchez FF, Tolosa E (eds) (1993) How to run a brain bank. *J Neurol Transm* Suppl 39.

EURAGE report (1987) Clinical, pathological and experimental opportunities for collaborative research on aging on the brain and dementia in the EEC countries and Switzerland.

Ravid R, Winblad B (1993) Brain banking in Alzheimer's disease: factors to match for, pitfalls and potentials. In Corain K *et al.*, (eds) *Alzheimer's Disease: Advances in Clinical and Basic Research.* John Wiley and Sons, New York, pp 213–18.

Swaab DF, Hanw J-J, Reynolds GP, Sorbi S (1989) Tissue banking and EURAGE. *J Neurol Sci* 93: 341–3.

Safety precautions in laboratories involved with dementia diagnosis and research

M. M. Esiri and J. H. Morris

A major concern of all laboratories involved in identifying neuropathological causes of dementia in human subjects is minimizing any danger of infection. It is also essential to eliminate or minimize any danger to health from the use of toxic chemicals in the post mortem room or laboratories. Precautions relating to the use of toxic chemicals must conform in the UK with the regulations governing the Control of Substances Hazardous to Health as recommended in Approved Codes of Practice (HMSO 1988, 1989).

The danger of infection at present arises principally in relation to the handling and processing of tissues from cases of *Creutzfeldt–Jakob disease* (*CJD*) and other *prion diseases* or *AIDS*. The agents concerned have very different biological properties necessitating different precautions. However, many common principles apply to the avoidance of contamination when dealing with potentially infective material. Details are laid out in recently published documents from the UK Health Advisory Committee (HMSO, 1991, 1994) and the American Neurological Association (1989) (see also Bell & Ironside, 1993). Because a risk of infection is not always recognized in cases in which it exists, high safety standards must be applied at all times. All those coming in contact with fresh human brain tissue should be immunized against hepatitis B virus.

All laboratories and post-mortem rooms must have written statements of the local safety policy which should be read by, and be always available to, all those working in or having access to these areas. These statements must be kept up to date, and regular inspections must be carried out to ensure that rules are being followed and equipment kept disinfected, clean and maintained adequately.

In the post-mortem room, all cadavers which present a risk of infection must be clearly labelled to indicate this and totally enclosed in a leak-proof body bag. Pathologists must wear protective clothing, waterproof gloves (two pairs may be preferred, or one pair over stainless steel mesh gloves) and a full face visor. No one with a significant cut or graze should undertake a post-mortem examination. If there is a substantial danger of infection, and for all post-mortem examinations, minor cuts or grazes should be fully covered by a waterproof dressing. If gloves are torn or cut, they should be replaced immediately. Any cuts sustained during a post-mortem examination should be encouraged to bleed and washed with running water. All such accidents must be reported. If there is a risk of infection, medical advice should be sought immediately.

Post-mortem examinations on cases in which there is a recognized danger of infection must only be performed by experienced staff in carefully controlled conditions, in an area specially designated for such examinations. The procedure must be unhurried, with a minimum of interruption. Three people should be present: the pathologist, an assistant and a circulator. Other post-mortem examinations should not be proceeding in the same room at the same time. The circulator observes, communicates, provides containers, warns of perceived dangers, e.g. from spillages and instruments, but remains uncontaminated. The skull should be opened at the end of the examination using a hand-saw, operated wearing stainless steel mesh gloves and preferably with a large, transparent, plastic bag fitted over the head and neck of the cadaver in which holes are made for the insertion of hands and saw. When the post-mortem examination is completed, protective clothing should be autoclaved before being laundered or disposed of by incineration, and contaminated work surfaces cleaned with detergent, followed by a suitable disinfectant. Instruments must be cleaned, disinfected and autoclaved. Chlorine-releasing agents are effective disinfectants to use against HIV infection. Sodium hydroxide is preferred against prions.

In the neuropathological laboratory, brains from cases of possible CJD should be sliced and handled in a Class I cabinet, i.e. an open-fronted exhaust protective cabinet from which airborne particles are retained on a filter. Such a cabinet is best housed in a separate containment room, level 3, on the door to which is posted a biological hazard warning notice (Health and Safety Executive, 1991 (HMSO, 1990)). Blocks from brain slices for histological processing should be placed in formic acid for at least 1 hour, following which they may be processed normally. Formic acid treatment has been found effectively to inactivate the CJD agent whilst retaining normal morphology of the tissue (Brown, Wolff & Gajdusek, 1990). Potentially HIV-infected material can be dealt with by wearing gloves at containment level 2 (HMSO, 1990, HMSO, 1991), at a designated, secluded and easily cleaned work bench which is always disinfected after use. All infected waste material must be autoclaved or disposed of by incineration. To destroy prions, autoclaving needs to take place at 134 °C for at least 18 minutes.

CJD has now been described in a histopathologist (Gorman *et al.*, 1992) and two histopathology technicians (Miller, 1988; Sitwell *et al.*, 1988). Thus, although the overall incidence of CJD in the medical and para medical professions does not differ significantly from that in the general population, these anecdotal cases indicate a need to ensure that appropriate precautions are taken by all who may come into contact with CNS material from such cases. Evidence from iatrogenically transmitted cases of CJD indicates that, if the prion agent is introduced in or near the brain, the incubation period for the disease is measured in months, whereas peripheral infection, of which a remote risk exists in pathology laboratories, can lead to incubation periods of years or decades (Brown, Preece & Will, 1992).

REFERENCES

American Neurological Association, 1989, Committee on Health Care Issues. Precautions in handling tissues, fluids and other contaminating materials from patients with documented or suspected Creutzfeldt–Jakob disease. *Ann Neurol* 19: 75–7.

Bell JE, Ironside JW (1993) How to tackle a possible Creutzfeldt–Jakob disease necropsy. *J Clin Pathol* 46: 193–7.

Brown P, Preece MA, Will RG (1992) Friendly fire in medicine: hormones, Homografts and Creutzfeldt–Jakob disease. *Lancet* 340: 24–7.

Brown P, Wolff A, Gajdusek DC (1990) A simple and effective method for inactivating virus infectivity from formalin-fixed tissue samples from patients with Creutzfeldt–Jakob disease. *Neurology* 40: 887–90.

Gorman DG, Benson DF, Vogel DG, Vinters HV (1992) Creutzfeldt–Jakob disease in a pathologist. *Neurology* 42: 463.

HMSO (1988) Control of substances hazardous to health regulations. *HMSO*, London.

HMSO (1989) Monitoring strategies for toxic substances – Guidance.

HMSO (1990) Categorisation of pathogens according to hazard and categories of containment. 2nd edn.

HMSO (1991) Safe working and the prevention of infection in clinical laboratories.

HMSO (1994) Health Services Advisory Committee. Precautions for work with human and animal transmissible spongiform encephalopathies. London.

Miller DC (1988) Creutzfeldt–Jakob disease in histopathology technicians. *N Engl J Med* 318: 853.

Sitwell L, Lach B, Atack E, Atack D (1988) Creutzfeldt–Jakob disease in histopathology technicians. *N Engl J Med* 318: 854.

Index

acetylcholinesterase 181, 221
acquired immunodeficiency syndrome
    (AIDS) 39, 40, 357, 367, 368,
    372–8
  neuropathology 374–7
  pathogenesis 377–8
Addison's disease 317
adrenoleukodystrophy 317, 320 (fig.)
adult onset neuronal ceroid lipofuscinosis
    (Kuf's disease) 316
adult polyglucosan body disease (Lafora
    disease) 316
affective disorders 2
ageing, normal
  sites with depletion of nerve cells 62
    (table)
  sites with no significant reduction of
    nerve cells 63 (table)
alcoholic dementia, primary 294–6
alcoholism 2, 40, 294–304
  cerebellar disease 50
Alexander's disease 315–16
aluminium 327
Alz-50 6
Alzheimer's disease 1, 2–3, 4–14, 38,
    70–110, 233
  amyloid 105, 110; neurotoxicity 106–7;
    tau association 109
  β-amyloid precursor protein 105–6
  β-amyloid protein 104–5
  apolipoproteins 104–5
  boxers developing 351–52
  brain slices 77–80
  brain weight 76–7
  cerebrovascular disease relationship 57
  cholinergic hypothesis 4–5
  chromosome 1 103, 109
  chromosome 14 95, 102–3, 109
  chromosome 19 103
  chromosome 21 101–2
  clinical diagnosis accuracy 37 (table)
  clinical features 2–3
  clinical studies 71–2
  clinico-pathological studies 72–3
  congophilic amyoid angiopathy 6–7,
    87–91, 93 (figs.), 94 (fig.)
  diagnostic criteria 95–7; CERAD 96–7,

    98, 99; Khatchaurian 96, 98; Tierney
    97, 98
  differential diagnosis 99–100
  Down's syndrome associated see Down's
    syndrome
  epidemiology 71–5
  external appearance of brain 77
  extrapyramidal signs 3, 177–8
  familial 39, 74; early onset 101–2
  first isocortical stage (Braak) 11
  genetic factors 74
  granulovascular changes 5–6
  hippocampal formation 1, 9
Ammon's horn sclerosis 408, 409
amnestic dementia (Korsakoff's psychosis)
    49
amnestic dementia of alcoholism
    (Korsakoff's syndrome) 50, 296
amphetamine abuse 164, 325
amphotericin B 324
amygdala 10, 10–11, 29
amyloid 105, 110
  deposition (congophilic angiopathy) 6–7,
    87–91
  neurotoxicity 106–7
  tau association 109
amyloid vascular deposits 63
β-amyloid precursor protein 6, 105–6, 110,
    130
  gene 130
β-amyloid protein 105–7, 110, 352
amyotrophic lateral sclerosis see
    parkinsonism dementia complex of
    Guam
anaemia 311
  sickle cell 311
angiotropic large cell lymphoma
    (malignant intravascular lymphoma)
    165
angular gyrus infarction 147
anterior cerebral artery infarct 147
anterograde amnesic syndrome 9
anti-parkinsonian medication 175, 176–7
apolipoproteins 104–5
argyrophilic plaques 61
assessment of microscopial changes 420–24
assessment of tissue volumes 415–17

  brain volume measurement 416
  cranial cavity measurement 416–17
  polyurethane cast method 417–20
  whole brain 415–16
astrocytoma 399
atherosclerosis 161
Auju people 195

Balint's syndrome 13
Baltic myoclonus (Unverricht–Lundborg's
    syndrome) 409–10
basal forebrain lesion 147
basal ganglia 29–31, 220–1
  physiology 221
basal nucleus of Meynert 29, 30 (fig.), 48,
    182
  cell loss 182
Behcet's syndrome 401–402
bilateral posterior cerebral infarction 147
Binswanger's encephalopathy 4, 144, 152–8
  clincial features 154–5
  computed tomography (CT) 155–7
  magnetic resonance imaging (MRI) 157
  neuroimaging 155–8
  pathogenesis 157–8
1,3-bis-(2-chloroethyl)-1-nitroso urea 325
bismuth salts 327
Boswell's patient 11
bovine spongiform encephalopathy 278
brain
  ageing changes compatible with normal
    mental function 60–6
  structural alteration 2
brain banks addresses of 429–33
brain biopsy 59–60
brain death 309
brainstem 32–3
brain tumours 2
broncho-pneumonia 307
Buerger's disease (thromboangiitis
    obliterans) 163

CADASIL 161–2
cancer chemotherapy 325
carbon monoxide poisoning 369
cardiac death 39
cardio-respiratory arrest 309

cardiovascular disease 144–7
 arterial wall changes 148–50
cat scratch disease 405
cerebellum 33–4, 309
cerebral amyloid angiopathies 260–73
 associated conditions 261 (table)
 type I familial amyloid polyneuropathy
  261 (table)
cerebral cortex 21–8
cerebral haemorrhage, cystatin-C reactivity
 263
cerebral hemiatrophy with contralateral
 cerebellar atrophy 409
cerebral syphilis 357
cerebral white matter 28
cerebrospinal fluid 40–1
 hydrodynamics 332
cerebrotendinous xanthomatosis 316
cerebrovascular disease 57
 dementia production 144–54
 progressive dementing syndrome
  production 144
cholecystokinin 181
choline acetyl transferase 185–6
chromosome 1 103, 109
chromosome 14 102–3, 109
chromosome 19 103
chromosome 21 102–3
chronic subdural haematoma 2
cisplatin 325
cocaine 164, 325
coeliac disease with dementia 412
cognitive deficits 3
cognitive function 1, 4
confusional state 2
congophilic angiopathy 159
consortium to establish a registry for
 Alzheimer's disease (CERAD) 40, 52,
 53, 96–7, 98, 99
corneal transplants 38
corpora amylacea 63
cortical atrophy 3
cortical Lewy body disease 182–8
 aetiology 187
 Alzheimer's disease relationship 185
 clinical syndrome 183
 clinico-pathological definition 186–7
 neurochemical findings 185–6
 neuropathological criteria 187 (table)
 Parkinson's disease relationship 186–7
 pathological differential diagnosis 187–8
corticobasal degeneration 316–17, 234,
 254–5
corticodentatonigral degeneration with
 neuronal achromasia 234
corticotrophin releasing factor 181
craniopharyngioma 399
Creutzfeldt–Jacob disease 37–8, 41
 familial 39, 281–2
 iatrogenic 277–8

cyclosporin 324–5
cystatatin-C 263
cytomegalovirus 53–4
cytosine arabinoside 325

dementia 2
 argyrophilic grains 255
 clinical assessment problems 174–5
 clinical features 3–4
 definition 2
 functional aetiologies 2
 lacking distinctive histology 4
 neuroanatomical basis 4
dementia with motor neuron disease
  250–2
dementia pugilistica 344–54
 Alzheimer's disease associated 351–52
 cerebellar damage 349
 cerebral hemispheres 350–2
 parkinsonian syndrome 350
 septum pellucidum abnormalities 346
  (fig.), 347–8
 substantia nigra degeneration 349–50
dentatorubro pallidoluysian degeneration
  (atrophy) 256
depression 2
domoic acid 327
dopamine 181, 186
Down's syndrome 122–31
 β/A4 protein deposition 127, 128, 129–30
 Alzheimer's disease associated 78, 101
 β-amyloid precursor protein 130; gene
  130
 arterial calcification 127
 atherosclerosis 127
 basal ganglia calcification 127
 brain changes 122–3
 chronology 129–31
 dementia 128–9
 neurochemical changes in the elderly 124
 glycoprotein deposition 127–8
 granulovacuolar neuronal degeneration
  127
 Hirano bodies 127
 neurofibrillary tangles 6, 124–6, 127
 neuronal fallout 123–4
 senile plaques 124–7
 vascular amyloidosis 127
drugs 324-6

embolic disease 161
encephalitis lethargica 369–72
 neuropathology 370–72
entorhinal cortex 9, 10, 21–2
epilepsy 408–10
 conditions giving rise to epilepsy and
  dementia 408 (table)
 neuropathology 408–10
 temporal lobe 409 (fig.)
epitopes 5

état criblé (Virchow–Robin spaces
 expansion) 63, 65 (fig.), 150–2
état lacunaire 151, 159–60
ethylene oxide 327–8
extrapyramidal signs 3, 177–8

Fabry's disease 323
familial amyloid polyneuropathy type 1
 261 (table)
familial amyotrophic chorea with
 acanthocytosis
 (neuroacanthocytosis; familial
  neuroacanthocytosis; Levine–Critchley
  syndrome) 234–5
familial cerebral amyloid angiopathy with
 deafness and ocular
 haemorrhage (Danish type) 261, 270–2
familial cerebral amyloid angiopathy with
 non-neuritic amyloid
 plaque formation (British type) 261
  (table), 266–70; neuro-imaging 267;
  neuropathology 267–70
familial hemiplegic migraine 162
familial oculo-leptomeningeal amyloidosis
 261
focal cognitive syndromes 4
focal neuronal gigantism 405
folate deficiency 315
foramen ovale, patent 39
frontal lobe atrophy 2, 3
frontal lobe degeneration of non-Alzheimer
 type 215
frontal lobe dementia 4
frontal lobe dysfunction 4
fronto-limbic dementia 354

Gaucher's disease type 1 318
Gerstmann–Sträussler–Scheinker disease
 213, 280–1
Gerstmann–Sträussler syndrome 53, 213
Gerstmann syndrome 367
giant cell (temporal) arteritis 163
glial nodule encephalitis 404
glioma 399–400
gliosis 151–2
globoid cell leukodystrophy (Krabbe's
 disease) 323–4
glutamate-N-methyl-D-aspartate 297
glycogen synthase kinase 108
GM$_1$ gangliosidosis 317–18, 320 (fig.)
GM$_2$ gangliosidosis 318
granulomatous angiitis of nervous system
 (isolated angiitis) 162–3
granulovacuolar degeneration 61–2
Guam 194–5

Hachinski ischaemic score 142–3
haematological conditions 311
heavy metals 326–7
hepatic disease 311–13

hepatic encephalopathy 301–303, 311, 314
      (figs.)
hereditary cerebral haemorrhage with
      amyloidosis – Dutch type 260, 261
      (table) 263–6
   amyloid chemistry 265–6
   genetics 265–6
   neuro-imaging 264
   neuropathology 264–5
hereditary cerebral haemorrhage with
      amyloidosis – Icelandic type 261
      (table), 262–3
hereditary dysphasic dementia 233–4
hereditary multi-infarct dementia 272–3
heroin 325–6
herpes simplex encephalitis 42, 357–62
   neuropathology 360–2
   pathogenesis 362
hippocampus 1, 9, 9–10, 21, 64 (fig.)
   anatomy 21–2
   cornu ammonis 22
   damage 309, 310 (fig.)
   dentate fascia 22
   isolation 10
   strata 22
Hirano body 5–6, 61–2, 196–7
histamine 297
histoblot method of PrP^{Sc} detection 293
Huntington's disease 3, 39, 219–35
   clinical aspects 221–2
   clinicopathological discrepancies 233
   concomitant neuropathologies 233
   epidemiology 220
   gene expression 232–3
   neuropathology 222–33; brainstem 232;
      cerebellum 232; cerebral cortex 231;
      coronal sections 223; external
      examination of brain 223; history
      219–20; hypothalamus 232;
      matrix-striosomes 231; neostriatal
      neurons 229–3; red nucleus 232; spinal
      cord 232; striatum 223–9; substantia
      nigra 231–2; subthalamic nucleus 232;
      thalamus 231; white matter 231
hydrocephalic dementia 3–4
hydrocephalus 332–42
   ex vacuo 332
   intermittently raised 334
   normal pressure 332–42; causes 335
      (table); classification 334; clinical
      features 335; diagnostic procedure
      337–82; neuropathology 335–8;
      prevalence 334–5
   obstructive, causes of 334 (table)
5-hydroxy-indoleacetic acid 181
hypercalcaemia 2
hypertension 154, 160–1
hyperviscosity syndromes 311
hypocalcaemia with calcification of basal
      ganglia 316–17

hypoglycaemia 313–14
hypoparathyroidism 316–17
hypothalamus 31–2
hypovitaminosis B$_{12}$ 2
hypoxia
   conditions associated with 308 (table),
      309–10
   effect on cerebral cortex 311, 313 (fig.)

immunoblot (Dot and Western) method of
      PrP^{Sc} detection 292
immunocytochemistry 53, 56 (fig.)
impaired subcortical functions 307
inflammatory conditions 401–405
inherited hepatolenticular degeneration
      (Wilson's disease) 311–13
intracranial artery thrombosis 161
intracranial neoplasms 398–400
isocortex pathological changes 11–12
isoform A 107
isolated angiitis of nervous system
      (granulomatous angiitis) 162–3

Jakai people 195
JC virus 53, 366–7

Kearns–Sayre syndrome 319–21
α-feto-glutarate dehydrogenase 296–7
Kii peninsula (Japan) 195
Kluver–Buck syndrome 205
Korsakoff's psychosis (amnestic dementia
      of alcoholism) 50, 296
Krabbe's disease (globoid cell
      leukodystrophy) 323–4
Kuf's disease (adult onset neuronal ceroid
      lipofuscinosis) 316
kuru 279–80

lactic dehydrogenase 41
lacunar disease 159
lacunes 63, 159
Lafora disease (adult polyglucosan body
      disease) 316
Lambert–Eaton myasthenia syndrome
      404
lead 328
left anterior temporal atrophy 33
Leigh's encephalopathy 321–22, 323 (fig.)
leptomeningeal carcinomatosis 399
lesion-deficit correlation 1
leu-enkephalin 181
leukoariosis 39
Levine–Critchley syndrome
      (neuroacanthocytosis: familial
      amyotrophic chorea with
      acanthocytosis; familial
      neuroacanthocytosis) 234–5
Lewy body 63, 178–81, 184 (fig.)
   normal elderly 180–1
   patients with dementia 180–1

Lewy body type dementia 1, 3, 63
limbic cortex neurons 182
limbic encephalitis see paraneoplastic
      syndrome
lipohyalinosis 159
liver cirrhosis 39
lobar atrophies: lesion–deficit correlation 1
locus ceruleus 182
lymphoma, intravascuolar (angiotropic)
      165, 399
lymphomatoid granulomatosis 164–5

magnetic resonance imaging (MRI) 39, 60
Marchiafava–Bignami disease 296, 303
Marinesco bodies 317
McLeod syndrome 234
measles virus 366
medial temporal limbic structures 9–10
medial temporal lobe lesions, amnesia
      associated 9
medication encephalopathy 2
medulla 33
meningeal thickening 40
meningioma 400, 402 (fig.)
mercury 328
metabolic conditions 308 (table)
metachromatic leukodystrophy 322–3
methyl bromide 328
methotrexate 325, 326 (fig.)
3-methoxy-4-hydroxyphenylglycol 181
midbrain 32
migraine, familial hemiplegic 162
mitochondrial cytopathies
      (encephalomyopathies) 319–21
mitochondrial
      myopathy–encephalopathy–lactic
      acidosis–stroke-like episodes (MELAS)
      319–21
mixed pathology 56–7
Morels laminar sclerosis 296
motor neurone disease 250–2
mucopolysaccaridosis type IIIB
      (San-filippo's disease) 319
multifocal leukoencephalopathy with
      calcification 412
multiple cavernous angiomas 165 (fig.)
multi-infarct dementia 137, 138, 145–7
multiple sclerosis 405–8
   aetiology 408
   differential diagnosis 407–8
   neuropathology 406–7
multiple system atrophy 50, 234, 256–7
myoclonic epilepsy 256
   with red fibres 319-21

necrotizing angiitis 325
necrotizing encephalitis 42
neorcortex 24–8
   Brodmann's areas 27
   glial cells 27

non-pyramidal cells 25–6
pyramidal cells 24–5
regional subdivision 27
vascular supply 27–8
neostriatum 3
neuritic plaque 65 (fig.)
neuroanthocytosis (familial amyotrophic
    chorea with acanthocytosis; familial
    neurocanthocytosis; Levine–Critchley
    syndrome) 234–5
neurofibrillary tangles 6, 61
    antipsychotic drugs promotion 392
    calcification 255–6
    in: Alzheimer's disease 6, 8, 10, 12, 78,
        82–4, 108; dementia pugilistica 349;
        Down's syndrome 6, 124–6, 127;
        parkinsonian dementia of Guam 6,
        195–6; Pick's disease 6, 213;
        post-encephalitic parkinsonism 6;
        progressive supranuclear palsy 6
neuroimaging 39
neurological examination 38–9
neuronal intranuclear inclusion disease
    317
neuronal loss 7, 181, 309
neuronal spheroids 63
neuropathy-atasia-retinitis
    pigmentosa-dementia syndrome
    (NARPS) 319–20
neuropil threads 6, 7–8
neurosyphilis 2, 378
Niemann–Pick disease 318–19
non-specific frontal lobe dementia 245–50
noradrenaline 181
nucleus basalis of Meynert (basal nucleus)
    29, 30 (fig.), 85–6

Opalski cells 313
opiates 325

paired helical filaments 107, 108
pancreatic disorders 313–14
paraneoplastic syndrome (limbic
    encephalitis) 38, 402–4
    aetiology 403–4
parietal lobe atrophy 3
parietal lobe infarct 147
parkinsonian dementia complex of Guam
    (amyotrophic lateral sclerosis)
    194–201, 351
    aetiology 199–201; cycad 199–200;
        genetics 199; infectious agents 194;
        toxic metals 200–1
    neuropathology 195–8; amyloid deposit
        198; congophilic angiopathy 198;
        neurofibrillary tangles 195–6; senile
        plaques 198
    overlap 198–9
Parkinson's disease 3
    Alzheimer's disease relationship 57–8

bradykinesia 176
cognitive deficits 176
dementia 175–7; clinical correlates
    176–7; pathological correlates 182
gait disturbance 176
late onset 176
lesion–deficit correlation 1
motor phenomena 175
neurochemical findings 181
neuropsychology 177
pathology 178–81; Lewy bodes 178–81;
    neuronal loss 181
problems of clinical ascertainment 175
symptoms 39
pellagra 303–4
perivascular parenchymal rarefaction
    151–2
periventricular low density 155–6
persistent vegetative state 309
Pick's disease 204–15, 234
    atypical 213
    clinical manifestations 204–5
    definition 211–13
    familial 39
    neurochemistry 210–11
    parietal predominance 215
    pathology 205–10; Pick bodies 209–10;
        Pick cells 209–10
    Pick–Alzheimer spectrum 213–14
    related conditions 213–15
pituitary adenoma 399
pneumocystic pneumonia 39
polycystic lipomembranous osteodysplasia
    with sclerosing leukoencephalopathy
    316
pons 33
porphyria 315
portal sysemic encephalopathy 301, 311
    MRI 303
post-encephalitic parkinsonism 369–72
    neuropathology 370–72
positron emission tomography 39, 60
post-mortem decay 426–7
post-mortem examination 39–59
    arrriving at final pathological diagnosis
        56
    brain parenchyma 45–52; amygdala 47;
        basal ganglia 48; brainstem 50;
        cerebellum 50–1; cortex 45–7;
        hippocampus 47; hypothalamus 49;
        locus ceruleus 50; medulla 50; pons
        50; stains 53; subacute nigra 50;
        subthalamus 49–50; thalamus 48;
        tissue block selection 51–2; white
        matter 47–8
    examination of brain slices 43
    external features 42–3
    extracranial organs 39–4
    fixed brain 41
    fresh brain 39–40

microscopic examination 54–6
mild pathological changes 58
no pathological features to account for
    dementia 58–9
pathological diagnosis of dementing
    disease in absence of history of
    dementia 59
retention of fresh frozen brain samples
    41
scheme of selection 52–4
spinal cord 40
ventricular system 43–5
volume changes 41–2
weight changes 41–2
prion disease 38, 277–87
    diagnosis 283–7
    infectious 277–80
    inherited 280–2; octapeptide coding
        repeats 282
    mice 280
    prion protein mutations 229 (fig.)
    sporadic 282–3
progressive multifocal
    leukoencephalopathy 47, 357, 366–9
    neuropathology 368–9
progressive subcortical gliosis of Neumann
    253–4
progressive supranuclear palsy 3, 44, 50,
    213, 233–4, 241–5
proline directed kinases 108
protein phosphatases 2A/2B 108
PrP, detecting novel mutations in 293
pseudodementia 2, 175
pseudo-Huntington's disease 256
pyruvate dehydrogenase complex 296–7

radiation necrosis 405
Ramsay Hunt syndrome 409–10
recreational drug abuse 325–6
renal failure, chronic 311, 313 (table)
right middle cerebral artery infarct 147
Rosetta stone 201

saccharide sequences 127
safety precautions in laboratories 434–5
Sanfillipo's disease (mucopolysaccharidosis
    type III) 319
sarcoidosis 401, 402 (fig.)
schizophrenia 385–93
    Alzheimer's disease frequency 391
    cytoarchitectural brain changes 386–90
    dementia 391–92
    gliosis 388 (table), 389–90
    macroscopic brain changes 385–6
    nature of disease 390–1
    neurodevelopmental model 390–1
    neuronal density 389
    neuronal disarray 389
    neuronal number 389
    neuronal size 389

schizophrenia (*cont.*)
  suggestions for neuropathological study 392
  synaptic alterations 389
  ultrastructural alterations 389
section magnification 425–6
section thickness 425–6
selegiline 177
senile plaques 5, 6–7, 8, 10, 12, 80–2
serotonin 181, 186
Shy–Drager syndrome 3
sickle cell anaemia 311
single photon emission tomography (SPECT) 39, 60
Sjogren's syndrome 405
slowly progressive aphasia with/without dementia 214
small vessel disease 147–8
somatostatin 181
space-occupying lesions 398–400
Spatz–Lindenberg disease 163
spongiform encephalopathies 26 (table), 272
spontaneous oral-facial dyskinesia 235
stage zero tangles 6
stains selection 53
stroke
  hereditary liability 161
  syndromes 39
subacute sclerosing pancephalitis 53, 213, 362–6
  aetio-pathogenesis 366
  neuropathology 364–6
subarachnoid haemorrhage 4
subcortical dementia syndrome 177

subcortical nuclei 3
subdural haematoma 398
subdural haematoma, acute/chronic 40
substance P met-enkephalin 151
substantia nigra 3, 23
superficial haemosiderosis of central nervous system 410–11
systemic lupus erythematosus 39, 163–4

tau 5, 6, 107–9, 127
  amyloid associated 109
  regulation 109
temporal (giant cell) arteritis 163
temporal lobe epilepsy, MRI 39
thalamus 31–2
  generation (dementia) 252
  infarction 147
thiamine deficiency 296–7
thiamine pyrophosphate 296
thio-TERA 325
thromboangiitis obliterans (Buerger's disease) 163
thyroid diseases 2
tissue fixation 424
tissue poisoning 424
toluene 328
toxic conditions 306 (table)
toxochoreoathetoid disease 256
toxoplasmosis 42
transjugular intrahepatic portal system 301
transketolase 296–7
trimethyl tin 328

ubiquitin 5, 127

'unidentified bright objects' 39
Unverricht–Lundborg syndrome (Baltic myoclonus) 409–10
uraemic encephalopathy 311

vascular dementia 4, 39–40, 137–69
  accuracy of clinical diagnosis 143
  aetiology 160–2; atherosclerosis 160–1; embolic disease 161; hypertension 160–1
  clinical criteria 142–3
  definition 140–1
  degree 141
  frequency 138–44; derivation 139; historical overview 138–9
  Hachinski ischaemic score 142
  mechanisms 145
  neuroimaging 141–2
  neuropathologic criteria 165–8
  severity rating scale 169
vasculitis 162–3
ventromedical frontal cortex 11–12
Virchow–Robin spaces expansion (état criblé) 63, 65 (fig.), 150–2
vitamin B_{12} deficiency 315

Wernicke–Korsakoff syndrome 296–301
  chronic 300
Whipple's disease 409 (fig.), 410 (fig.), 411–12
white matter damage 309–10
white matter small vessel disease 158–9
Wilson's disease (inherited hepatolenticular degeneration) 311–13